Sensible ECG Analysis

To KTK–
I agree, it was always *unconditional.*

For John A. Handal, M.D.
who taught me always to first treat the patient, not the test results.

Sensible ECG Analysis

Kathryn Monica Lewis, RN, BSN, PhD
Phoenix, Arizona

Edited by
Kathleen A. Handal, MD, DABEM
Scottsdale, Arizona

Delmar Publishers

an International Thomson Publishing company ITP®

Albany • Bonn • Boston • Cincinnati • Detroit • London • Madrid
Melbourne • Mexico City • New York • Pacific Grove • Paris • San Francisco
Singapore • Tokyo • Toronto • Washington

NOTICE TO THE READER

Publisher does not warrant or guarantee any of the products described herein or perform any independent analysis in connection with any of the product information contained herein. Publisher does not assume, and expressly disclaims, any obligation to obtain and include information other than that provided to it by the manufacturer.

The reader is expressly warned to consider and adopt all safety precautions that might be indicated by the activities described herein and to avoid all potential hazards. By following the instructions contained herein, the reader willingly assumes all risks in connection with such instructions.

The publisher makes no representations or warranties of any kind, including but not limited to, the warranties of fitness for particular purpose or merchantability, nor are any such representations implied with respect to the material set forth herein, and the publisher takes no responsibility with respect to such material. The publisher shall not be liable for any special, consequential, or exemplary damages resulting, in whole or in part, from the readers' use of, or reliance upon, this material.

Cover design: TDB Publishing Services

Delmar Staff
Publisher: Susan Simpfenderfer
Acquisitions Editor: Dawn Gerrain
Developmental Editor: Debra Flis
Project Editor: Stacey Prus
Art and Design Coordinator: Mary Colleen Liburdi
Production Coordinator: John Mickelbank
Marketing Manager: Katherine Hans

Printed in Canada
For more information, contact:

Delmar Publishers
3 Columbia Circle, Box 15015
Albany, New York 12212-5015

International Thomson Publishing Europe
Berkshire House
168-173 High Holborn
London, WC1V7AA
United Kingdom

Nelson ITP, Australia
102 Dodds Street
South Melbourne,
Victoria, 3205 Australia

Nelson Canada
1120 Birchmont Road
Scarborough, Ontario
M1K 5G4, Canada

International Thomson Publishing France
Tour Maine-Montparnasse
33 Avenue du Maine
75755 Paris Cedex 15, France

International Thomson Editores
Seneca 53
Colonia Polanco
11560 Mexico D. F. Mexico

International Thomson Publishing GmbH
Königswinterer Straße 418
53227 Bonn
Germany

International Thomson Publishing Asia
60 Albert Street
#15-01 Albert Complex
Singapore 189969

International Thomson Publishing Japan
Hirakawa-cho Kyowa Building, 3F
2-2-1 Hirakawa-cho, Chiyoda-ku,
Tokyo 102, Japan

ITE Spain/Paraninfo
Calle Magallanes, 25
28015-Madrid, Espana

1 2 3 4 5 6 7 8 9 10 XXX 06 05 04 03 02 01 00 99

Library of Congress Cataloging-in-Publication Data
Lewis, Kathryn, RN
Sensible ECG analysis / Kathryn Lewis, Kathleen Handal.
p. cm.
Includes bibliographical references and index.
ISBN 0-7668-0520-4
1. Electrocardiography. I. Handal, Kathleen A. II. Title.
RC683.5.E5L45 1999
616.1'207547--dc21

99-29634
CIP

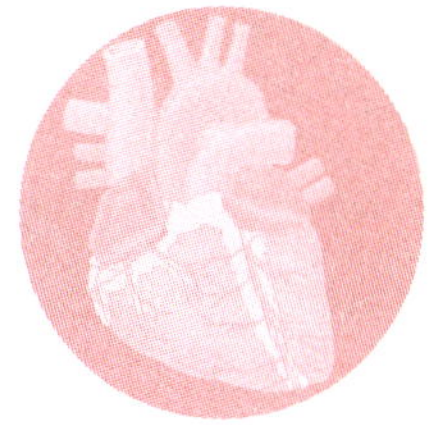

Contents

CHAPTER 5

The Junctional Mechanisms 63

CHAPTER 6

CHAPTER 7

Foreword

Heart disease is the leading cause of death in the United States. We have come a long way in our understanding of the physiology of the heart and the pathophysiology of heart disease. As our knowledge base has been expanded, modified, and corrected, the clinical and out-of-hospital field has made tremendous advances in the practical application of electrocardiography. This has directly translated into saving lives and preventing the overt complications of heart disease. In *Sensible ECG Analysis*, Kathryn Lewis, RN, BSN, PhD, and Kathleen A. Handal, MD, DABEM, take what can be a very complicated, difficult-to-understand area of medicine and transform it into a practical, applicable body of knowledge. At a time when science has become so incredibly complex, it is a breath of fresh air to have access to such a text that distills out the essence of what is "sensible" and practical.

Sensible ECG Analysis carefully and concisely guides the learner and practitioner through the anatomy, physiology, and electrophysiology of the heart, and then proceeds into the area of understanding the ECG, normal and abnormal, before progressing into rhythm disturbances. Each rhythm disturbance is analyzed through practical rhythm strip recognition and is appropriately dealt with in regards to cause, consequences, and intervention as it applies to the patient. Doctors Lewis and Handal then provide a wonderful overview to 12-lead ECG evaluation. It is imperative that the modem field provider recognizes the presence of an acute myocardial infarction. Understanding the 12-lead ECG is vital for making such a diagnosis. This allows the provider to initiate appropriate measures immediately, while in the field. The chapter on pacemakers and the self-assessment exercises round out the reader's journey through the world of electrocardiography. The *Sensible ECG Analysis Instructor's Manual* provides the seasoned practitioner with the tools necessary to teach this sensible approach to ECG analysis.

In a world of medical precision and intense legal scrutiny, and as we enter the second millennium, it is imperative that the field practitioner understands the fine points and intricacies of ECG and rhythm strip interpretation as they directly apply to stabilizing patients and saving lives. I have found no better method to help achieve the necessary education and skills than that which the authors present in this outstanding treatment of ECG analysis.

—Robert A. Friedman, MD, FAAFP

Preface

The electrocardiograph (ECG) is a tool, a sign, an extension of the history and physical examination. In a patient who presents with chest pain, the accurate interpretation of the ECG is vital.

For the most part, chest pain signals cardiac compromise due to a perfusion deficit. This interpretation is one tool that will formulate the basis of a treatment plan with the goal of reperfusion. Time is critical and time is not on the side of the health care provider. The learner of ECG rhythm analysis should value and defend the sense of urgency for rapid and accurate interpretation of the ECG. This is the foundation for subsequent implementation of interventions that protect the window of opportunity for reperfusion.

Because the ECG is such a useful tool, it should be mastered by all who are entrusted with the care of the cardiac patient. The increased interest in the cardiac arrhythmias has brought greater insight into the pathology underlying normal and abnormal ECGs, and a plethora of books of greater complexity on the subject.

Sensible ECG Analysis makes no pretenses of enabling the reader to master all the infinite intricacies of electrophysiology. Most individuals can plant a seed and watch it grow without the intricate knowledge of horticulture. Those who read, interpret, and monitor patients can make sensible use of the ECG without the complexity of physics.

The language of ECG is not difficult, just different. In order to speak the language one must practice. Most people learn a language by conversing freely without indepth knowledge of linguistics. Individuals learn the language of ECG by simple, repetitive practice as well as observing and listening to patients.

The ECG reflects the heart and all its functions. It is a window to the magnificent process of electrical activation and subsequent life-sustaining pulses. *Sensible ECG Analysis* is designed to help the practitioner read an ECG and realize what that recording implies about the heart. An ECG also allows monitoring the heart's response to interventions.

CHAPTER ORGANIZATION

This text is written for health professionals who use the ECG as a tool to assess patient progress, or lack of, and to monitor and document response to interventions. Anatomy, basic electrophysiology, and timing techniques are explained. Each arrhythmia is described and accompanied by key terms, etiology, clinical implications, and anticipated treatment. A systematic approach to the analysis and interpretation of each arrhythmia is explained. Helpful summaries of the characteristics of each of the arrhythmias are provided. Practical self-assessment exercises are included with detailed answer keys. References to medications and algorithms to provide the reader with further insight into clinical applications for the patient in cardiac crisis are also included.

TO THE LEARNER

ECG rhythm interpretation contributes to the differential diagnosis and overall care of the patient.

The traditional ECG is an accurate, noninvasive tool that is vital in the identification and differential diagnosis of the patient in cardiac compromise. Accurate interpretation by the practitioner provides accurate, moment-to-moment insight. We have written this text to help you master the steps you need to accurately interpret the ECG when you are responsible for monitoring a patient and deciding the appropriate care and intervention.

We have designed the text in a specific format, which, if followed will help you master the skills necessary for accurate interpretation of each arrhythmia. The introductory chapters will provide baseline insight into cardiac anatomy and electrophysiology. Wave forms and timing techniques are explained as they reflect the heart's function. Each arrhythmia is introduced, described, and explained.

The ECG tracings are taken from patients whose clinical problems, signs, and symptoms were documented and reflect the content for each chapter. There are many practice strips, with detailed answers for your ready reference. There are also simple self-assessment exercises. Once you have completed the practice, analyze your answers, and compare them with the answer key. If they differ from those provided, compare the specific differences and review the chapter before moving on.

As you progress, you may be tempted to study directly from the answer key rather than come up with your own interpretation. Do not do this. The sample practice strips are an important part of the learning process—a step that should be followed carefully.

The key to mastering ECG rhythm analysis is consistent application of the steps to interpretation. Be sure to master each chapter before moving on to the next. Developing the foundation blocks of information is essential. Once you have completed this text, you should be able to use everything you have learned to help with decisions and care and correctly apply your skills. YOU are the critical link providing insight and clues vital to the care of the patient in cardiac compromise.

ACKNOWLEDGMENTS

The accumulation of knowledge and insight is not a solitary process. Since 1977, I have learned from patients, families, and various mentors. Mary Boudreau Conover has been my teacher, counselor, and guide through my growth and development in cardiac care since the seventies. Dr. Marriott gave me the strength always to question "why" and never to accept the norm. Dr. Kathleen Handal, who never takes anything for granted, prodded me out of procrastination. Many thanks for her editing and determination for perfection. Her motto "Always the Best" became my banner.

Andy Yee, R-Pharm, EMT-Basic, has doggedly searched down the rhythms he believed would be helpful to the learners and the patients they will ultimately serve. Dan Donahue, NREMT-P, labored to catalogue actual scenarios, answered field questions, and was my steadfast friend and advocate.

My thanks to the monitor techs who filled envelopes with strips and data each week. My undying gratitude to the students who provided the acid test for each version of this work since its inception in 1977.

REVIEWERS

The authors and Delmar would like to acknowledge the following individuals who reviewed the manuscript and provided several valuable suggestions for improvement:

Joanne Ceimo, MD, FACC
Cardiologist
Scottsdale, Arizona

Terry DeVito, RN, M.Ed, EMT-P, CEN
Assistant Professor and Coordinator, EMS Education
Capital Community Technical College
Hartford, Connecticut

Carol Eckert, RN, MSN, TNS
Former CEN, CCRN
Director, Nursing Education
Bellevue Area College
Belleville, Illinois

Ann Hudgins, RN, BSN, EMT-P
Assistant Professor
UT Southwestern Medical Center
Dallas, Texas

Carol Hurdelbrink, RN, BSN
EMS/Trauma Director
North Suburban Medical Center
Thornton, Colorado

Dr. Karen Minchella, CMA
Consulting Management Associates, LLC
Fraser, Michigan

John Stasic, BAEE
Medtronic Corporation
Tempe, Arizona

Susan L. Woods, PhD, RN
Professor, Biobehavioral Nursing and Health Systems
University of Washington
Seattle, Washington

CHAPTER 1

Review of the Heart's Anatomy and Function

Premise To know the heart's mechanical function and purpose is to recognize signs and symptoms of its malfunction.

Objectives

After reading the chapter and completing the Self-Assessment Exercise, the student should be able to

1. describe the position of the heart within the body
2. identify the structures and functions of the heart and its blood vessels
3. identify the phases of systole and diastole

Key Terms

atrial kick
cardiac output
chest pain
endocardium
epicardium
heart rate
myocardium
perfusion
stroke volume

Introduction

Most students of ECG are not enchanted with the typical review of cardiac muscle and functions. However, a review is necessary to maintain perspective of cardiac **perfusion**. The ECG will relate problems of ischemia in various surfaces of the heart. The practitioner will read the ECG, recall the surface of the heart visualized by the ECG and the responsible coronary blood supply in jeopardy, and realize the implications in terms of what can happen next with this patient. All this provides a sound basis for patient care decisions.

perfusion The distribution of oxygenated blood

REVIEW OF CARDIAC FUNCTION

Myocardial contraction and subsequent ejection of blood are a direct result of electrical activation. Electrical activation is complete and accurate if the heart muscle and the conduction system imbedded within are well perfused and oxygenated.

In simplest terms, the function of the heart is to pump blood to the lungs for oxygenation and then to pump that blood back into systemic circulation. This process requires blood volume and the timeless, persistent muscular contraction of

cardiac output

The product of heart rate and stroke volume

heart rate

The number of contractions, or how fast the heart beats

stroke volume

The amount of blood ejected with each heart beat

chest pain

The term used by patients to describe pain, discomfort, burning, pressure, tightness, heaviness, aching, fullness, hard to breathe, or difficulty getting one's breath

heart muscle. When there is malperfusion of cardiac muscle, there are problems with electrical function, cardiac output, and systemic circulation.

Cardiac output is the product of heart rate and stroke volume. Variations in cardiac output can be produced by altering the heart rate or the stroke volume. **Heart rate** is the number of contractions, or how fast the heart beats. Heart rate is primarily determined by the integrity of the heart's electrical conduction system and the influence of the body's autonomic nervous system as it tries to identify and respond to changes and needs of the body. **Stroke volume** is the amount of blood ejected with each heart beat. It is primarily determined by the efficient contraction of cardiac muscle and the blood volume returning to the heart.

Normally, the body compensates for increases and decreases in stroke volume and heart rate, so that as one increases, the other decreases. If the demands of the body's tissues for oxygen are not met due to a decreased cardiac output, the body will display signs and symptoms, for instance, chest pain, dizziness, altered levels of consciousness, near-syncopal episodes, changes in skin temperature and hydration, and decreased urinary output. For the purposes of this book, **chest pain** is used to describe a range of subjective terms that the patient may use. These terms include pain, discomfort, burning, pressure, tightness, heaviness, aching, fullness, hard to breathe, and difficulty getting one's breath. Diminished circulation through the pulmonary system will result in progressive hypoxia, and, if left untreated, the body begins a spiral decline.

When symptoms develop because of a drop in heart rate and the body exhibits the above signs, the patient is said to be symptomatic, that is, hypotensive and hypoperfusing. When the heart muscle is damaged or injured as with infarction, the heart's pumping ability may fail, stroke volume will decrease, and heart rate will increase. Unfortunately, any change in cardiac output requires functioning oxygenated tissue and an increase in myocardial oxygen demand. A poorly perfused myocardium cannot respond to this increased debt, and the problem intensifies.

The Heart's Mechanical Structures

The right atrium and ventricle differ in function and musculature. The right atrium is a low-pressure receptacle, receiving blood from the systemic circulation, and is a thin-walled muscular structure. The right ventricle is thicker than the atrium, to accommodate the pressures necessary to eject blood to the pulmonary circulation. Despite the differences, they act as a single unit to move blood from the great veins to the pulmonary circulation.

The left atrium and ventricle act similarly to move oxygenated blood from the lungs to the high-pressure systemic circulation. The left atrium is a low-pressure receptacle, receiving blood from the pulmonic circulation, and is a thin-walled muscular structure. The left ventricle is thicker than the left atrium and right ventricle because the left ventricle must accommodate the pressures necessary to eject blood to the systemic circulation. Tension in the left ventricular tissue reflects the pressure against which it must pump. Systemic vascular resistance can cause an increase in the size and thickness of the left ventricle. Figure 1-1 illustrates right and left ventricular structures in relation to their intake and outflow structures and to the lungs.

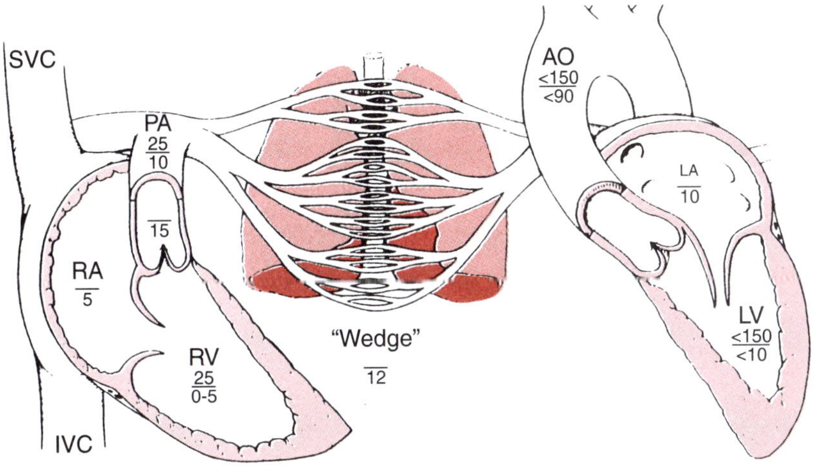

Figure 1-1 Right and left atrial and ventricular structures in relation to their intake and outflow structures and to the lungs. Note the differences in pressures within the right and left ventricles.

Cardiac Position and Movement

The terms *right* and *left* heart are not descriptive of their position in the body. The right ventricle is anterior, in front of the left and occupies a position immediately behind the sternum, whereas the left ventricle is rotated so that it faces toward the left side and is more posterior in the thorax.

The heart is suspended and secured in the pericardial cavity by its attachments to the great vessels. The heart is located in the center of the chest, within the mediastinum between the lungs (Figure 1-2). Approximately one-third of the heart lies to the right of the midline, and two-thirds of the heart lies to the left of the midline. The heart is superior to the diaphragm, with the apex located to the left of the central portion of the diaphragm. The base of the heart is located superiorly, posteriorly, and to the right of the midline at about the level of the second intercostal space.

As you can see, the heart is protected anteriorly by the sternum and the rib cage and posteriorly by the vertebral column and the rib cage. The apex is free to move, and in fact, during ventricular contraction, dimensional changes take place within

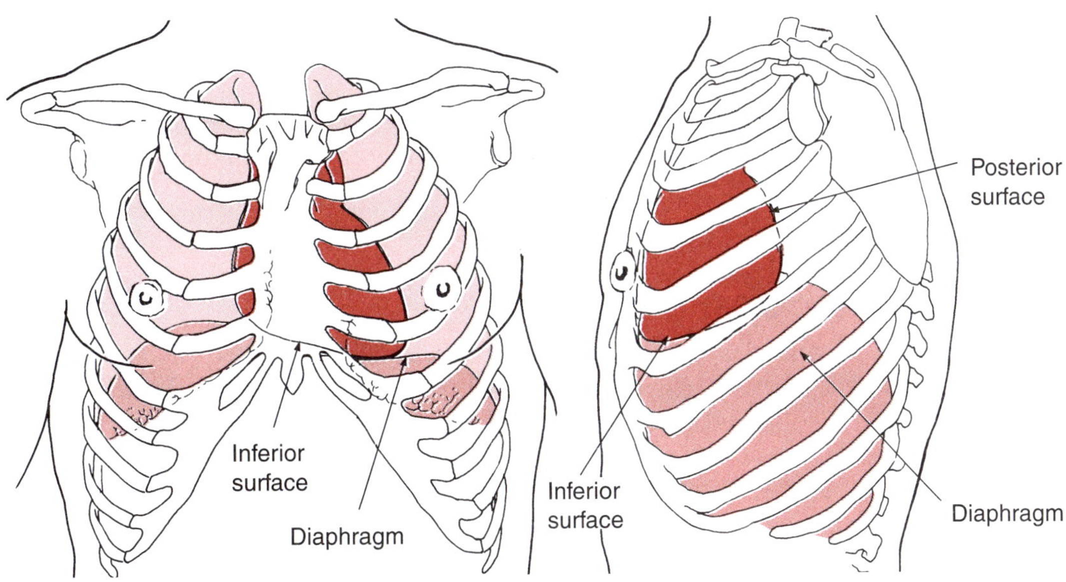

Figure 1-2 The position of the heart within the body. The heart is located in the mediastinum, superior to the diaphragm with the bulk of the left ventricle to the left side and posterior.

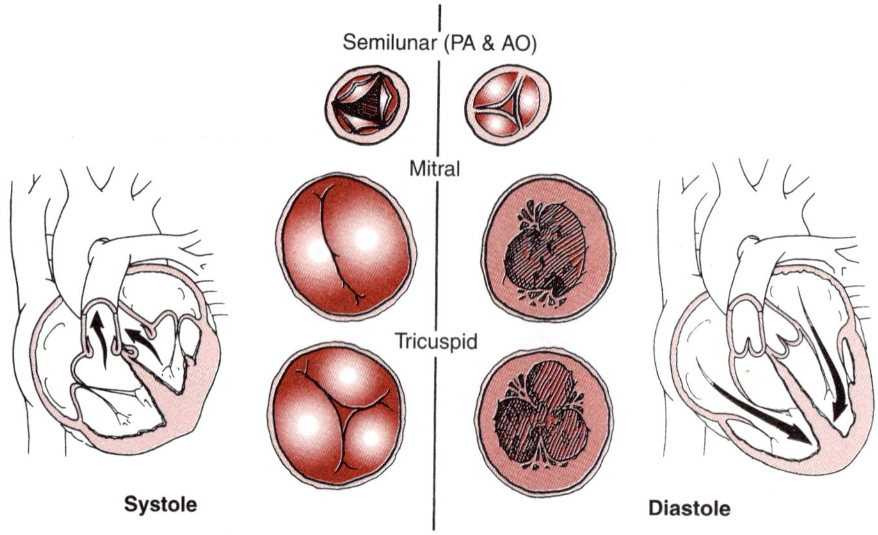

Figure 1-3 A schematic representation of the position of the cardiac valves during ventricular systole and diastole

the ventricle, causing the apex to move forward and to strike against the left chest wall in the area of the left intercostal space. This characteristic thrust is felt by the examiner as the apical pulse. The placement of the heart within the rib cage gives rise to the position of the ECG chest-wall electrodes to best view the heart's surfaces.

The Cardiac Valves

There are four delicate, resilient, but strong valves that guard the entrance and exit of each ventricle (Figure 1-3). Even though they function passively, they greatly enhance the movement of blood by preventing backflow. There are no valves between the veins and their entrance into the atria. The heart always must accept the blood that comes to it. Even if the ventricles cannot eject all the blood during systole, blood continues to enter the heart via the atria. This constant flow of blood into the heart will cause the atria to distend and stretch. This abnormal stretch will give rise to various ECG patterns and arrhythmias.

There is a point in ventricular diastole when all the valves are open, and the pressure within the entire cardiovascular system is the same. Just at the end of ventricular diastole, in the microsecond prior to ventricular systole, the ventricles tense. It is at this point that the coronary arteries are in greatest jeopardy. They cannot perfuse since they are imbedded in this tense and rigid muscular structure.

The semilunar valves, so named for their crescent shape, are situated between the ventricles and their respective arteries. The pulmonic (PA) valve is located between the right ventricle and the pulmonary artery; the aortic (AO) valve is located between the left ventricle and the aorta. The aortic and pulmonic valves open completely during ventricular ejection/systole and close completely during ventricular filling/diastole. Figure 1-3 illustrates the heart's valves during ventricular systole and diastole. Note the apparent bulging of the valves during ventricular systole.

There is a slight enlargement of the aorta and the pulmonary artery in the area of the AO and PA valves. This enlargement provides space behind the open AO valve cusps so that the leaflets do not occlude the openings/orifices of the coronary arteries. This space favors the development of *eddy currents* (Figure 1-4) that hold the valve cusps away from the arterial wall in such a way that they will be easily caught and closed by the backflow of blood at the end of systolic ejection (Little 1985).

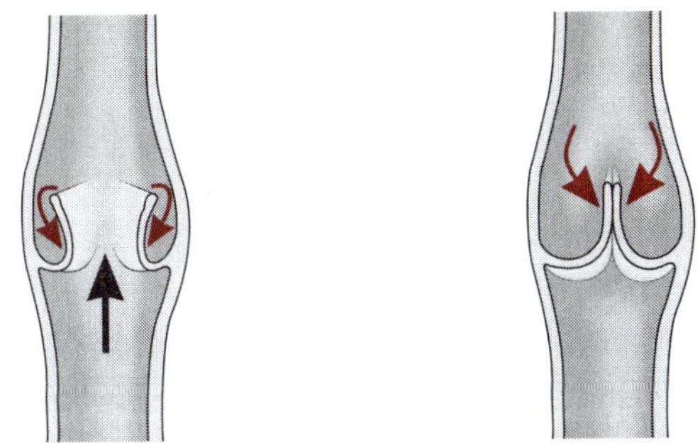

Figure 1-4 A schematic representation of the eddy currents in the aortic valve during ventricular systole and diastole. The enlargement (A) provides space behind the open AO valve cusps so that the leaflets do not occlude the coronary artery orifices in ventricular systole. The eddy currents (B) act to hold the cusps away from the wall of the aorta in ventricular systole and are easily caught and closed at the end of ventricular systole and during ventricular diastole.

The structure of the mitral and tricuspid (AV) valves controls the flow of blood into the ventricles. The valve cusps are extensions of the chordae tendinae, which are, in turn, extensions of the papillary muscles. Papillary muscles are specialized extensions of the myocardium. Ventricular contraction distorts the valves, which are larger than their openings. This disparity in size allows for complete closure during ventricular systole. Sometimes there is a great disproportion in size, which causes an abnormal movement (called a *prolapse*) of the valve into the atrium.

The mitral valve has two cusps and is located between the left atrium and ventricle; the tricuspid valve has three cusps and is located between the right atrium and ventricle.

Cardiac Muscle

The wall of the heart is composed of three anatomically distinct layers:

1. the outer layer or **epicardium**
2. the middle muscle layer or muscular **myocardium**
3. the inner layer or **endocardium**.

The epicardium continues with the outer covering of the ventricles and contains some small nerve branches and the main coronary blood vessels. The endocardium consists of tissue layers that make it somewhat thicker than the rest of the heart. The myocardial layer contains many nerve fibers and sensory endings. These are more abundant in the atria than in the ventricles.

epicardium
The outer layer of the heart

myocardium
The middle muscle layer of the heart

endocardium
The inner lining of the heart

The Atria. The atria are reservoirs of blood and are very distensible. They are collapsible when partially filled and are usually quite elastic when overfilled. The atrial capacity of the normal adult is 160 ml on the right and about 140 ml on the left. During ventricular systole, forward movement of blood into the ventricles is stopped because of the closed AV valves. At the end of ventricular diastole, the atria contract, and blood is added to the already well-filled ventricles. This addition of

atrial kick
The amount of blood added to ventricular diastole with atrial contraction

blood is **atrial kick**. In specific ECG abnormalities, the loss of atrial kick will ensue and the patient will display signs and symptoms of the deficit, such as dizziness, fatigue, and other signs of hypotension and hypoperfusion.

The right atrium has more extensions of the myocardial layer (trabeculae) than the left, perhaps to facilitate the greater pressures from venous flow on the right, that is, superior and inferior venae cavae and the coronary sinus.

The Ventricles. The ventricles are the major force behind perfusion. The more circular left ventricle is designed to support the highly resistant systemic circulation. It is quite effective in developing and maintaining high intracardiac pressures to maintain that circulation. The bellow-shaped right ventricle supports moving blood from the systemic circulation into the low-pressure pulmonary circulation.

The walls of the ventricles are similar in structure to the atria, and for ease of study, the layers are repeated here. There are three anatomically distinct layers:

1. outer epicardium
2. the muscular myocardium
3. the inner endocardium.

The ventricular myocardium is much thicker than that of the atria and is arranged in a much more complicated sequence of layers and bundles. The muscle bundles are *trabeculae* and are extensions of the myocardium. The dense myocardium is thicker on the left, and the trabecular layer is thicker on the right.

The ventricular septum is the thickest part of the ventricular wall and is common to the right and left ventricular chambers and has trabeculation on both sides.

There are two primary muscle groups, superficial and deep spiral (Figure 1-5). The superficial muscles have their origin in the cardiac ring that separates the atria from the ventricles. They wrap around so that they exert a wringing effect during

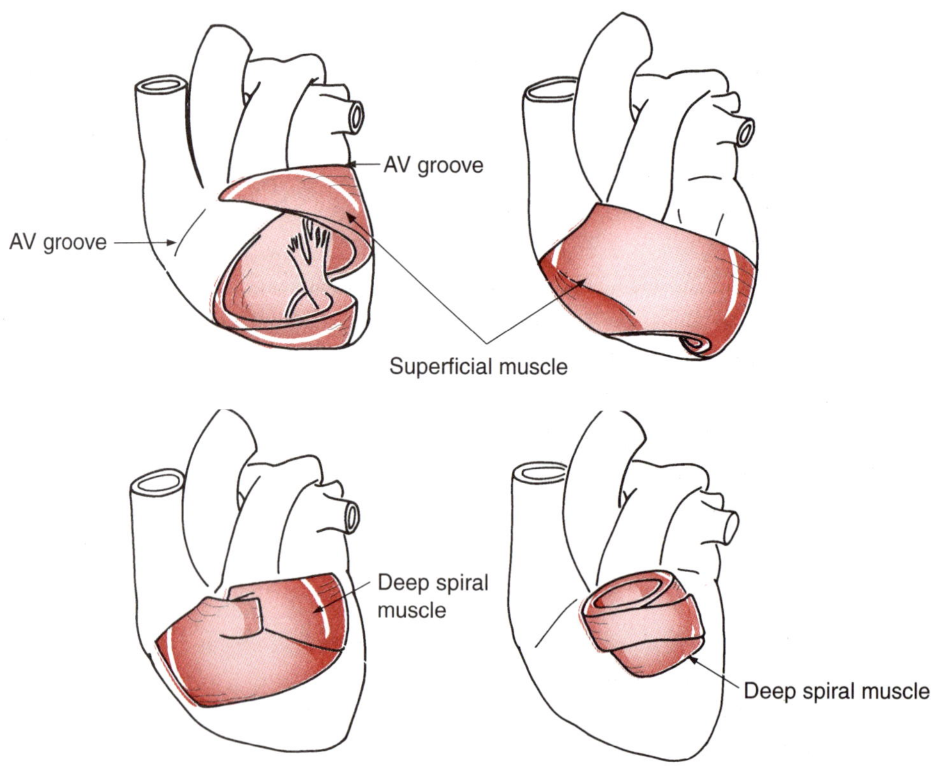

Figure 1-5 Layers of muscles of the right and left ventricles. Two groups of fibers surround the outside of both ventricles and their origin in the atrioventricular (AV) groove. The deep spiral muscle (lower left) also has its origin in the AV groove and encircles both ventricles. The deep spiral muscle (lower right) is specific to the left ventricle.

muscular contraction. The deeper spiral muscles are arranged as spirals and coils in clockwise and counterclockwise fashion. The deep bulbospiral muscle on the left is responsible for the forceful ejection of blood from the left ventricle during ventricular systole.

Figure 1-5 illustrates how the fibers leave their origin at the root of the pulmonary artery and the aorta and insert into the papillary muscles and trabeculae. Between the origin and insertion there is a 360-degree path down to the apex and then back onto the inside of the heart at its base.

This is a great simplification of a very complex matrix that supports maximum projection and emptying of blood in ventricular systole and maximum filling of blood in ventricular diastole.

Knowledge of the muscle groups and their winding configurations will give insight into why, in right inferior myocardial infarction, left ventricular output can be greatly affected.

Ventricular Systole

The spiral arrangement of the ventricular myocardium is adapted to propelling blood flow. During the early stages of ventricular contraction, the inflow tract from atria to apex shortens, and the outflow tract from apex to aorta lengthens, thus making the left ventricle more spheroid. The ventricular septum is activated early on and provides a rigid *prop*, around which the heart will wring, twist, and thrust in an effort to move the blood out the outflow tract. During this time, the heart rotates somewhat to the right, and the left ventricle is brought forward.

Ventricular contraction (systole) and the associated rapid increase in ventricular pressures promptly close the mitral and tricuspid (AV) valves. The AV valves bulge into the atria, and ventricular pressures rise rapidly as the contraction process begins to squeeze the blood contained inside the ventricle against the closed AV valves. Ventricular pressure continues to increase. As it rises above aortic pressure, the aortic valve cusps are forced open, and the period of rapid ventricular ejection begins.

During the remainder of ventricular systole, ventricular pressure falls below aortic pressure, and a negative pressure gradient develops across the aortic valve. Due to its forward momentum, blood continues to be ejected from the ventricle during this period, in spite of the reversed pressure gradient, but the rate of ejection decreases rapidly.

The fact that blood continues to move forward during this period appears paradoxical, but the total energy of ventricular blood is still higher than the total energy level of the blood in the aorta. About 0.17 of a second after the onset of the phase of reduced ejection, forward movement of blood out of the ventricles stops, and the flow momentarily reverses as blood attempts to regurgitate into the ventricle. This backflow will *catch* the aortic valve cusps, and they are promptly closed. It is at this time that the coronary arteries begin to fill.

Ventricular Diastole

Within about 0.06 to 0.08 of a second after the closure of the aortic valve, ventricular volume is stabilized, and the mitral and tricuspid (AV) valves are still closed. Blood cannot leave or enter the ventricles. This is the period of isovolemic relaxation. During this time, pressure within the ventricles drops rapidly, and relaxation of the ventricular myocardium begins. At the same time, the curve of the AV valves begins to flatten out. When ventricular pressure falls below atrial pressure, the mitral cusps bulge toward the ventricles. At the end of isovolemic relaxation, the ventricular pressures fall below that of the atria. Traction on the valve cusps by the chordae tendinea during diastole plays a role in valve opening.

Opening of the AV valves permits blood that has collected in the atria to rush into the relaxing ventricles; this is the period of rapid ventricular filling early in ventricular diastole. At this point, ventricular pressures are low, and blood is literally sucked into the ventricles. Ventricular filling continues until the atrial and ventricular pressures are similar. After electrical activation, atrial contraction squeezes additional blood into the ventricles. Intraventricular pressures increase, and the process of ventricular depolarization and subsequent contraction begins again.

Figure 1-6 illustrates the phases of ventricular diastole and systole. Note the position of the valves during early and late filling stages and the change in the size of the ventricles. Notice too, the position of the cardiac valves during the phases ranging from ventricular filling to contraction.

The right ventricle pumps blood at 25 to 32 mm Hg pressure into the lungs for oxygenation and for release of carbon dioxide. The left atrium receives oxygenated blood from the lungs. The blood then passes into the left ventricle, which pumps at about 120 mm Hg pressure into the arterial system. Externally, the anterior and posterior intraventricular sulci contain the coronary blood vessels and a variable amount of fat. The muscular layers of the ventricle are developed so that the muscle mass to the right ventricle is considerably less than that of the left ventricle. This variance in muscle mass is the result of the difference in pressures between the muscular chambers. Although each ventricle pumps essentially the same amount of blood, the major difference in structure reflects the difference in function.

Coronary Artery Perfusion

Like other organ systems, the heart has its own blood supply. However, unlike other organ systems, coronary artery perfusion is affected by the diastolic phase of the cardiac cycle. Coronary artery perfusion is affected by the unique position at the beginning of the aorta, just behind the aortic cusps. While the right and left sides of the heart receive oxygenated blood from the coronary arteries, the timing for optimal perfusion differs.

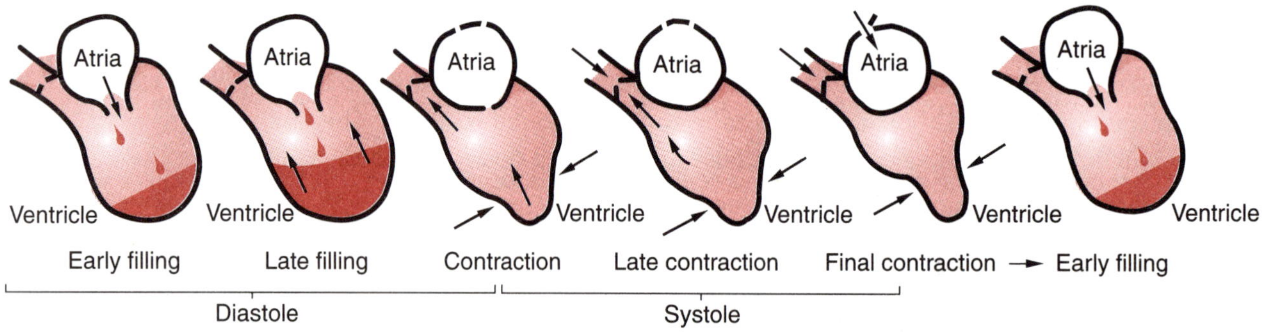

Figure 1-6 Schematic representation of the events in ventricular diastole and systole. During ventricular diastole, the AO and PA valves are closed so that blood only enters the ventricles from the atria. Atrial systole occurs during late ventricular filling (diastole) and contributes to the boost of blood volume in the ventricles just prior to ventricular systole (atrial kick).

For example, the right ventricular myocardium receives a flow of oxygenated blood from the coronary circulation almost continuously throughout the cardiac cycle. Even during ventricular systole, the right ventricle generates lower systolic pressure, which allows for some coronary filling. The left ventricular myocardium receives oxygenated coronary blood flow only during the diastolic phase of the cardiac cycle, probably because the left ventricle exerts systolic pressure equal to or greater than aortic pressure. As a result, intramyocardial tension and pressure hamper blood flow within the myocardium, particularly to the subendocardial layers.

The coronary arteries are also responsible for blood supply to the electrical conduction system. The right coronary artery has its origin behind a cusp of the aortic valve. It proceeds downward and perfuses the right anterior and posterior surfaces of the heart. The posterior descending branch of the right coronary artery also emits septal branches that perfuse the posterior one-third of the ventricular septum and a terminal portion of the infero-posterior division of the left bundle branch, a part of the heart's ventricular electrical conduction system.

The right coronary artery is responsible for about 55 to 60 percent of the blood supply to the sinus node, the major electrical pacemaker of the heart (Guyton 1990; Hurst 1989; Mandel 1980; Little 1985). In about 90 percent of individuals, the posterior descending branch of the right coronary artery perfuses the electrical conduction system at the AV junction. In the remaining 10 percent, dual blood supply from the right posterior descending branch of the right coronary artery and the anterior descending branch of the left coronary artery perfuse the heart's ventricular electrical conduction system.

The common portion of the left coronary artery after its origin from the aorta and before the bifurcation into the left anterior descending (LAD) and circumflex arteries is called the left main trunk (LMT). Clinicians often call this the *widow maker* because obstruction here predisposes to a high incidence of sudden death. The LAD is usually larger than the circumflex.

LAD disease causes loss of a large amount of muscle mass and parts of the electrical conduction system. The LAD is frequently implicated in sudden cardiac death, predominantly in adult males.

The left circumflex branch winds around the left ventricle dividing the left atrium and left ventricle. The extent of perfusion of the left circumflex to the right atrium varies. The left circumflex supplies about 40 percent of perfusion to the sinus node.

Figure 1-7 demonstrates the relative position of each of the major branches of the coronary arteries. Note large amounts of muscle mass dependent on the left anterior descending coronary artery (LAD).

As blood is perfused through the coronary circulation system, oxygen and nutrients are delivered to myocardial tissue; substrate, carbon dioxide, and metabolic waste products are removed. The deoxygenated blood is collected by smaller cardiac veins that empty into the great cardiac vein, coronary sinus, and finally the right atrium. The venous blood from the posterior aspect is drained into the middle cardiac vein. The remaining blood empties directly into the right ventricle by way of the small Thebesian veins.

Adequate perfusion of the coronary circulation is directly dependent on blood volume and the time in ventricular diastole. The coronary arteries are in jeopardy during ventricular systole and must distend and refill during ventricular diastole. Therefore, heart rate and blood volume have an integral part in maintaining coro-

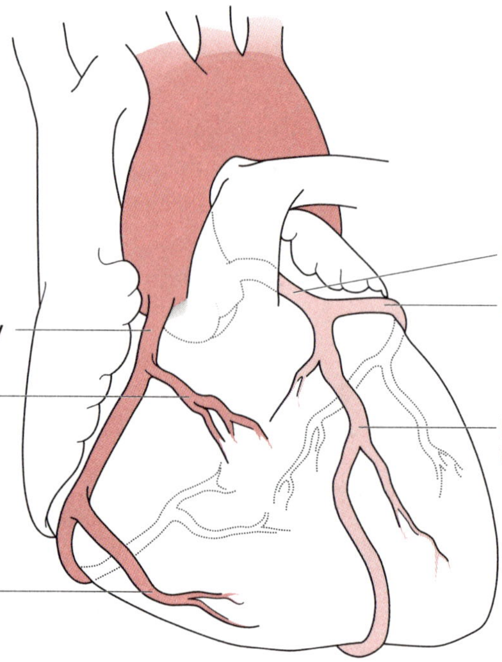

Figure 1-7 Right and left coronary arteries as they exit from the ascending aorta and cross-ventricular muscle mass.

nary artery perfusion. To alter either for a prolonged period of time would hamper myocardial perfusion with great consequence to myocardial function.

Summary

In this chapter, we have come to learn and appreciate the heart's function and purpose, in order to comprehend the magnitude of the signs and symptoms of its malfunction. It is important for us to visualize the landmarks of the surfaces of the heart and the coronary arteries responsible for perfusion to those surfaces.

As practitioners, we will read the ECG, recall the surface of the heart visualized by the various leads of the ECG, and deduce which coronary blood supply is in jeopardy. From this we should anticipate probable complications and plan patient care decisions. This appreciation and insight will separate practitioners from those who rely solely on an automatic ECG rhythm-identification machine for patient care decisions.

Self-Assessment Exercise

Fill in the Blanks

Complete the statements, and then compare your answers with those in the back of the book.

1. The heart consists of right and left sides. The right and left sides of the heart differ in _______________ and _______________.

2. The right ventricle delivers unoxygenated blood from _______________ circulation to the _______________.

3. The left ventricle delivers _______________ blood from the _______________ to the _______________.

4. In comparison, the musculature of the left ventricle is _______________ than the right since it is a high-pressure system projecting blood to the _______________.

5. The _______________ valve lies between the right atrium and the _______________ ventricle.

6. The _______________ valve lies between the left atrium and _______________ ventricle.

7. Blood exiting the right ventricle passes through the _______________ valve to the _______________. Blood exiting the left ventricle passes through the _______________ valve to the _______________.

8. Within the thorax, the heart is _______________ and positioned so the right ventricle is more _______________. The left ventricle is therefore in a more _______________ position.

9. The right coronary artery has its origin behind a cusp of the _______________ and proceeds _______________ and perfuses the right _______________ and _______________ surfaces of the heart. The right coronary gives a branch to the AV node at about the same level of the posterior descending branch. The right coronary perfuses the right atrium and both the _______________ and _______________ nodes.

10. The posterior descending branch of the right coronary artery also emits branches that perfuse the ventricular septum posteriorly. These are called the _______________ branches. These branches supply a portion of the _______________, the posterior third of the septum, and a portion of the inferio-posterior division of the left-bundle branch.

11. The left coronary artery also has its origin behind an aortic cusp. The left coronary divides into two branches, the _______________, and the _______________.

12. The anterior descending branch perfuses the anterior two-thirds of the ventricular _______________, a major portion of the _______________, and the anterosuperior division of the _______________.

13. The lateral branch, also called the _______________, winds around the left ventricle, dividing the left atrium and left ventricle. The extent of perfusion of the left posterior ventricle varies between individuals. The left circumflex also perfuses the _______________.

References

Aronson, R. The hemodynamic consequences of cardiac arrhythmias. *Cardiovascular reviews and reports.* New York: le Jacq Publishing Co.; 1981.

Berne, R. M., & Levy, M. N. *Cardiovascular physiology* (4th ed.). St. Louis, MO: C. V. Mosby; 1981.

Goldberger, E. *Textbook of clinical cardiology.* St. Louis, MO: C. V. Mosby; 1982.

Goode, P. Davis, Jr., Park, Edwards. *The heart: The living pump.* New York: Torstar Books, Inc.; 1984.

Michaelson, C. R. (Ed). *Congestive heart failure.* St. Louis, MO: C. V. Mosby; 1983.

Sokolow, M. & McIlroym, M. B. *Clinical cardiology* (2nd ed.). Los Altos, CA: Lange Medical Publications; 1979.

Tartora, G. J. *Introduction to the human body: The essentials of anatomy and physiology.* New York: HarperCollins; 1994.

CHAPTER 2

Electrophysiology and the ECG Recording

Premise There can be electrical activity and no mechanical response, but there can never be mechanical response without electrical activation.

Objectives

After reading the chapter and completing the Self-Assessment Exercise, the student should be able to

1. identify and describe the four properties critical to electrical activity
2. identify the structures of the heart's electrical conduction system
3. begin to relate cardiac perfusion deficits with electrical malfunction

Key Terms

absolute refractory period
action potential
automaticity
conductivity
contractility
depolarization
ectopy
electrode
excitability
lead
myocardial cells
nonrefractory phase
refractoriness
relative refractory period
repolarization
specialized cells

Introduction

Electrical activity precedes mechanical activity (contraction). Electrical activation describes the events that result in the contraction and relaxation of cardiac muscle, thus sustaining perfusion of the body and the heart itself. This electrical reaction causes chemical reactions and an electrical chain of events within cardiac muscle that are ultimately displayed on the electrocardiograph, measured, and assessed.

action potential
Abrupt phasic changes in the electrical charges of the cell membrane, including polarization, depolarization, and repolarization

depolarization
Electrical activation of the heart tissue due to spread of the electrical impulse

ELECTROPHYSIOLOGY OF THE HEART

Action potential describes the electrolyte exchanges that occur across the cell membrane during depolarization and the four phases of repolarization. **Depolarization**

is electrical activation of myocardial cells. It is the process by which the inside of the cell becomes less negative. There are mechanisms by which specific cells depolarize.

1. In atrial and ventricular cells, there is a rapid influx of sodium into the cell.
2. In the His-Purkinje system, there is a slow, time-dependent decrease in potassium permeability and an increase in sodium permeability.
3. In the sinus node and AV nodes there is a slow inward flow of calcium.

Depolarization is a very active process. Unfortunately, ischemia can exist and not affect the wave forms that reflect depolarization. Unless an ischemic or injury process directly affects an electrical conduction pathway, it will not be visualized in a depolarization wave form.

repolarization
The process by which a cell, after being discharged, returns to its state of readiness

Repolarization describes the process by which the cells return to the resting level. Repolarization is rapid at first, reaches a plateau, and then a longer, rapid surge occurs, until the resting state is reached.

The Phases of the Cardiac Cycle

The phases are described as follows:

Phase 0 Rapid depolarization. As a change in cellular permeability occurs, sodium rushes into the cell, making the cell more positive. This action produces the characteristic upstroke in the action potential.

Phase 1 Initial repolarization. This is the phase in which the rapid influx of chloride inactivates the inward pumping of sodium.

Phase 2 The plateau. During this time, a slow inward flow of calcium occurs, while the flow of potassium is slowed considerably.

Phase 3 Final rapid depolarization. During this phase, there is a sudden acceleration of the rate of repolarization as the slow calcium current is inactivated and the outward flow of potassium is accelerated.

Phase 4 Diastolic depolarization. There is a difference in activities during this phase for working cells and pacemaker cells. In pacemaker cells, there is a time-dependent fall in outward potassium current with a rapid sodium influx, causing depolarization to be self-initiated.

Diastolic depolarization is very rapid in the cells of the sinus node, less rapid in the bundle of His, and very slow in the terminal fascicles of the bundle branches. Nonpacemaker (working) cells remain in the steady state until their membranes are acted on by another stimulus. Figure 2-1A illustrates action potential and electrolyte movement. Figure 2-1B illustrates the difference between action potential in pacemaker and working cells.

myocardial cells
Cells which make up the bulk of the heart's muscle and are the actual contractile units of the heart. These cells must be able to respond to electrical stimulus.

specialized cells
Cells with four specific properties that govern their function: automaticity, excitability, conductivity, and contractility. These cells make up the heart's electrical conduction system.

Properties of Cardiac Muscle

There are two types of cardiac cells. In combination, they are responsible for the mechanical and electrical activity of the heart. First we will discuss the **myocardial cells**, which make up the bulk of the heart's muscle and are the actual contractile units of the heart. These cells must be able to respond to electrical stimulus.

The other group of cells are **specialized cells**, which make up the heart's electrical conduction system. The specialized cells have four specific properties that govern their function: automaticity, excitability, conductivity, and contractility.

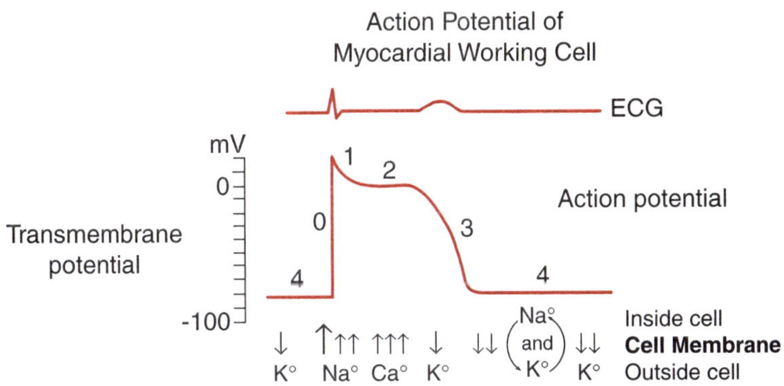

Figure 2-1A Action potential of working myocardial cells. Electrolyte exchanges occur across the cell membrane during action potential.

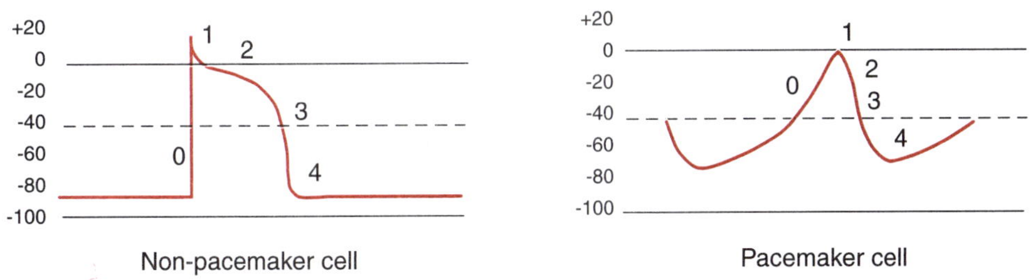

Figure 2-1B Schematic representation comparing action potential of pacemaker and nonpacemaker (working) myocardial cells.

Automaticity is the ability of a cell to reach potential and *generate* an action potential without being stimulated. This property is attributed to the pacemaker cells. In pacemaker cells, there is a regular, predictable fall in potassium concentration during electrical diastole. The potassium leak and the increased permeability to sodium cause the threshold to be reached and an action potential to occur at regular, usually predictable intervals. The current is then transmitted along all the myocardial cells.

automaticity
The ability of a cell to spontaneously generate an impulse without being externally stimulated. Cells that possess automaticity at a predictable rate serve as pacemakers.

Excitability is the ability of a cell to reach threshold and *respond* to a stimulus. The smaller the amount of required stimulus, the more excitable the cell. The greater the amount of required stimulus, the less excitable the cell. Cardiac cells become irritable because of the difference in ion concentration. This degree of irritability determines their degree of excitability or responsiveness. Ischemia and hypoxia will enhance excitability and to some extent promote premature, competitive behavior, or **ectopy**.

excitability
The capacity of a cell to respond to a stimulus

ectopy
When cells compete with pacemaker cells; occurs early in cardiac cycle

Conductivity is the *transmission* or propagation of electrical impulses from cell to cell. Inherent to each cell is the capacity for transmission. There is a difference in the rate of transmission for atrial and ventricular cells.

conductivity
The property of cardiac muscle that describes the ability to transmit an impulse

For instance, from the time the sinus node discharges an impulse, preferential conduction through atrial tissue is roughly 0.08 second, followed by a delay of 0.12 to 0.20 second within the AV node. Subsequent activation of the bundle branch system takes place in only 0.02 second; total ventricular activation is usually 0.10 second or less. These electrical events are translated to the ECG as specific wave forms.

Because of the anatomical interconnection of myocardial muscle fibers, the stimulation of a cardiac cell is facilitated by the many lateral and end-to-end connections within that muscle. Thus, the electrical current can flow from cell to cell and laterally using these interconnections.

contractility
The ability of the heart to react to electrical conduction with organized response; the mechanical response to depolarization

Contractility is the ability of cardiac muscle fibers to shorten and *contract* in response to the electrical stimulation. Contractility is the mechanical response to the other properties just described.

refractoriness
The ability of myocardial tissue to reject an impulse. This capability exists in various stages or degrees.

absolute refractory period
The phase of refractoriness when the cells are unresponsive to a stimulus

relative refractory period
The phase of refractoriness when some cells may respond normally to a stimulus, but others may not

nonrefractory phase
The final phase of refractoriness when all cells are repolarized and ready to respond in a normal fashion

Another property is one of **refractoriness**, which is the ability to reject an impulse or remain unresponsive to a stimulus. Refractoriness is divided into three phases:

1. One is the **absolute refractory period**, during which time the cells cannot respond to the stimulus. The term is synonymous with depolarization and is a mechanism that protects the heart from all other ectopic impulses.
2. The **relative refractory period** (RRP) describes the time when only a strong stimulus can cause depolarization. The relative refractory period is when repolarization is almost complete, and some cells can respond, although not entirely in a normal fashion. So some may respond normally, some in a bizarre fashion, and some not at all.

   There is a time during the RRP when the cells are most *vulnerable*. There are enough cells able to respond, although in a disorganized manner. When this occurs, serious, life-threatening arrhythmias can occur.
3. Last is the **nonrefractory phase**, when all cells are repolarized and ready to respond in a normal fashion.

The length of time for each of the refractory periods can vary between normal individuals and also is affected by medications, recreational drugs, disease, electrolyte imbalance, myocardial ischemia, and myocardial injury.

THE NERVOUS SYSTEM CONTROL OF THE HEART

The autonomic nervous system controls the visceral functions of the body. There are divisions responsible for the heart, smooth muscles, and the glands. There are two divisions, the sympathetic and the parasympathetic systems. The sympathetic nerves originate in the spinal cord between the first thoracic and second lumbar vertebrae. They supply both the atria and ventricles, but primarily the ventricles. The chemical mediators of the sympathetic system are the hormones *norepinephrine* and *epinephrine*, which have the effect of enhancing excitability and increasing the force of contraction. There is also a modest increase in the rate of discharge in the sinus node. Norepinephrine has a minor effect on the heart; its major effect is on blood vessels.

The parasympathetic nerves leave the central nervous system through the cranial and sacral spinal nerves. The vagus is the parasympathetic nerve controlling the heart, primarily the atria. Stimulation of the vagus causes the release of the hormone acetylcholine. The effects of parasympathetic stimulation are slowing of the rate of discharge of the sinus node, a decrease in atrial and AV nodal conduction,

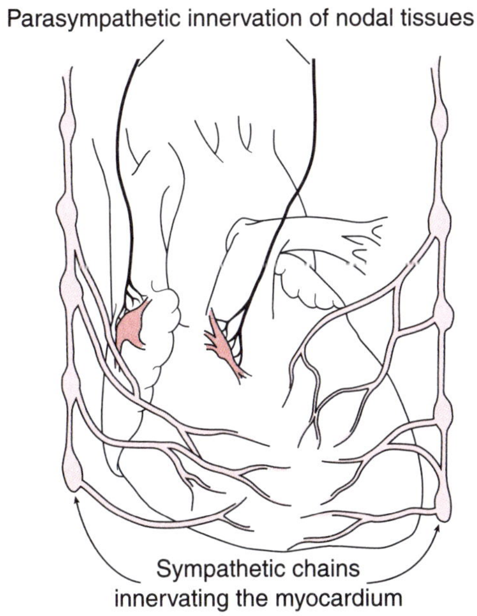

Figure 2-2 Autonomic nervous system innervation of nodal tissue and the myocardium by the parasympathetic (vagus) nerve fibers and the sympathetic chains

and minimally, a decreased transmission through the Purkinje fibers. Figure 2-2 illustrates parasympathetic and sympathetic innervation of the heart.

THE ELECTRICAL CONDUCTION SYSTEM

The heart's own electrical conduction system consists of the following structures (Figure 2-3):

1. the sinus node
2. atrial tissue
3. the AV junction
   - The AV junction consists of the AV node and the bundle of His down to where it begins to branch. The regions that constitute the AV junction are divided according to cell types: atrial-nodal (AN) region, nodal (N) region, and the nodal-His (NH) region (Figure 2-4).
     a. The AV node delays oncoming impulses to afford uniform conduction to the bundle of His and onto the ventricular conduction system.

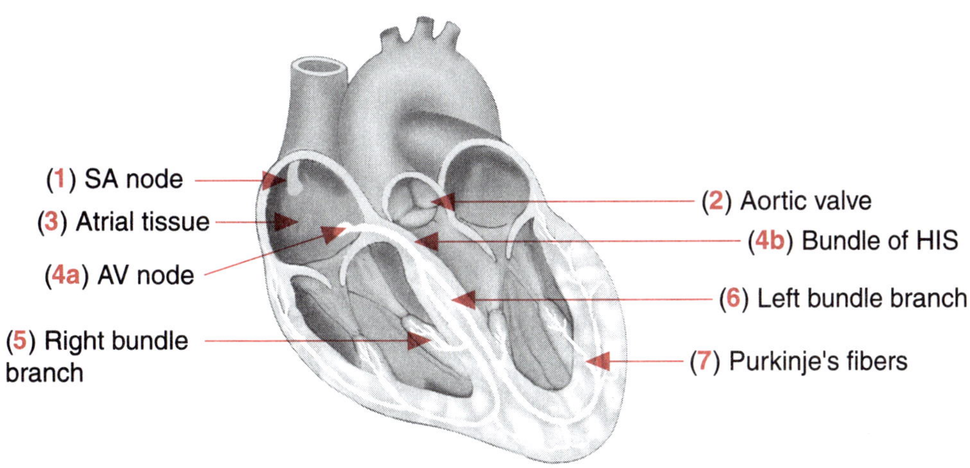

Figure 2-3 The position of the structures of the heart's electrical conduction system: (1) sinus node, (2) aortic valve, (3) atrial tissue, (4a) AV node, and (4b) bundle of His, (5) right bundle branch, (6) left bundle branch, (7) Purkinje system

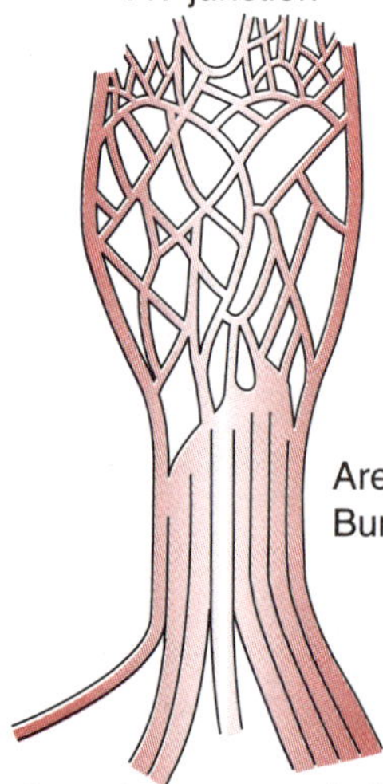

Figure 2-4 Schematic representation of the AV junction, demonstrating the entrance fibers into the AV node, orientation of the AV node to the bundle of His, and the entrance fibers into the intraventricular septum

b. The bundle of His has two capabilities:

— One is simple conduction of the impulse as it comes through from the AV node. An impulse that originates within the bundle of His is conducted through the ventricular bundle branches, resulting in a narrow QRS complex, not unlike a sinus-induced QRS complex.

— The other capability is generating an impulse forward to the ventricles and retrograde (backward) back up to the atria. For some time it was thought that the AV node functioned as a pacemaker, but the work of Sherf and James (1985) determined that there are no rapid-sodium channels within the AV node necessary for predictable pacemaker function. The pacing function within AV junctional tissue is referred to by convention as *junctional.*

4. the penetrating portions of the bundle branch system
   - the right bundle branch
   - the left bundle branch system
     a. left anterior fascicle
     b. left posterior fascicle
5. the Purkinje system

Normally, the sinus node governs the physiologic heart rate. The sinus node reaches potential more quickly than the rest of the cardiac tissue and is referred to as the *pacemaker.* A pacemaker is a cell or group of cells that generates an impulse at a predictable rate of speed.

There is no recording on conventional ECG that represents SA node depolarization. Such depolarization can be inferred only from subsequent atrial activation (Mudge 1986). Following SA node depolarization, the atrial tissue is activated and is directed inferiorly to the AV node by preferential conduction and from the right atrium to the left atrium via Bachman's bundle. Preferential conduction also occurs in the left atrium.

The next area to be activated is the AV node, which is situated at the floor of the right atrium near the atrial septum. After physiologic delay at the AV node, the impulse is transmitted past the bundle of His and onward through the fascicles of the bundle branch system into the Purkinje system.

During the final stages of myocardial contraction, repolarization is initiated. In normal ventricular tissue, the wave of repolarization starts in the last area to be depolarized and travels in a direction opposite that of depolarization. The forces of repolarization move more slowly, and the magnitude of electrical potential at any given moment is considerably less than the forces of depolarization. Repolarization is a passive process and is greatly affected by ischemic and hypoxic tissue. As a result, recordings of the repolarization are smaller and wider than those of the depolarization wave.

Summary of Electrophysiology

1. A wave of depolarization that moves toward the positive electrode records an upright deflection on the ECG.
2. Depolarization moving toward the negative electrode records a negative deflection.
3. A wave of depolarization that moves perpendicular to the exploring electrode will record a biphasic wave of depolarization.
4. The deflection of the wave of repolarization should be similar to that of depolarization. If there is upright recording of depolarization, the wave of repolarization also should be positive.

These explanations provide some insight into depolarization and repolarization and how those wave forms are depicted on an ECG lead. But the heart is a three-dimensional structure, and forces of depolarization must therefore be viewed using multiple exploring electrodes that reconstruct the various dimensions of depolarization.

THE ELECTROCARDIOGRAPH

The word **lead** can be confusing in ECG. Sometimes it means the wires that connect the ECG to the patient. Correctly, a *lead* or *lead system* is an electrical picture of a heart's surface. We will simply use the term *lead.*

lead
An electrical picture of the heart's surface

A lead has a positive and negative component. Each lead looks at a specific surface of the heart from the point of view of the positive **electrode** in that lead. Impulses that travel toward the positive electrode are seen as positive deflections in that lead. Impulses that travel away from the positive electrode are seen as negative deflections in that lead.

electrode
The conductor used to establish electrical contact with the body

The standard 12-lead ECG system utilizes five electrodes, one for each limb and a floating electrode on the chest wall. The system is categorized into three lead systems: standard limb leads, augmented leads, and precordial (chest) leads. Most monitoring systems utilize these three leads.

The initial six leads are I, II, III, AVR, AVL, and AVF. These are termed the limb leads because they are derived from electrodes attached to the arms and legs. The limb leads explore the electrical activity of the heart in the frontal plane. The other six leads explore forces of depolarization in the horizontal plane. The frontal plane is the two-dimensional surface visualized by looking directly at the anterior chest, and the horizontal plane is the view of the heart as seen from across the section of the chest.

Standard Limb Leads

Leads I, II, and III record myocardial activity within the frontal plane or the surfaces of the heart. They are positioned in such a way as to record the electrical potential between the sites of two electrodes. Leads I, II, and III are equidistant from the center of the heart's electrical activity. For the purposes of quick reference to the heart's electrical activity, most monitoring systems utilize those three leads.

With conventional electrode placement, changes in the assignment of polarity are internal to the ECG machine. It is necessary to know the assignment of polarity so that an intelligent assessment of heart function is possible, and changes in function can be visualized and understood.

The negative electrode is placed on the right side of the chest, about the level of the first and second intercostal space; the positive electrode is placed inferior to the left apex of the heart below the rib cage to the left. The indifferent electrode is on the left side of the chest, about the level of the first and second intercostal space. The indifferent electrode will assume (+) or (–) polarity with the lead assignment. By convention, in some monitors the negative electrode is white, the indifferent is black, and the positive electrode is red. In newer models, with 12-lead ECG capability, the limb leads are identified with uppercase letters and placed on the corresponding wrists and ankles.

Figure 2-5 shows each lead against a line drawing of the torso and the view of the heart surface.

Lead I records the action potential between the left arm and the right arm (Figure 2-5A). The positive electrode of this lead is on the left shoulder and visualizes the left lateral surface.

Lead II records the potential between the right arm and the left leg (Figure 2-5B). The positive of this lead is on the left torso, just below the rib cage. Lead II visualizes activity on the left inferior and apical surfaces of the heart.

Lead III records the potential between the left arm and the left chest (Figure 2-5C). Although the positive of this lead is still on the left torso, this lead visualizes activity on the inferior surface. Changes in lead III may reflect proximal right coronary artery disease.

Leads I and III are mirror images of each other. An impulse or deflection on ECG flowing toward the positive electrode in lead I is seen as negative in lead III;

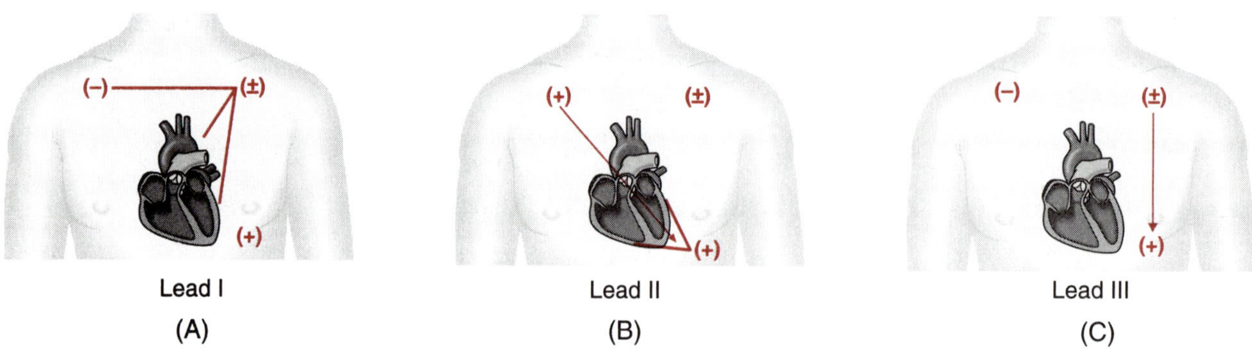

Figure 2-5 The position of the electrodes and the lead systems as they visualize the surfaces of the heart. (A) shows lead I. The positive of this lead is on the left shoulder and visualizes electrical activity on the left side of the heart. (B) shows lead II. The positive of this lead is on the left torso below the rib cage and visualizes activity on the left inferior surface. (C) shows lead III. This lead system visualizes the right inferior surface.

similarly, impulses that flow toward the positive electrode in lead III are seen as negative in lead I. Another term for this concept is *reciprocal.*

POINTS TO REMEMBER

1. The right arm is the negative pole, and the left leg is positive in the lead systems I and II. During this time, the electrode on the left arm is indifferent.
2. In lead system III, the left arm is negative.

Augmented Leads

Leads AVR, AVL, and AVF are designed to record the potential from the cavity of the heart to the limb lead of the positive electrode in that lead system. The amplitude in these leads must be increased about 50 percent, thus the term *augmented.* This is a programmed function within the monitoring device.

Lead AVL visualizes the heart from the point of view of the left shoulder and primarily looks at the left free wall. Lead AVR visualizes the heart from the point of view of the right shoulder and primarily looks at the cavity of the heart. Lead AVF visualizes the heart from the point of view of the foot and primarily looks at the inferior surface of the heart.

The Precordial (Chest) Leads

Lead V_1 is located over the fourth intercostal space to the right sternal border and looks specifically at the right bundle branch system.

Lead V_2 is located over the fourth intercostal space to the left sternal border and looks at the right anterior surface.

Lead V_3 is located between V_2 and V_4 and looks at the right anterior septal surface.

Lead V_4 is located at the fifth intercostal space on the midclavicular line and looks at the left anterior surface.

Lead V_5 is located at the fifth intercostal space on the anterior-axillary line and looks at the left ventricle.

Lead V_6 is located at the fifth intercostal space on the midaxillary line and looks at the lateral surface. Figure 2-6 shows the precordial points on the rib thorax (Figure 2-6A) and an illustration of the precordial leads as they reflect the surface of the myocardium (Figure 2-6B).

This is a good time to describe the lead MCL_1. This is a popular bipolar chest lead that simulates V_1. It is a modification of the chest lead where the positive electrode is on the chest and the negative electrode is on the left arm. The position of the electrodes for MCL_1 is illustrated in Figure 2-7 and shows the position of the electrode at the right sternal border between the fourth and fifth intercostal spaces, the same as in precordial lead V_1. The negative electrode does not change from the original placement; recall it is indifferent in lead II, positive in lead I, and negative in MCL_1. MCL_1 may be helpful in visualizing some wave forms, is a helpful tool and should not be used as the sole differential in some tachycardias.

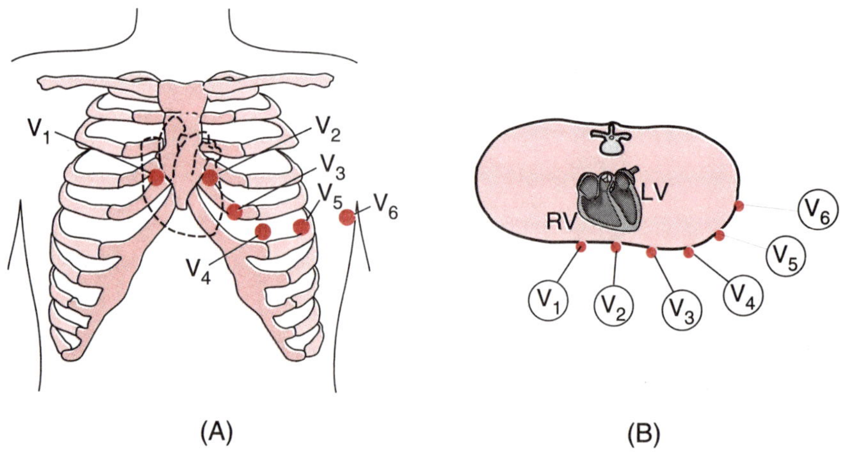

Figure 2-6 (A) The position of the electrodes on the rib thorax, and (B) the precordial leads as they reflect the surface of the myocardium

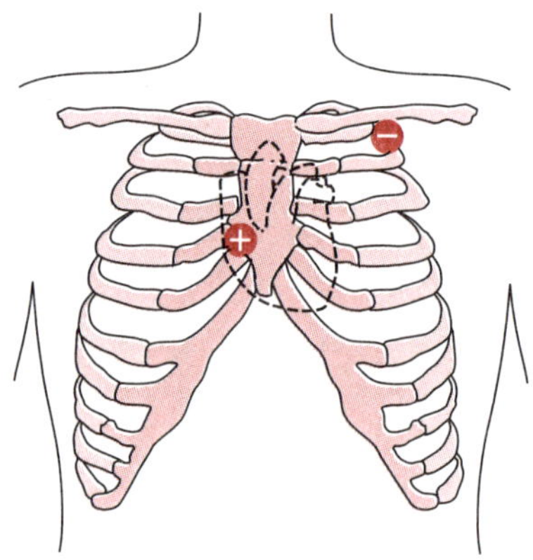

Figure 2-7 The position of the electrodes for the monitoring system MCL_1

Calibration

There is a limited amount of information to be derived from the amplitude of each of the wave forms and complexes, provided the monitor is properly calibrated. A standard signal of 1mV should move the stylus vertically ten small blocks (or two larger blocks).

When the monitor is properly calibrated, or standardized, the amplitude of wave forms can reflect changes in heart muscle, for example, hypertrophy.

Occasionally, it becomes necessary to "increase the gain," a common phrase meaning to increase the amplitude of the recording. This increase in amplitude may cause confusion with ECG rhythm analysis, since increased electronic "noise" or artifact will distort the ECG recording and confuse interpretation. Figure 2-8 shows the ECG paper and calibration markings or deflections for easy reference.

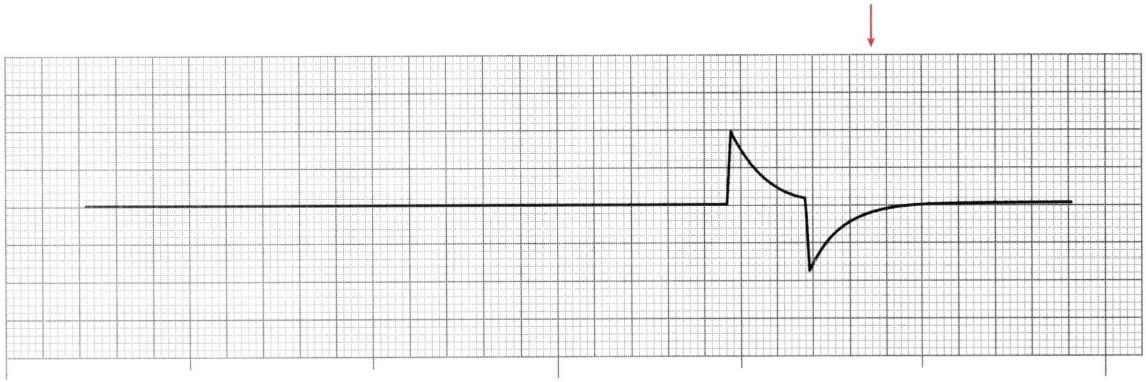

Figure 2-8 ECG paper and the deflections made during calibration

Artifact

Artifact describes confusing additions to the ECG tracing that prevents accurate interpretation. Artifact can be caused by somatic tremor over the torso and abdomen, patient movement, respiratory exursion, shivering, and seizures. A common artifact is 60 Hertz (60 cycle) interference from alternating current (AC) generators in close proximity to the patient.

Increasing the amplitude often distorts the ECG as increased electronic "noise" may distort the wave forms and confuse interpretation.

Summary

The heart's complex electrical activity can be affected by medications, drugs, and disease. The electrical activity is amplified to be displayed and assessed by the electrocardiograph (ECG), a series of complex electrical functions. The ECG is made of electrodes and lead systems that simply view the surfaces of the heart from the point of view of the positive electrode in a lead system. To know the position of the electrode in a lead, and the view of the heart displayed by that lead, gives insight into the function and perfusion of the heart.

Self-Assessment Exercise

Fill in the Blanks

Complete the statements, and then compare your answers with those in the back of the book.

1. The heart has both ____________ and ____________ activities.
2. The ability to spontaneously generate an impulse is called ____________.
3. The ability to respond to an impulse is called ____________.
4. The ability to transmit an impulse is called ____________.

5. The ability to contract is called ____________ .

6. Finally, without ____________ , there can be no ____________ .

The structures of the heart's conduction system are:

7. ____________ ,

8. ____________ ,

9. ____________ , which consists of two structures,

10. the ____________ and the ____________ .

11. The impulse continues down into the ventricles via the ____________ , which is thicker and slower in conduction.

12. The impulse also travels down the ____________ , which divides into the ____________ and the ____________ .

13. Finally, the system terminates in the ____________ .

14. Lead III is the ____________ of lead I.

15. Lead I visualizes the ____________ .

16. Lead II visualizes the ____________ .

17. Lead III visualizes the____________ .

18. Lead V_1 visualizes the____________ .

19. Lead V_2 visualizes the____________ .

20. Lead V_3 visualizes the____________ .

21. Lead V_4 visualizes the____________ .

22. Lead V_5 visualizes the____________ .

23. Lead V_6 visualizes the____________ .

References

Brown, K. R. & Jacobson, S. *Mastering dysrhythmias*. Philadelphia: F.A. Davis; 1988.

Conover, M. B. *Understanding electrocardiography: Arrhythmias and the 12-lead ECG* (7th ed.). St. Louis, MO: Mosby-Year Book, Inc.; 1996.

Goldberger, E. *Textbook of clinical cardiology*. St. Louis, MO: C. V. Mosby; 1982.

CHAPTER 3

Wave Forms and Measurements on the ECG

Premise Counting time, measuring lines and deflections, analyzing the wave forms that give witness to heart function, and doing it consistently—that's what the ECG is all about.

Objectives

After reading the chapter and completing the Self-Assessment Exercises, the student should be able to

1. use the ECG graph to identify and measure wave forms
2. measure time and plot out wave forms and complexes
3. determine heart rate and rhythm
4. begin a systematic approach to ECG rhythm analysis
5. relate the ECG wave forms to the heart's electrical activity

Key Terms

amplitude
complex
duration
elevation
interval
inverted
millivolt
negative
positive

Key Wave Forms

P, Q, R, S, T, and U
PR segment
PR interval
QRS complex
ST segment
QT interval

Introduction

The ECG is a graph of wave forms and lines, taken over a period of time. This myriad of complexes must be named, identified, and related to heart function to determine if the wave form depicted is representative of normal or abnormal function. The ECG will provide the basis for patient care decisions, and that is the exciting part of ECG analysis.

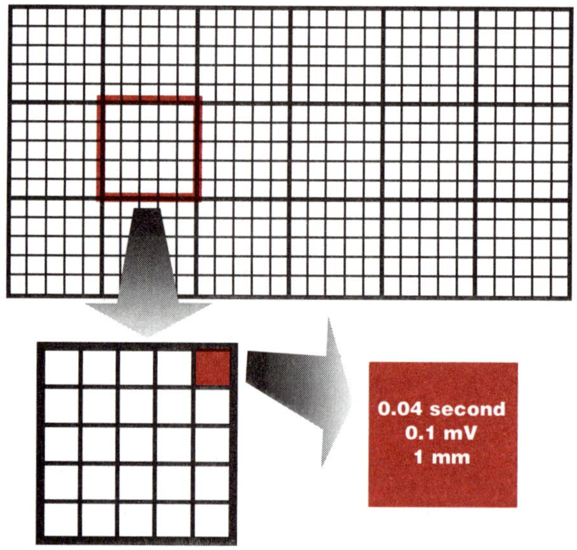

Figure 3-1 The ECG monitoring paper, with the blocks enlarged to illustrate the minimum units of measurement. The smallest of the blocks has three values: 0.04 second in duration (horizontal measurement), 0.1 mV in amplitude (vertical measurement), and 1 mm in height (also a vertical measurement). Five blocks on the horizontal would measure 0.20 second. Five blocks on vertical would measure 5 mm and/or 0.5 mV. Note the darker lines that delineate five of the smallest blocks.

MEASURING AN ECG RECORDING

All ECG monitors run at a standard rate and use paper with standard squares. Each small square is equal to 0.04 second. Each large square is made up of five small squares equal to 0.20 second. There are five large squares per second and 300 per minute. So, in an ECG event, such as a wave form representing ventricular activity, the QRS, occurring once every large square, is occurring at a rate of 300 per minute.

Amplitude or voltage is measured on the vertical, and each of the smallest blocks measures 0.1 **millivolt** (0.1 mV). The same small block measures height; each block measures 1 millimeter (1 mm). Diagnostic ECG devices should be standardized so that l mV is equal to 10 mm. Figure 3-1 shows the large ECG square with the minimum units of measurement highlighted: 0.04 second, 1 mm, and 0.1 mV.

amplitude
The maximum departure of the wave from the average value

millivolt
One thousandth of a volt

duration
The time it takes for a wave to begin and end

Estimating heart rate and evaluating **duration** and amplitude of wave forms are critical tasks in assessing the ECG. Once one gains insight into the purpose and design of the ECG recording, the calculations become easier with practice.

There are small vertical lines on the upper margins of most ECG paper. There are 15 of the larger blocks between these margin lines, and therefore they are placed 3 seconds apart (0.20 x 15 = 3.00 second) and (0.20 x 30 = 6.00 second). In Figure 3-2, ECG paper shows the markers indicating three- and six-second intervals.

CALCULATING RATE

Time is measured on the electrocardiograph moving from left to right across the ECG paper. Heart rate can be calculated in two ways—first, with very rapid and regular rates. Remember this sequence: If the interval occurs every

4 small squares, the rate is 375 per minute
5 small squares, the rate is 300 per minute
6 small squares, the rate is 250 per minute
7 small squares, the rate is 214 per minute
8 small squares, the rate is 188 per minute
9 small squares, the rate is 168 per minute
10 small squares, the rate is 150 per minute.

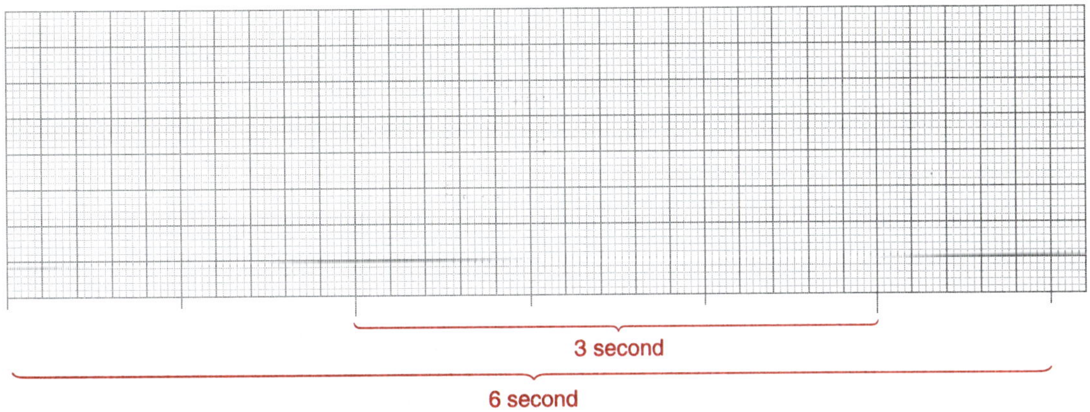

Figure 3-2 ECG monitoring paper showing markers indicating three- and six-second intervals. There are 15 blocks in three second, and 30 blocks in six second.

With more reasonable rates, if the interval occurs every

1 large square, the rate is 300 per minute
2 large squares, the rate is 150 per minute
3 large squares, the rate is 100 per minute
4 large squares, the rate is 75 per minute
5 large squares, the rate is 60 per minute
6 large squares, the rate is 50 per minute

This method of calculation is shown in Figure 3-3 with ECG paper and an ECG rhythm. Counting the number of large squares (blocks) between QRS complexes and dividing into 300 provides the estimated rate.

MEASURING WAVE FORMS

The electrical activity of the heart is depicted by wave forms and segments electronically inscribed onto lined paper. On this paper, there is a baseline from which wave forms are inscribed and the direction of the inscription is described as positive (above the baseline) or negative (below the baseline).

A single wave form begins and ends at the baseline. If the wave form continues past the baseline, it takes on another identity. For instance, a **positive** wave form

positive
A wave inscribed above the baseline

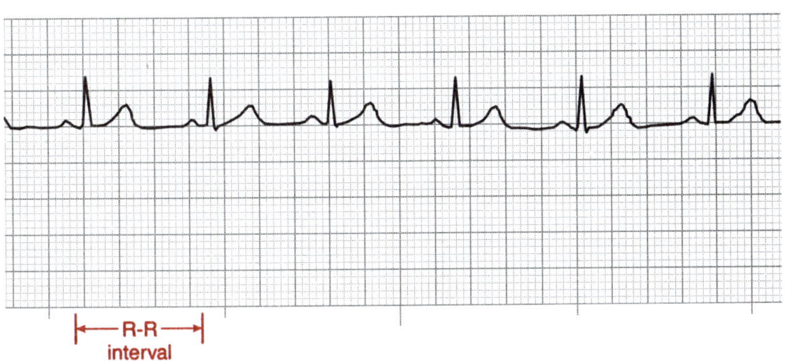

Figure 3-3 ECG recording with markers denoting the number of large squares (blocks) between the QRS complexes (R-R interval). Since there are three such blocks between QRS complexes, dividing 3 into 300 provides the estimated rate of 100 per minute.

negative
A wave inscribed below the baseline

R continues downward past the baseline and continues to become a **negative** wave form, *S*. Notching of a wave form while on the same side of the baseline does not imply two different wave forms. Sometimes the notching of a wave form reflects a disturbance in the electrical conduction pathway through the muscle. At other times, it is merely the manner in which the wave form is written.

In ECG terminology, lines are called *segments*. Segments may deviate from the baseline. When they deviate above the baseline they are elevated; when they deviate below the baseline, they are depressed. A wave form and a segment is an **interval**. Two or more wave forms together are a **complex**.

interval
A wave form plus a segment

complex
A group of wave forms

The wave forms are usually written as uppercase letters—P, Q, R, S, T, and U—for example QRS or PR. If a wave form is less than 5mm then the lowercase is used; for example, rS would indicate that the R wave is less than 5 mm and the S wave is greater than 5 mm.

Each wave form represents electrical depolarization for a specific part of the heart. The appearance of each has a predictable direction, duration, and amplitude for the normal heart. Deviations from the normal appearance will contribute, in part, to interpretation of the entire ECG rhythm analysis.

Remember the flow of electrical current begins in the sinus node, through atrial tissue, pausing at the level of the AV node, passes through the bundle of His continuing onward through the bundle branch system, terminating in the Purkinje fibers. Each of these events is represented with an ECG wave form.

The P Wave

Any single depolarization of the atria will cause a deflection known as a P wave. The duration of the P wave is no more than 0.11 second and represents the time of depolarization of both atria. The amplitude of the P wave is about 0.2 to 0.3 mV. Any increase in duration and amplitude may reflect atrial abnormalities related to hypertension, valvular disease, or congenital heart defects.

If an impulse originates within the sinus node, the resulting atrial depolarization will trace an upright, predictable, positive P wave that normally measures about 2.5 mm in height and 0.08 second in duration.

inverted
Upside down or reversed; a negative wave form

If depolarization occurs in a retrograde fashion from the AV nodal/bundle of His (NH) region of the bundle of His, the P wave will be negative or **inverted**. If depolarization occurs from anywhere in the atria, the P wave will assume a different-looking configuration from sinus-induced P waves, and the rhythm of the sinus P waves will be disturbed and reset. Figure 3-4A shows the P wave in relation to the QRS. Figures 3-4B and 3-4C depict the various P wave configurations based on their point of origin.

The PR Interval

The PR interval has two parts: the P wave and the PR segment. The PR segment is the time of activation of the His-Purkinje system. The PR interval measures 0.12 to 0.20 second, three to five small blocks. The P wave is usually 0.08 second, and the PR segment usually measures 0.12 second. In Figure 3-5A, the PR segment is highlighted. In Figure 3-5B, the PR interval is highlighted as it is calculated from the

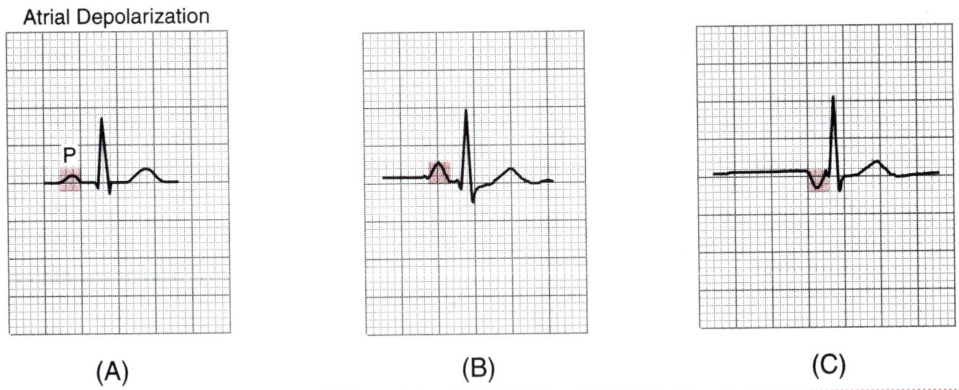

Figure 3-4 (A) The relationship of the P wave (shaded) to the QRS complex. (B) A (+) P wave that is sinus in origin. (C) A (-) P' wave that is junctional in origin. The negative P' indicates the retrograde atrial depolarization from inferior to superior in direction.

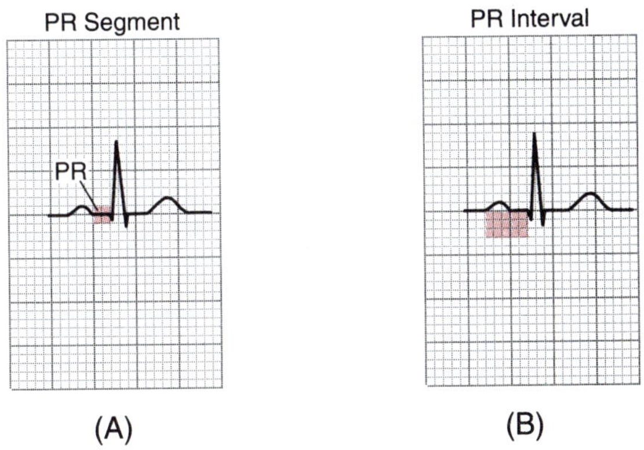

Figure 3-5 (A) The PR segment (shaded) of the PR interval. (B) The measurement of the PR interval to include the P wave and the PR segment. The PR segment is seldom referred to separately from the PR interval unless describing the phenomenon of AV block.

beginning of the P wave to the beginning of the QRS complex regardless of the direction of the P wave and the wave forms making up the QRS.

The QRS Complex

The QRS complex represents ventricular depolarization or how long the impulse takes to spread through the ventricles. The QRS complex (Figure 3-6) is made up of 1, 2, or 3 wave forms in any of the following combinations: The first negative deflection is a Q wave (Figure 3-7).

The first positive deflection is an R wave (Figure 3-8).

R waves can only be positive. If there is a second R wave it is *R prime* (Figure 3-9).

The S wave is a negative (-) deflection following the Q or R wave (Figure 3-10). S waves can only be negative. If there is a second S wave, it is *S prime.*

QS is the term describing the configuration of the QRS when only Q and S waves are present (Figure 3-11). By convention, any combination of Q, R, and S waves is called a QRS complex.

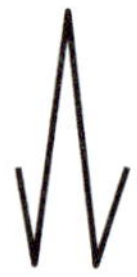

Figure 3-6 QRS complex with Q, R, and S wave forms

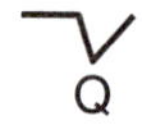

Figure 3-7 Q wave form of the QRS complex

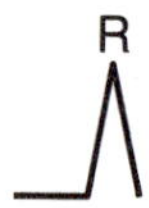

Figure 3-8 R wave form of the QRS complex

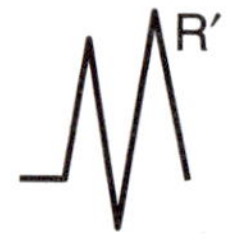

Figure 3-9 R′ wave form of the QRS complex

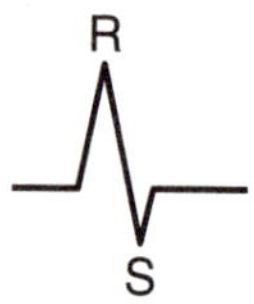

Figure 3-10 S wave form of the QRS complex

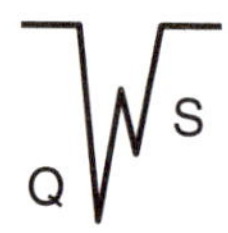

Figure 3-11 QRS complex with Q and S wave forms

The QRS measures less than 0.10 second when the ventricles are stimulated from a supraventricular source such as the sinus node, an atrial or junctional ectopic. When a QRS occurs from within the ventricles, the QRS morphology changes. The QRS will appear different than normally occurring QRSs; the direction of the wave of depolarization will be opposite from the direction of repolarization. For example, an R wave will be followed by an inverted T wave and, if the ventricular induced QRS is a QS or negative wave form, it will be followed by a positive T wave. Ventricular-induced QRS wave forms are frequently, but not always, greater than 0.12 second in duration. Figure 3-12 A through C shows the morphology and measurements of QRS complexes from sinus, atrial, and junctional sources in comparison to one that occurs from within ventricular tissue (Figure 3-12 D). Figure 3-12 E and F show the beginning and end points of measurements of QRS complexes based on their morphology.

The ST Segment

The ST segment represents the window between ventricular depolarization and repolarization. Depolarization is an active, dynamic process that follows a specific pathway. It is very quick in comparison to repolarization, which is a passive, longer process, directly dependent on oxygenated tissue.

The ST segment is a most sensitive visualization of heart muscle. If there are ischemic or injury processes within the heart, they will be seen in the ST segment in the lead facing the ischemic or injured area.

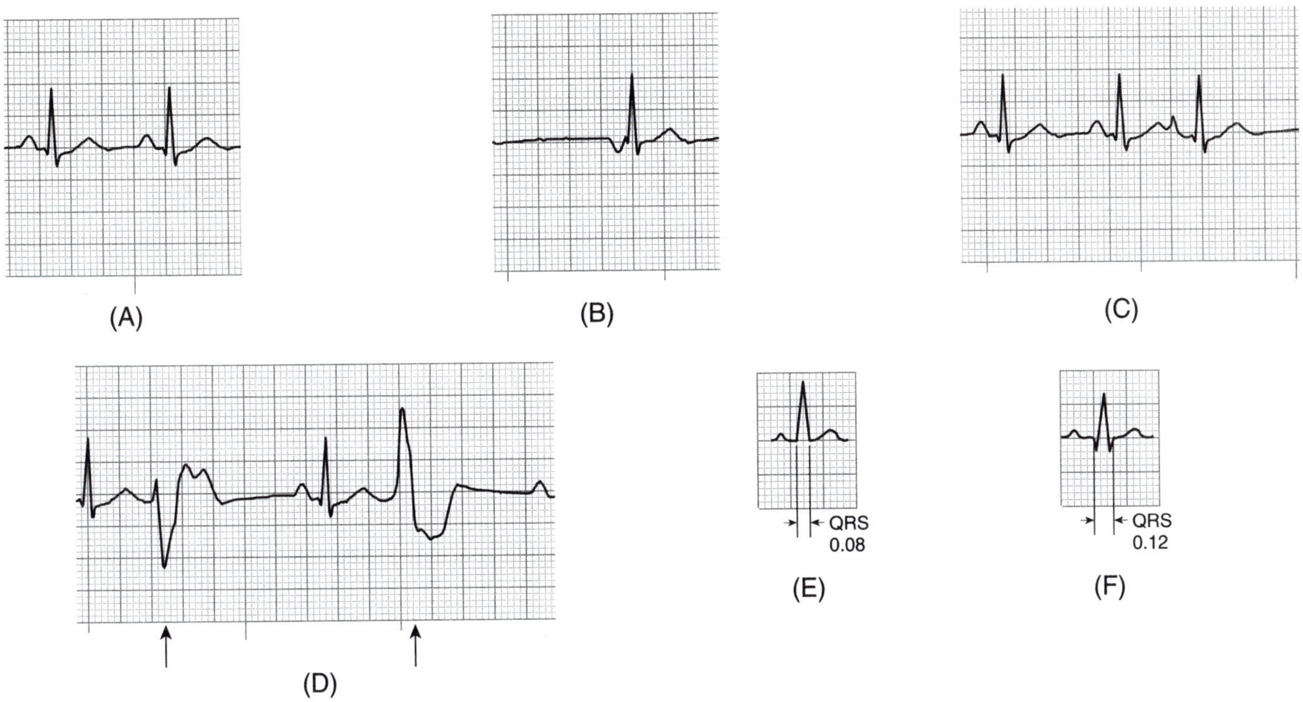

Figure 3-12 QRS complexes that are sinus (A), junctional (B), atrial (C) and ventricular (D) in origin. Note the similarity between QRS complexes that are supraventricular in origin. This happens because most of the time, the current flow through the ventricular conduction is the same. The QRS that is ventricular in origin (Figure 3-12 D) is clearly different since the ectopic impulse does not depolarize using the ventricular conduction system. (E) shows the measurement of a QRS that consists only of an R wave; (F) shows the measurement of the QRS with all three ventricular wave forms.

The ST segment is normally at the baseline, or isoelectric. It may be elevated or depressed with myocardial injury, ischemia, ventricular aneurysm, or some medications. The ST segment extends from the end of the QRS (J point) to the beginning of the T wave. A normal ST segment may be elevated (above the baseline) for 1 to 2 mm. An **elevation** greater than 2 mm is suspicious of myocardial hypoxia, ischemia, or injury in the lead facing the problem area. Confirmation of a questionable ST segment elevation would be done using another lead or group of leads visualizing the same or adjacent surface.

elevation
Deviation of the ST segment above the baseline

A straight, horizontal ST segment above or below the baseline is highly significant of ischemia. Ventricular systole occurs at the time seen as the very beginning of the ST segment. Figure 3-13 A, B, C, D displays some of the ST segment variations.

The T Wave

The T wave is an asymmetrical wave form that represents ventricular repolarization, rest, and recovery. T waves following P waves represent atrial repolarization but are not usually seen. When they are, they appear to distort the T wave and the resulting T wave amplitude is increased or additive; that is, the amplitude of the P and the amplitude of the T make for an enlarged T wave.

T waves are asymmetrical but are not notched (unless distorted by a prematurely occurring P wave); they may be positive or negative. They are usually about 0.5 mV in amplitude. They are sometimes of such low amplitude that it is difficult to see and/or read. Figure 3-14 A, B, and C illustrates examples of the T wave.

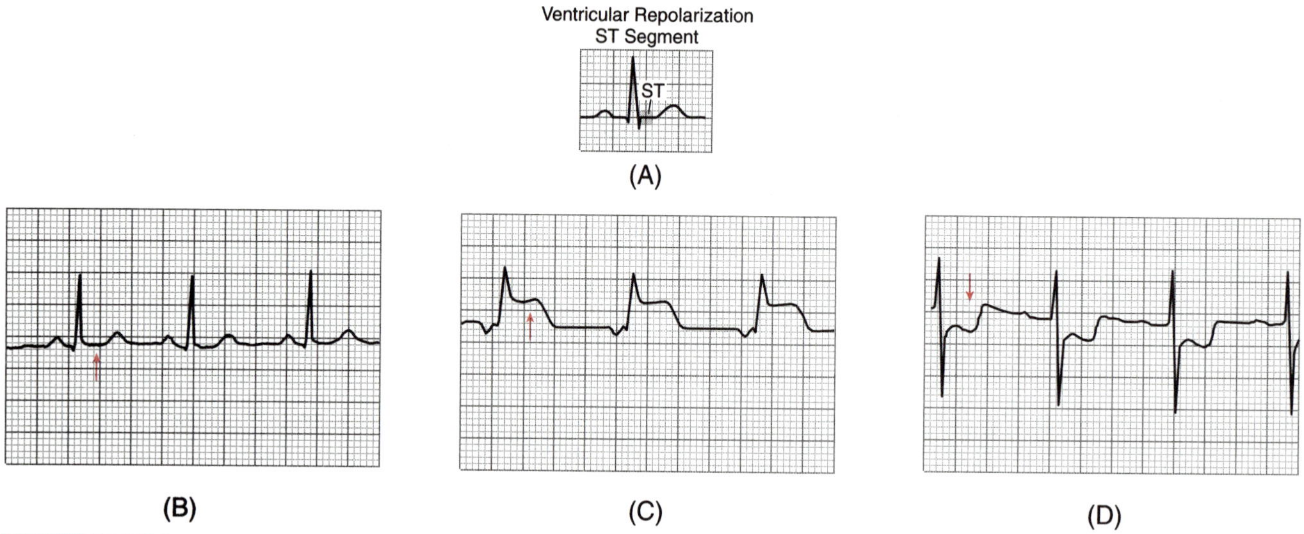

Figure 3-13 (A) The ST segment highlighted within cardiac complex. Note the variations in ST segments in (B) at the baseline. (C) shows 3 mm ST segment ↑, (D) shows 3 mm ST segment ↓.

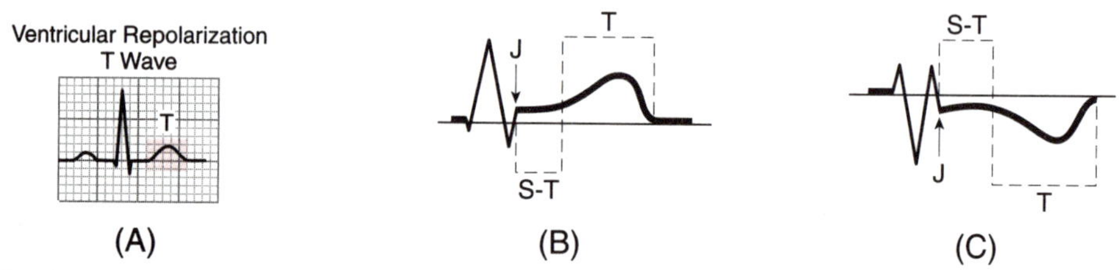

Figure 3-14 (A) The T wave representing ventricular depolarization. (B) Measuring the T wave with ST segment elevation and, (C) measuring an inverted T wave with ST segment depression.

The QT Interval

The QT interval represents total ventricular activity, depolarization (QRS) and repolarization (ST segment and the T wave). The time for ventricular repolarization is proportional to heart rate. That is, the faster the heart rate, the faster repolarization should occur, and thus the shorter the QT interval. With slower heart rates, the QT is longer. It is important to realize that the QT can change with some cardiac drugs that alter action potential and refractory times.

The normal QT measures about 0.36 to 0.44 second and varies between males and females and with age. There is a cumbersome formula to calculate the corrected QT interval for heart rate, but a simpler rule is that the QT should be about 40% of the measured R-R interval. Figure 3-15 illustrates a QT interval and abnormal variations.

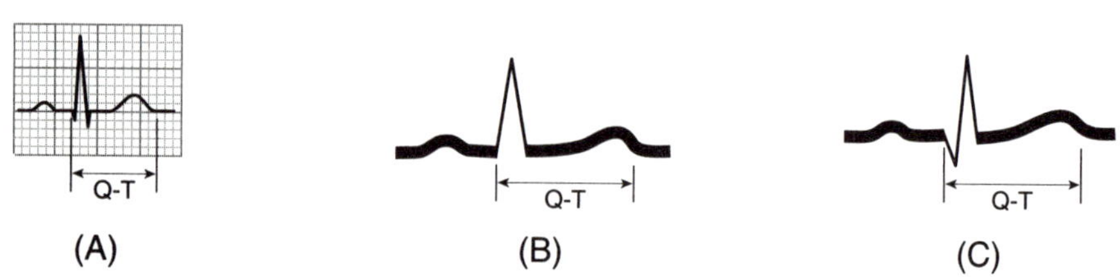

Figure 3-15 (A) The QT interval highlighted within the cardiac complex. (B) and (C) show the measurement based on the wave forms that make up the QRS complex.

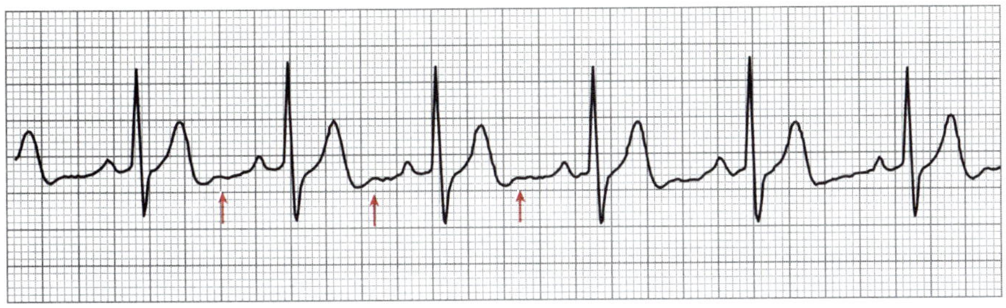

Figure 3-16 The U wave highlighted (arrow) within the cardiac complex. U waves plot only with other U waves, just as P waves plot with Ps, and QRS plots with the QRS complex.

The U Wave

The U wave follows the T wave and is the same polarity as the T wave. It is usually of low voltage and not often seen. Its true origin and mechanism are unknown, but it does become prominent in some electrolyte disturbances, with some medications and with heart disease. Figure 3-16 demonstrates a U wave.

Summary

The ECG wave forms represent the electrical activity in specific areas of the heart. Each wave form or complex has a predictable appearance, amplitude, and duration. Recognizing the normal and the consistent application of the principles of measurement will provide a foundation for sound arrhythmia analysis. Figure 3-17 is a

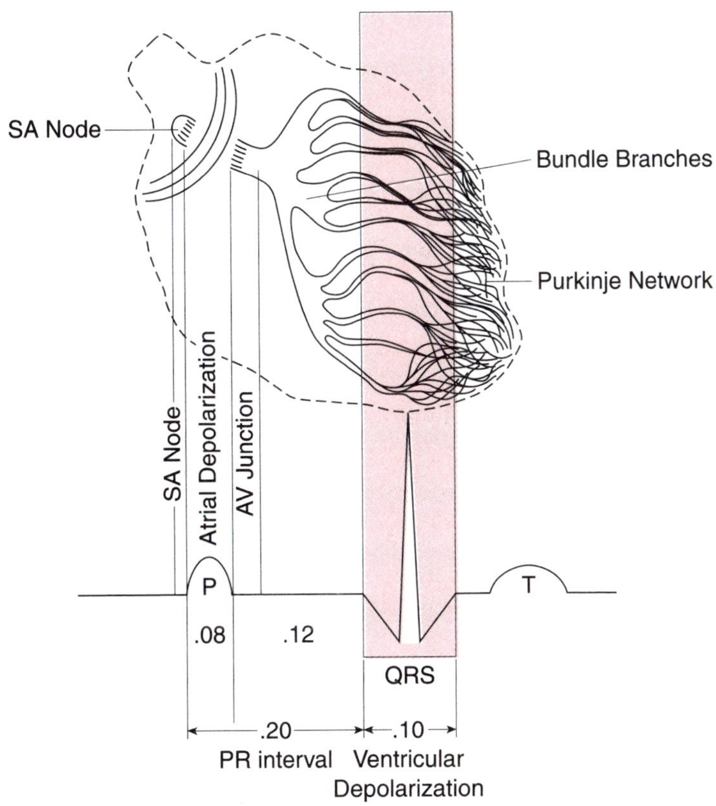

Figure 3-17 Schematic representation of the relationship of the myocardial conduction system to the ECG measurements

schematic summarizing the association of ECG wave forms and the electrical conduction system. It will take time, but the practitioner must commit this to memory. Any deviation from normal may represent pathology. *To know the normal is to recognize the abnormal!*

Table 3-1 is a summary of the wave forms and their measurements. Table 3-2 is a quick reference for calculating rate using the large boxes, 0.20 second. Table 3-3 is a quick reference guide for calculating rate using the smallest boxes, 0.04 second.

Table 3-1 Summary of ECG wave forms and measurements

The P Wave

- Represents atrial depolarization
- Measures 0.08 second and 2–3 mm in amplitude
- Shape is usually symmetrical and upright.
- May be notched in appearance
- P' (P prime) indicates atrial depolarization from an atrial or junctional source.

PR Interval

- Total supraventricular activity; activation of the His-Purkinje system
- 0.12–0.20 second
- The PR segment very importantly represents AV nodal delay and measures about 0.12 second.

QRS Complex

- Represents ventricular depolarization
- When supraventricular in origin, the QRS measures greater or equal to 0.10 second and 1–1.5 mV in amplitude.
- When ventricular in origin, the QRS measures greater than 0.10 second, and the amplitude is often greater than the normal QRS, and the QRS will be opposite in direction from the T wave.

ST Segment

- Represents early ventricular repolarization
- Measures less or equal to 0.12 second and may be angular, depressed, or elevated
- Deviations may reflect ischemia.

T Wave

- Represents completed ventricular repolarization
- Measures less or equal to 0.20 second and measures 5–6 mm; may be positive or negative
- Rarely distorted or notched. Atrial repolarization may alter the shape of the T wave. This is *Ta distortion.* The *T* meaning repolarization, and the *a* meaning of the atria.
- Asymmetrical

U Wave

- A positive or negative deflection following the QRS
- Most of the time is flat and unseen

QT Interval

- Total ventricular activity, 0.24–0.38 second
- Affected by ventricular rate and certain medications and electrolytes

Table 3-2 Calculating heart rate by counting the number of large squares between two consecutive QRS complexes and dividing into 300

Distance between two QRS complexes (# of large boxes)	Estimated rate per minute
1	300
1 1/2	200
2	150
2 1/2	125
3	100
3 1/2	86
4	75
4 1/2	67
5	60
5 1/2	55
6	50
6 1/2	46
7	43
7 1/2	40
8	37
8 1/2	35
9	33
9 1/2	32
10	30

Table 3-3 Calculating heart rate by counting the number of small squares between two consecutive QRS complexes and dividing into 1500

Distance between two QRS complexes (# of small boxes)	Estimated rate per minute
4	375
5	300
6	250
7	214
8	187
9	166
10	150
11	136
12	125
13	115
14	107
15	100
16	94
17	88
18	83
19	79
20	75

HOW TO LOOK AT AND ANALYZE THE WAVE FORMS

A clear, organized and consistent approach is necessary to accurately analyze the ECG wave forms. Abnormalities of cardiac rhythms are particularly easy to work out, and the key is the P wave.

1. Plot out P waves, calculating rate and rhythm.
2. Plot out QRS complexes, calculating rate and rhythm.
3. Confirm the association between each P wave and the QRS complex.

Labeling the ECG

The ECG rhythms are usually labeled with two terms. The first term indicates the source of the energy, the pacemaker. The second term indicates the effects of the conduction on heart rate or rhythm.

For example, sinus rhythm is interpreted as the sinus being the pacemaker, and the effect is heart rate between 60 and 100 beats per minute. Junctional tachycardia implies the pacemaker is in the AV junction and the rate is greater than 100 beats per minute. An example follows:

Sinus	Tachycardia at 110 per minute
pacemaker site	rate/rhythm/event

In the case of the back-up pacemakers, the inherent rate range for the AV junction is 40 to 60 per minute, and the ventricular escape rate range is 20 to 40 per minute. When each of these accelerates but remains less than 100 beats per minute, the term *accelerated* precedes it. Thus, an AV junctional rate of 75 will be *accelerated junctional rhythm at 75 per minute;* a ventricular pacer at 80 will be *accelerated ventricular rhythm at 80 per minute.*

It is important to qualify each identification with the specific rate per minute. This information coupled with the patient's vital signs, level of consciousness, and overall presentation will provide the greatest insight into the arrhythmia and guide interventions.

HOW TO ASSESS A MONITOR PATTERN

1. Determine if the rhythm is supraventricular or ventricular in origin. If the QRS is 0.10 second or less, it is likely supraventricular in origin, that is from the sinus node, from within the atria or from the AV junction.
2. Look to the left of the QRS. Look for a P for every QRS. If the QRS is 0.10 second or less, look to the left of it. If the P wave is
   a. (+) it's probably sinus in origin
   b. (-) or absent and the QRS is regular, it's probably junctional
   c. (+) and premature, it's atrial in origin
3. Is the PR interval consistent? Remember, atrial activation (P wave) is usually followed by ventricular activation (a QRS complex), and there is normally one P wave for each QRS complex.
4. Analyze if different complexes are premature (early) or escape (late). Plot out the P waves:

   a. If P waves plot out regularly, the ectopic is probably ventricular in origin.
   b. If P waves do not plot out regularly, the ectopic is probably supraventricular in origin, most likely, atrial.

5. Calculate the rate:
   a. Plot P to P and QRS to QRS at the baseline, *not* peak to peak. Some QRS complexes are notched or otherwise altered by artifact and make the peak-peak method inaccurate.
   b. If Ps and/or QRSs are regular, divide the number of large boxes between two regularly occurring wave forms and divide into 300.
   c. In rapid rates, divide the number of small boxes between two regularly occurring wave forms and divide into 1,500.
6. Describe any other deviation:
   a. ST segment elevation or depression
   b. T wave changes such as inversion
   c. widening of the QRS
   d. change in rhythm, sudden or gradual

Measuring ventricular rate and rhythm involves plotting wave forms. For instance, when plotting ventricular rate, the practitioner will measure from the beginning of the QRS, whatever its configuration, to the next QRS at the baseline. When plotting the measurements, it is important to remain at the baseline. Some QRS complexes are notched or distorted, or the baseline may vary, and measuring from peak to peak is inaccurate.

Summary

The ECG is a graphic representation of the heart's electrical functions, a myriad of wave forms and lines that depict the electrical activity of the heart. The ECG gives valuable insight into the status of the heart. Correct identification of the wave forms describes changes in the heart, the status of the patient, and often contributes to a specific treatment plan.

Much of the information in this chapter must be committed to memory, which will provide the basis for analysis. While there are tools of reference to help with the interpretation, persistent practice with measurements of complexes by the human hand and eye cannot be replaced.

The practitioner must be able to determine if the wave form is representative of normal or abnormal function, make the appropriate interpretation, and correlate all this with clinical findings. This is the exciting part of ECG rhythm analysis.

Self-Assessment Exercises

Matching

Find the phrase in the right column that matches the numbered word or phrase in the left column, and compare your answers with those in the back of the book.

____ 1. Automaticity	A. Ability to respond to an electrical impulse
____ 2. Conductivity	B. Ability to transmit an impulse
____ 3. Diaphragm	C. Cells that generate an impulse at a predictable rate of speed
____ 4. Diastole	D. Cells that generate an impulse in competition with pacemaker cells
____ 5. Ectopic	E. Inner lining of the heart, continuous with the entire cardiovascular system
____ 6. Endocardium	F. Contraction phase of the heart's cycle
____ 7. Epicardium	G. Extensions of myocardial muscle; papillary muscles are an example
____ 8. Excitability	H. Decreased perfusion of oxygenated blood
____ 9. Ischemia	I. Filling phase of the heart's cycle
____ 10. Left Anterior Descending Coronary Artery (LAD)	J. Larger chambers of the heart
____ 11. Left Circumflex Coronary Artery	K. Middle muscle layer of the heart
____ 12. Myocardium	L. Outermost layer of the heart
____ 13. Pacemaker	M. Perfuses the heart's inferior surface, SA and AV nodes
____ 14. Perfusion	N. Perfuses the heart's anterior surface, the septum, and part of the ventricular electrical conduction system
____ 15. Right Coronary Artery	O. Perfuses the heart's posterior and, distally, the inferior surface
____ 16. Septum	P. Delivery of oxygenated blood
____ 17. Sternum	Q. Landmark for the anterior surface of the heart
____ 18. Systole	R. Landmark for the inferior surface of the heart
____ 19. Trabeculae	S. Separates left from right ventricle
____ 20. Ventricles	T. The term that describes spontaneous initiation of an impulse
	U. Visualizes the left free wall
	V. Visualizes the true posterior surface

ECG Rhythm Identification Practice

For each of the ECG practice rhythms:

1. Identify the P, Q, R, S, T (and U waves if any are seen).
2. Calculate the measurement and rates asked for in each strip.
3. When complete, compare your answers with those in the back of the book.

Figure 3-18

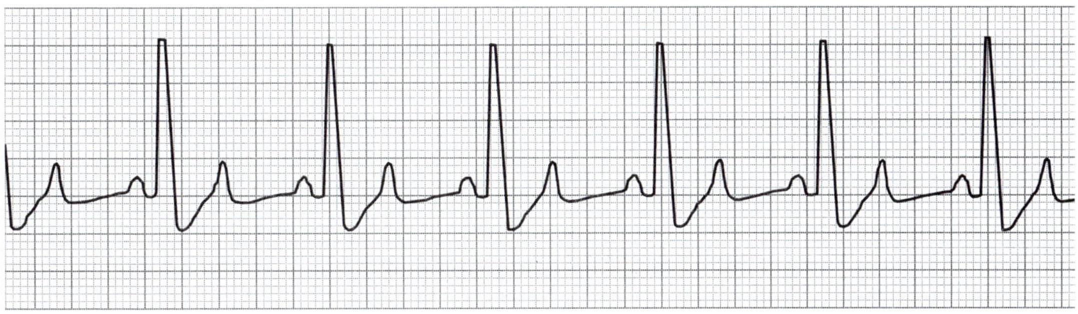

1. Identify the P, Q, R, S, T, U waves.
2. Look to the left of the QRS, and identify each P wave.
   Is the P wave (+) or (-) __________?
3. QRS (ventricular) rate/rhythm ____________.
4. P (atrial) rate/rhythm ______________.
5. PR interval ______________.

Figure 3-19

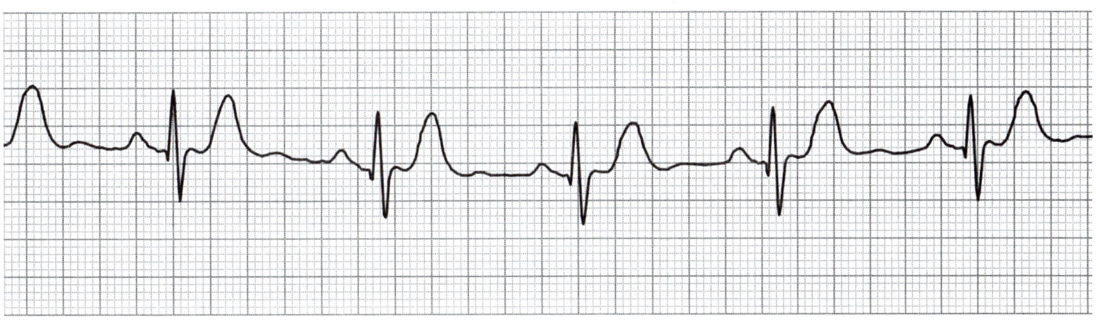

1. Identify the P, Q, R, S, T, U waves.
2. Look to the left of the QRS, and identify each P wave.
   Is the P wave (+) or (-) __________?
3. QRS (ventricular) rate/rhythm ____________.
4. P (atrial) rate/rhythm ______________.
5. PR interval ______________.

Figure 3-20

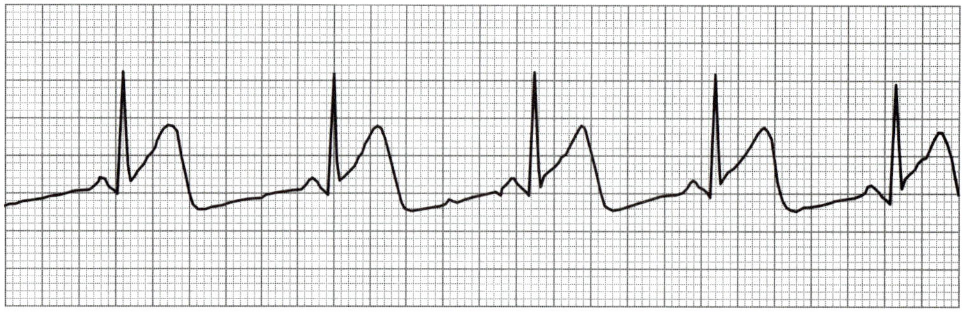

1. Identify the P, Q, R, S, T, U waves.
2. Look to the left of the QRS, and identify each P wave.
   Is the P wave (+) or (-) __________?
3. QRS (ventricular) rate/rhythm ____________.
4. P (atrial) rate/rhythm ______________.
5. PR interval ______________.

Figure 3-21

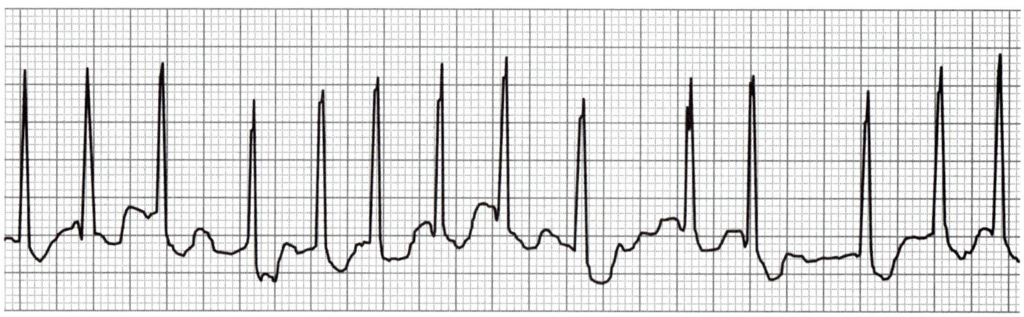

1. Identify the P, Q, R, S, T, U waves.
2. Look to the left of the QRS, and identify each P wave.
   Is the P wave (+) or (-) __________?
3. QRS (ventricular) rate/rhythm ____________.
4. P (atrial) rate/rhythm ______________.
5. PR interval ______________.

Figure 3-22

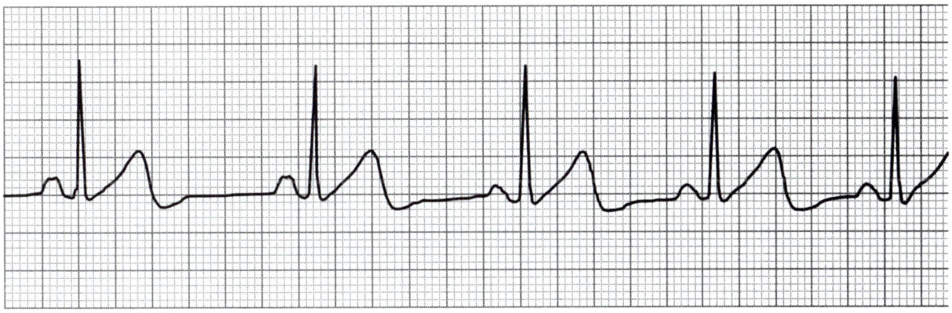

1. Identify the P, Q, R, S, T, U waves.
2. Look to the left of the QRS, and identify each P wave.
   Is the P wave (+) or (-) __________?
3. QRS (ventricular) rate/rhythm ____________.
4. P (atrial) rate/rhythm ______________.
5. PR interval ______________.

Figure 3-23

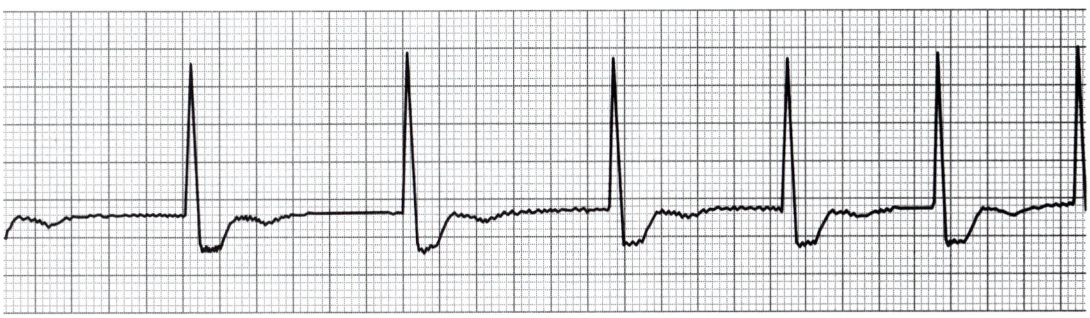

1. Identify the P, Q, R, S, T, U waves.
2. Look to the left of the QRS, and identify each P wave.
   Is the P wave (+) or (-) __________?
3. QRS (ventricular) rate/rhythm ____________.
4. P (atrial) rate/rhythm ______________.
5. PR interval ______________.

Figure 3-24

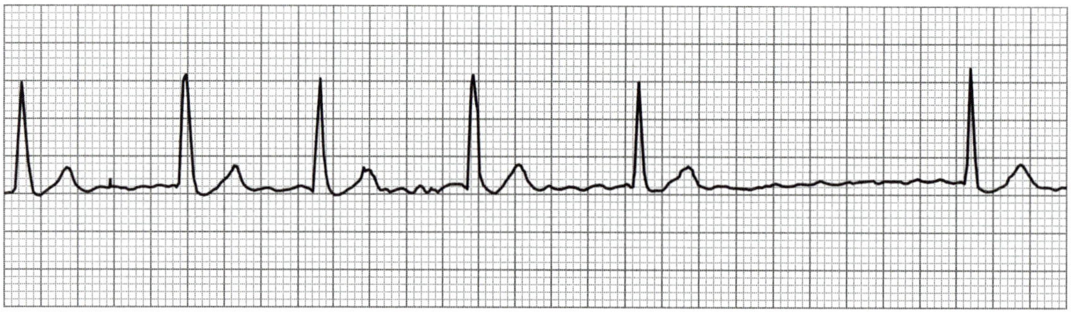

1. Identify the P, Q, R, S, T, U waves.
2. Look to the left of the QRS, and identify each P wave.
   Is the P wave (+) or (-) __________?
3. QRS (ventricular) rate/rhythm ___________.
4. P (atrial) rate/rhythm ______________.
5. PR interval ______________.

Figure 3-25

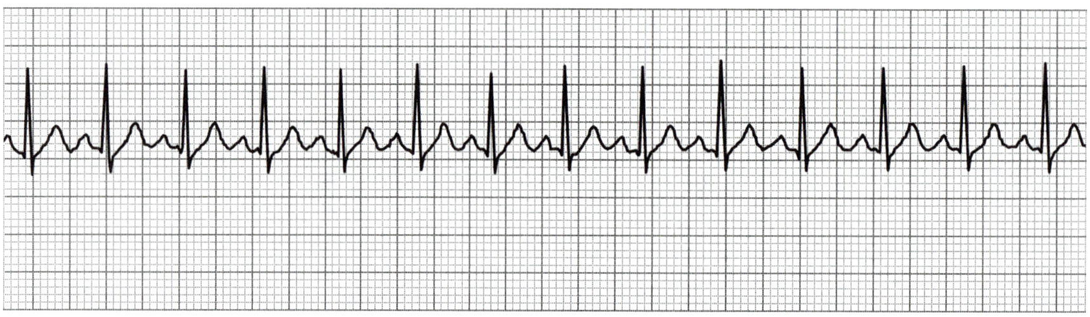

1. Identify the P, Q, R, S, T, U waves.
2. Look to the left of the QRS, and identify each P wave.
   Is the P wave (+) or (-) __________?
3. QRS (ventricular) rate/rhythm ___________.
4. P (atrial) rate/rhythm ______________.
5. PR interval ______________.

References

Conover, M. B. *Nurse's pocket guide to electrocardiography* (3rd ed.). St. Louis, MO: C. V. Mosby; 1994.

Conover, M. B. *Understanding electrocardiography: Arrhythmias and the 12-lead ECG* (7th ed.). St. Louis, MO: Mosby-Year Book, Inc.; 1996.

Marriott, H. J. *Practical electrocardiography* (8th ed.). Baltimore: Williams and Wilkins; 1988.

CHAPTER 4

The Sinus Mechanisms

Premise Abnormalities of heart rhythm are easy to figure out. The key is to find the P wave.

Objectives

After reading the chapter and completing the Self-Assessment Exercises, the student should be able to

1. plot out P waves, calculating rate and rhythm
2. plot out QRS complexes, calculating rate and rhythm
3. confirm the association between each P wave and the QRS complex
4. determine if the rhythm is appropriate to the patient
5. interpret the configuration and morphology using more than one ECG lead
6. select the appropriate intervention

Key Terms

arrhythmia
bradycardia
hypoperfusion
rhythm
SA arrest
SA block
tachycardia

Introduction

Normally, the heart can and will depolarize spontaneously and rhythmically. The rate will be controlled by the pacemaker that depolarizes at the highest rate. The sinus (SA) node normally has the highest frequency of discharge. Subsequent depolarization of atrial tissue will write a P wave on ECG. If the impulse succeeds in traveling through the AV junctions and activating the ventricles, a normal QRS complex (0.10 second) will follow. Variations in the sinus mechanisms have to do with rate and rhythm. As long as the sinus fires and atrial tissue responds, the process recurs normally at a given rate of speed. The clue is to look to the left of each QRS and find a single, positive P wave for each normal QRS—that is the sinus mechanism.

In order to accurately identify the rhythm, specific criteria must be evaluated. In each of the mechanisms, the criteria will be addressed in a consistent manner, so the reader can develop a consistent pattern of identification.

All monitors have the capability to look at the heart from various leads. Portable monitors used in the prehospital have at least three leads available to those practitioners. As practitioners suspect ischemia and hypoxia in surfaces of the heart, we can select lead systems that best visualize the surfaces, deduce the responsible coronary artery, and project the anticipated complications.

SINUS RHYTHM

rhythm
Recurring movement or fluctuation pattern

In order to describe the **rhythm** of the heart as sinus rhythm (the impulse originating in the sinoatrial [SA] node, the normal pacemaker of the heart) without qualifications, the indicated criteria must be met:

1. P Wave: The P waves are positive (upright) and uniform in lead II. Every P wave is followed by a QRS complex.
2. PR Interval: The PR interval (from the beginning of the P wave to the beginning of the QRS complex) is constant and consistently between 0.12 and 0.20 second.
3. QRS Complex: The QRS complex duration is 0.10 second or less. Every QRS complex is preceded by a single, predictable, positive P wave.
4. QRS Rate: A *normal* predictable heart rate is between 60 and 100 per minute in the adult patient. There is very little variance in rhythm.
5. QRS Rhythm: The rhythm is regular. Sinus rhythm is the standard against which most dysrhythmia are measured, compared, and analyzed.

Figure 4-1 shows a single, positive P wave for each QRS complex, and the PR interval is consistent. The heart rate is between 60 and 100 beats and rhythmic.

Figure 4-2 consists of two leads from the same patient. In the lead II, the P wave is barely visible, but present. When you are not sure that P waves exist, be persistent in your efforts and select a different lead. Comparing leads I, II, and III you will usually see visible P waves more prominently in at least one other lead.

SINUS TACHYCARDIA

tachycardia
Heart rate greater than 100 beats per minute

Tachycardia means fast (tachy) heart (cardia), a rate greater than 100 beats per minute. Recall that the word *sinus* appearing before the word *tachycardia* indicates that the origin of the rhythm is the SA node, the normal pacemaker of the heart.

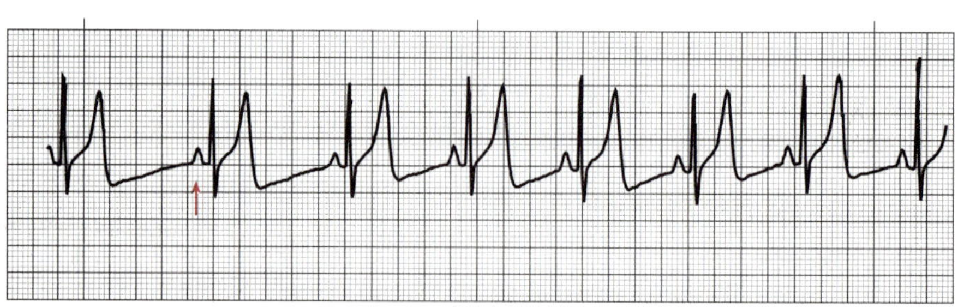

Figure 4-1 An ECG tracing showing one (+) P wave to the left of each QRS complex; the PR interval is consistent and the heart rate is between 60 and 100 per minute. These computations represent a sinus mechanism.

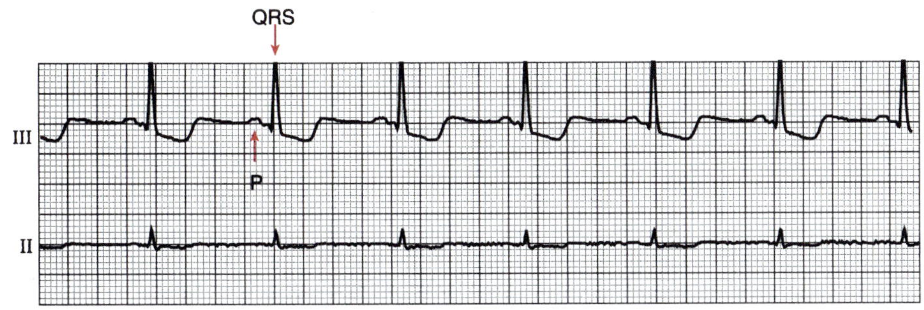

Figure 4-2 An ECG tracing from a patient showing simultaneous leads. Note the difference in the ECG wave forms as depicted in two leads. Note that III depicts the wave forms more clearly. This example illustrates that reliance on only one lead is a disservice to the patient as well as the individual interpreting the ECG tracing.

If all the criteria for a sinus mechanism have been fulfilled but the heart rate is greater than 100 beats per minute, the rhythm is called *sinus tachycardia.* The range for a sinus tachycardia is usually 100 to 180 beats per minute. The sinus node rarely exceeds 180 per minute, although rates up to 200 per minute have been seen with exertion. ECG characteristics for sinus tachycardia are as follows:

1. P Wave: The P waves are positive and uniform in lead II. Every P wave is followed by a QRS complex.
2. PR Interval: The PR interval is normal between 0.12 and 0.20 second and is constant from beat to beat.
3. QRS Complex: The QRS complex duration is 0.10 second or less. Every QRS complex is preceded by a P wave.
4. QRS Rate: The rate is constant above 100 (100 to 160) per minute.
5. QRS Rhythm: The rhythm is regular.

Figure 4-3 is an ECG of sinus tachycardia.

Causes of Sinus Tachycardia

Normal body function (physiologic) tachycardia is common for infants at about 120 to 130 beats per minute. In the adult, sinus tachycardia results from the body's needs for increased perfusion as with exercise and emotions, such as fever, pain, fear, anger, and anxiety.

Sinus tachycardia is a sign of physiologic stress, such as hypovolemia, hyperthyroidism, or any condition that causes an increased sympathetic stimulation.

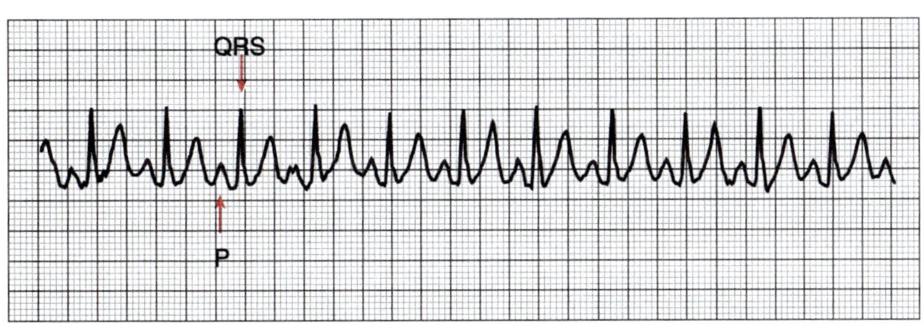

Figure 4-3 An ECG tracing showing one (+) P wave to the left of each QRS complex; the PR interval is consistent and the heart rate is greater than 100 per minute. These computations represent a sinus tachycardia.

Other pathologies causing sinus tachycardia are congestive heart failure, cardiogenic shock, pulmonary embolism, valve disease, hypertension, myocardial ischemia, injury, and infarction.

Medications such as atropine and beta adrenergic drugs can cause sinus tachycardia. Drugs that cause vasodilation may have sinus tachycardia as a side effect. These include nitroglycerin, morphine, furosemide (lasix), and some antihistamines.

Drug abuse and illegal drugs cause sinus tachycardia. An example is opiate intoxication such as heroin, cocaine, and methamphetamines, in various forms and combinations. Other examples are crystal methamphetamine known as *crack* or *rock* (smokable cocaine) methamphetamine, *white crosses* (speed) and *black beauty*, a form of methamphetamine.

Look-alike drugs made up of mega doses of caffeine such as GHB, also known as ecstacy or the rape drug, cause sinus tachycardia, as do marijuana and *shurm*, marijuana soaked in formaldehyde. PCP, a horse tranquilizer, and MDA, an elephant tranquilizer, are taken to enhance and create incredible human strength.

If sinus tachycardias persist as a result of any of these conditions, coronary perfusion may be in jeopardy and ischemia and injury will occur. The injury pattern may be seen in some leads and not in others.

For instance, if right coronary perfusion is in jeopardy, there will be ST elevation in leads II and III. However, if ischemia and injury occur in the left free wall or some aspect of the anterior surface lead II may not show any changes, but ST elevation will be a significant finding in lead I, and ST depression will be seen in lead III.

Intervention

When assessing the patient, determine if the circumstances are appropriate to the rhythm/rate presented. Consider how much of a deviation this rate is from the patient's normal physiologic resting rate.

Patient care begins with initial assessment, past medical history, focused history, and physical exam in an effort to identify the cause. For patients with chest pain or pressure or with those patients whose clinical presentation indicates they are compromised by the tachycardia, treatment usually begins with high-flow oxygen therapy.

Place the patient on an ECG monitor to determine if the tachycardia is indeed sinus in origin. Assess more than one monitoring lead for signs and symptoms of ischemia and injury. ECG rhythm analysis also should include a 12-lead ECG.

For patients with chest pain or pressure, consider pain relief with nitroglycerin or morphine sulfate according to local protocol. Otherwise, be supportive and continue to identify and treat the underlying cause. Treatment may include appropriate antidotes whenever possible for offending drugs.

Figure 4-4 is an example of sinus tachycardia in an adult allegedly using methamphetamine. Figure 4-5 is an example of sinus tachycardia in an exercising adult.

bradycardia

Slow heart. A disorder in heart rate where the ventricular rate is below 60 per minute.

SINUS BRADYCARDIA

Bradycardia means slow (brady) heart. If the heart rate is under 60 beats per minute, but all the criteria for a sinus mechanism have been fulfilled, the rhythm is known as *sinus bradycardia*. The ECG characteristics of sinus bradycardia are as follows:

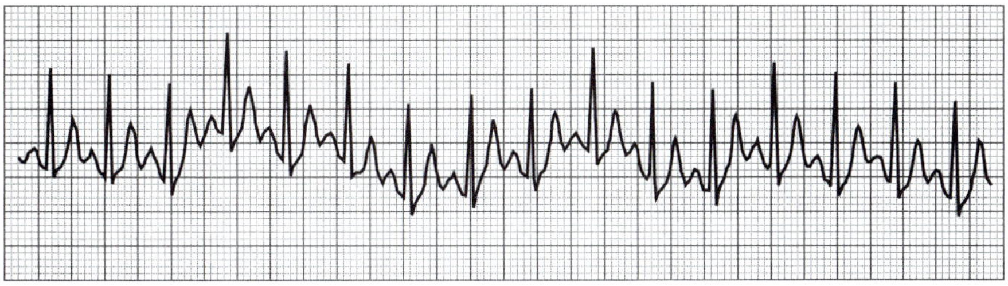

Figure 4-4 An ECG tracing showing sinus tachycardia from an adult allegedly using methamphetamine. Note the wandering baseline caused by rapid respirations and patient movement.

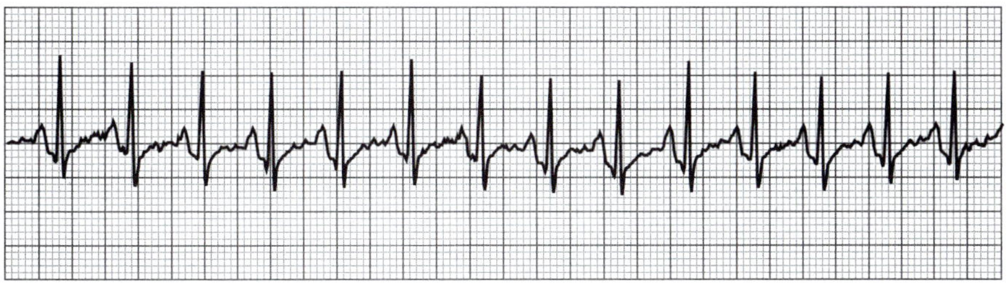

Figure 4-5 An ECG tracing from an exercising adult. Note there is a single (+) P wave to the left of each QRS complex; the rate is 150 per minute.

1. P Wave: The P waves are positive and uniform in lead II. Every P wave is followed by a QRS complex.
2. PR Interval: The PR interval is normal between 0.12 and 0.20 second and is constant from beat to beat.
3. QRS Complex: The QRS complex duration is 0.10 second or less. Every QRS complex is preceded by a P wave.
4. QRS Rate: The rate is constant below 60 per minute, with little variance.
5. QRS Rhythm: The rhythm is regular.

Figure 4-6 is an ECG of sinus bradycardia.

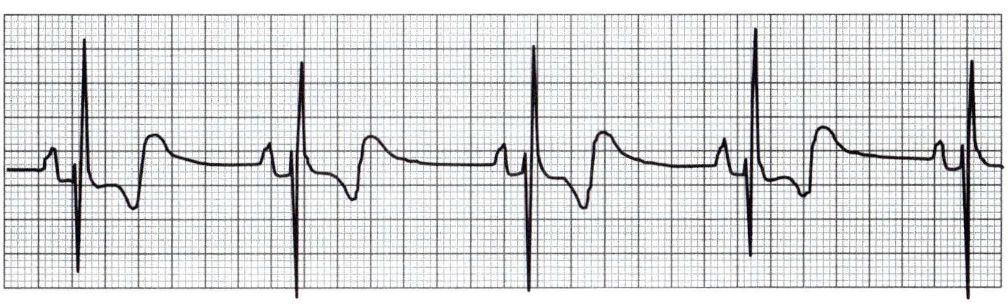

Figure 4-6 An ECG tracing showing one (+) P wave to the left of each QRS complex; the PR interval is consistent and the heart rate is less than 60 per minute. These computations represent a sinus bradycardia.

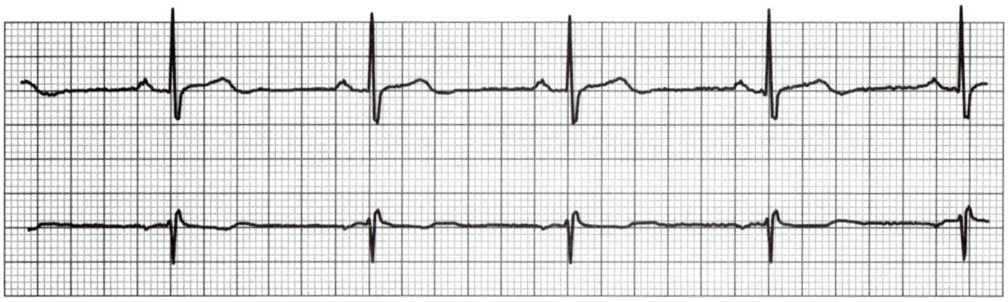

Figure 4-7 An ECG tracing showing sinus bradycardia in two leads from a conditioned adult.

Causes of Sinus Bradycardia

hypoperfusion
Deficiency in circulation of oxygenated blood

A slow heart rate indeed may be the norm for physically conditioned individuals or may be considered a normal variant. Often, a sinus bradycardia is seen with increased vagal tone and often not accompanied with hypotension nor **hypoperfusion**. Sinus bradycardia also is seen in conditioned athletes and during sleep patterns. Sinus bradycardia is seen in conditions of hypothermia and some thyroid conditions such as myxedema.

When sinus bradycardia is unexpected and does not fit the situation, care should be directed toward assessment and intervention to increase the rate to a level that provides reasonable perfusion. The optimal rate will vary from patient to patient.

Intervention

Patient care begins with initial assessment, which includes past medical history and detailed physical exam. Determine if the rate is physiologic or compromising to the patient. If the patient is symptomatic and hypotensive and has other signs of hypoperfusion, immediate intervention is necessary. The goal is to improve perfusion by increasing heart rate.

Two available modalities are medications (Atropine) and electronic pacing. There is always the risk that a sudden change in heart rate after Atropine may cause an increase in myocardial oxygen debt and further compromise the patient.

For any patient with chest pain or pressure, place the patient on an ECG monitor to identify the arrhythmia. Nonphysiologic bradycardia may be the only initial ECG sign that the patient has proximal right coronary artery disease, affecting sinus node function. Assess more than one monitoring lead for signs and symptoms of ischemia and injury. ECG rhythm analysis should also include a 12-lead ECG.

Figure 4-7 shows simultaneous leads of sinus bradycardia in a conditioned adult. In Figure 4-8 sinus bradycardia from a patient who complained of chest pressure.

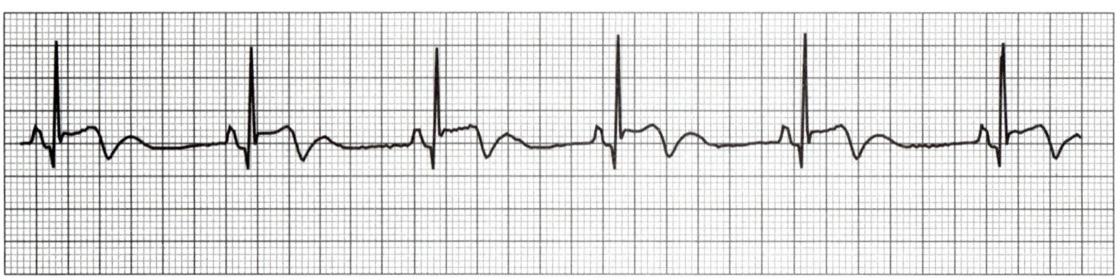

Figure 4-8 An ECG tracing from a patient with chest pressure. Note the ST segment elevation and T wave inversion indicative of myocardial ischemia/injury. The presence of Q waves in this patient is suspicious. Serial ECGs and comparisons with old records would help differentiate a normal variant from Q waves that represent myocardial infarction.

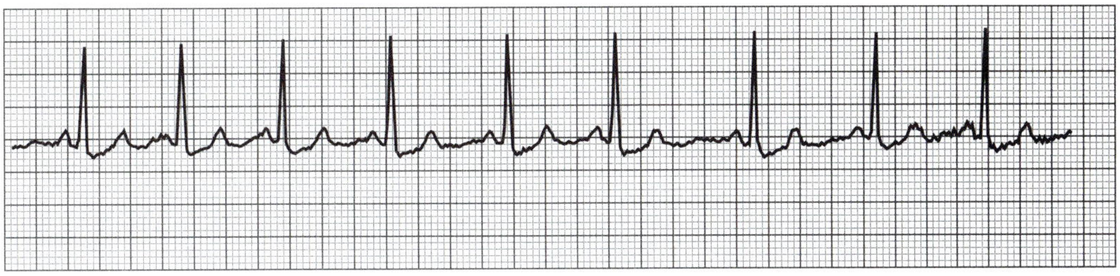

Figure 4-9 An ECG tracing showing one (+) P wave to the left of each QRS complex; the PR interval is consistent, but the heart rate varies. These computations and the irregularity represent a sinus arrhythmia. It is helpful to report the rate range. In this patient it is about 66 to 100 per minute.

Note the consistent appearance of the positive P wave to the left of each QRS in all strips. Note also the ST elevation in lead II indicating possible ischemia and/or injury (see Chapter 11).

SINUS ARRHYTHMIA

In sinus **arrhythmia**, the impulse has its origin in the sinus node and subsequent conduction is normal. The rhythm of impulse formation, and thus the heart's response, is irregular; (ar-) irregular (-rhythmia) rhythm. The PR intervals are consistent, but the PP and RR intervals are continually changing. The heart rate varies from about 53 to 68 beats per minute, about a 10 percent variation. The ECG characteristics of sinus arrhythmia are as follows:

arrhythmia
Disorder of heart rate or rhythm

1. P Wave: The P waves are positive and uniform in lead II. Every P wave is followed by a QRS complex.
2. PR Interval: The PR interval is normal between 0.12 and 0.20 second and is constant from beat to beat.
3. QRS Complex: The QRS complex duration is 0.10 second or less. Every QRS complex is preceded by a P wave.
4. QRS Rate: The rate varies by more than 10 percent.
5. QRS Rhythm: The rhythm is irregular due to the changing rate.

Figure 4-9 is an ECG showing sinus arrhythmia. Note the gradual increase and decrease of heart rate.

Causes of Sinus Arrhythmia

Sinus arrhythmia is not a disease, nor does it reflect a disease. It is a natural response and meets all the criteria described under sinus rhythm except for the variation in rhythm, naturally associated with the respiratory cycles. It is commonly seen in adolescents.

Intervention

Unless the arrhythmia is accompanied with a bradycardia that causes hypotension and hypoperfusion, no intervention is necessary. If such is the case, begin patient care as for sinus bradycardia.

Figures 4-10 and 4-11 are examples of sinus arrhythmia. Note that despite the irregularity, there is a consistent appearance of the positive P wave to the left of each QRS in all strips.

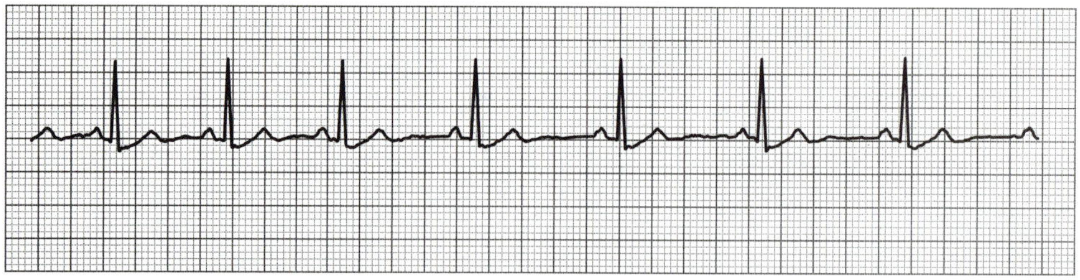

Figure 4-10 An ECG tracing of sinus arrhythmia 67 to 86 per minute.

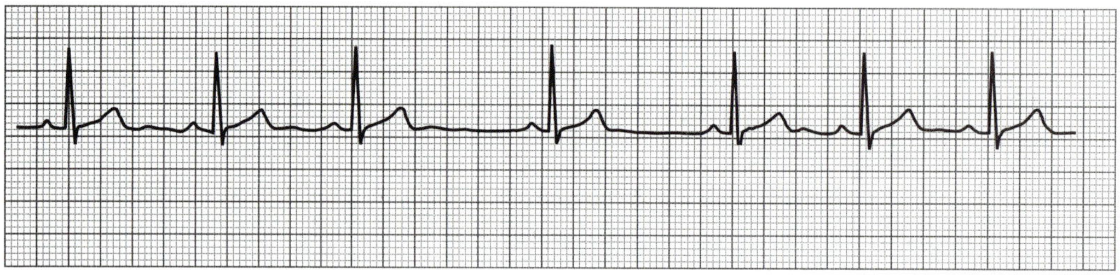

Figure 4-11 An ECG tracing of sinus arrhythmia 54 to 71 per minute.

SINUS ARREST

SA arrest

An event caused by a sudden failure of the SA node to initiate a timely impulse

Sinus or **SA arrest** is an event caused by a sudden failure of the SA node to initiate a timely impulse. In sinus arrest, multiples of PQRST complexes are missing, sometimes two, sometimes three or four. There does not have to be a pattern to the frequency of occurrences. In other words, a patient can have periods of SA arrest, missing two or three PQRST complexes. This may not recur for several minutes or hours, and then an episode of missing five complexes recurs.

If the period of arrest is more than one cycle length, physiologically another pacemaker should take over and initiate a new rhythm. In most cases, it is the AV junction. This will be discussed in Chapter 5. The ECG characteristics of sinus arrest are as follows:

1. P Wave: Since the SA node has ceased functioning, no sinus P waves are visible.
2. PR Interval: The PR interval is normal between 0.12 and 0.20 second and is constant from beat to beat.
3. QRS Complex: The QRS complex duration is 0.10 second or less. After the arrest, if the escape rhythm is supraventricular, the QRS will remain the same. If the escape rhythm is ventricular, the resulting QRS will be greater than 0.10 second and appear different than the dominant, supraventricular (narrow) QRS.
4. QRS Rate: Report the overall dominant sinus rate, qualify the length of the arrest (the period of time between QRS complexes containing the arrest period), and report the escape rate.
5. QRS Rhythm: The rhythm is regular. An escape rhythm may be regular or irregular, according to the site of the escape pacemaker.

Figure 4-12 is an ECG tracing that is an example of sinus arrest.

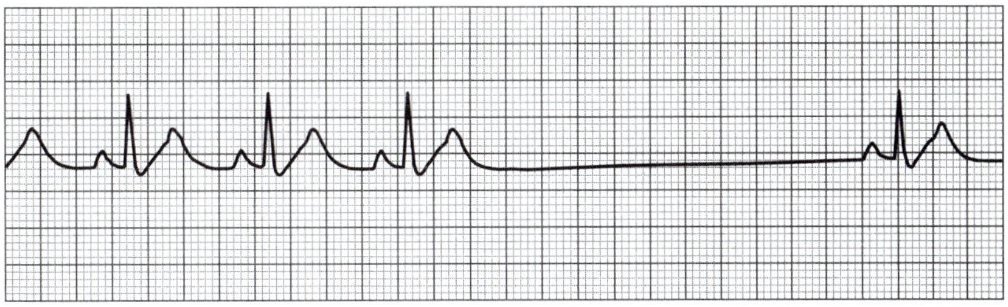

Figure 4-12 An ECG tracing showing one (+) P wave to the left of each QRS complex; the PR interval is consistent, and the heart rate is within normal limits prior to the event of SA arrest. Count the number of large squares between the QRS complexes containing the arrest. Multiply by 0.20 (the value of one large square) for the estimated period of arrest, about 2.76 seconds.

Causes of Sinus Arrest

Sinus arrest reflects a problem within the SA node, usually as a result of proximal right coronary artery disease. If that condition exists, the ability of the AV junctional escape mechanism also may be affected. Sinus arrest also can be seen with sleep apnea.

Intervention

Patients are treated based on the degree of hemodynamic compromise. On initial assessment, the patient may complain only of near-syncopal episodes. As with all cases of patient compromise, care begins with documenting past medical history, focusing on medications, and a physical exam.

Begin with high-flow oxygen therapy, and place the patient on a monitor. Include a 12-lead ECG. If SA arrest occurs frequently, an electronic pacemaker may be implanted. Medical direction may recommend the use of Atropine as a temporizing measure until a pacemaker is implemented.

Figure 4-13 is an example of SA arrest in a 51-year-old male during a sleep apnea episode.

Figure 4-14 is an example of SA arrest in an 82-year-old male patient who complained of frequent episodes of syncope. The patient was unresponsive to Atropine, responded well to transcutaneous pacing (TCP), and eventually had pacemaker implantation.

SA block
An event in which the SA node initiates the impulse, but the propagation over atrial tissue is blocked, so the atria are not depolarized.

SINOATRIAL (SA) BLOCK

SA block is also called *sinus exit block.* SA block is an event and not always reflective of disease within the sinus node. In SA block, the SA node initiates the impulse, but the

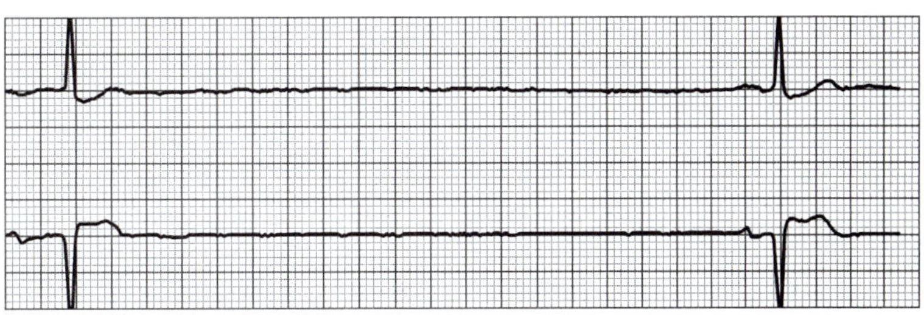

Figure 4-13 An ECG tracing from a 51-year-old patient showing sinus arrest during a sleep apnea episode

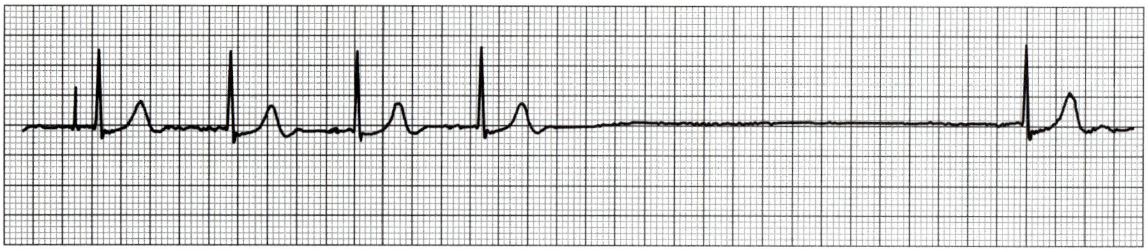

Figure 4-14 An ECG tracing from an 82-year-old patient showing sinus arrest. The patient required insertion of an electronic pacemaker.

propagation over atrial tissue is blocked, so the atria are not depolarized. Therefore, there is no P wave nor QRS complex. SA block represents a failure of transmission of the impulse over atrial tissue. The ECG characteristics of SA block are as follows:

1. P Wave: The P waves are positive and uniform in lead II. However, an entire cycle (P, QRS, and T) is missing. The SA node initiates an impulse, but it is not propagated through the atria; it is blocked, and hence there is no P wave. The pause is a multiple of the regular cycle length.
2. PR Interval: The PR interval is normal between 0.12 and 0.2 second and is constant from beat to beat except during the pause, when an entire cycle is missing. Also, the PR interval may be slightly shorter following the pause.
3. QRS Complex: The QRS complex duration is 0.10 second or less except during the pause, when an entire cycle is missing.
4. QRS Rate: The rate may be constant or varying, according to the number and position of the missing cycles. The R-R interval is a multiple of the regular cycle length.
5. QRS Rhythm: The rhythm may be regular or irregular, according to the number and position of the missing cycles.

Figure 4-15 is an ECG tracing showing SA block. In this example, the sinus P waves plot out. The *X* indicates the missing PQRST complex. The R-R interval of the SA block is equal to twice the normal R-R interval.

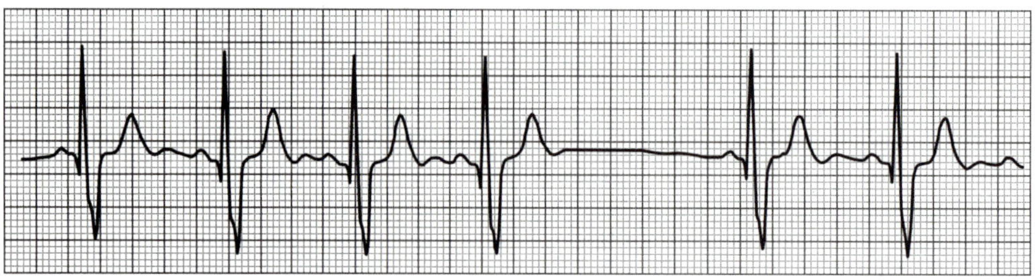

Figure 4-15 An ECG tracing showing one (+) P wave to the left of each QRS complex; the PR interval is consistent, and the heart rate is within normal limits prior to the event of SA block. Plot out the P waves and measure the R-R interval of the SA block. Note that the long P-P interval is equal to two P-P intervals. The ECG also shows U waves and broad terminal S waves in the QRS complex.

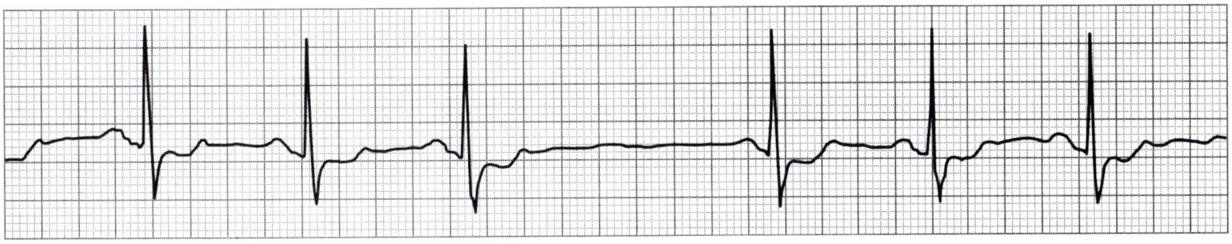

Figure 4-16 An ECG tracing showing SA block

Causes of SA Block

SA block is most commonly caused by medications, such as quinidine, acetylcholine, and excessive potassium ingestion. Excessive vagal stimulation also may cause SA block; this is episodic and may only be documented if the patient is on a monitor.

Intervention

Unless the underlying rhythm is slow, intervention is supportive and focused on identifying the cause. This involves performing an initial assessment and completing a focused history with special attention to cardiac conditions and medication ingestion. SA block is rarely life threatening.

Figure 4-16 is an example of SA block. Note the schematic, which shows how the P waves plot through the event without disturbing the cadence of the sinus rhythm.

Summary

Normally, the sinus node dominates heart rhythm and does so for a lifetime. An arrhythmia is present when the heart rate is too slow, too fast, or irregular, or when depolarization does not propagate over atrial tissue, and, finally, when the SA node fails to produce a stimulus at all.

In each of the sinus mechanisms, the visible P wave will be positive and precede each QRS. Where there is no P wave, there is no atrial depolarization.

Most of the sinus arrhythmias are explainable, and the patients tolerate minor deviations. In most instances, identifying and treating the cause remedies the arrhythmias. When the patient situation is complicated with persistent bradycardia and accompanying hypotension and hypoperfusion, treating the patient with a slow rate is appropriate.

Table 4-1 is a summary of the sinus mechanisms and the ECG components to help differentiate the rhythms.

Table 4-1 Summary of the ECG configurations of the sinus mechanisms and the proposed interventions

Sinus	Rhythm	Bradycardia	Tachycardia	Arrhythmia	Exit Block	Sinus Arrest
P waves	(+)/QRS	(+)/QRS	(+)/QRS	(+)/QRS	(+)/QRS	(+)/QRS
P-R Interval	0.12–0.20 sec	0.12–0.20 sec	0.12–0.20 sec	0.12–0.20 sec	0.12–0.20 sec	0.12–0.20 sec
QRS duration	≤0.10	≤0.10	≤0.10	≤0.10		
Rate/minute	60–100	<60	>100	60–100		
Rhythm	regular	regular	regular	irregular	regular except for the event	regular except for the event
Event			gradual onset	gradual change	misses one beat; sinus plots through; cadence is regular	misses more than one beat; rhythm after is irregular and slow
Rx		Consider Atropine, fluids, dopamine for perfusion; Pace (TCP)	ID & Rx cause such as pain or pressure, fever, anger, anxiety, dehydration, hypovolemia, medications, and/or drug use/abuse	only with bradycardia and patient is hypotensive and hypoperfusing	only if it persists; increases in frequency and duration; associated with a slow rate; hypotensive and hypoperfusing	only if it persists; increases in frequency and duration; associated with a slow rate; hypotensive and hypoperfusing

Self-Assessment Exercises

Fill in the Blanks

Complete the statements and then compare your answers with those in the back of the book.

SINUS RHYTHM	SINUS BRADYCARDIA	SINUS TACHYCARDIA
1 (+) P plus QRS	1 (+) P plus QRS	____________
PRI: 0.12–0.20 second	____________	____________
QRS: 0.10 second or less	____________	____________
RATE: 60–100 per minute	____________	____________
RHYTHM: regular	____________	regular

SINUS RHYTHM	SINUS ARRHYTHMIA	SINUS BLOCK
1 (+) P plus QRS	1 (+) P plus QRS	____________
PRI: 0.12–0.20 second	____________	____________
QRS: 0.10 second or less	____________	____________
RATE: 60–100 per minute	____________	____________
RHYTHM: regular	____________	regular

ECG Rhythm Identification Practice

For the following rhythms fill in the blanks and then check your answers with those in the back of the book.

Figure 4-17

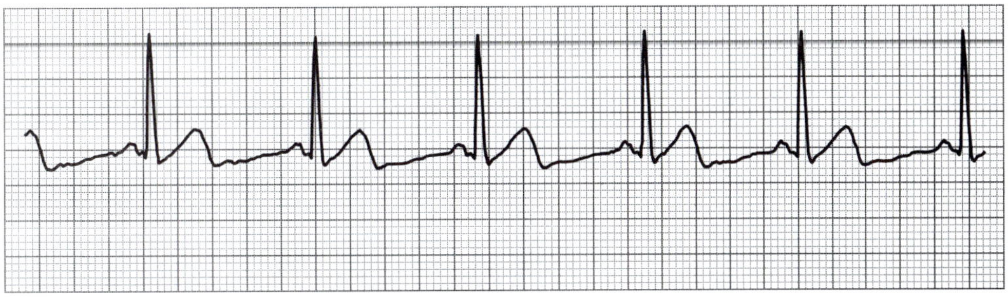

QRS duration ______________ QT ____________

Ventricular rate/rhythm ____________________

Atrial rate/rhythm ________________________

PR interval ______________________________

Identification ____________________________

Symptoms ________________________________

____

Treatment ________________________________

Figure 4-18

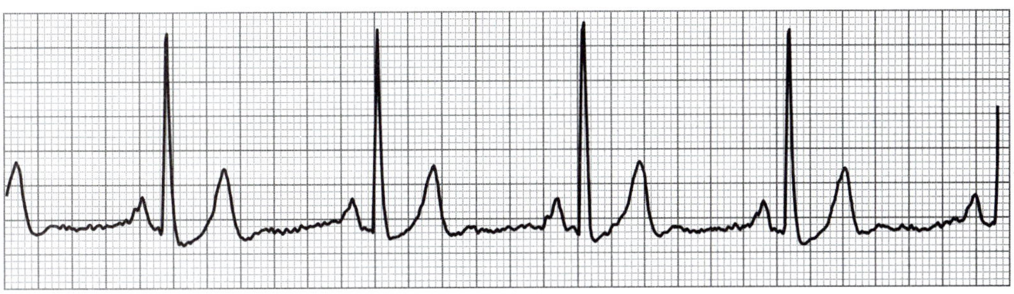

QRS duration ______________ QT ____________

Ventricular rate/rhythm ____________________

Atrial rate/rhythm ________________________

PR interval ______________________________

Identification ____________________________

Symptoms ________________________________

____

Treatment ________________________________

Figure 4-19

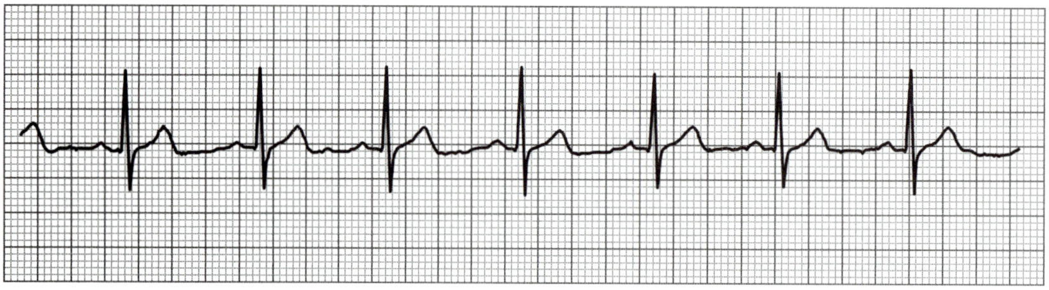

QRS duration ________________ QT ____________

Ventricular rate/rhythm ________________________

Atrial rate/rhythm ____________________________

PR interval __________________________________

Identification ________________________________

Symptoms ____________________________________

____

Treatment ____________________________________

Figure 4-20

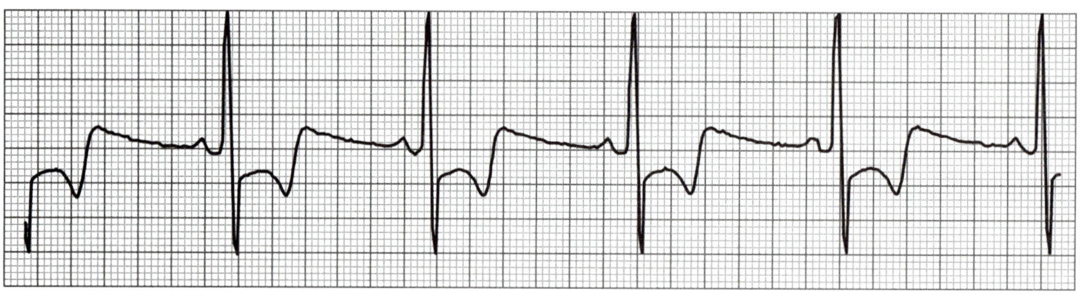

QRS duration ________________ QT ____________

Ventricular rate/rhythm ________________________

Atrial rate/rhythm ____________________________

PR interval __________________________________

Identification ________________________________

Symptoms ____________________________________

____

Treatment ____________________________________

Figure 4-21

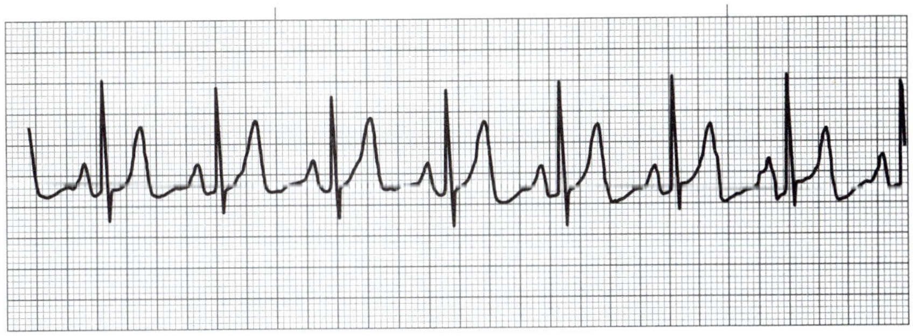

QRS duration ____________ QT ____________
Ventricular rate/rhythm ____________
Atrial rate/rhythm ____________
PR interval ____________

Identification ____________
Symptoms ____________
____
Treatment ____________

Figure 4-22

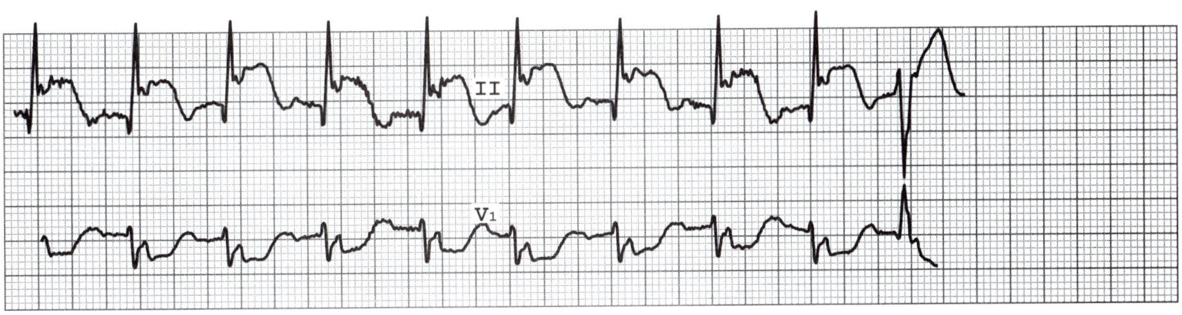

QRS duration ____________ QT ____________
Ventricular rate/rhythm ____________
Atrial rate/rhythm ____________
PR interval ____________

Identification ____________
Symptoms ____________
____
Treatment ____________

Figure 4-23

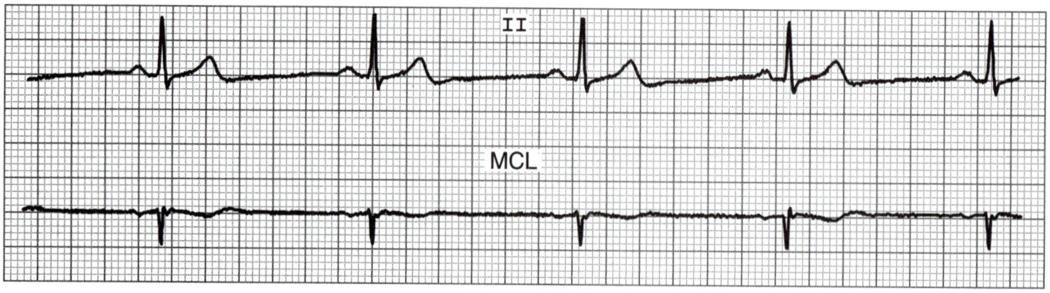

QRS duration ______ **QT** ______
Ventricular rate/rhythm ______
Atrial rate/rhythm ______
PR interval ______

Identification ______
Symptoms ______
______
Treatment ______

Figure 4-24

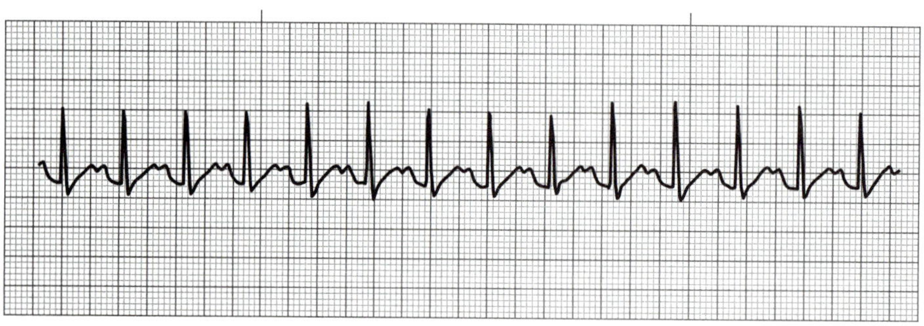

QRS duration ______ **QT** ______
Ventricular rate/rhythm ______
Atrial rate/rhythm ______
PR interval ______

Identification ______
Symptoms ______
______
Treatment ______

Figure 4-25

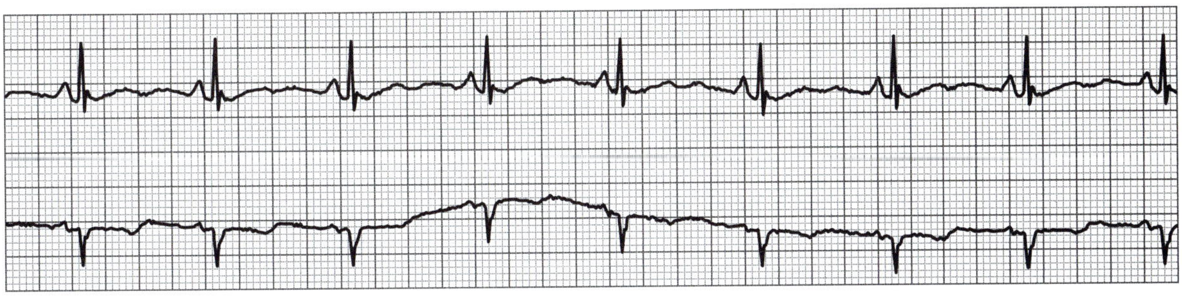

QRS duration ________________ QT ____________

Ventricular rate/rhythm ________________________

Atrial rate/rhythm ____________________________

PR interval ___________________________________

Identification ________________________________

Symptoms ____________________________________

____

Treatment ____________________________________

Figure 4-26

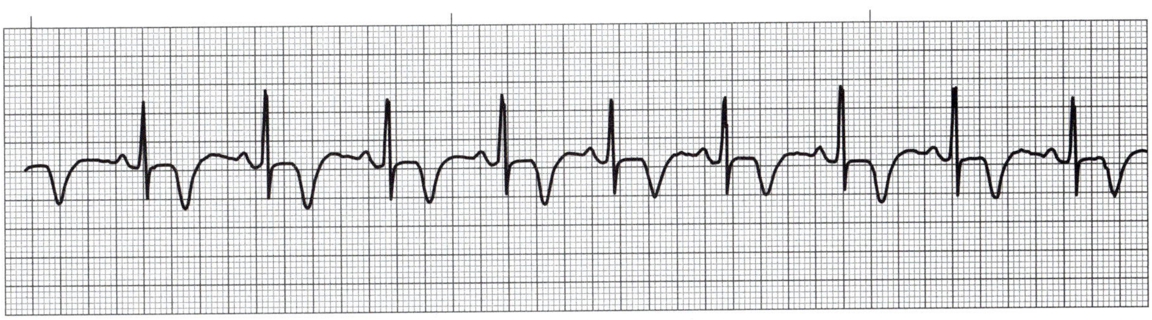

QRS duration ________________ QT ____________

Ventricular rate/rhythm ________________________

Atrial rate/rhythm ____________________________

PR interval ___________________________________

Identification ________________________________

Symptoms ____________________________________

____

Treatment ____________________________________

Figure 4-27

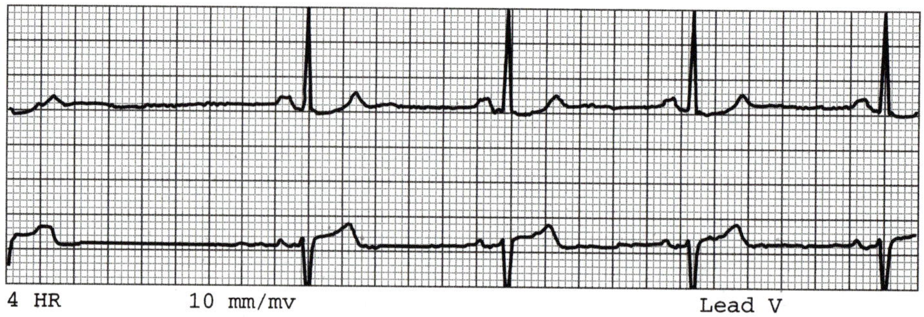

QRS duration ______________ QT ______________
Ventricular rate/rhythm ______________
Atrial rate/rhythm ______________
PR interval ______________

Identification ______________
Symptoms ______________
____
Treatment ______________

Figure 4-28

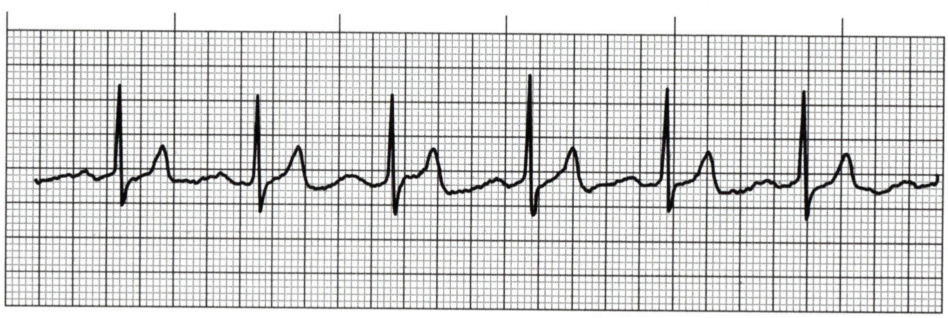

QRS duration ______________ QT ______________
Ventricular rate/rhythm ______________
Atrial rate/rhythm ______________
PR interval ______________

Identification ______________
Symptoms ______________
____
Treatment ______________

Figure 4-29

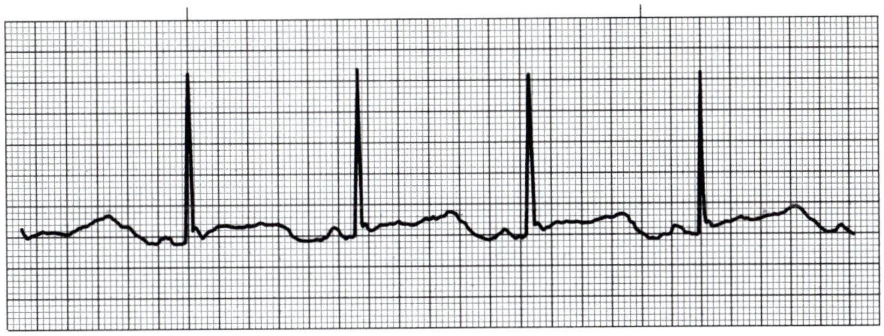

QRS duration ________ QT ________

Ventricular rate/rhythm ________

Atrial rate/rhythm ________

PR interval ________

Identification ________

Symptoms ________

____

Treatment ________

Figure 4-30

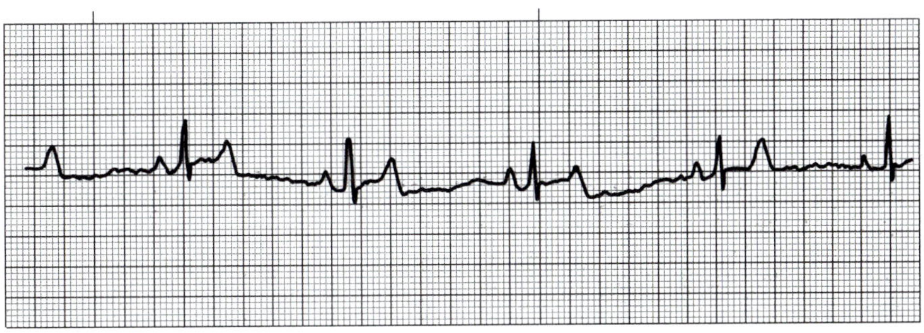

QRS duration ________ QT ________

Ventricular rate/rhythm ________

Atrial rate/rhythm ________

PR interval ________

Identification ________

Symptoms ________

____

Treatment ________

References

Conover, M. B. *Nurse's pocket guide to electrocardiography* (3rd ed.). St. Louis, MO: C. V. Mosby; 1994.

Conover, M. B. *Understanding electrocardiography: Arrhythmias and the 12-lead ECG* (7th ed.). St. Louis, MO: Mosby-Year Book, Inc.; 1996.

Conover, M. B., & Wellens, H. J. *The ECG in emergency decision making*. Philadelphia: W. B. Saunders; 1993.

Goldberger, E. *Textbook of clinical cardiology*. St. Louis, MO: C. V. Mosby; 1982.

Mandel, W. J. (Ed). *Cardiac arrhythmias: Their mechanisms, diagnoses and management* (2nd ed.). Philadelphia: Lippincott; 1987.

Marriott, H. J. *Practical electrocardiography* (8th ed.). Baltimore: Williams and Wilkins; 1988.

Marriott, H. J., & Conover, M. B. *Advanced concepts in arrhythmias* (2nd ed.). St. Louis, MO: C. V. Mosby; 1989.

CHAPTER 5

The Junctional Mechanisms

Premise: The difference between sinus and junctional rhythms is the shape and direction of the P wave.

Objectives

After reading the chapter and completing the Self-Assessment Exercises, the student should be able to

1. recognize the change in direction of the P wave
2. differentiate between sinus and junctional P waves
3. differentiate between ectopic and escape junctional mechanisms
4. identify the causes for the junctional mechanisms
5. select the appropriate intervention

Key Terms

escape beat
junctional rhythm
junctional (AV) tachycardia
P prime (P′)
premature junctional complex (PJC)
retrograde atrial depolarization

Introduction

When the sinus node fires, a single positive predictable P wave should precede each QRS with a consistent PR interval. While there are variations in rate and rhythm, the relationship of P wave, PR interval, and the QRS complex remain consistent.

When the sinus node fails to function, the next possible pacemaker to respond lies within the AV junction. The conduction into the ventricles is usually without problem, and the resulting QRS shows little or no difference from a sinus-induced QRS.

The AV junction can function as a back-up or escape pacemaker, generating an impulse at a predictable and satisfactory rate. The AV junction also can function as an ectopic, challenging the sinus node by generating an impulse and taking control of heart rate.

The differential diagnosis between these two supraventricular pacemakers is dependent on the analysis of the P wave. Since cause and interventions are similar for each of the junctional mechanisms, they will be discussed after the ECG characteristics.

JUNCTIONAL MECHANISMS

For some time, it was thought that the AV node functioned as a pacemaker. James (1974) determined that there are no rapid-sodium channels within the AV node known to be necessary for predictable pacemaker function.

An impulse that originates within the nodal-His (NH) region of the bundle of His is conducted through the ventricular bundle branches and results in a narrow QRS complex, not unlike a sinus-induced QRS complex. By convention, the pacing function within AV junctional tissue is referred to as *junctional*. Any P wave that is other than from the sinus node is referred to as **P prime** or **P′**. Figure 5-1 is a graphic illustration of the position of the P′ in three variations of a junctional mechanism.

P prime (P′)
Label for any ectopic P wave, other than a sinus impulse

Cause

The junction rarely functions in competition with the sinus node because its primary role is that of a back-up pacemaker since it is normally depolarized with each sinus beat. When the sinus fails, or when the sinus impulse is blocked within the AV node, the bundle of His may reach potential and generate an impulse. This is termed an **escape beat**. If the His bundle sustains the role of pacemaker it is termed a **junctional rhythm**.

escape beat
The development of latent pacemakers to stimulate the heart when there is sinus-node slowing or arrest. The atria, AV junction, or ventricles may be the site of a single complex or a sustained rhythm

junctional rhythm
The point at which the bundle of His is able to sustain the role of back-up pacemaker when the sinus node is blocked or has failed

ESCAPE JUNCTIONAL COMPLEX

An escape beat is one that comes after a delay in the cardiac cycle. There is a pause, as with SA block or SA arrest, and at the conclusion of the delay is a narrow QRS with a retrograde P′ before, during, or after the QRS, or the P′ may not be visible at all. An escape junctional beat occurs because the sinus has failed to maintain control and the

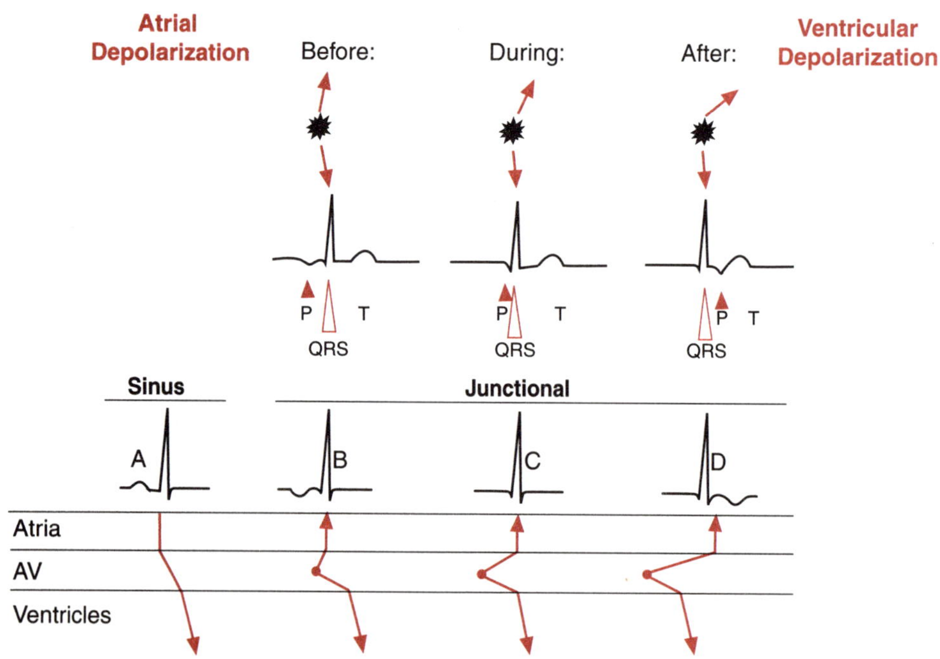

Figure 5-1 Sinus and junctional induced complexes. Note the (+) P to the left of the QRS in a sinus mechanism, and (A) one showing one (-) P′ wave to the left of each QRS complex, (B) indicating a junctional mechanism. (C) shows a QRS complex without a visible P wave and (D) shows a (-) P′ buried within the ST segment. The schematic above and below the ECG depicts the retrograde depolarization of the atria from the junctional site.

junction, not having been stimulated by a sinus-induced wave front, reaches its potential and discharges. If the condition persists, the escape beat can take over the pacemaking function. This is the junctional rhythm previously described.

The P′ wave may be completely or partially hidden within the preceding T wave or greatly enhance the amplitude and distort the preceding T wave. The P′ waves can be seen before, during, or after the QRS complexes and are inverted (negative) in leads II, III, and aVF.

The position of the P′ wave depends on the following:

1. The atria are depolarized before the ventricles. The P′ wave is inverted in lead II with a short (0.12 second or less) P′R interval.
2. The atria and the ventricles may or may not be depolarized simultaneously. The P′ wave is then hidden within the QRS complex and is not visible on the electrocardiogram.
3. The atria are depolarized after the ventricles. The P′ wave is then inverted in lead II, following the QRS complex.
4. When no P′ waves are visible, a fourth possibility exists: the atria are not depolarized because retrograde conduction is blocked. The QRS complex is 0.10 second or less, with normal ventricular depolarization.

Figure 5-2 A and B are ECG tracings showing two examples of sinus mechanisms, each with an escape junctional complex. Note in each example the long pause, ending with a narrow QRS that is similar to the sinus QRSs. However, in each example, there is no sinus-induced P wave prior to the escape junctional QRS complexes. In each example, the QRS complexes do not vary in configuration or size despite the difference in point of origin. Recall that impulses that have an origin above the ventricles typically conduct normally with a narrow QRS as a result.

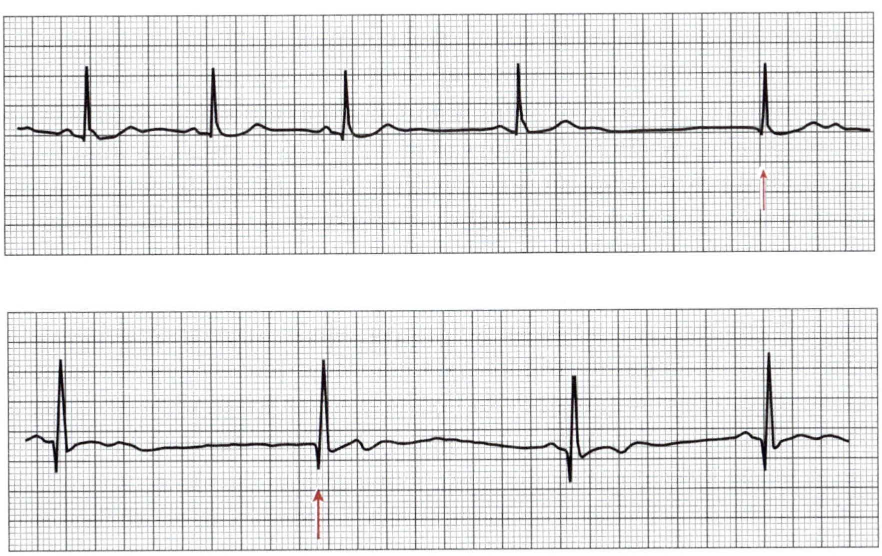

(A) (B)

Figure 5-2 Two ECG tracings showing (A) one (+) P wave to the left of each QRS complex; the PR interval is consistent, and the heart rate is within normal limits. The heart rate visibly slows until a long pause of about 1.6 second. The next complex is a QRS without the visible sinus P wave to the left. This is the *junctional escape beat.* (B) shows a (+) P plus a QRS (a sinus beat), a pause, a QRS with no visible P wave (the junctional escape beat), and a return to a sinus bradycardia. In each example, note that the configuration and measurement of the QRS complex do not vary despite the difference in origin.

Cause

Remember the role of the junctional pacer is that of a back-up when the sinus fails, or the sinus-induced wave forms fail to conduct through AV junctional tissue.

Intervention

There is no reason to interfere with a junctional escape mechanism. The practitioner must be suspicious as to *why* the junction took over as a pacer. There is always concern for underlying proximal right coronary artery disease that often results in sinus arrest.

Junctional Rhythm

The junction is capable of providing a consistent and predictable heart rate. When the junction becomes the dominant pacemaker, the single impulse origination in the junction can travel in two directions.

The ventricles are depolarized normally, since the impulse spreads through the bundle of His to the bundle branches and then through to the Purkinje network, leading to ventricular depolarization, Therefore, the QRS complexes are normal in duration, 0.10 second or less. However, the atria are depolarized in a manner opposite to that of normal. This is known as **retrograde atrial depolarization**. This retrograde atrial depolarization is reflected on the ECG by a negative (downward, inverted) P′ wave in lead II.

retrograde atrial depolarization
The reverse direction; inferior to superior

In order to describe a rhythm as junctional in origin, the following criteria must be met:

1. P′Wave: The P′ that is junctional in origin is negative (-) and visible in front of, within, or after the QRS. Whichever occurs, the position is consistent.
2. P′R Interval: When the inverted (-) P′ waves are visible before the QRS complexes, PR interval is relatively short, about 0.12 second.
3. QRS Complex: The QRS complex duration is 0.10 second or less.
4. QRS Rate: The inherent rate is constant and ranges between 40 and 60 per minute.
5. QRS RHYTHM: Junctional rhythm is regular at any rate range.

Figure 5-3 is an ECG of a junctional rhythm. Note that there are no P waves for any QRS complex.

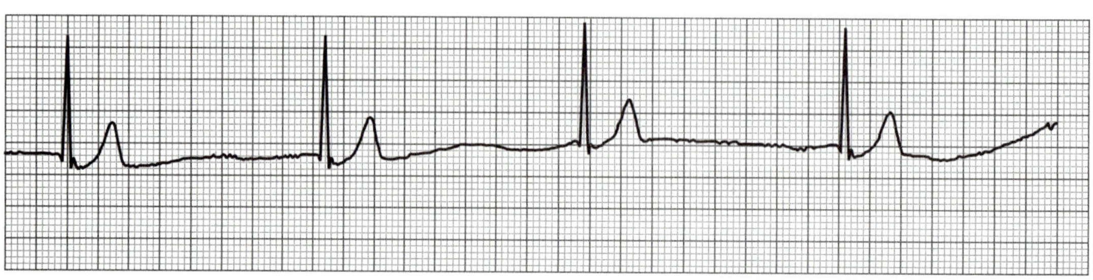

Figure 5-3 An ECG tracing showing a narrow QRS complex but no preceding P wave. This indicates a junctional rhythm.

PREMATURE JUNCTIONAL COMPLEX

In the case of a **premature junctional complex (PJC)**, the P′ wave may be completely or partially hidden within the preceding T wave or greatly enhance the amplitude and distort the preceding T wave. The P′ waves can be seen before, during, or after the QRS complexes and are inverted (negative) in leads II, III, and aVF. The following is a summary of the ECG characteristics of junctional escape beats and PJCs.

premature junctional complex (PJC)

A discharge of an ectopic focus from the area of the bundle of His within the AV junction that causes premature atrial depolarization. Represented on the ECG as a negative (-) P'.

1. P′ Wave: The P′ that is junctional in origin is negative (-) and visible in front of, within, or after the QRS. Whichever occurs, the position is consistent.
2. P′R Interval: When the P′ occurs prior to the QRS, the P′R interval may be normal or prolonged and often differs from the PR interval of the dominant rhythm.
3. QRS Complex: The QRS complex duration is 0.10 second or less, most of the time. If the resulting QRS changes configuration and is greater than 0.10, this reflects the degree of refractoriness of the conduction tissue.
4. QRS Rate: The inherent sinus rate is constant.
5. QRS Rhythm: In the case of the PJC, the regularity of the basic rhythm is disturbed. In the case of an escape beat, there is a long pause that ends with the escape junctional beat.

Figures 5-4, 5-5, and 5-6 are examples of sinus mechanisms with PJCs. Figure 5-5 is an example of the P′ prior to the premature QRS; Figure 5-6 has no visible P′

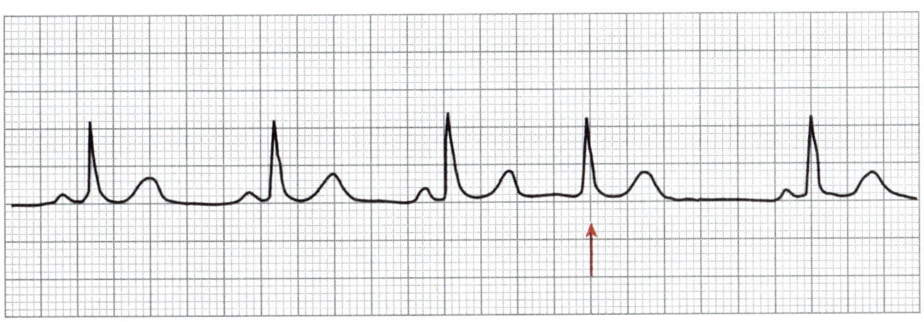

Figure 5-4 An ECG tracing showing one (+) P wave to the left of each of three sinus beats. The fourth QRS complex is similar to the sinus QRSs but is early (premature) and has no P wave. The sinus P waves do not plot through the event.

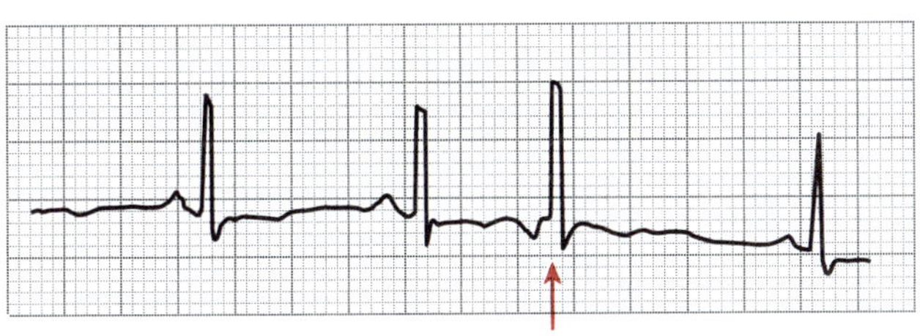

Figure 5-5 An ECG tracing showing one (+) P wave to the left of each of first two sinus beats. The third QRS complex is similar to the sinus QRSs but is early (premature) and has a (–) P' preceding. The sinus P waves do not plot through the event. This would be described as sinus rhythm at 77 per minute with a PJC.

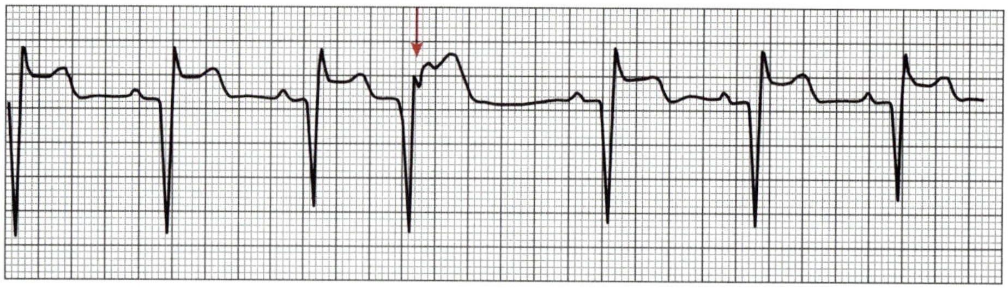

Figure 5-6 An ECG tracing showing a (+) P wave for each of two clearly visible QRS complexes, indicating a sinus mechanism. The fourth QRS is clearly premature, but there is no (+) P prior to the QRS. There is a negative deflection within the ST segment of the premature complex, which may indicate the retrograde conduction to the atria. The sinus P waves do not plot through the event, but resume cadence afterward. There is 3 to 4 mm ST segment elevation and deep Q waves (18 mm and 0.06 second). These findings may indicate proximal right coronary artery disease with ischemia, injury, and necrosis. The ECG interpretation would be sinus rhythm at 67 per minute with a PJC, 3 to 4 mm ST segment elevation, and Q waves at 18 mm and 0.06 second.

before the premature QRS but the P′ is visible within the ST segment of the ectopic QRS. In each of the examples, the sinus P wave does not plot through the events, indicating a disruption in normal, predictable sinus/atrial activity.

Cause of PJCs

PJCs may be idiopathic or symptomatic of digitalis excess. Excessive sympathetic stimulation may also cause PJCs.

Intervention

Assess the patient's clinical signs and symptoms, questioning medical and medication history, allergies, and vital signs.

ACCELERATED JUNCTIONAL RHYTHM

Accelerated junctional rhythm is the term used when the junctional rate is between 60 and 100 beats per minute. The ECG characteristics are as follows:

1. P′ Wave: The P′ that is junctional in origin is negative (-) and visible in front of, within, or after the QRS. Whichever occurs, the position is consistent.
2. P′R Interval: When the inverted (-) P′ waves are visible before the QRS complexes, PR interval is relatively short, about 0.12 second.
3. QRS Complex: The QRS complex duration is 0.10 second or less.
4. QRS Rate: When the junctional rate accelerates to greater than 60, it is identified as accelerated junctional rhythm.
5. QRS Rhythm: Junctional rhythm is regular at any rate range.

Figure 5-7 is an example of an accelerated junctional rhythm. Note that the heart rate is faster than 60 per minute and yet very regular; this is the hallmark of a junctional pacemaker.

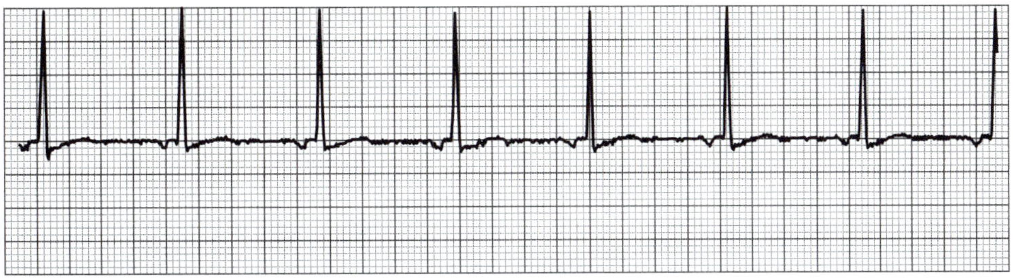

Figure 5-7 An ECG tracing showing a regular, narrow QRS with a (-) P′ to the left of each QRS. The QRS rate is 67 per minute. The ECG interpretation would be accelerated junctional rhythm at 60 per minute.

Cause of Accelerated Junctional Rhythm

The junction can accelerate for the same reasons as the sinus or with digitalis excess.

Intervention

It is rarely necessary to intervene, except to document signs, symptoms, and patient medical and medication history.

JUNCTIONAL TACHYCARDIA

The ECG characteristics for **junctional tachycardia** are similar to those of a junctional rhythm and accelerated junction rhythm, with the exception of rate. In junctional tachycardia, the rate is 100 to 140 beats per minute. Figure 5-8 is an ECG showing junctional tachycardia. The rate is rapid at 125 per minute, and the rhythm is very regular. If this were sinus tachycardia, the rate is not so fast that a P wave would be easily seen preceding the QRS.

junctional (AV) tachycardia
Rhythm originating from the AV junction at a rate above 100 per minute.

Summary of Causes of Junctional Mechanisms

Junctional escape beats and junctional rhythms make up a passive escape rhythm that takes control when sinus rate is too slow, during excessive vagal stimulation, acute myocardial infarction, or episodes of SA block or SA arrest. Junctional escape beats, single occurrences of a junctional-induced QRS, are often seen after premature atrial complexes (PACs) or premature ventricular complexes (PVCs).

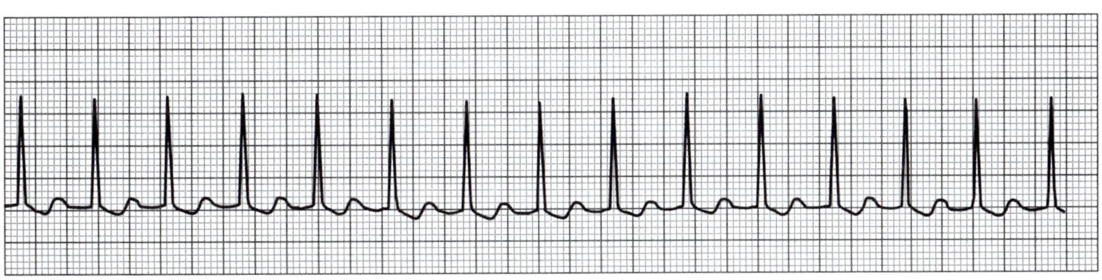

Figure 5-8 An ECG tracing showing narrow QRS with no identifiable P wave to the left of the QRS. The QRS rate is 125 per minute. This is probably junctional tachycardia at 125 per minute.

A junctional escape rhythm can occur when there is no conduction through the AV node (complete AV block), most commonly when the source of the block is at the level of the AV node. This can occur with acute myocardial infarction and with right coronary artery occlusion or spasm.

Enhanced automaticity in the AV junction causes PJCs. *Accelerated junctional rhythm* is the term that describes an AV junction rhythm faster than 60 and less than 100 beats per minute. *Junctional tachycardia* is the termed used when the junctional rate is greater than 100 beats per minute and rarely exceeds 130 beats per minute. Episodes of junctional tachycardia also may occur after open heart surgery. Enhanced automaticity within the AV junction is usually the result of digitalis toxicity but may occur with metabolic disturbances.

Digitalis toxicity has catastrophic consequences. Sadly, the signs of toxicity can go unnoticed or attributed to other maladies, even in the face of therapeutic blood levels. AV junctional ectopics and junctional rhythms of increasing rates are some of the ECG signs of toxicity. While the patient's heart rate is within normal limits, the patient has a myriad of signs and symptoms often attributed to long-standing chronic complaints. These include gastrointestinal (GI) disturbances and visual complaints. Psychiatric symptoms range from agitation to feeling listless and apathetic. Nervousness, loss of memory, nightmares, feelings of paranoia, weakness, and fatigue are common complaints, uncorrected with other therapies or interventions.

INTERVENTION

Most patients tolerate a junctional escape rhythm. However, the situation should not be taken for granted. If the patient is compromised by slow rate, for instance, decreased levels of perfusion, or the occurrence of premature ventricular complexes (PVCs), consider the use of medications to accelerate the rate. The AV junction can respond to vagal blocking and may accelerate to a more satisfactory rate, or the sinus node will accelerate and regain control.

The initial assessment and history should focus on medication history and compliance. Of interest too is whether or not the patient borrowed medication, such as digitalis preparations. This does occur, and the patient does not perceive this as a wrong thing to do. The presence of a PJC may be the first indication of the enhanced automaticity provoked by digitalis toxicity.

When the heart rate is within normal limits, there is no reason to intervene, other than cataloging signs and symptoms for further study by the responsible physician. When the heart rate is slow, and the patient is symptomatic, hypotensive, and hypoperfusing, the tendency is to treat with medications to increase heart rate.

If digitalis is a suspected cause for the bradycardia, the accelerated junctional rhythm, and/or the junctional ectopics, supportive therapy until the patient can be treated for the digitalis toxicity is in order. This would include preparing for transcutaneous or transvenous pacing.

Vagal maneuvers can help differentiate the narrow QRS tachycardias, if the patient's symptoms warrant. Medications may be useful, but when the patient is considered hemodynamically compromised, synchronized cardioversion should be considered.

Summary

When the sinus node falters or fails, the AV junction can function as a back-up pacemaker or be ectopic, challenging the sinus node by generating an impulse and taking control of heart rate from 60 to 130 beats per minute. The difference between junctional and sinus mechanisms is the polarity of the P waves.

Care of the patient includes detailed physical exam and a medical history focusing on medications, specifically digitalis preparations. Clinical intervention solely to treat a bradycardia in a patient who is not compromised is rare. If the patient is compromised, an electronic pacemaker may be required.

Table 5-1 is a summary of the ECG configurations of junctional mechanisms.

Table 5-1 Summary of ECG configurations of junctional mechanisms.

	Junctional Escape Beat	Junctional Rhythm	Accelerated Junctional Rhythm	Junctional Tachycardia	Premature Junctional Complex (PJC)
P waves	(-) or none	(-) or none	(-) or none	(-) or none	(-) or none
P-R interval	<0.12 sec	<0.12 sec	<0.12 sec	<0.12 sec	<0.12 sec
QRS duration	0.10	≤0.10	≤0.10	≤0.10	≤0.10
Ventricular rate per minute		40–60	60–100	>100	
Ventricular rhythm		regular	regular	regular	
Intervention	?med Hx ?digitalis	if the patient is symptomatic with the slow rate, consider: atropine, fluids, dopamine, TCP	?med Hx ?digitalis	?med Hx ?digitalis	?med Hx ?digitalis

Self-Assessment Exercises

Matching

Find the phrase in the right column that matches the numbered word or phrase in the left column, and compare your answers with those in the back of the book.

____	1. 0.10 second	a. P wave
____	2. 0.08 second	b. QRS complex
____	3. 0.12–0.20 second	c. PR interval
____	4. 0.36–0.44 second	d. QT interval

Fill in the Blanks

Complete the statements, and then compare your answers with those in the back of the book.

SINUS RHYTHM	SINUS BRADYCARDIA	JUNCTIONAL RHYTHM
1 (+) P plus QRS	1 (+) P plus a QRS	____________
PRI 0.12–0.20	0.12–0.20	____________
QRS equal to or less than 0.10	equal to or less than 0.10	____________
Rate 60–100 per minute	less than 60 per minute	____________
Rhythm regular	regular	____________

ECG Rhythm Identification Practice

For the following rhythms fill in the blanks and then check your answers with those in the back of this book.

Figure 5-9

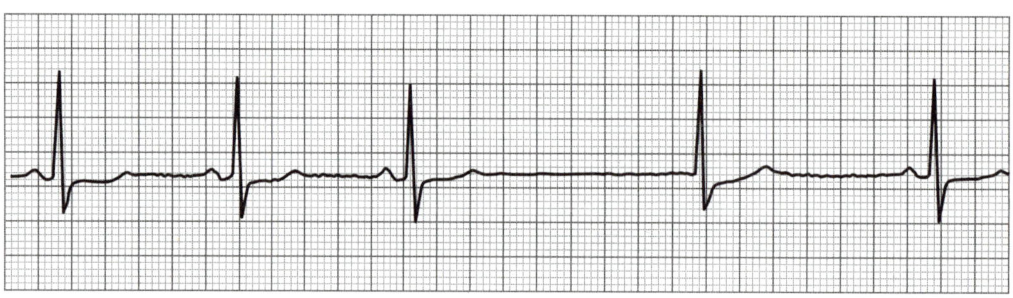

QRS duration ____________ QT ____________

Ventricular rate/rhythm ____________

Atrial rate/rhythm ____________

PR interval ____________

Identification ____________

Symptoms ____________

____

Treatment ____________

Figure 5-10

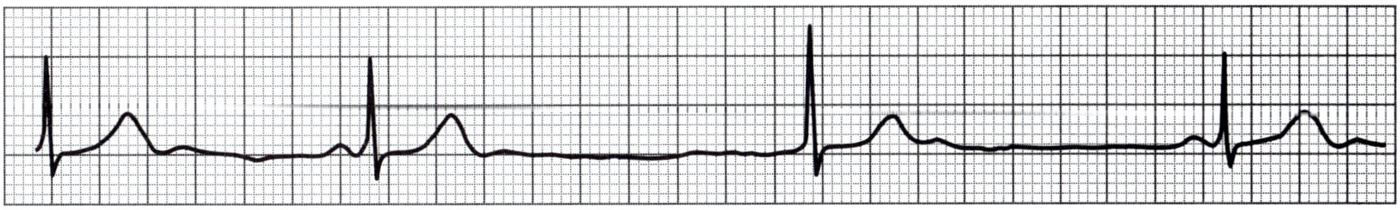

QRS duration ______________ QT __________
Ventricular rate/rhythm ______________________
Atrial rate/rhythm __________________________
PR interval ________________________________

Identification ______________________________
Symptoms ___________________________________
____
Treatment ___________________________________

Figure 5-11

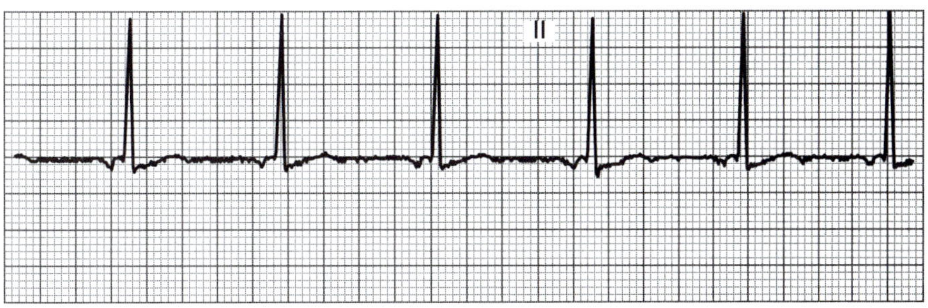

QRS duration ______________ QT __________
Ventricular rate/rhythm ______________________
Atrial rate/rhythm __________________________
PR interval ________________________________

Identification ______________________________
Symptoms ___________________________________
____
Treatment ___________________________________

Figure 5-12

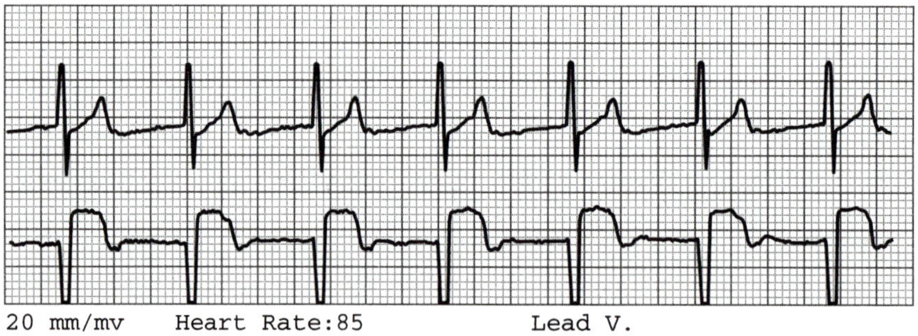

QRS duration ________________ QT ____________

Ventricular rate/rhythm ________________________

Atrial rate/rhythm ____________________________

PR interval __________________________________

Identification ____________________________________

Symptoms ____

____

Treatment ____

Figure 5-13

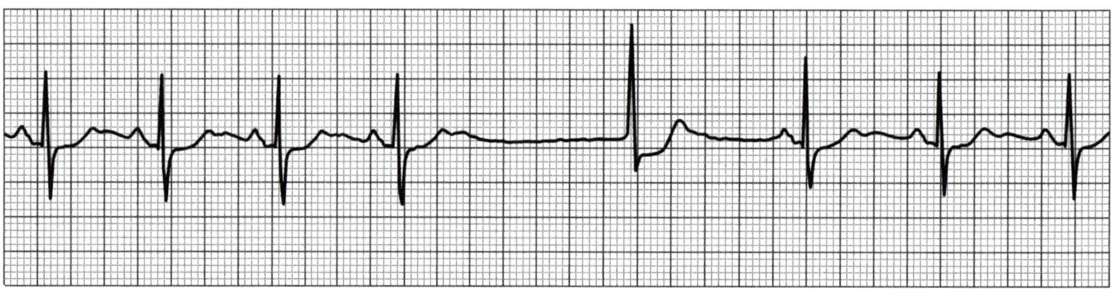

QRS duration ________________ QT ____________

Ventricular rate/rhythm ________________________

Atrial rate/rhythm ____________________________

PR interval __________________________________

Identification ____________________________________

Symptoms ____

____

Treatment ____

Figure 5-14

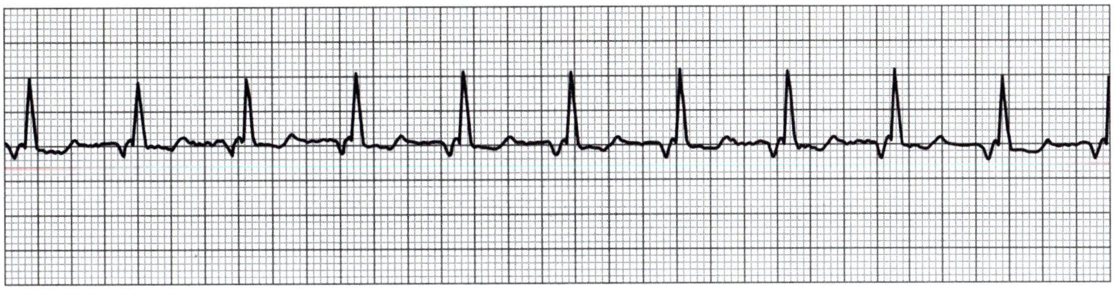

QRS duration ________________ QT ______________

Ventricular rate/rhythm ______________________

Atrial rate/rhythm __________________________

PR interval ________________________________

Identification ______________________________

Symptoms ________________________________

____

Treatment ________________________________

Figure 5-15

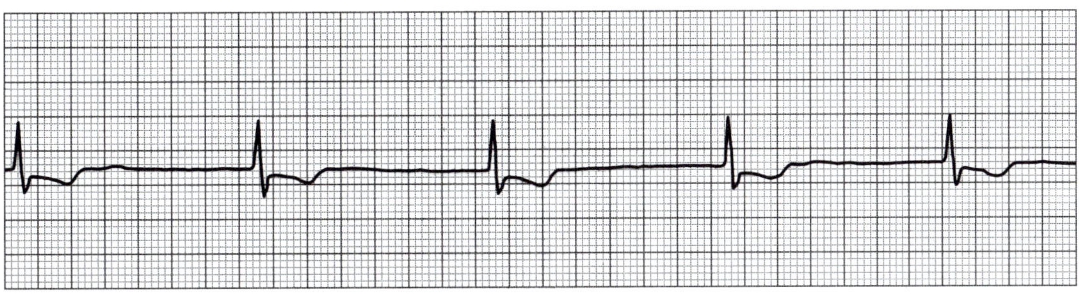

QRS duration ________________ QT ______________

Ventricular rate/rhythm ______________________

Atrial rate/rhythm __________________________

PR interval ________________________________

Identification ______________________________

Symptoms ________________________________

____

Treatment ________________________________

Figure 5-16

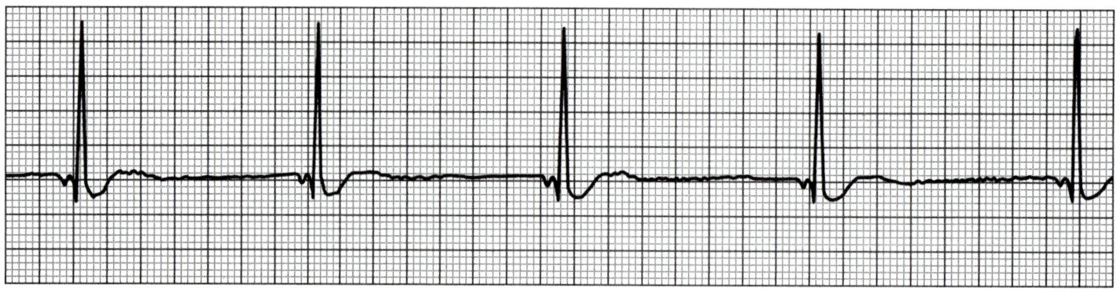

QRS duration ________________ QT ____________

Ventricular rate/rhythm ______________________

Atrial rate/rhythm __________________________

PR interval ________________________________

Identification ________________________________

Symptoms ___________________________________

____

Treatment ___________________________________

Figure 5-17

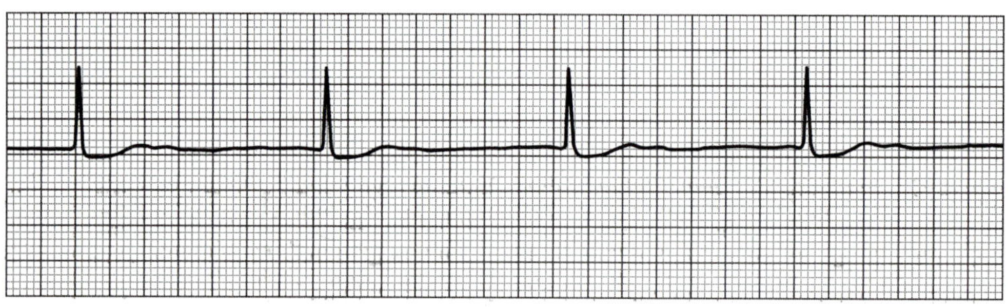

QRS duration ________________ QT ____________

Ventricular rate/rhythm ______________________

Atrial rate/rhythm __________________________

PR interval ________________________________

Identification ________________________________

Symptoms ___________________________________

____

Treatment ___________________________________

References

Conover, M. B. *Nurse's pocket guide to electrocardiography* (3rd ed.). St. Louis, MO: C. V. Mosby; 1994.

Conover, M. B. *Understanding electrocardiography: Arrhythmias and the 12-lead ECG* (7th ed.). St. Louis, MO: Mosby-Year Book; 1996.

Conover, M. B. & Wellens, H. J. *The ECG in emergency decision making*. Philadelphia: W. B. Saunders; 1993.

Goldberger, E. *Textbook of clinical cardiology*. St. Louis, MO: C. V. Mosby; 1982.

Mandel, W. J. (Ed). *Cardiac arrhythmias: Their mechanisms, diagnoses, and management* (2nd ed.). Philadelphia: Lippincott; 1987.

Marriott, H. J. *Practical electrocardiography* (8th ed.). Baltimore: Williams and Wilkins; 1988.

Marriott, H. J., & Conover, M. B. *Advanced concepts in arrhythmias* (2nd ed.). St. Louis, MO: C. V. Mosby; 1989.

CHAPTER 6

The Atrial Mechanisms

Premise The key to recognizing an atrial ectopic is to remember a few concepts:

1. the sinus cannot be premature
2. atrial ectopics are premature
3. sinus P waves plot through unless disturbed by atrial ectopics

Objectives

After reading the chapter and completing the Self-Assessment Exercises, the student should be able to

1. identify the ECG characteristics of the atrial mechanisms
2. differentiate atrial from junctional ectopics
3. identify and describe the mechanisms for atrial tachycardia, reentrant tachycardias, atrial flutter, and fibrillation
4. list the significant clinical findings in the unstable patient
5. identify and describe the mechanical, pharmacologic, and electrical interventions used in the atrial arrhythmias

Key Terms

bigeminy	paroxysmal
ectopic	reentry
fibrillation	stable
flutter	unstable

Introduction

The QRS complex provides information about the origin of the impulse responsible for the ventricular complex. The origin may be from a supraventricular source or from the ventricles. Analysis of the P wave and calculation of atrial rate and rhythm provide the information for the differential diagnosis of the supraventricular arrhythmias.

The atrial arrhythmias are manifestations of abnormal electrical activity in the atria. Atrial stretch, hypoxia, drugs, medications, and chemical imbalance are factors that contribute to enhanced or triggered automaticity, resulting in an atrial **ectopic**.

ectopic
Originating from a site other than the sinus node. Cells that compete with pacemaker cells.

A clinical concern is the grave potential for debilitating tachycardias and the formation of mural emboli.

PREMATURE ATRIAL COMPLEX (PAC)

A sinus-induced QRS presents with a single positive predictable P wave preceding each and every QRS with a consistent PR interval. A junction-induced QRS may present with either a single, negative predictable P wave preceding each QRS, or a single, negative predictable P wave following each and every QRS or no visible P wave at all.

In the case of atrial ectopy, a P′ will occur; however, the P′ will be positive. The intrinsic sinus rhythm will be disturbed, and sinus P waves will not plot through rhythmically, but the QRS complex is usually 0.10 or less, since the impulse will be conducted normally.

Premature atrial complexes (PACs) occur when an ectopic atrial pacemaker propagates an impulse before the next normal sinus beat. The ectopic atrial beat is usually easily identified. The morphology of the QRS complex will be narrow and relatively unchanged. The preceding P′:

- will be early or premature
- may vary in size and configuration from the sinus P waves

Finally, PACs disrupt the regularity and rhythm of the sinus rhythm. The sinus P waves will not plot through the premature event since the premature depolarization will affect sinus activity. When the sinus node regains control, the rhythm and regularity will be restored. The ECG characteristics of PACs are as follows:

1. P′ Wave: The configuration of the P wave of the PAC differs from that of the dominant rhythm. If the PAC is early, the P′ wave may be completely or partially hidden within the preceding T wave or greatly enhance the amplitude and distort the preceding T wave.
2. P′R Interval: The P′R interval may be normal or prolonged and often differs from the PR interval of the dominant rhythm. Repeated PACs may not have consistent P′R intervals as compared to each other.
3. QRS Complex: The QRS complex duration is 0.10 second or less, most of the time, if the resulting QRS changes configuration, is greater than 0.10, and reflects the degree of refractoriness of the conduction tissue.
4. QRS Rhythm: The regularity of the sinus rhythm is disturbed by the PAC. It may be quite irregular when there are many PACs. Most of the time, the observer can plot through the P waves and determine that sinus rhythm (regularity) is disturbed.
5. QRS Rate: The rate depends on the basic rhythm and the number of PACs.

Table 6-1 A grid for assessing the sources of a narrow QRS complex

1. Look to the left of the QRS	
2. Look at the P waves:	
It is *Sinus*	if there is 1 (+) P for each QRS
It is *Junctional*	if there is (–) P in front of or after each QRS or no P at all
It is *Atrial*	Tachy = very regular Flutter = flutter waves you can count Fib = junk—no identifiable Ps, QRS irregular

Table 6-1 describes a way of differentiating the supraventricular mechanisms.

Figure 6-1 is an ECG tracing illustrating a sinus rhythm with a premature atrial ectopic. To differentiate atrial from junctional ectopic, use the grid from Table 6-1. Use the grid to the left of the ECG, and, by process of elimination, identify the source of the ectopic.

An atrial ectopic may not successfully conduct into the ventricles. The ability to conduct is a matter of timing and opportunity. For instance, if the PAC finds the AV node or the bundle branches completely refractory, the impulse will not conduct into the ventricles. This is a *blocked* or *nonconducted* PAC.

The position of the atrial P′ may be hidden within the ST segment or T wave and usually can be recognized when there is an alteration of T wave morphology. For instance, when the amplitude of the T wave changes suddenly, or appears notched, the cause is a premature P′ superimposed on that T wave.

Figure 6-2 is an ECG tracing of a sinus rhythm with two nonconducted PACs. Note the increased amplitude of the T waves just prior to the pause in the rhythm. The P′ created an additive influence on that T wave. The P′ did not conduct into the ventricles; therefore, there was no QRS, and this absence of conduction created the pause seen in the tracing.

Figure 6-3 is an ECG tracing of a sinus rhythm with a nonconducted PAC, causing a sudden pause in the cadence of the sinus rhythm. The pause is followed by junctional escape beats. In this tracing, the P′ is visible in the ST segment. The

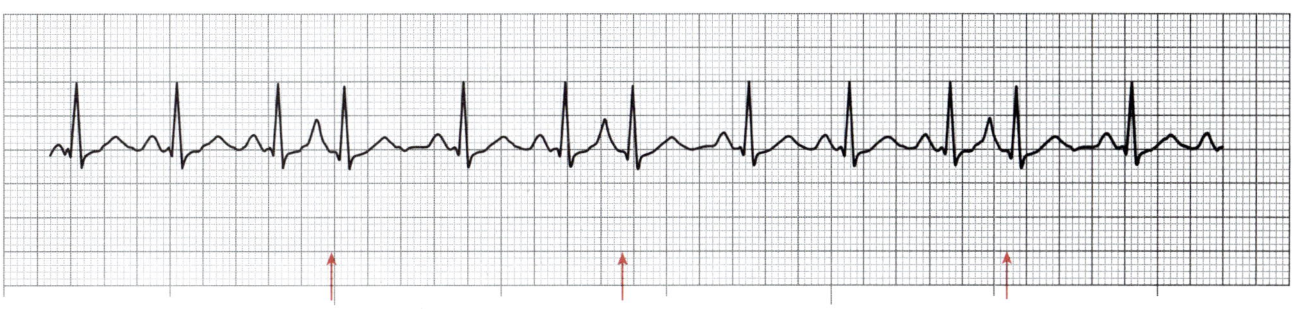

Figure 6-1 An ECG tracing showing one (+) P wave to the left of each of the first three sinus beats, a sinus rhythm at 96 per minute. The next QRS complex is similar to the sinus QRSs but is premature and has a (+) P′ superimposed on the previous T wave. The sinus P waves do not plot through the event. The PACs recur (arrow) each time, disturbing sinus rhythm. The ECG interpretation would be sinus rhythm at 96 per minute with frequent PACs.

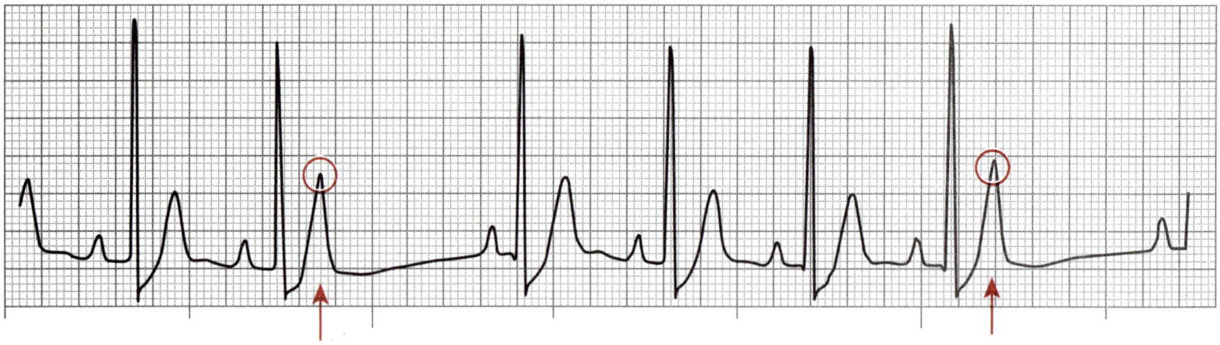

Figure 6-2 An ECG tracing showing one (+) P wave to the left of each of the first two sinus beats, a sinus rhythm. There is a sudden pause in the cadence of the sinus mechanism. Look back at the last T wave and note the increased amplitude. The height of the T wave is a combination of P- and T-wave amplitudes. The sinus P waves do not plot through the event, and the cadence of the sinus rhythm resumes at about 75 per minute. The ECG interpretation would be sinus rhythm at 75 per minute with frequent, nonconducted PACs.

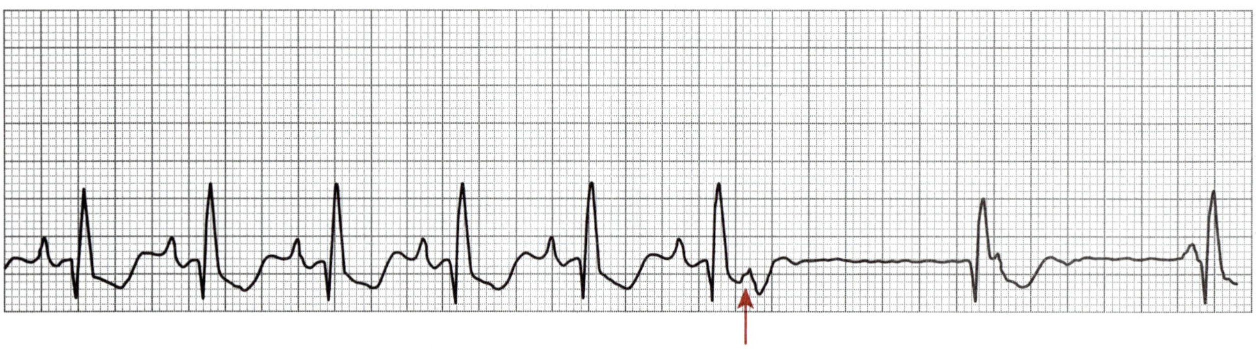

Figure 6-3 An ECG tracing showing one (+) P wave to the left of each of the first six sinus beats, a sinus rhythm. There is a sudden pause in the cadence of the sinus mechanism. Look back at the ST segment and note the appearance of the P′. The sinus P waves do not plot through the event. An escape junctional rhythm is the source of the last two QRSs. The ECG interpretation would be sinus rhythm at 86 per minute with a nonconducted PAC, followed by a junctional escape rhythm at 50 per minute.

PAC did not conduct into the ventricles, and this created the pause seen in the tracing. There is a junctional escape mechanism for two beats, which is not uncommon following atrial ectopics. Sinus P waves seem to be surfacing, and perhaps as the sinus accelerates, it will capture and conduct as it did earlier in the tracing.

Causes of PACs

PACs may be of no consequence or may result in the many variations of atrial arrhythmias. However, PACs often warn of impending heart failure. One must assess the patient circumstances, questioning medical history and medications taken by the patient that are prescribed or borrowed.

The most significant causes for PACs are atrial distention as with heart failure, ischemia resulting from proximal right coronary artery disease, digitalis excess, pericarditis, ingestion of stimulants, and caffeine and recreational drug use and drug abuse. Other causes of atrial stretch include conditions such as chronic lung disease, which results in increased pulmonary vascular resistance.

Atrial ectopy also can occur in the third trimester of pregnancy. At this time, the mother's blood volume has increased by 50 percent. In addition, the perfusion of the fetus and placenta results in increased peripheral vascular resistance. The increased workload can cause an increase in heart size, distention, and ventricular hypertrophy. It is not unusual then for the atria to stretch to accommodate the increased workload that has occurred over a rather short period of time. Atrial stretch promotes excitability and enhances automaticity.

Once the infant and placenta are delivered, accompanied by blood loss, there is a significant, sudden decrease in blood volume and peripheral resistance. The sudden diminished volume can leave behind a boggy atria, which gives rise to the atrial ectopic. Until the mother's heart size, blood volume, and peripheral resistance return to normal, the potential for atrial arrhythmias can continue.

Cause of the Nonconducted PAC

Whether or not a PAC conducts and results in a QRS is opportunistic. Remember, the process of depolarization reflects the flow of an electrical current to all the cells along the pathway of conduction. The cells then return to their original resting state by the process of repolarization. Ventricular repolarization is complete at the end of the T wave, permitting a new impulse to start the process again. A new impulse, occurring before the peak of the T wave, finds the ventricular conduction system unable to accept it since the impulse tries to conduct during the ventricular absolute refractory period. Although the downslope of the T wave is still within the refractory period, an impulse may be conducted under certain circumstances. This is the relative refractory period. If no conduction is possible, the PAC is blocked, that is, not conducted.

Whenever there is a sudden change in QRS rhythm, look to the preceding ST segment and T wave. If there is a change in morphology in the ST segment or the T wave *and* the sinus P waves do not plot through the event, a PAC occurred but was unable to conduct into the ventricles, thus no QRS complex.

If the premature atrial impulse finds one or more of the bundle branches or fascicles *partially* refractory, the impulse may be conducted with delay. The result is a wider QRS complex, conducted differently or *aberrantly* following the P′ wave (see Chapter 7).

1. The most common cause of the unexpected change in sinus rhythm is a PAC.
2. The most common cause of the unexpected pause in sinus rhythm is a nonconducted PAC.
3. The most common cause of sudden distortion of a T wave is the superimposed P′ of the PAC.

ATRIAL BIGEMINY

Bigeminy is when every other beat is an ectopic beat. When a PAC follows every sinus beat, that, is sinus, PAC, sinus, PAC, and so on, the result is *atrial bigeminy*, as noted in Figure 6-4.

bigeminy
An ECG rhythm where every other beat is an ectopic

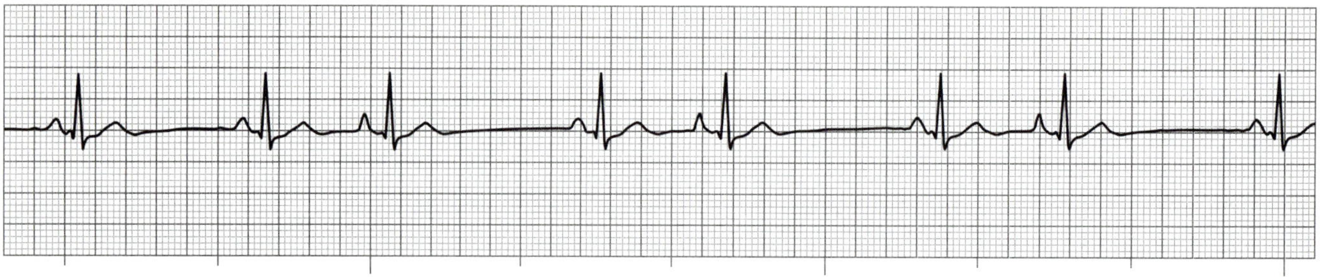

Figure 6-4 An ECG tracing showing a sinus mechanism with one (+) P for each QRS. However, not all the P waves are similar. In fact, there appear to be premature QRS complexes, each with a premature P′ waves creating a pattern; every other beat is an ectopic. When every other beat is an ectopic, this is *bigeminy*. In this case, the ectopic has its origin in the atria. Thus, the ECG interpretation would be sinus rhythm at 86 per minute with *atrial* bigeminy.

It is possible to have nonconducted atrial bigeminy and misdiagnose the rhythm as sinus bradycardia. When there is a sudden change to a bradycardia, take care to assess the T waves. There will be a distortion of the T waves just prior to the bradycardia, indicating the P′ occurring at the time.

Causes of Atrial Bigeminy

Atrial bigeminy is not common and may occur in patients as the first sign of congestive heart failure. Assess the patient for signs and symptoms of peripheral edema, sudden weight gain, adventitious lung sounds.

WANDERING ATRIAL PACEMAKER (WAP)

Wandering atrial pacemaker (WAP) is an old term referring to a change of the pacemaker from sinus to another supraventricular focus. It usually occurs as a result of slowing of sinus rate. When pacemaker dominance is shared by more than one pacemaker, P waves of varying configuration result. Thus, the title *wandering pacemaker*. Pacemaker dominance can be shared by the SA node, the AV junction, and/or an atrial focus identified by a variation in P wave polarity.

For example, following a sinus complex, there may be junctional complexes, atrial complexes, among sinus beats; the size and shape of the P or P′ waves and the respective P′R intervals will probably vary. There are no premature beats. The most common occurrence is when the sinus and junction share dominance at similar rates.

It is more accurate to read and report the ECG from left to right, identifying the source of the rhythm, that is, sinus @ (rate) → junctional @ (rate) → sinus. Provide clinical input assessing the patient, the overall rate, and perfusion.

The ECG characteristics of WAP include:

1. P Wave: The configuration of the P wave varies according to the pacemaker, and pacemaker dominance is shared by more than one pacemaker, that is sinus, atrial, and/or junctional.

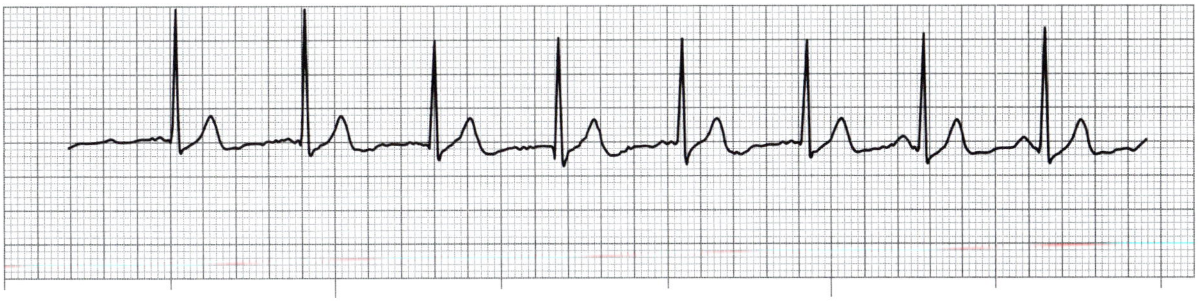

Figure 6-5 An ECG tracing showing a narrow QRS complex of similar configuration. In the beginning, there were no P waves preceding the QRSs. As the rhythm progresses, (+) P waves are seen in the last two complexes. The sinus rate is faster than the junction; therefore, the sinus takes control. The ECG interpretation would be accelerated junctional rhythm at 75 per minute progressing to sinus at 86 per minute. In some texts, this might be described as a "wandering atrial pacemaker." It is more correct to describe the rhythm variations. It is also important to question why the junction accelerates and why the sinus node defers and to take careful notes of the patient's medical and medication history.

2. PR Interval: The PR interval depends on the dominant pacemaker. The PR interval of the sinus beats is between 0.12 and 0.20 second, and the P′R interval of the junctional beats is 0.12 second or less and constant from beat to beat.
3. QRS Complex: The QRS complex duration is 0.10 second or less.
4. QRS Rate: The rate may vary with the shifting pacemaker sites.
5. QRS Rhythm: The rhythm will be slightly irregular with the shifting pacemaker sites.

Figure 6-5 is an example of a shift from junctional to sinus mechanisms. Note in the beginning of the tracing, the QRS complexes have no P waves preceding them. The last three QRS complexes each have (+) P waves preceding them.

The clinical significance of WAP occurs when the result is a bradycardia and the patient is hypotensive and hypoperfusing. The shift from sinus to junctional rhythm usually occurs when the sinus slows. With no impulse coming through the AV junction, the pacemaker there reaches potential and discharges an impulse. The significance to the practitioner is to determine why the sinus slowed down.

Occasionally, the AV junction will accelerate in competition with the sinus. Enhanced automaticity within junctional tissue may be due to digitalis.

ATRIAL TACHYCARDIA

In atrial tachycardia, an atrial ectopic discharges a stimulus at a rate of 130 to 250 beats per minute. Fortunately, the AV node therapeutically delays many of the impulses, and the resulting ventricular rate is usually reasonable. The ventricular rhythm can be regular or irregular. Figure 6-6 is an example of atrial tachycardia. Note the rate of the (+) P′ waves, so the atria are in tachycardia at 136 beats per minute. Clearly the ventricles are not responding for each P′ impulse. The difference in atrial and ventricular rates is due in part to the therapeutic delay within the AV node.

MULTIFOCAL ATRIAL TACHYCARDIA

There may be multiple different atrial foci that depolarize the atria at different and rapid rates. The difference is an arrhythmia characterized by atrial tachycardia, with

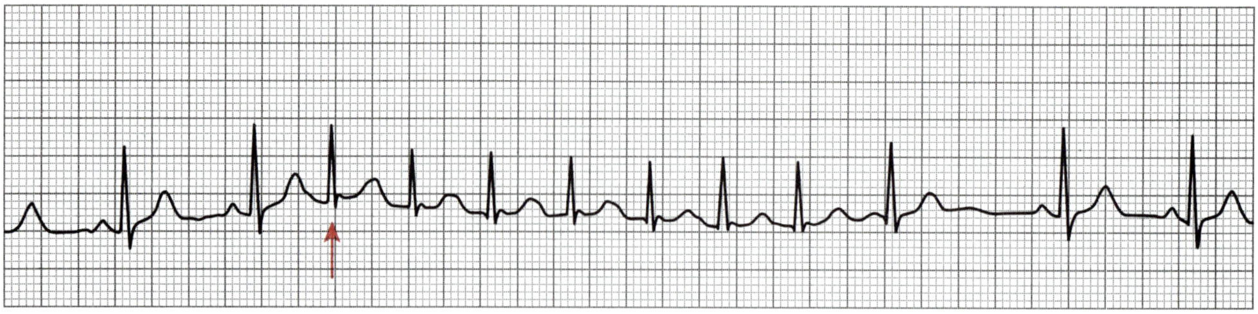

Figure 6-6 An ECG tracing showing a narrow QRS complex of similar configuration throughout. Plotting out the P waves, the atrial rate is 86 per minute for the first two complexes. The rate changes suddenly. Note the PAC (arrow) at the beginning of the tachycardia. The rate here is 136 per minute, and T waves are distorted and lumpy indicating the atrial ectopics. The rate changes again, beginning with a pause and reverting to a sinus rhythm. The visible sudden onset and end of the tachycardia is called *paroxysm.* The identification is sinus at 86 → atrial tachycardia (PAT) at 136 per minute → sinus at 86 per minute. The sinus P waves do not plot through this event.

a variation in both P′ contour and the rate of atrial depolarization, *multifocal atrial tachycardia* (MAT). The atria are discharging at very rapid rates, 150 to 250 beats per minute. The ventricular rate will be slower and irregular.

At first glance, it may be difficult to differentiate MAT from atrial **fibrillation**. In MAT, while morphology of the P′ waves changes, they recur in a pattern and are often negative/positive in configuration. Multifocal or chaotic atrial tachycardia is seen in patients with severe chronic obstructive pulmonary disease. Figure 6-7A and B are examples of multifocal atrial tachycardia.

fibrillation
Chaotic electrical cardiac activity that is unable to stimulate coordinated cardiac contractions. As a result, the pumping activity of the atria and/or ventricles is lost. The ECG inscribes an irregular and wavy baseline.

PAROXYSMAL ATRIAL TACHYCARDIA

An atrial ectopic focus may develop a rapid rate of depolarization, thus creating a tachycardia. When this arrhythmia is seen to appear and disappear suddenly, it is referred to as **paroxysmal** atrial tachycardia. If the AV node supports the rhythm, every atrial impulse will be conducted through to the ventricles.

paroxysmal
A tachycardia that results from an atrial ectopic. More correctly termed paroxysmal supraventricular tachycardia.

1. P′ Wave: Begins abruptly, at rates of 150 to 160; a visible P′ may be seen and differs in configuration from the sinus P wave. At more rapid rates, however, the P′ is hidden in the preceding T wave and may not be seen as a separate entity.

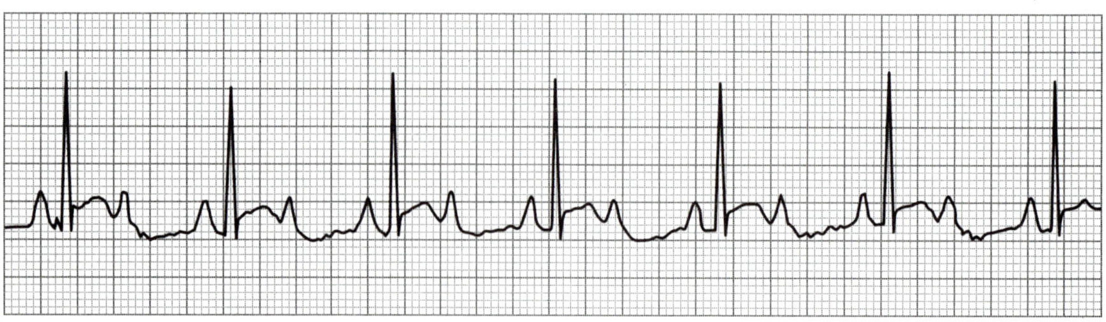

Figure 6-7A An ECG tracing showing a narrow QRS complex of similar configuration. The P waves plot through at a rate of 100 per minute. The ventricular response (QRS rate) is not as fast. The rhythm interpretation would be atrial tachycardia with a ventricular rate at 67 per minute, with 2–3 mm ST segment elevation.

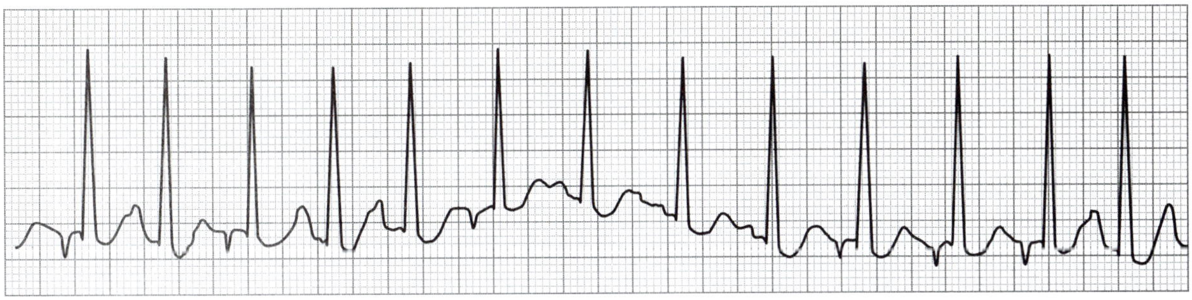

Figure 6-7B An ECG tracing of an example of MAT with P waves that are both (-) and (+), each with varying PR intervals. This is easily confused with atrial fibrillation.

2. P′R Interval: While the sinus PR interval is between 0.12 and 0.20 second and is constant from beat to beat, the P′R interval of the atrial tachycardia will be different than sinus but consistent. At rapid rates, the P′R interval is difficult to measure.
3. QRS Complex: The QRS complex duration is 0.10 second or less. Every sinus QRS complex is preceded by a P wave. The QRS of the atrial tach may be normally or abnormally conducted, depending on the degree of ventricular refractoriness.
4. QRS Rhythm: Atrial tachycardia starts suddenly and is very regular.
5. QRS Rate: The rate is very regular.

Figure 6-8 is an example of atrial tachycardia. The sudden change in the rhythm begins with the PAC. The tachycardia is regular.

Causes of Atrial Tachycardia

Atrial tachycardias may be idiopathic or can be precipitated by sympathetic stimulation, as in anxiety, ingestion of caffeine, smoking, or excessive alcohol intake. The patient "feels" the sudden start of an atrial tach, whereas the increase in heart rate in sinus tach often goes unnoticed.

Young adults sometimes have attacks of atrial tachycardia that break spontaneously. The tachycardiac also can occur, with adults in early stages of menopause or climacteric.

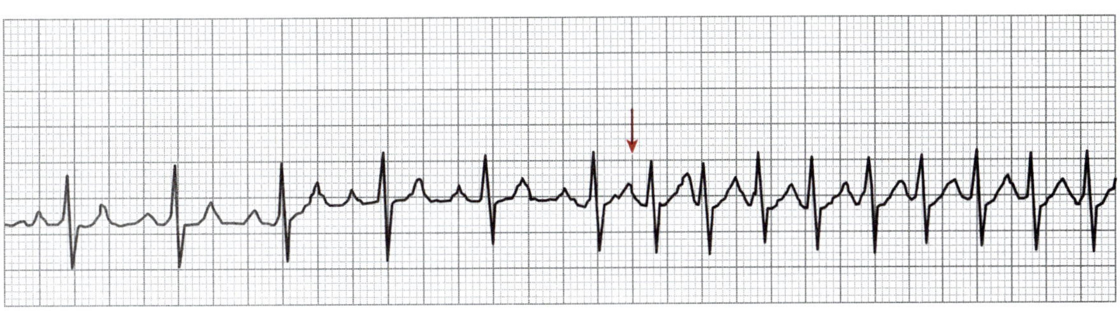

Figure 6-8 An example of the onset of atrial tachycardia. In the beginning, the tracing shows a sinus rhythm at 100 per minute. A PAC (arrow) begins the sudden change in rate at 188 per minute.

SUPRAVENTRICULAR TACHYCARDIA

The term *supraventricular* has several connotations. First is the category of rhythm—that is, the origin is above (supra) the ventricles (ventricular). Hence, the term. Supraventricular (SVT) also denotes the condition where an atrial ectopic has taken control over the atria, and the AV node unwittingly supports the tachycardia.

The three (3) most common mechanisms are

- AV nodal reentry: A retrograde P wave coincidental with abnormal, narrow QRS (most common)
- Concealed bypass tract: No evidence of heart disease, a younger, healthy patient, but QRSs are wide—no clinical evidence of preexistent BBB.
- SA nodal/atrial reentry: Presence of P′ waves before the narrow QRS—and in the presence of organic disease.

reentry
The ability of an impulse to reexcite the same region through which it has previously passed

Reentry is defined as the ability of an impulse to reexcite some region of the atria through which it has already passed. Reentry usually occurs when an impulse deviates into a circular conduction pathway, forming a loop.

There are dual pathways in the AV node of differing conduction rates and refractory levels, which when activated separately support a reentrant tachycardia. These independent AV pathways are parallel and are capable of bidirectional conduction. The beta pathway is characterized by faster conduction but a longer period of refractoriness. The alpha pathway is characterized by slower conduction but a faster period of refractoriness, as shown in Figure 6-9. The PAC enters the AV node and is blocked in the fast (beta) pathway but passes antegradely down the slow pathway into the ventricles and in a retrograde fashion back up into the atria using the rapid pathway. The return of the current to the atria produces an atrial echo beat, and if this circuit is sustained, the ventricles will respond in a reciprocal fashion.

Like atrial tachycardia, SVT with AVN reentry begins abruptly. At the onset, the tachycardia is preceded by a prolonged P′R interval. This mechanism establishes the reentry circuit. The P′ waves may distort the QRS. However, there should be no alteration of the QRS amplitude (QRS alternans).

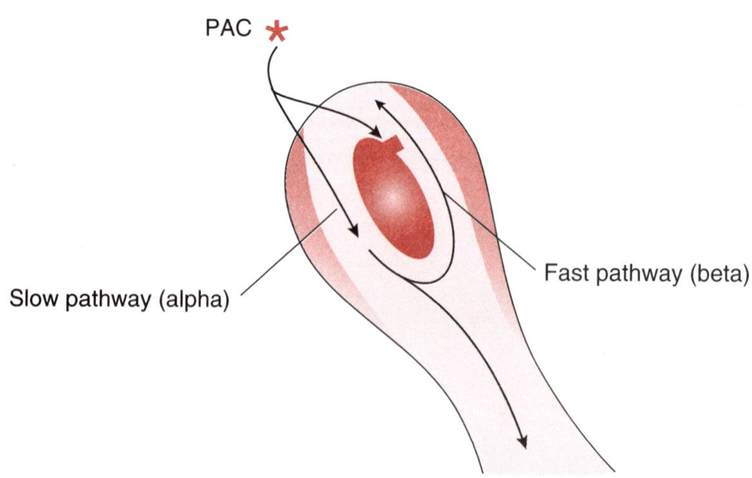

Figure 6-9 The AV node and the dual pathways, alpha and beta. A PAC enters the AV node, proceeding down the alpha pathway to the ventricles. During this time, the impulse crosses over, activates, and conducts back up into the atria.

Two AV nodal reentrant tachycardias can result: one accessing the fast path downward and the slow path in a retrograde fashion (fast-slow) often seen in children; and the other accessing the slow path downward and the rapid path in a retrograde fashion (slow-fast). Since it uses the slow pathway for return to the atria, the RP′ is longer than the P′R interval. The slow-fast is almost always triggered by a PAC associated with a prolonged P′R interval preceding it. Sometimes the P′ is often lost or blended into the narrow QRS and impossible to see.

Many small potential circuits (microcircuits) normally exist within a conduction system, such as the AV node, atrial and ventricular tissue where the terminal Purkinje fibers attach to cardiac muscle.

Macrocircuits or larger circular pathways also may form. These circuits are at least partially composed of cardiac conduction tissue. An example of this phenomenon would be a circuit formed by a congenital accessory pathway or by AV node microcircuits, which are functionally grouped together into two major pathways. Figure 6-10 is composed of three sketches. The first is the AV node showing normal conduction. The second shows an atrial ectopic with AV nodal reentry. The third shows the Kent bundle as a potential pathway for conduction.

Normally, the impulse travels through the conduction fibers in an *even* and *synchronous* manner and collides with itself in the potential circuits. However, conditions of ischemia can affect selected portions of these conduction fibers, altering their speed of conduction. These cells recover slowly from previous impulses and may not conduct new approaching impulses. When the block occurs, there is an abrupt stop to the tachycardia.

An altered circuit may be partially or totally refractory. If the circuit is partially refractory in only one direction, the impulse will be blocked from transmitting in that direction.

When the impulse is blocked in one direction through a pathway, it is a *unidirectional* block. When an impulse encounters refractory tissue, the impulse detours away from the blocked area, deviating around the conduction pathway, forming a loop. Impulse transmission then becomes asynchronous.

The impulse enters the ischemic area in a *retrograde* direction and is conducted through ischemic tissue slowly. Remember that ischemic cells are slow cells and

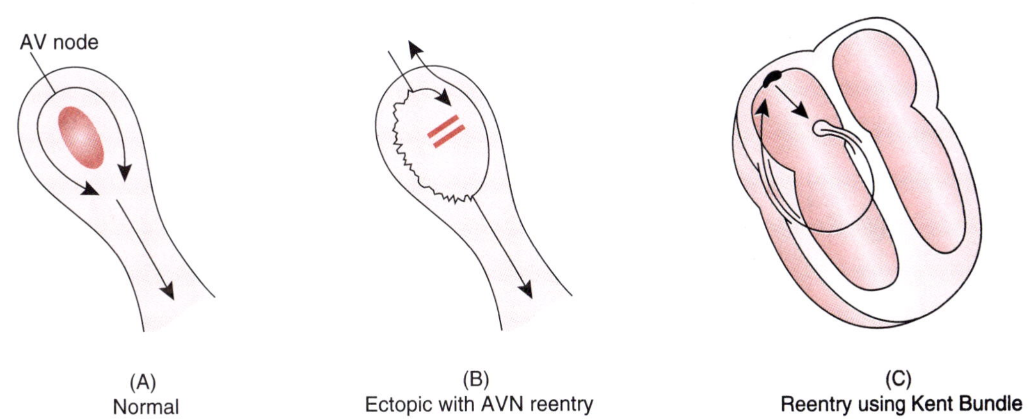

Figure 6-10 Three examples of AV conduction: (A) normal AV conduction, (B) a PAC and AV nodal reentry, and (C) a reentry circuit using the accessory Kent bundle

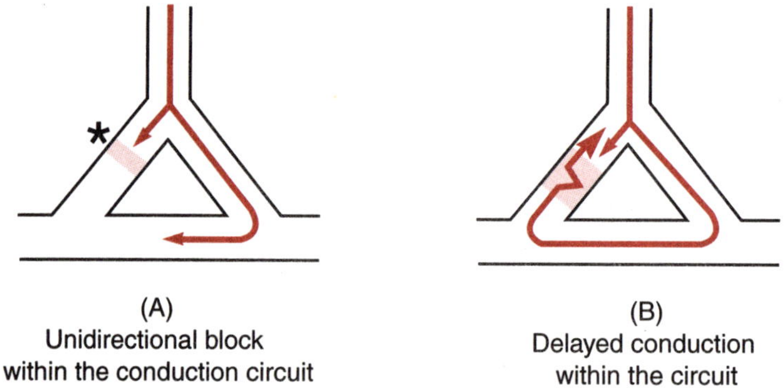

Figure 6-11 (A) Reentry with unidirectional block, and (B) delayed conduction of the reentry circuit.

have prolonged refractory periods. If tissue surrounding the previously blocked area has recovered sufficiently to be excitable, the emerging impulse will reenter the adjacent tissue. As a result, an original impulse will now reexcite or depolarize the area through which it has just passed. Figure 6-11A and B illustrate the concept of unidirectional block and subsequent reentry.

If the reentrant impulse exits early in repolarization, when the disparity in recovery is still pronounced, the impulse may recycle within the circuit, producing a *chain-reaction response.* The response often disintegrates into chaotic activity.

The ECG characteristics of SVT with AV nodal reentry are as follows:

1. P Wave: P waves, because of the overall rate, cannot be clearly delineated to establish the diagnosis as sinus, atrial, or junctional.
2. P′R Interval: P waves are not easily seen; therefore, there is no measurable P′R interval.
3. QRS Complex: The QRS complex duration is 0.10 second or less.
4. QRS Rate: The rate is greater than 150 per minute.
5. QRS Rhythm: The rhythm is very regular.

Figure 6-12 is an example of SVT with AV nodal reentry. Note the sudden onset, the narrow QRS, and the rapid rate.

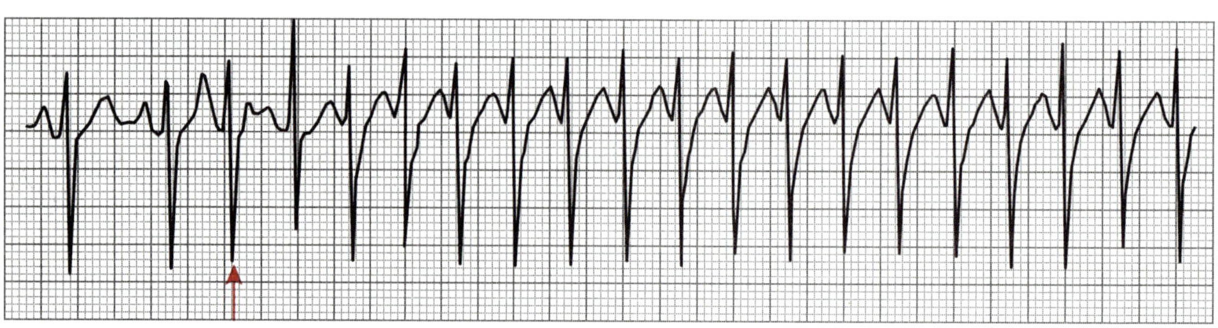

Figure 6-12 An ECG tracing showing a sinus tachycardia, a PAC progressing to a narrow-complex tachycardia at 214 per minute.

Causes and Consequences of the SVTs

SVTs can be seen in patients with organic heart disease of any type, and chronic lung and liver diseases. "Drug abuse" as described in sinus tachycardia can precipitate the tachycardias. SVT and PAT in patients with limited cardiac reserve may precipitate angina pectoris or congestive heart failure. SVT and PAT may also occur in the presence of little or no structural heart disease.

Patient history and chief complaints include sudden onset, feelings of breathlessness, a full feeling in the neck and ringing in the ears, palpitations, dizziness, and hypotension. The observer should expect a change in vital signs. A sudden increase in pulse rate sometimes to 188 or more beats per minute can understandably cause a decrease in cardiac output. The degree of drop will vary between patients. The patient's tolerance to the arrhythmia and drop in blood pressure will provide a sense of urgency in choosing an intervention.

The patient's level of consciousness is an excellent indicator of the patient's ability to tolerate the arrhythmia. While the sudden onset causes anxiety and apprehension, the patient is usually responsive and alert. Any deviation where the patient is slow to respond or has any altered level of consciousness (LOC) is **unstable** and is cause for immediate intervention.

unstable

Signs of cardiopulmonary dysfunction that may jeopardize life

Intervention in Supraventricular Tachycardias

Ectopic impulses generated as a result of reentry are usually precipitated by fast rates, and recovery time is limited. Many times, the tachycardia will resolve spontaneously or after sedation. When it does not, increasing vagal tone will exert a braking effect on the conduction velocity through the AV junction. Recall that the vagus is part of the parasympathetic nervous system, and the mediator is acetylcholine. The AV node is richly supplied with autonomic nerves and is especially sensitive to acetylcholine. Stimulating the vagus causes acetylcholine release, which delays conduction and increases refractoriness in the AV node.

There are several ways of increasing vagal tone. For example, the patient can be encouraged to try *Valsalva's maneuver,* which is straining or bearing down as long as possible as if having a bowel movement; or direct the patient to place a hand against the mouth and blow down as hard as possible for as long as possible. Figure 6-13 is an ECG from a patient responding to vagal maneuver. Note the sudden change in ventricular response.

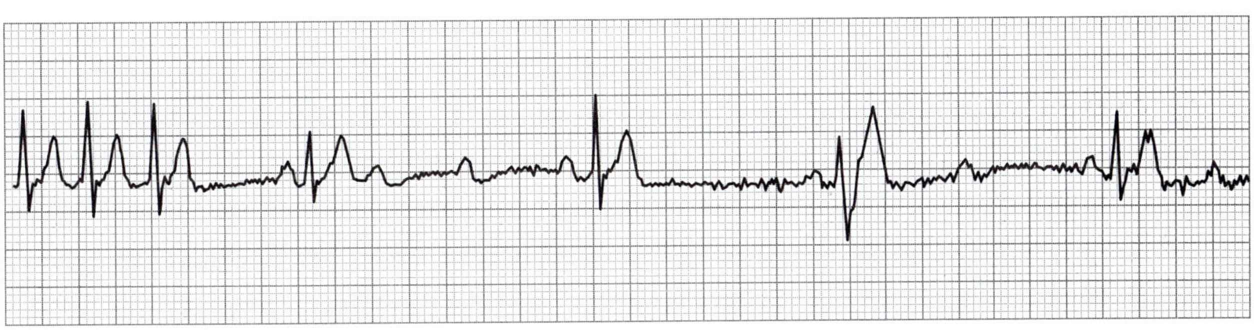

Figure 6-13 An ECG tracing showing atrial tachycardia and the sudden slowing of atrial and ventricular rates during a documented vagal maneuver.

In noncompromised patients, provoking gagging by placing a finger or catheter down the throat increases vagal tone. However, emesis may result and compromise the airway. Similarly, caution should be used when simulating a dive reflex. This can be done by placing a cold, wet towel over the center portion of the face. This maneuver also increases vagal tone.

Deep, profound coughing is another maneuver, but it must be very deep and hard. Pressure on the eyeball is not an acceptable maneuver. It is rarely effective, and may cause retinal detachment. If it did work, it was probably because the patient gasped in fear of enucleation.

Carotid sinus massage (CSM) may be employed by the physician as a method of terminating the arrhythmia. Prior to this maneuver, the physician should assess for carotid bruit. Absence of bruit is not a foolproof method for ruling out plaque formation or stenosis. Any history of dizziness or transient ischemic attacks (TIAs) and presence of carotid bruit on either side are contraindications for CSM.

Carotid sinus massage should never be applied for longer than five seconds and used with great care in patients over 65 years. CSM can provoke SA arrest. CSM may result in either an abrupt temporary slowing (not gradual as with sinus tachycardia) or no effect at all.

Several medications can be used to treat atrial tachycardias. If an offending drug is the cause, using the appropriate antidote while efficiently managing the airway is the treatment of choice.

If the diagnosis is a reentrant tachycardia, use of drugs that decrease conduction velocity and increase refractoriness of AV node is in order. These may include adenosine and verapamil.

Figure 6-14 is a continuous ECG tracing from a 20-year-old male with SVT in whom adenosine was used. Note the sudden change in rhythm. The patient experienced a sudden, "overwhelming rush of relief" with the change in rhythm.

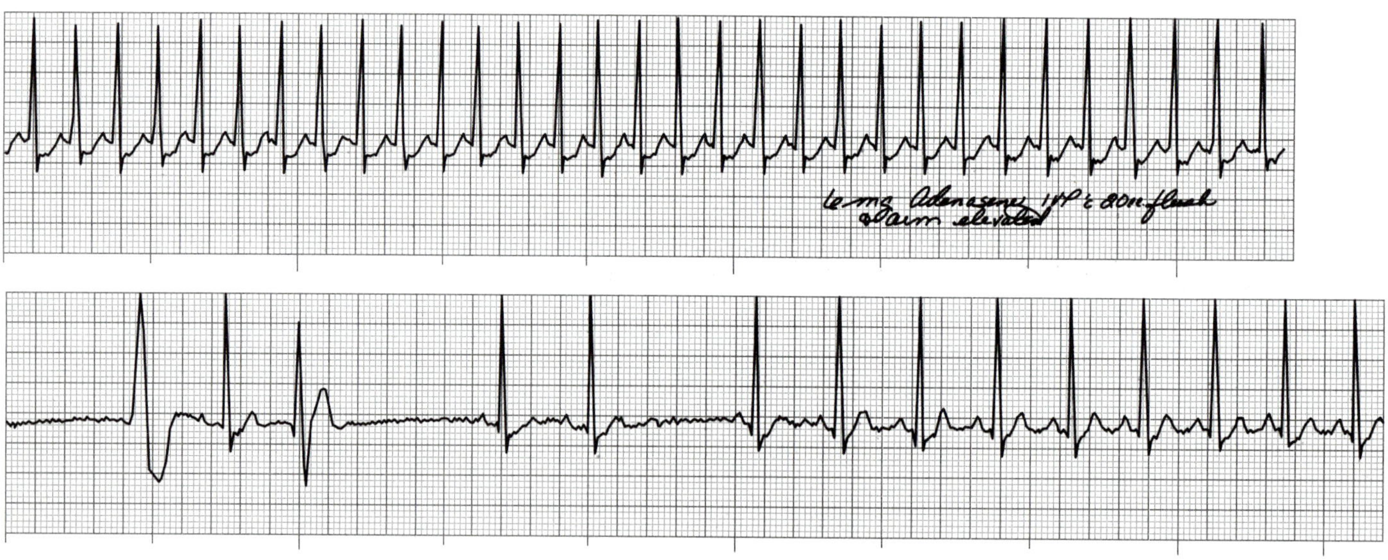

Figure 6-14 Continuous ECG tracing from a 20-year-old male who complained of increased heart rate for four hours while playing softball. He presented in the Emergency Department with chest pain and diaphoresis. The patient stated that this happens frequently, but he usually corrects the situation by holding his breath. Adenosine 6 mg was administered. This is an example of the variations of rhythms that occur after adenosine. The changes—which range from brief periods of asystole, apparent AV conduction delay, and ventricular ectopy—were transient.

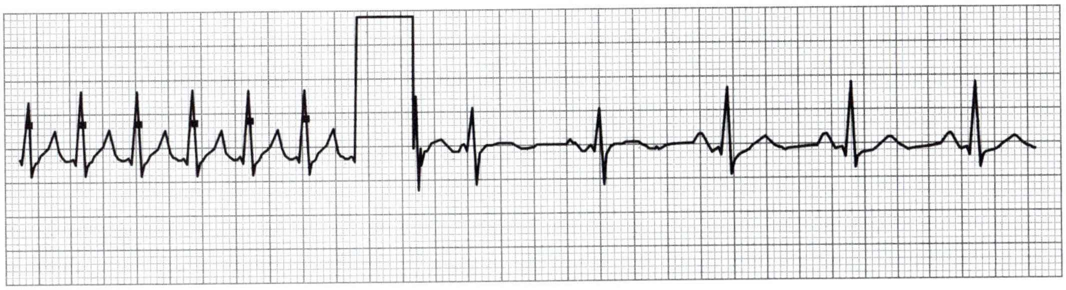

Figure 6-15 An ECG tracing showing SVT converted with synchronized cardioversion. Note the marks indicating synchrony on each of the QRS complexes. There is a 2 mV deflection indicating the delivery of electrical current. Note that the initial deflection coincides with the expected QRS complex.

Emergency cardioversion is employed to depolarize the atria and return the patient to a more organized rhythm. Synchronized cardioversion is the delivery of electrical current simultaneously with the QRS complex to avoid delivering a depolarizing current to the ventricles during the vulnerable period when the heart is susceptible to fibrillation. The peak of the vulnerable period, the time when it is most susceptible, is 0.20 to 0.30 seconds to the left of the peak of the T wave. The initial energy setting is usually 50 to 100 Joules. The patient should be sedated whenever possible. Figure 6-15 is an ECG tracing showing the conversion from SVT to sinus using synchronized cardioversion.

ATRIAL FLUTTER

One consequence of PACs is the occurrence of atrial **flutter**. A common mechanism is a reentry circuit within the right atrium. Atrial depolarization will be seen as sharp, positive deflections at a rate of 200 to 300 per minute. The atrial P′ waves are referred to as *flutter* or *ff* waves. In atrial flutter, the rapid atrial rate may take on a sawtooth appearance (Figure 6-16), but this is not critical to the definition. The ventricular rate and rhythm are a direct reflection on the AV node's ability to slow down the impulses coming to it. Remember that the physiological function of the AV node is to therapeutically delay conduction and protect ventricular response.

flutter
Ectopic electrical activity that stimulates a cardiac chamber in a rapid, yet organized fashion

When atrial flutter is new to the patient, it often presents with a ventricular rate of about 150 per minute. In other words, every other atrial impulse is conducted through to the ventricles. The arrhythmia is often termed *atrial flutter with two-to-one conduction*. The atrial flutter waves will plot through regularly.

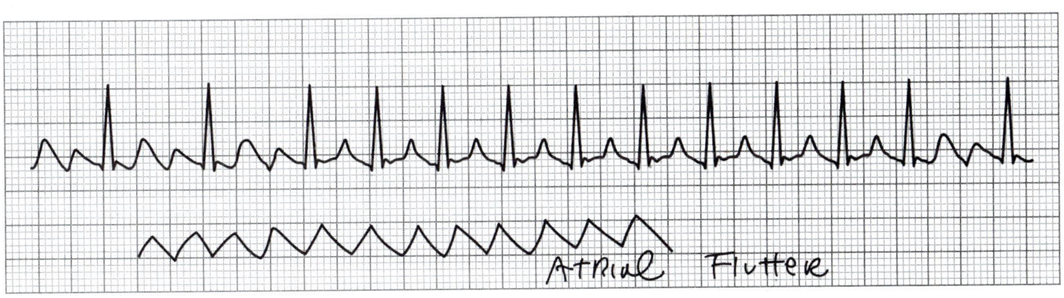

Figure 6-16 An ECG tracing showing a narrow QRS-complex tachycardia with varying ventricular rate. Note the *flutter* waves as they can be plotted out across the tracing. The flutter waves cause occasional distortions in the QRS complex.

Atrial flutter with 2:1 block can be misdiagnosed as sinus tachycardia. However, in sinus tach, the P and T waves are usually distinctly different from each other and do not plot through regularly. In other words, Ps plot with Ps, and Ts plot with Ts, but the T-P-T is not rhythmic and regular. Also, looking at the negative deflections, one can plot out the flutter waves more easily.

Another clue to differentiate sinus tachycardia at 150 beats per minute from atrial flutter with 2:1 AV block is finding the P′ midway between the QRS complexes. One should suspect there are additional Ps within the QRS complex and in fact be able to detect the P Primes (P′). The alteration in morphology of the QRS by P′ is *Ta* distortion.

Finally, the patient complains of a sudden onset of the rapid rate and feelings of weakness and dread, which do not occur with sinus tachycardia. The ECG characteristics of atrial flutter are as follows:

1. ff Waves: Atrial depolarization is regular.
2. P′R Interval: The P′R interval of the ff waves is usually 0.24 to 0.40 second and constant with the QRS.
3. QRS Complex: The QRS complex duration is 0.10 second or less, most of time. If the resulting QRS changes configuration and is greater than 0.10, which reflects the degree of refractoriness of the conduction tissue, the ff waves will distort the QRS and T waves.
4. QRS Rate: Ventricular rate depends on AV conduction velocity.
5. QRS Rhythm: The ventricular response may be regular or irregular depending on AV conduction.

Figure 6-17A and B are examples of atrial flutter from patients with various forms of therapy.

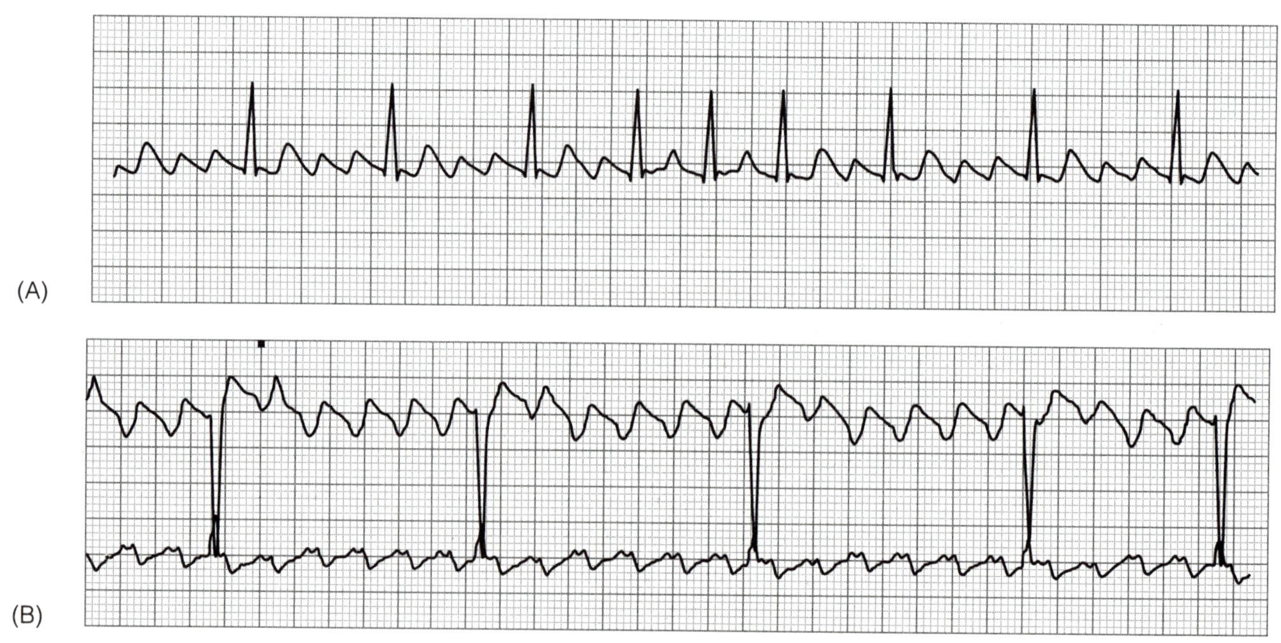

Figure 6-17 (A) ECG showing new-onset atrial flutter in a patient, and (B) a continuous ECG tracing from a patient with recurrent atrial flutter. The patient was taking lanoxin 0.25 mg daily, for 37 days.

Causes and Consequences of Atrial Flutter

Atrial flutter is never considered a normal variant. Patients must be assessed to determine the etiology. Atrial flutter is common in adults over 40 years of age with chronic heart disease, chronic hypertension, and myocardial ischemia. Atrial flutter is also seen in patients with valvular heart disease, acute myocardial infarction, hypoxia, quinidine excess, and pulmonary embolus, and in patients with chronic pulmonary and hepatic diseases.

AV conduction delay results in a reasonable ventricular rate in most instances. If not, and the patient is compromised, mechanical, pharmacologic, or electrical interventions may be employed. Beware of atrial flutter with a slow, regular rhythm less than 60 per minute—consider there is AV block, and the junction has taken over as the pacemaker to the ventricles. In this dysrhythmia, the flutter-QRS interval will vary.

Intervention in Atrial Flutter

Treating patients with atrial flutter depends on their clinical condition. In some patients, the atrial flutter will convert spontaneously once the offending condition is under control. In others, administration of high-flow oxygen may be sufficient to cause the rhythm to revert back to sinus. Others may require medications and even cardioversion.

Digitalis has two effects on atrial flutter. First, it slows conduction in the AV node, thereby slowing the ventricular response. Digitalis also tends to increase the rate of atrial depolarization, which may cause the atrial flutter to convert to sinus rhythm or even atrial fibrillation.

ATRIAL FIBRILLATION

Another consequence of PACs is the occurrence of atrial fibrillation, a chaotic and erratic depolarization state within the atria. In contrast to atrial flutter, atrial fibrillation is one of the most commonly seen arrhythmias. The rate of atrial depolarization cannot be measured, as it often exceeds 300 to 600 per minute and the results in a chaotic baseline. The atrial P′ waves are referred to as *fib* or *ff* waves. Atrial kick is lost as the atria are quivering, and there is no organized atrial contraction.

The irregular fibrillatory waves are usually easy to recognize and sometimes referred to as *coarse* atrial fibrillation (Figure 6-18A). In other cases, the fibrillation is of such low amplitude that it is referred to as *fine* atrial fibrillation (Figure 6-18B).

Assessment of the tracings to determine the arrhythmia will help the practitioner with the identification. For example, in Figure 6-18A and B, the QRS complexes are narrow, indicating a supraventricular origin. However, there are no identifiable P waves with consistent PR intervals, so the rhythm is not sinus in origin.

Next, the QRS rhythm in both examples is irregular, so it cannot be identified as junctional in origin. The only other option for the origin of narrow QRS is atrial. There are no *flutter* waves, so, by process of elimination, the rhythms are both atrial fibrillation. The ventricular rate range should be reported to provide an indication of the therapeutic blocking ability of the AV node.

The *coarse* or *fine* appearance of the fibrillatory waves has no clinical relevance.

In atrial fibrillation, the AV node is bombarded by hundreds of atrial ectopics, at varying rates and amplitudes. The AV node therapeutically and randomly con-

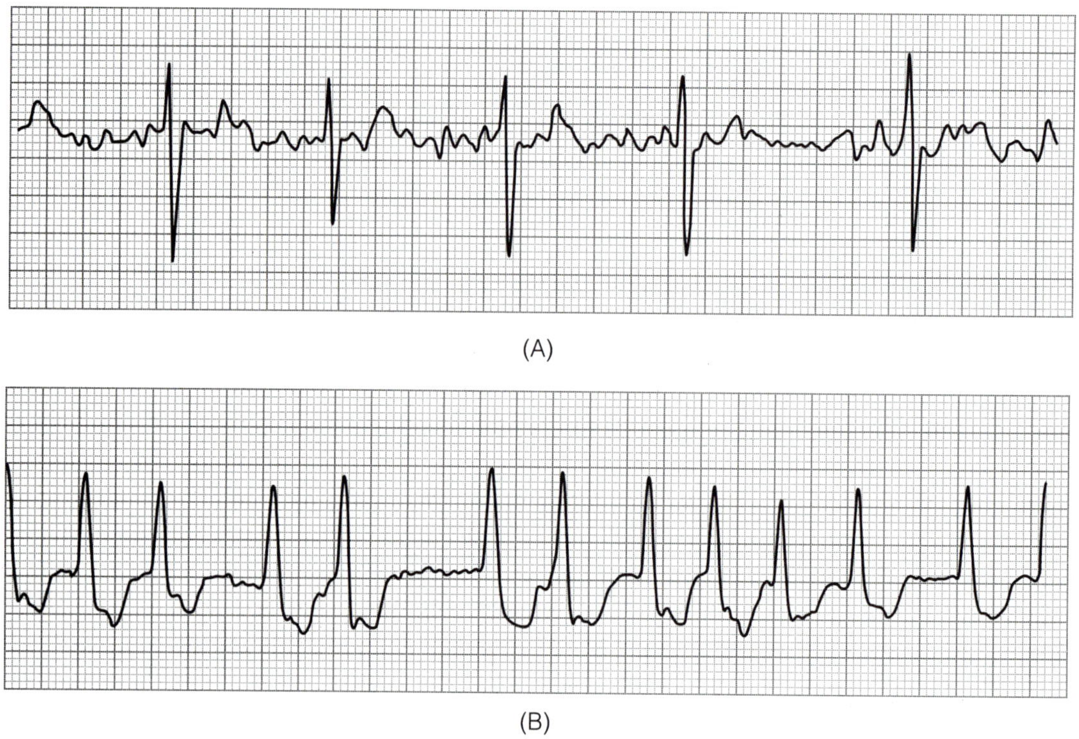

Figure 6-18 (A) ECG tracing showing narrow QRS complex with an irregular rhythm. The chaotic pattern between the QRS complexes is the atrial fibrillation. This *coarse* pattern is easily seen. (B) ECG tracing from a patient with narrow QRS complex with an irregular rhythm. Similar to (A), there are no identifiable P waves nor a consistent PR interval. The baseline between QRS complexes is finely distorted. This is *fine* atrial fibrillation. There is 5 to 6 mm ST segment depression.

ducts impulses at a varying rate of speed, so the ventricular response is irregular. When atrial fibrillation is new to the patient, the atrial rates are immeasurable, and the ventricular rhythm is irregular and very rapid. A rapid ventricular rate may compromise the patient. It is important to note the ventricular rate, as well as the patient's medication and medical history, when reporting this arrhythmia. The ECG characteristics of atrial fibrillation are as follows:

1. ff Waves: Atrial depolarization is erratic and irregular.
2. PR Interval: There is no PR interval.
3. QRS Complex: The QRS complex duration is 0.10 second or less most of the time, if the resulting QRS changes configuration and is greater than 0.10 and reflects the degree of refractoriness of the conduction tissue. The atrial fib waves will often distort the QRS and T waves.
4. QRS Rate: The rate depends on AV conduction time. Calculate and report the ventricular rate range.
5. QRS Rhythm: The ventricular response is irregular. If the QRS rhythm is regular, there is AV block, and the source of the QRS is usually junctional in origin. This irregularity frequently occurs with digitalis toxicity.

Causes and Consequences of Atrial Fibrillation

Atrial fibrillation rarely occurs in healthy subjects. It should never be considered a normal variant. Patients must be assessed to determine the cause. Atrial fibrillation occurs with ischemic heart disease, hypertensive heart disease, chronic pulmonary and valvular diseases, and congestive heart failure. Patients with coronary artery disease may develop paroxysmal atrial fibrillation in the course of acute myocardial infarction. However, atrial fibrillation may develop as a consequence of atrial dilatation (stretch) secondary to chronic congestive heart failure as well as the diseases mentioned.

For example, patients with hypertensive heart disease typically develop left ventricular and left atrial enlargement due to years of sustained high blood pressure. Patients with thyrotoxicosis may develop atrial fibrillation with very rapid ventricular rates. Atrial fibrillation can occur with cardiac inflammatory diseases and pulmonary embolism.

In some patients, atrial fibrillation occurs paroxysmally, and as such lasts for only minutes, hours, or days. In other cases, the atrial fibrillation may persist for months and years. Paroxysmal atrial fibrillation is occasionally precipitated by emotional stress, excessive alcohol consumption, or excessive straining with vomiting.

Beware of atrial fibrillation with very slow ventricular rates (Figure 6-19). If atrial fibrillation presents with a slow, regular rhythm less than 70 per minute—consider there is AV block. The atria and ventricles are in dissociation, meaning atrial and ventricular function is separate and independent. In this example, the junction has taken over as the pacemaker to the ventricles.

There are many significant consequences to atrial fibrillation. These include the predictable loss of atrial "kick," diminished cardiac output, and coronary perfusion. This is complicated by rapid ventricular rates. The faster the ventricular rate, the more cardiac output will be decreased. A significant drop in cardiac output can cause congestive heart failure, hypotension, and even cardiogenic shock and myocardial ischemia and infarction.

Chronic atrial fibrillation, even when *controlled*, meaning a reasonable ventricular rate, can result in a significant complication, the creation of a mural thrombus. The thrombi are formed by platelet aggregation in the fibrillating atria, as well as with any underlying inflammation that may exist. A mural thrombus can break off and embolize at any time, especially when the rhythm is converted to normal sinus rhythm.

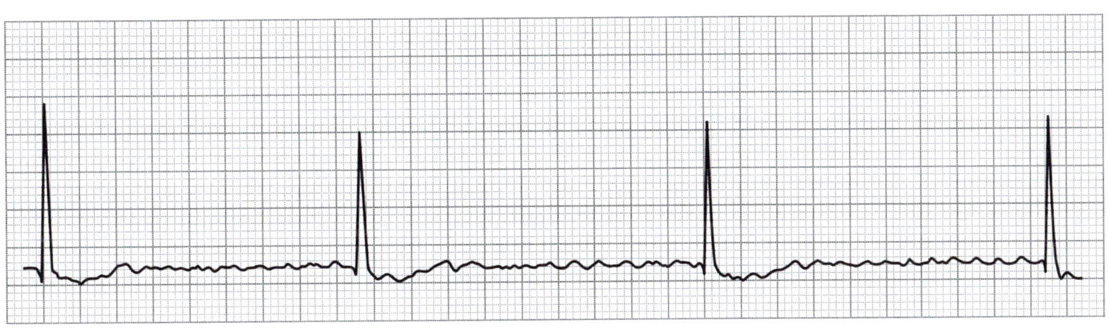

Figure 6-19 An ECG tracing from a patient in atrial fibrillation with an escape junctional rhythm. Note the regularity of the narrow QRS complex. The ECG identification would be atrial fibrillation with an escape junctional rhythm at 36 per minute.

This sudden conversion to normal atrial contraction may cause the dislodgement of all or part of the thrombus, leading to pulmonary embolus, peripheral embolus, and stroke. For this reason, some patients with atrial fibrillation are on anticoagulants, or at least aspirin, to prevent platelet aggregation.

Interventions in Atrial Fibrillation

Atrial fibrillation with rapid ventricular rate requires intervention. The pharmacologic interventions with atrial fibrillation are similar to those discussed in atrial flutter, and the mainstay for treating the patient is digitalis.

Accurate medical history, including medication history, is critical. Patients on digitalis need to be assessed to determine if indeed the digitalis has caused the symptoms and debilitation.

Treatment with medications generally takes hours or days. Some patients may never convert back to sinus rhythm. If the cause of the atrial fibrillation is the result of chronic disease, the huge, dilated atria may have become incapable of normal depolarization.

With the relatively new onset of atrial fibrillation with cardiac compromise, and where ventricular rate is rapid and irregular, electrical conversion may be the treatment of choice.

Summary

Arrhythmias that are supraventricular in origin come from above the ventricles but probably occur because of atrial ectopics. Differentiation among the various sources of supraventricular tachycardia is based largely on rate and how it starts off. Table 6-2 provides a simple tool for differentiation of the source of the narrow QRS arrhythmia by assessing the P waves.

Atrial arrhythmias are clinically significant because they often result in a rapid ventricular response which will increase oxygen consumption, compromise cardiac output, and thus decrease coronary blood flow. Atrial contribution to cardiac output is lost, and most atrial arrhythmias indicate underlying problems such as congestive heart failure, hypoxemia, hypoxia, drug toxicity, stress, or sinus node dysfunction.

With the refinement of physiologic testing, there are more and more explanations, each with its specific terminology. The basic clinical implications are the same: when the ventricular rate is too fast to maintain effective perfusion, the patient is unstable and must be treated immediately.

Table 6-2 Differentiation of the source of the narrow QRS by assessing P waves

Look at the P waves:	
Sinus:	1(+) P for each QRS
Junctional:	(–) P′ in front or behind each QRS or no P at all
Atrial:	a different (+) P′ in front of the QRS

Table 6-3 ECG characteristics of the various atrial mechanisms.

	PAC	Flutter	Fibrillation	Tachycardia	SVT with AVN Reentry	SVT with Aberrancy
P waves	(+)/QRS (+)no/QRS	usually sawtooth >250/min	unable to identify	sometimes 1:1 with the QRS; sometimes independent RP>PR rate <250	within the QRS; distorts the QRS at its beginning or at its end	(+) with a PAC at the beginning of the tach
PR interval	different					0.12–0.20 second
QRS duration	≤ 0.10	≤ 0.10	≤ 0.10	≤ 0.10	≤ 0.10	confused with a PVC >0.10
Ventricular rate/minute		60-100 usually	60-100 when controlled with medication	>100	>150/minute often >180/minute	>100/min
Ventricular rhythm		regular or irregular	irregular Beware if regular or slow	regular starts suddenly	regular	regular except for the event
Rx	question cause Caffeine, atrial stretch, meds, drugs, normal variant	question meds question COPD Depends on the ventricular rate and patient tolerance	question meds question COPD question DIG Depends on the ventricular rate and patient tolerance	vagal maneuver Verapamil or Adenosine Synch cardioversion	vagal maneuver Verapamil or Adenosine Synch cardioversion	vagal maneuver Synch cardioversion

stable
The absence of chest pain, syncope, or other signs of cardiopulmonary compromise

Reentrant tachycardias can be interrupted by the delivery of a medication designed to slow conduction and/or increase the refractoriness of the pathway. The patient may present as being **stable** that is, not compromised. For example, the patient's level of consciousness (LOC) and blood pressure are not significantly altered. The patient may describe feelings of palpitation with SVT and atrial flutter and fib that are new to the patient. If this is the case, the provider can continue with assessment of medical and medication history and supportive care.

Occasionally the patient will present with an altered or diminished LOC, hypotension, and hypoperfusion. This is described as being *unstable.* Clearly the sense of urgency for intervention is greater in the unstable patient. Usually the care is directed to slowing the ventricular response. This involves administration of medications that will slow AV conduction. If the patient is dangerously affected, then electrical intervention is in order.

Self-Assessment Exercises

Matching

Find the phrase in the right column that matches the numbered word or phrase in the left column, and compare your answers to those in the back of the book.

____ 1. narrow QRS, regular, ventricular rate 190+	A. atrial flutter
____ 2. narrow QRS, rate 150, (+)P′ halfway between the QRS complexes	B. atrial fibrillation
____ 3. negative P′ in front of each narrow QRS	C. junctional rhythm
____ 4. no identifiable P waves, irregular narrow QRS	D. junctional tachycardia
____ 5. sudden onset, sudden stop of narrow QRS tachycardia	E. paroxysmal atrial tachycardia
	F. sinus tachycardia
	G. SVT

Fill in the Blanks

Complete the statements, and then compare your answers with those in the back of the book.

SINUS RHYTHM	JUNCTIONAL RHYTHM	PREMATURE ATRIAL COMPLEX
1 (+) P + QRS	1(-) P′ + QRS or no P	________________
PRI 0.12–0.20	0.12 or less	________________
QRS 0.10 or less	0.10 or less	________________
QRS rate: 60–100 per minute	40–60 per minute	________________
QRS rhythm: regular	regular	________________

ATRIAL TACH	SINUS TACH	JUNCTIONAL TACHYCARDIA
________________	P wave = 1(+) P + QRS	________________
________________	PRI = 0.12–0.20 second	________________
________________	QRS = 0.04–0.10 second	________________
________________	QRS rate = 100–150	________________
________________	QRS rhythm = regular	________________

ECG Rhythm Identification Practice

For the following ECG tracings, fill in the blanks and then check your answers against those in the back of the book.

Figure 6-20

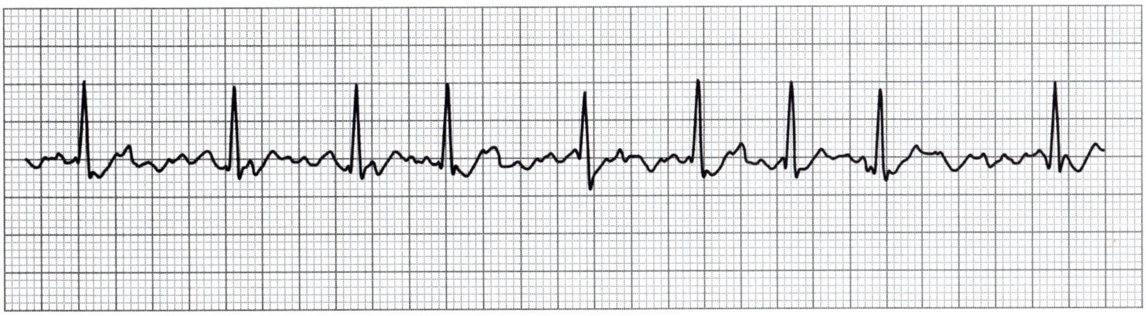

QRS duration ________________ QT ______________
Ventricular rate/rhythm __________________________
Atrial rate/rhythm ______________________________
PR interval _____________________________________

Identification ___________________________________
Symptoms _______________________________________
____
Treatment ______________________________________

Figure 6-21

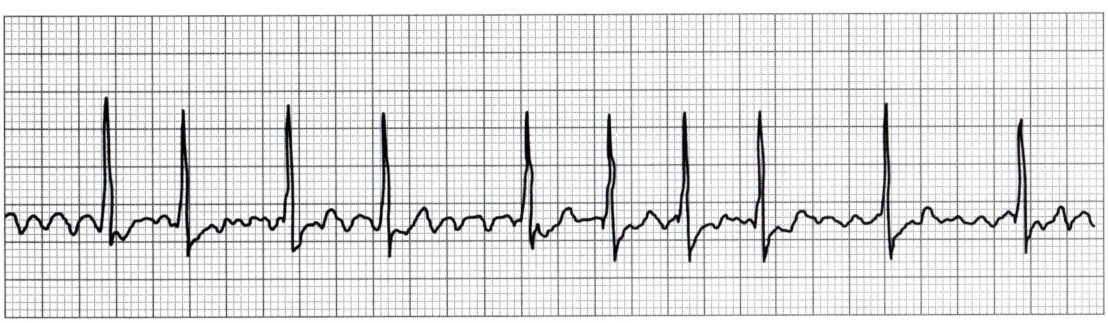

QRS duration ________________ QT ______________
Ventricular rate/rhythm __________________________
Atrial rate/rhythm ______________________________
PR interval _____________________________________

Identification ___________________________________
Symptoms _______________________________________
____
Treatment ______________________________________

Figure 6-22

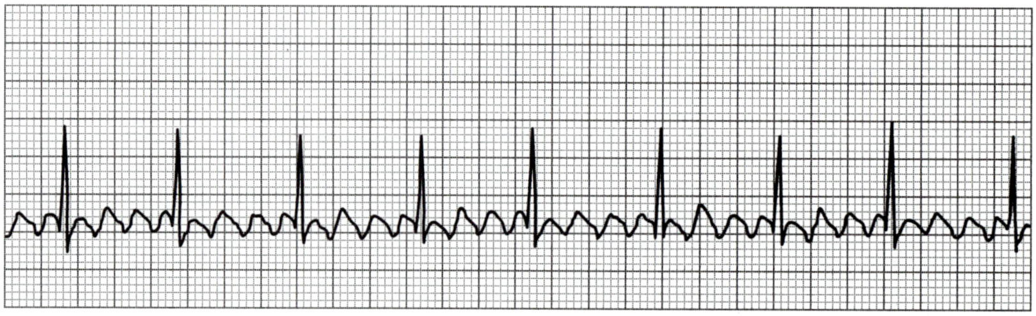

QRS duration ______________ QT ___________

Ventricular rate/rhythm ____________________

Atrial rate/rhythm ______________________

PR interval __________________________

Identification ____________________________

Symptoms ________________________________

____

Treatment ________________________________

Figure 6-23

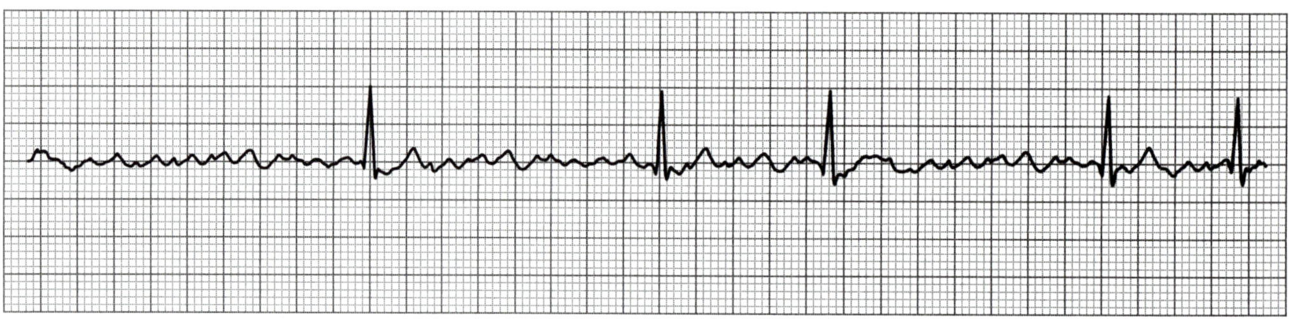

QRS duration ______________ QT ___________

Ventricular rate/rhythm ____________________

Atrial rate/rhythm ______________________

PR interval __________________________

Identification ____________________________

Symptoms ________________________________

____

Treatment ________________________________

Figure 6-24

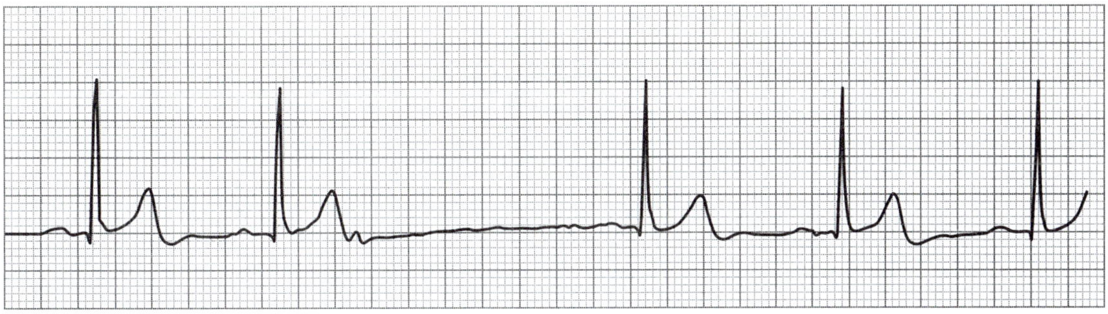

QRS duration ______________ QT ____________

Ventricular rate/rhythm ______________________

Atrial rate/rhythm __________________________

PR interval ________________________________

Identification ______________________________

Symptoms _________________________________

____

Treatment _________________________________

Figure 6-25

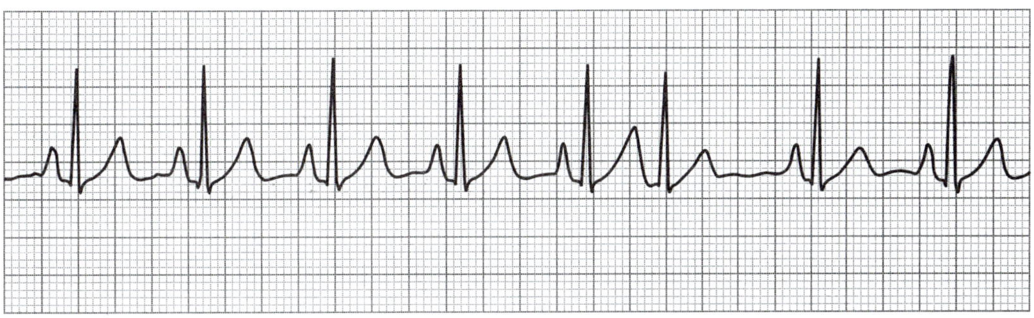

QRS duration ______________ QT ____________

Ventricular rate/rhythm ______________________

Atrial rate/rhythm __________________________

PR interval ________________________________

Identification ______________________________

Symptoms _________________________________

____

Treatment _________________________________

Figure 6-26

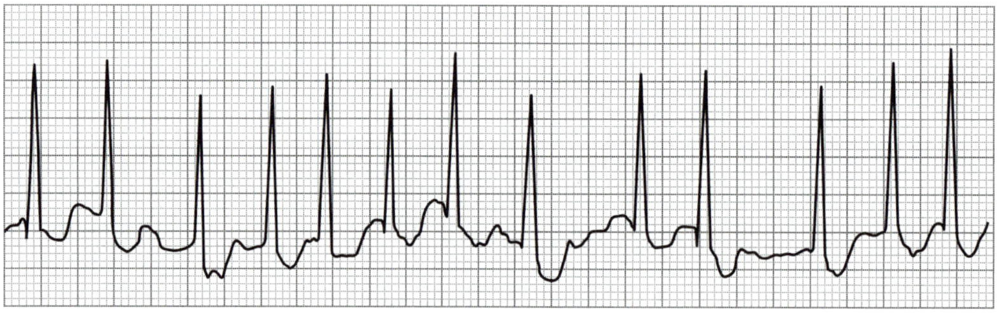

QRS duration ________ **QT** ________
Ventricular rate/rhythm ________
Atrial rate/rhythm ________
PR interval ________

Identification ________
Symptoms ________
____
Treatment ________

Figure 6-27

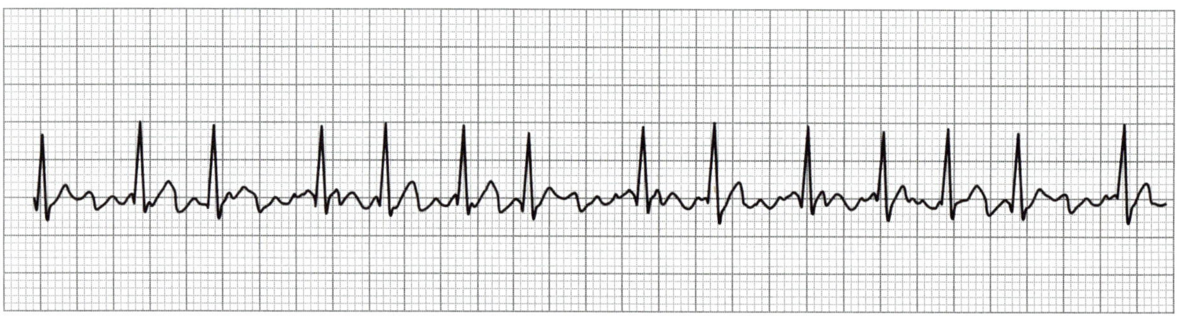

QRS duration ________ **QT** ________
Ventricular rate/rhythm ________
Atrial rate/rhythm ________
PR interval ________

Identification ________
Symptoms ________
____
Treatment ________

Figure 6-28

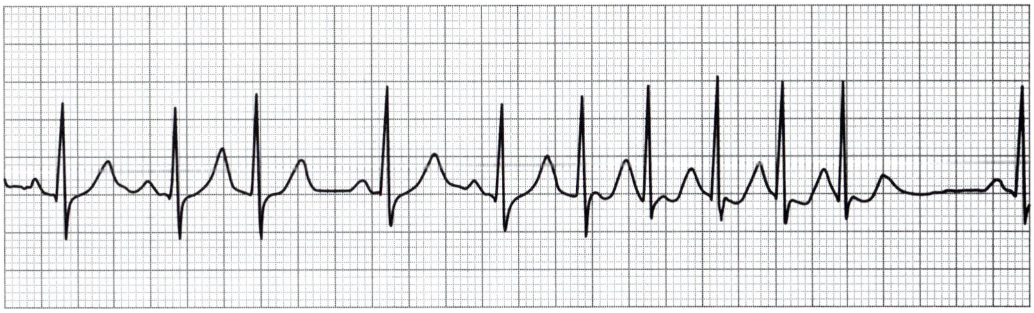

QRS duration ______________ QT ____________

Ventricular rate/rhythm ______________________

Atrial rate/rhythm __________________________

PR interval ________________________________

Identification ______________________________

Symptoms ________________________________

____

Treatment ________________________________

Figure 6-29

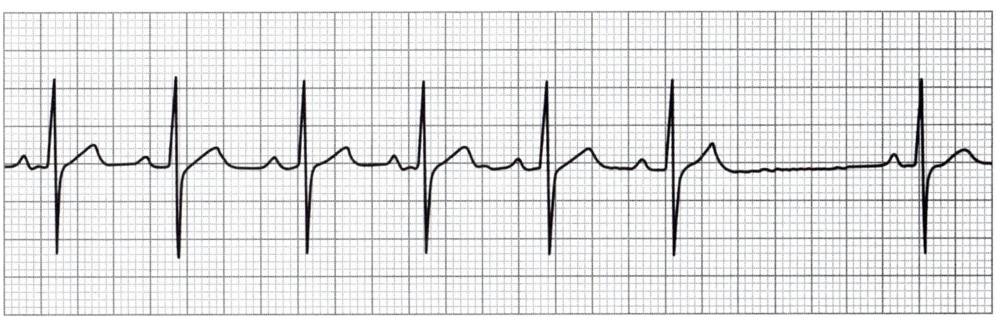

QRS duration ______________ QT ____________

Ventricular rate/rhythm ______________________

Atrial rate/rhythm __________________________

PR interval ________________________________

Identification ______________________________

Symptoms ________________________________

____

Treatment ________________________________

Figure 6-30

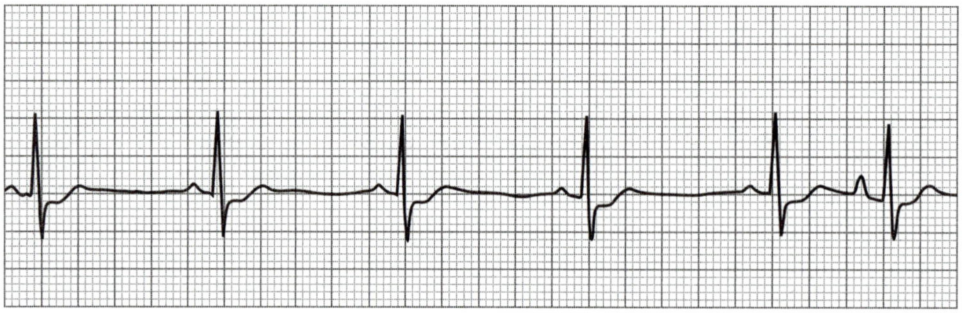

QRS duration ________________ QT ____________

Ventricular rate/rhythm ________________________

Atrial rate/rhythm ___________________________

PR interval ________________________________

Identification __________________________________

Symptoms ______________________________________

____

Treatment ______________________________________

Figure 6-31

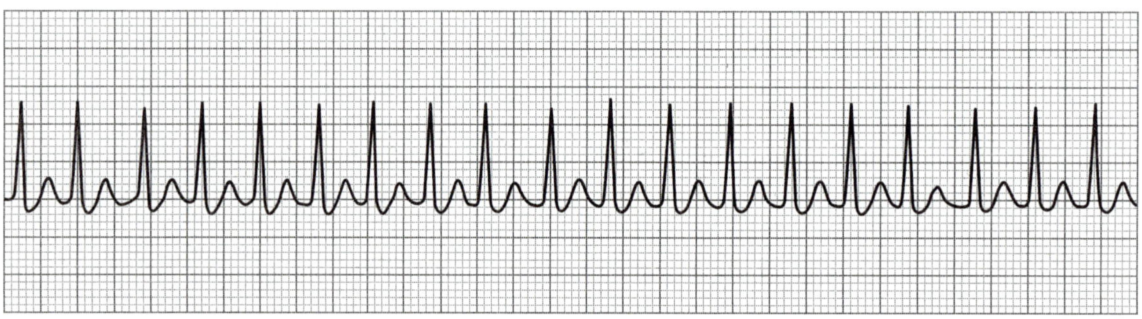

QRS duration ________________ QT ____________

Ventricular rate/rhythm ________________________

Atrial rate/rhythm ___________________________

PR interval ________________________________

Identification __________________________________

Symptoms ______________________________________

____

Treatment ______________________________________

Figure 6-32

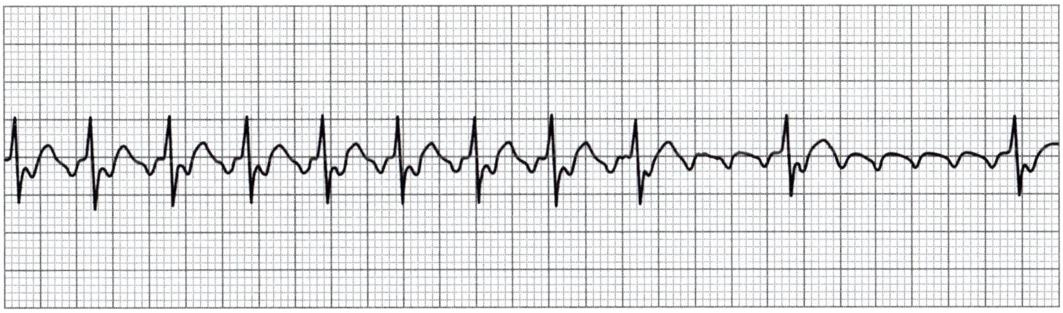

QRS duration ______________ QT ____________

Ventricular rate/rhythm ______________________

Atrial rate/rhythm __________________________

PR interval ________________________________

Identification ______________________________

Symptoms _________________________________

____

Treatment _________________________________

Figure 6-33

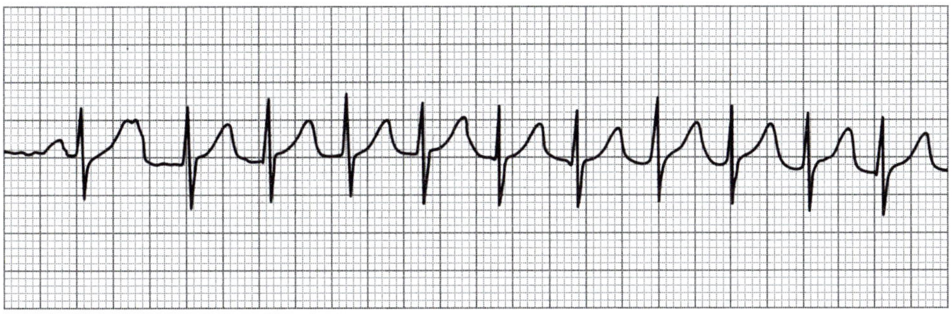

QRS duration ______________ QT ____________

Ventricular rate/rhythm ______________________

Atrial rate/rhythm __________________________

PR interval ________________________________

Identification ______________________________

Symptoms _________________________________

____

Treatment _________________________________

References

Conover, M. B. *Nurse's pocket guide to electrocardiography* (3rd ed.). St. Louis, MO: C. V. Mosby; 1994.

Conover, M. B. *Understanding electrocardiography: Arrhythmias and the 12-lead ECG* (7th ed.). St. Louis, MO: Mosby-Year Book; 1996.

Conover, M. B. & Wellens, H. J. *The ECG in emergency decision making*. Philadelphia: W. B. Saunders; 1993.

Emergency Cardiac Care Subcommittee and Subcommittees, American Heart Association. Guidelines for cardiopulmonary resuscitation and emergency cardiac care. *JAMA*. 1994.

Goldberger, E. *Textbook of clinical cardiology*. St. Louis, MO: C. V. Mosby; 1982.

Mandel, W. J. (Ed). *Cardiac arrhythmias: Their mechanisms, diagnoses and management* (2nd ed.). Philadelphia: Lippincott; 1987.

Marriott, H. J. *Practical electrocardiography* (8th ed.). Baltimore: Williams and Wilkins; 1988.

Marriott, H. J., & Conover, M. B. *Advanced concepts in arrhythmias* (2nd ed.). St. Louis, MO: C. V. Mosby; 1989.

Sung, R. J. et al. *Supraventricular tachycardia; mechanisms and treatment.* Cardiovascular clinics. Vol. 11, No. 27, 1980.

Wellens, H. J. & Durrer, D. *Electrical stimulation of the heart in the study and treatment of the tachycardias.* Baltimore: University Park Press, 1987.

Wolff, G.S., et al. The fast-slow form of AV nodal reentrant tachycardia in children. *American Journal of Cardiology*, Vol. 43, 1181; 1989.

Wu, D. & Denes, P. Mechanisms of paroxysmal supraventricular tachycardia. *Archives of Internal Medicine*,135–437; 1985.

Wu, D., et al. Clinical, electrocardiographic and electrophysiologic observations in patients with PSVT. *American Journal of Cardiology*, Vol. 41, 1045; 1978.

CHAPTER 7

The Ventricular Mechanisms

Premise ● Any QRS different from a normally occurring QRS will be considered ventricular until proven otherwise.

Objectives

After reading the chapter and completing the Self-Assessment Exercises, the student should be able to

1. recognize the difference between QRSs that are supraventricular and ventricular in origin
2. name the PVC in terms of its position in the cardiac cycle
3. differentiate between ectopic and ventricular escape mechanisms

Key Terms

end-diastolic	R-on-T
idioventricular	trigeminy
interpolated	uniform
multiform	ventricular bigeminy

Introduction

Previous chapters have dealt with *supra*ventricular arrhythmias; those rhythm disturbances that arise either in the sinus node, the atria, or the AV junction, with normal ventricular depolarization. In this chapter, we will deal with ectopics and arrhythmias that have their origin in ventricular tissue and cause abnormal ventricular depolarization.

The cells of normal ventricular musculature and conduction tissue are fast cells, due to the rapid influx of sodium. Slow cells are so named since they have extended refractory periods, conduct, and recover more slowly. Ectopic cells may be fast or slow and in the presence of pathology fast cells may be converted to slow cells and contribute to ectopic formation and conduction defects.

Disturbances in conduction may produce ectopic impulses by the process known as *reentry*. Reentry is defined as the ability of an impulse to re-excite some region of the heart through which it has already passed. Reentry usually occurs when an impulse deviates around a circular conduction pathway forming a loop. There are many such potential circuits within ventricular conduction tissue where terminal Purkinje fibers attach to cardiac muscle.

When such circuits and ectopic formation occurred in atrial tissue, the AV node usually protected the heart from rapid and chaotic rates. With ventricular ectopy, the vigilance of the practitioner, early recognition, and intervention are the only protection for the patient.

PREMATURE VENTRICULAR COMPLEX (PVC)

A PVC is a manifestation of abnormal electrical activity arising within the ventricles. PVCs are a common manifestation and frequently encountered and are regarded suspiciously since they often reflect myocardial ischemia and injury. More common problems and issues surround ventricular ectopy. The most significant factors contributing to the development of the triggered automaticity in the ventricles are:

adrenergic drugs
caffeine
congestive heart failure
electrolyte disturbances
hypertension
hypertrophy
hypokalemia, usually as a result of tissue hypoxia
hypovolemia
hypoxia
medications such as digitalis, isoproterenol, dopamine, epinephrine
myocardial stretch
rapid rates, insufficient to provide adequate perfusion
slow rates, insufficient to provide adequate perfusion
stress
tissue infarction

Recognizing the PVC

An impulse whose origin is within ventricular tissue and is outside the normal ventricular conduction system creates a QRS that is different from any supraventricular QRS. The QRS will have an increased amplitude with a T wave of opposite polarity to the QRS. For instance, a positive QRS will be followed by a negative T wave. Similarly, a negative QRS will be followed by a positive T wave.

The QRS morphology of the PVC is usually but not always greater in amplitude and wider than the dominant QRS. Ventricular activation that begins at a site of the ectopic ventricular focus travels across ventricular muscle mass instead of using the His-Purkinje system. Depolarization then takes longer, resulting in a broad (greater than 0.10 second) QRS complex. Figure 7-1 is an illustration of the formation of a ventricular ectopic. Figure 7-2 is an ECG tracing of a sinus rhythm with a PVC.

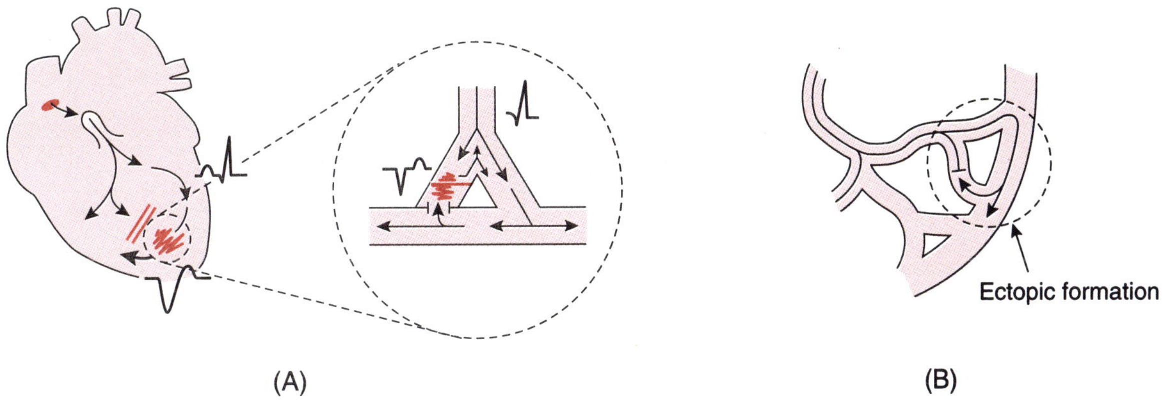

Figure 7-1 (A)The formation of a ventricular ectopic. An overall view of the conduction system with unidirectional block at a site in ventricular tissue. (B) A closer view of the focus of ventricular ectopic formation.

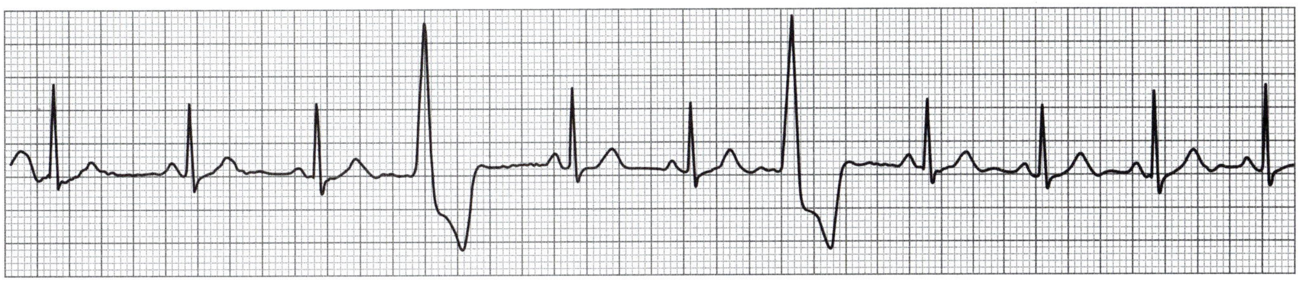

Figure 7-2 An ECG tracing of rhythm and two premature ventricular complexes (PVCs). Note the difference in morphology in the QRS complexes: the QRS of the premature complex is different from the dominant QRSs since it does not use the ventricular conduction pathways. The premature, ventricular QRS is opposite from its T wave. The sinus P waves plot through the events as sinus cadence is undisturbed. The PVCs are similar to each other and are ***uniform*** in appearance. The ECG interpretation would be sinus at 86 per minute with frequent, uniform PVCs.

Characteristics of a Ventricular Ectopic

Remember, the *P* in *PVC* means *premature*, so, by definition, a PVC will be seen to occur *prior* to normally conducted beats.

1. P Wave: That of the underlying rhythm.
2. PR Internal: That of the underlying rhythm.
3. QRS Complex: The QRS complex is different from the dominant rhythm and often appears bizarre in appearance compared with the normal QRS complexes.

   Often the QRS/T is greater in amplitude and duration than the dominant QRSs. However, PVCs can occur and present with diminished amplitude and narrow duration.

   The T wave of the PVC is opposite from its QRS in orientation than a PVC of supraventricular origin.
4. QRS Rate: The rate is that of the underlying rhythm.

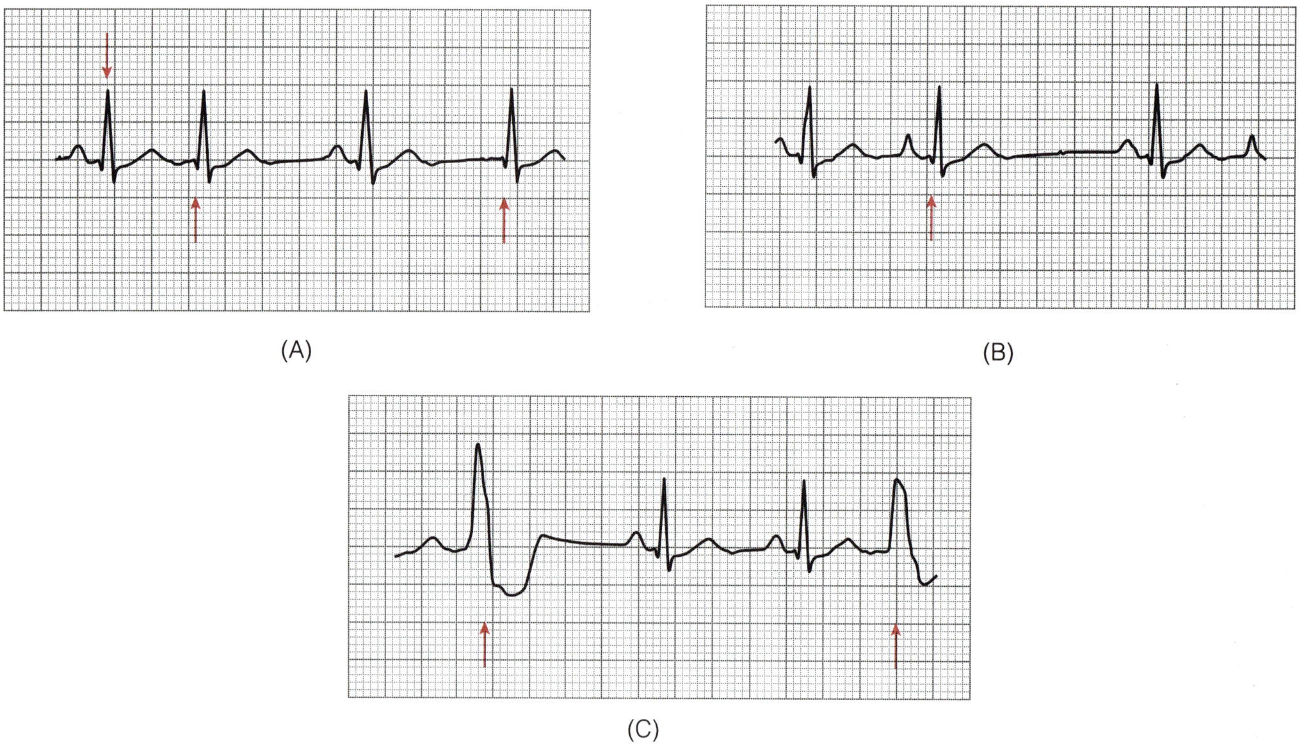

Figure 7-3 An ECG tracing showing (A) a sinus-induced QRS followed by a PJC → sinus, followed by a junctional escape beat. (B) sinus with PACs; and (C) sinus with PVCs. In (A) and (B), all the QRS complexes are similar as each uses the bundle branch system normally. In (C), the QRS complex of the PVC is different, and that QRS is opposite from its T wave. The PVC occurs within the ventricular musculature, outside the bundle branch system causing the abnormal configuration.

5. QRS Rhythm: The rhythm is that of the underlying rhythm, and its regularity will be disturbed by the PVC.

Figure 7-3 is a comparison of QRS configurations that are sinus, atrial, junctional in origin and PVCs.

Narrow, Complex PVCs

PVCs originating within the intraventricular conduction system will be narrower than PVCs that occur outside the bundle branch system. This is because the bundle branch system will support the conduction in a different but relatively normal fashion. For a fascicular PVC, the initial wave form and the direction of the QRS will alter, depending on which fascicle is the origin.

For instance, an anterior fascicular PVC will have an inferior, rightward direction and will appear positive in lead II and negative in lead I. A posterior fascicular PVC will have a superior leftward direction and will appear negative in lead II and positive in lead I.

In either instance, the fascicular PVC will have an rSR′ configuration in precordial lead V_1 since the impulse originates within the left ventricular fascicles, and the right bundle branch will be the last to be activated. Figure 7-4A is a graphic of the ECG and ventricular conduction system showing the formation of the PVC in the left anterior fascicle (LAF) of the left bundle branch and the resulting wave forms

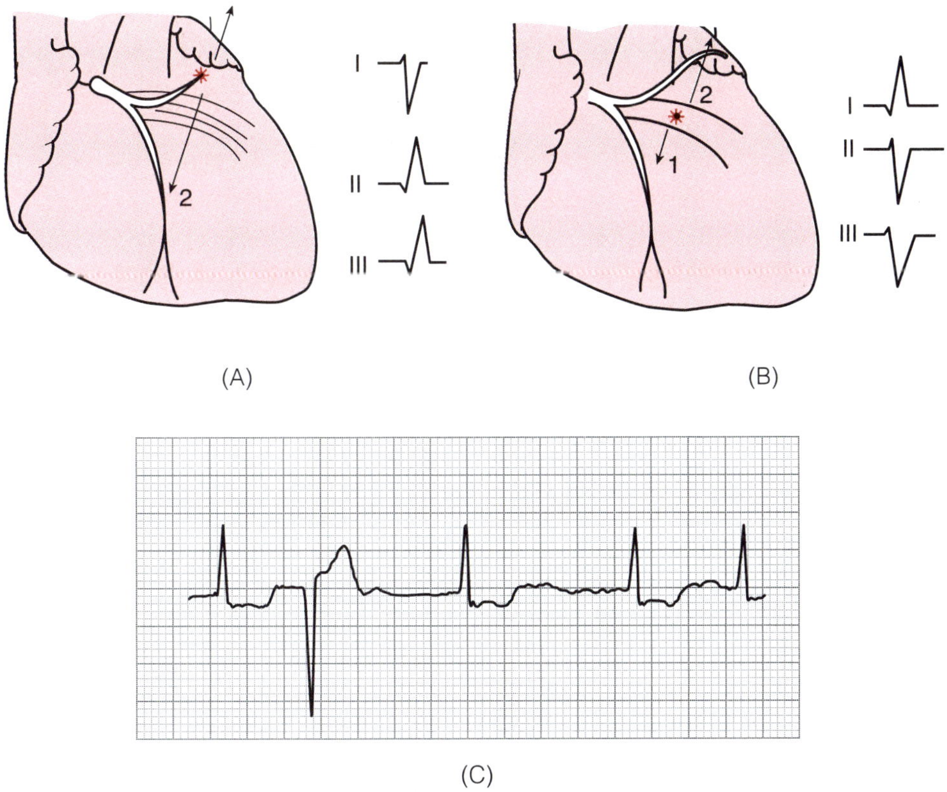

Figure 7-4 (A) The origin of a left anterior fascicular PVC and how it is visualized on ECG limb leads I, II, and II. (B) Another example of the direction of current flow of a PVC whose origin was in the area of the left posterior fascicle. (C) The ECG interpretation would be atrial fibrillation, 67 to 100 per minute, 2 mm ST segment depression and with a narrow-complex PVC. (This was confirmed on 12-lead ECG.)

in leads I and II. Figure 7-4B is a graphic of the ECG and ventricular conduction system showing the formation of the PVC in the left posterior fascicle (LPF) of the left bundle branch, and the resulting wave forms in leads I and II. Figure 7-4C is an ECG tracing of atrial fibrillation and a narrow-complex, fascicular PVC, confirmed on 12-lead ECG.

Variations in PVCs

PVCs are described by their occurrence within the cardiac cycle.

Premature Ventricular Complex with Full Compensatory Pause. A PVC is frequently characterized by a so-called compensatory pause. The interval between the QRS complex before the PVC and the complex following the PVC is twice that of the regular cycle interval. This occurs when the PVC does not interfere with the pacemaking activity of the SA node. The sinus P waves following the PVC are not always visualized since they occur during the previous complex's refractory period. Mathematically, the distance between the sinus beat that precedes the PVC, and the sinus beat that follows the PVC is equal to the sum of two consecutive sinus intervals. Figure 7-5 consists of ECG tracings illustrating a PVC with full compensatory pause.

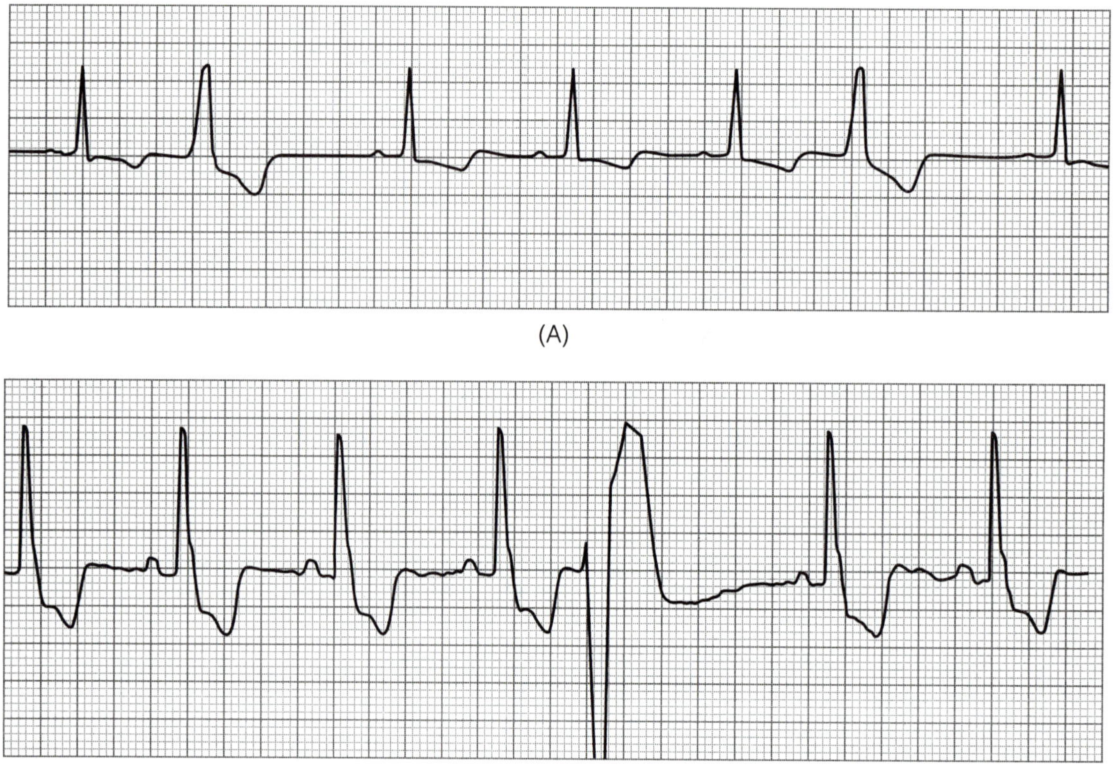

Figure 7-5 ECG tracings (A) and (B) each illustrate sinus rhythm with a PVC with compensatory pause. Note that the R-R interval containing the PVC is twice the previous R-R interval. Sinus P waves plot through as sinus cadence is undisturbed. The ECG interpretation for (A) would be sinus rhythm at 67 per minute with inverted T waves and a PVC. The ECG interpretation for (B) would be sinus at 71 per minute, with 5 to 6 mm ST segment depression and a PVC.

end-diastolic
A PVC occurring at the end of, or just after a sinus P wave

End-Diastolic PVC. When a PVC occurs at the end or just after a sinus P wave, it is **end-diastolic**. Remember, a sinus P wave is the last electrical event in ventricular diastole (that is, it occurs at the end of diastole, hence its name). Although the P wave preceded the PVC, it is *not* the cause of the QRS complex.

An end-diastolic PVC is considered a safe PVC in terms of perfusion and of electrical malfunction within the heart. It occurs far from the T wave and it can generate cardiac output of 90 to 95 percent normal. Figure 7-6 is an illustration of sinus rhythm with an end-diastolic PVC.

interpolated
A PVC occurring between two consecutive sinus beats

Interpolated PVC. When a PVC occurs between two consecutive sinus beats, it is an **interpolated** PVC. The sinus node depolarized at its inherent rate, and there are QRS complexes after each sinus beat. The PVC is sandwiched between two normal sinus complexes. These are often digitalis induced.

The PR interval following the interpolated PVC is typically conducted with a prolonged PR segment. This altered conduction occurs as a result of AV node delay because of refractoriness, and the sinus is simply waiting its turn. Another less frequent cause is retrograde penetration by the PVC. This phenomenon cannot be proven on the EKG and is only inferred. It is sometimes referred to as *concealed*

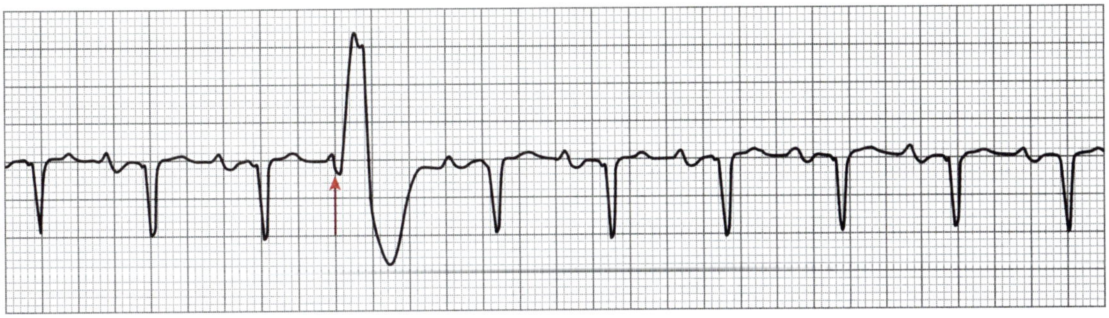

Figure 7-6 An ECG tracing showing sinus at 100 per minute with an end-diastolic PVC. Note the presence of the PVC just after the sinus P wave. The PR interval is 0.24 second indicating AV node delay.

conduction. This prolongation of the PR segment may help differentiate an interpolated PVC from artifact. Figure 7-7 is an example of a sinus mechanism with an interpolated PVC.

Uniform PVCs. When PVCs originate in one focus, they are usually **uniform** in configuration in a given lead. The formation of a reentrant ectopic impulse is closely related to the conduction of the preceding impulse. Thus, the PVC will occur within a fixed distance from the original impulse. This is known as *fixed coupling* and is commonly seen.

uniform
Similar in appearance, size, and amplitude

Intraventricular reentry may cause the exact coupling. This may occur because the normal impulse is conducted in one direction, and then, very slowly through a depressed segment of tissue, it emerges to reactivate normal tissue. If this interval is the same after each normal beat, the relationship will be established and seen as fixed coupling.

Afterdepolarization occurs when ventricular tissue is diseased or if the patient is on digitalis preparations. These after potentials follow the previous action potential, and if they reach their threshold, they will produce a PVC with exact coupling.

Uniformity in appearance and fixed coupling does not guarantee that the impulse comes from the same focus. It is possible for one focus, firing in the same

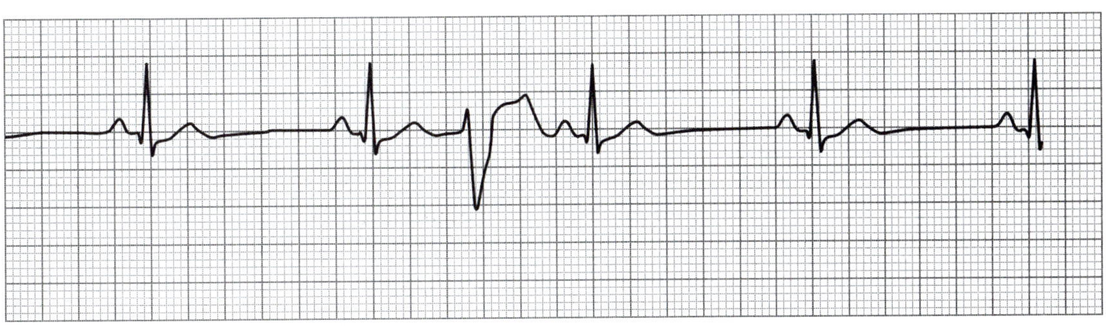

Figure 7-7 An ECG tracing showing sinus bradycardia with an interpolated PVC. Note that the sinus P waves plot through undisturbed. The ECG interpretation would be sinus bradycardia with 1 to 2 mm ST segment depression and an interpolated PVC.

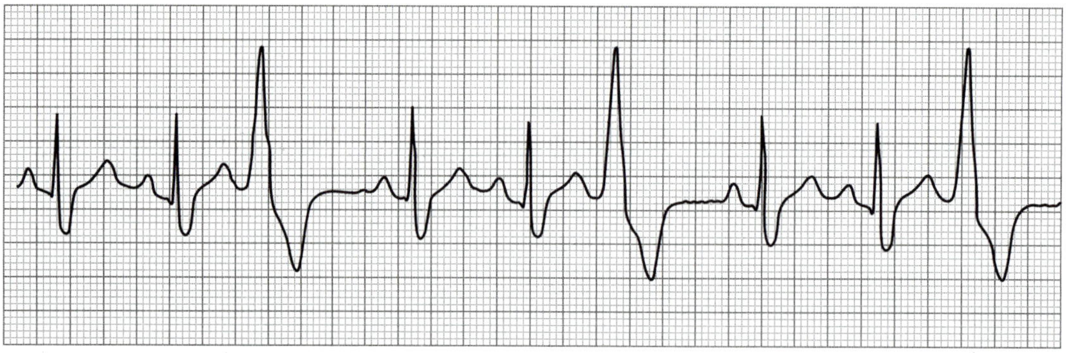

Figure 7-8 An ECG tracing showing sinus rhythm at 86 per minute with 2 mm ST segment elevation and frequent uniform PVCs. Notice that the distance between the normal QRS and the PVC is similar in each instance.

direction, in close proximity to another focus to generate a PVC that is very similar. Figure 7-8 is an ECG showing frequent uniform PVCs.

multiform

Ectopic beats with different shapes, presumed to result from different sites of origin. May be a single focus but following a different pathway when activating the ventricles.

Multiform PVCs. PVCs may originate in more than one focus, or a PVC may reenter (and exit) from the same focus, but depolarization occurs in a different direction. When this occurs, the PVC takes on a different appearance. The term **multiform** is recommended since a single focus can take different pathways through the ventricles and result in different QRS configurations. Just as similarity in PVC morphology does not guarantee the same focus, differences in PVC morphology do not guarantee multiple foci. Figure 7-9 is an ECG showing the multiple PVCs of different QRS morphology.

Couplets or Paired PVCs. *Pairs* or *couplets* are two closely coupled PVCs in a row. A couplet should not be confused with *coupling*, which refers to the relationship of the PVC to the previous normal beat. Couplets are dangerous since the second PVC can fall on refractory tissue and cause ventricular fibrillation. Figure 7-10 is an ECG tracing showing the occurrence of paired PVCs.

bigeminy

An ECG rhythm where every other beat is an ectopic

Ventricular Bigeminy. Ventricular **bigeminy** is the occurrence of every other beat as an ectopic. When this occurs, a normal beat is followed by a PVC, and the PVC is coupled with the previous QRS. The mechanism for this is thought to be

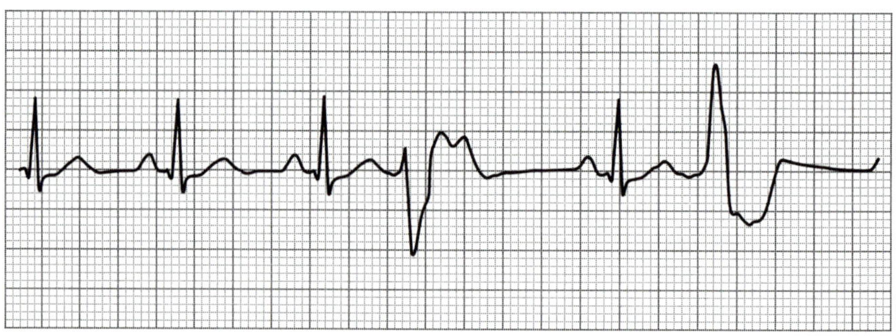

Figure 7-9 Note the difference between the PVCs. The ECG interpretation would be sinus rhythm about 78 per minute with frequent multiformed PVCs.

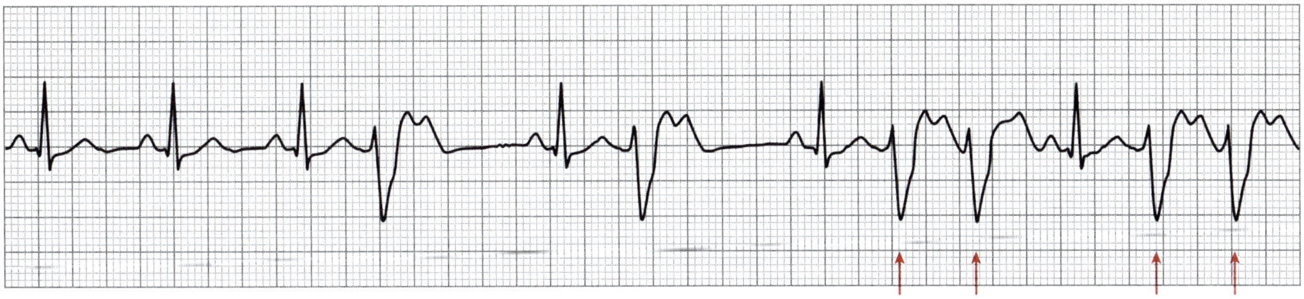

Figure 7-10 An ECG tracing showing sinus rhythm with frequent uniform PVCs and two examples of ***paired*** PVCs or ***couplets***. Couplets indicate the beginning of reentry and are regarded as dangerous to the patient.

reentry or afterdepolarization that may be caused by digitalis toxicity. Ventricular bigeminy can be an isolated occurance in an otherwise healthy person.

Trigeminy occurs when every third beat is a PVC. In ventricular bigeminy or trigeminy the underlying rhythm can be sinus, atrial, or junctional in origin.

trigeminy
An ECG rhythm where every third beat is an ectopic

Ventricular bigeminy is often seen in patients on digitalis preparations. Figure 7-11 consists of ECG tracings from the same patient showing ventricular bigeminy (A) and trigeminy (B).

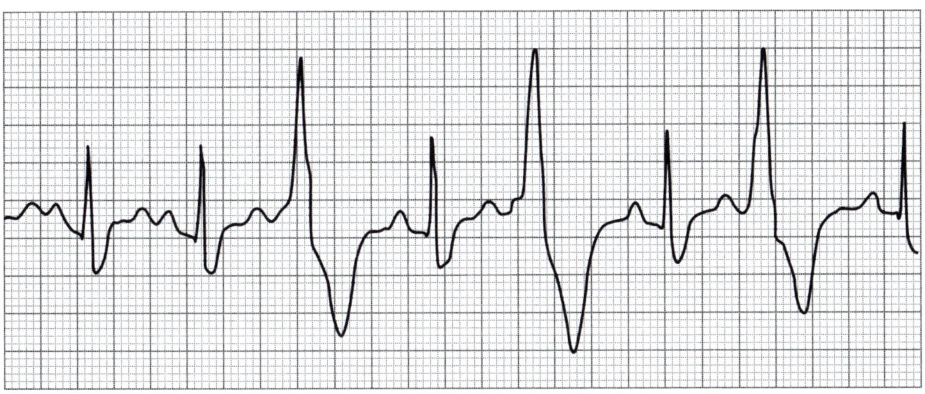

(A)

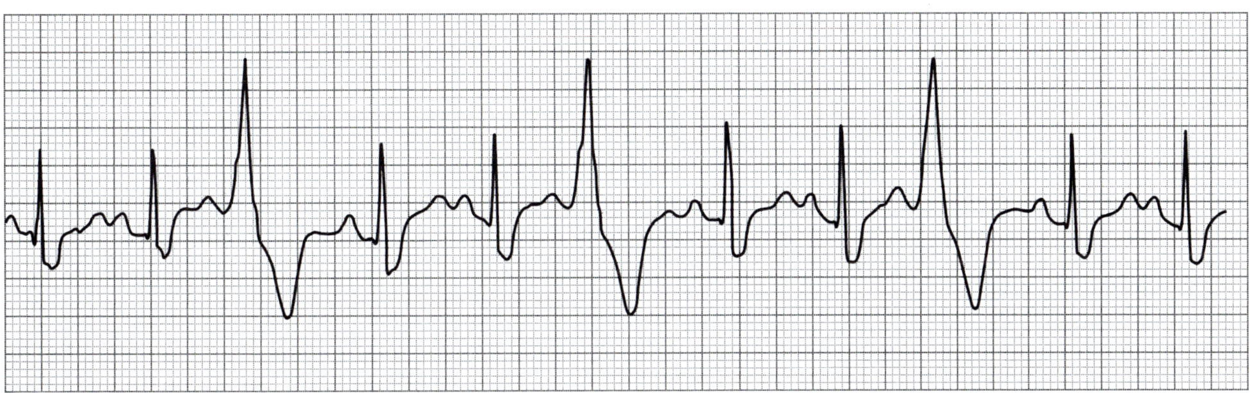

(B)

Figure 7-11 A continuous ECG tracing from a patient illustrating (A) ventricular ***bigeminy*** (every other complex is a PVC), and (B) ***trigeminy*** (every third complex is a PVC). There is 5 mm ST segment elevation.

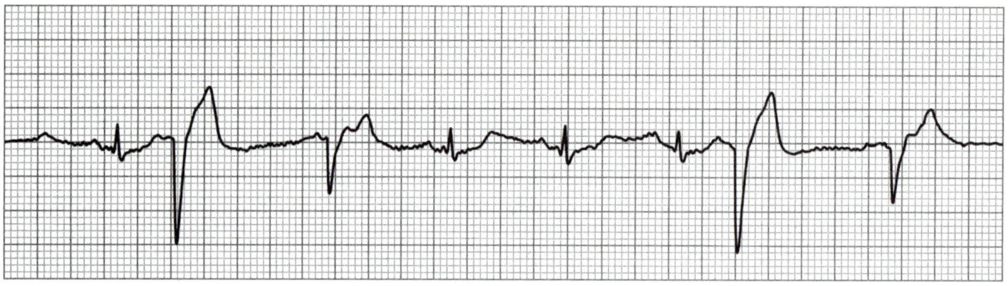

(A)

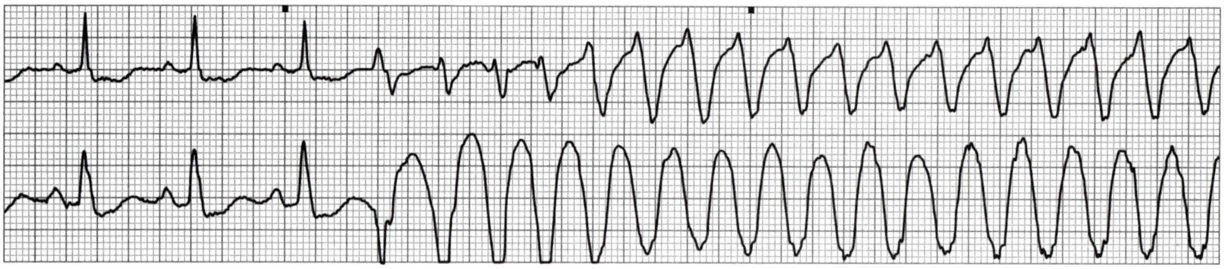

(B)

Figure 7-12 Two examples of R-on-T PVCs. (A) is an ECG tracing showing sinus rhythm with frequent R-on-T PVCs in a 61-year-old male with chest pain. Note that the PVCs are narrow, perhaps fascicular in origin. This patient later developed ventricular fibrillation. (B) is an ECG tracing from a 55-year-old patient who developed ventricular tachycardia. The patient responded to antiarrhythmic medication and was reportedly successfully reperfused.

R-on-T

When a PVC occurs so prematurely that it lands on the prior T wave (the ventricle's vulnerable period of repolarization). Ventricular fibrillation may result.

R-on-T Phenomenon. The **R-on-T** phenomenon is the close coupling of the premature beat with the preceding beat. The R wave of the PVC is superimposed onto the T wave of the preceding beat. Recall that 0.02 to the right of the peak of the T wave is a vulnerable period, with the ability of a premature beat to initiate a dangerous and often a catastrophic arrhythmia. Figure 7-12 is an example of ECG tracings with R-on-T PVCs.

Intervention

Assessment of the patient in whom ventricular ectopy is apparent, questioning the presence of chest pain, medical history, and medication regimen provides a basis for interventions. Providing pain relief and reassessing the presence and frequency of the ectopics will help with the decision to use antiarrhythmia therapy. Most antiarrhythmic medications inhibit the fast sodium channels. Arrhythmias that are unresponsive to the usual therapy may be arising in slow rather than fast automatic cells. In such cases, slow channel (calcium) antagonists may be more effective.

MONOMORPHIC VENTRICULAR TACHYCARDIA

When three or more PVCs occur in a row, and their rate exceeds 100 beats per minute, the arrhythmia is labeled *ventricular tachycardia*. Ventricular tachycardia may break through in spite of adequate sinus rate and often occurs suddenly. It is usually initiated by a PVC that is distinctly premature, but it can occur without any warning. When the ECG shows only ventricular tachycardia, it is described as sustained ventricular tachycardia or sustained V-tach. Figure 7-13 is an ECG tracing showing ventricular tachycardia. The ECG characteristics of ventricular tachycardia are as follows:

1. P Wave: P waves may not be distinguishable during ventricular tachycardia, although atrial activity, dissociated from ventricular activity, may not be affected.
2. PR Interval: Atrial activity is dissociated from ventricular activity, a PR interval is not measurable.
3. QRS Complex: The QRS complex duration is usually greater than 0.12 second and bizarre in appearance. The T wave may not be easily identified from the QRS complex.
4. QRS Rate: The ventricular rate is between 100 and 170 per minute. Three or more consecutive PVCs constitutes ventricular tachycardia.
5. QRS RHYTHM: The rhythm is regular or very slightly irregular.

An ectopic pacemaker in the ventricle often produces a wide-complex tachycardia. Ventricular tachycardia may terminate spontaneously. The more rapid the

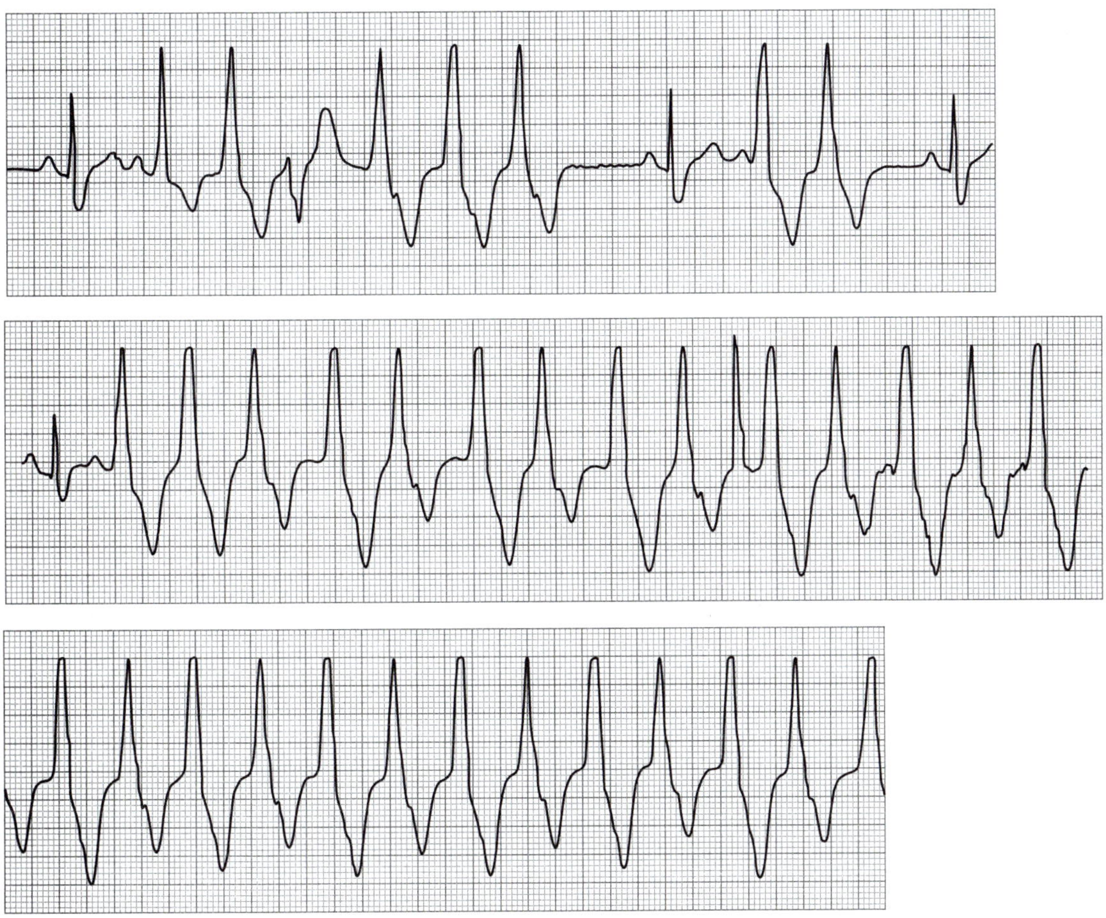

Figure 7-13 Continuous ECG tracing from a patient with sinus rhythm, frequent, paired PVCs, episodes of ventricular tachycardia, and, finally, the ventricular tachycardia sustains itself. Sinus P waves are sometimes visible and can be plotted out. Sinus cadence is independent of the ventricular tachycardia. As the tachycardia rate increases, the P waves become indistinct.

ventricular tachycardia, the greater the incidence of instability. Ventricular tachycardia of greater than 170 per minute is often an unstable situation.

Intervention. When ventricular tachycardia persists, and the patient is hemodynamically stable, antiarrhythmic medications such as lidocaine may be employed. If the rhythm does not convert, or if the patient were considered unstable, then electrical cardioversion may be required to terminate the arrhythmia.

All wide-complex tachycardia should be treated as ventricular tachycardia until proven otherwise. The initial intervention for wide-complex tachycardia is as though the rhythm is ventricular tachycardia until 12-lead ECG and clinical analysis are completed.

INTERMITTENT VENTRICULAR TACHYCARDIA

During sinus, atrial, or junctional rhythms, there may be a *run* or *salvo* of 3 PVCs in a row. For instance, one may see three PVCs in a row—that is, a burst of ventricular tachycardia—then two more sinus beats, followed by more PVCs. Figure 7-14 is an illustration of two rhythms each with episodes or runs of ventricular tachycardia.

POLYMORPHIC VENTRICULAR TACHYCARDIA—TORSADES DE POINTES (TdP)

Torsade is a form of ventricular tachycardia that creates a spindlelike pattern on the ECG. For example, there will be QRS complexes of one polarity followed by beats of the opposite polarity separated by beats of an intermediate form. The alteration

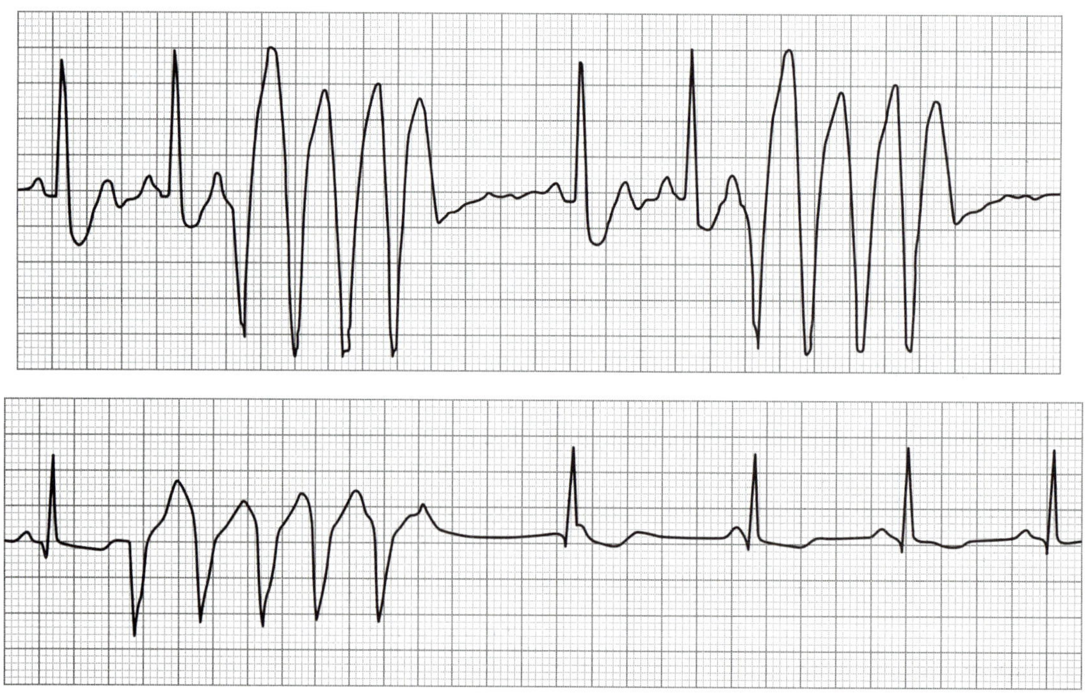

Figure 7-14 Two ECG tracings, each showing sinus mechanisms with *runs* of ventricular tachycardia, each beginning with R-on-T PVCs.

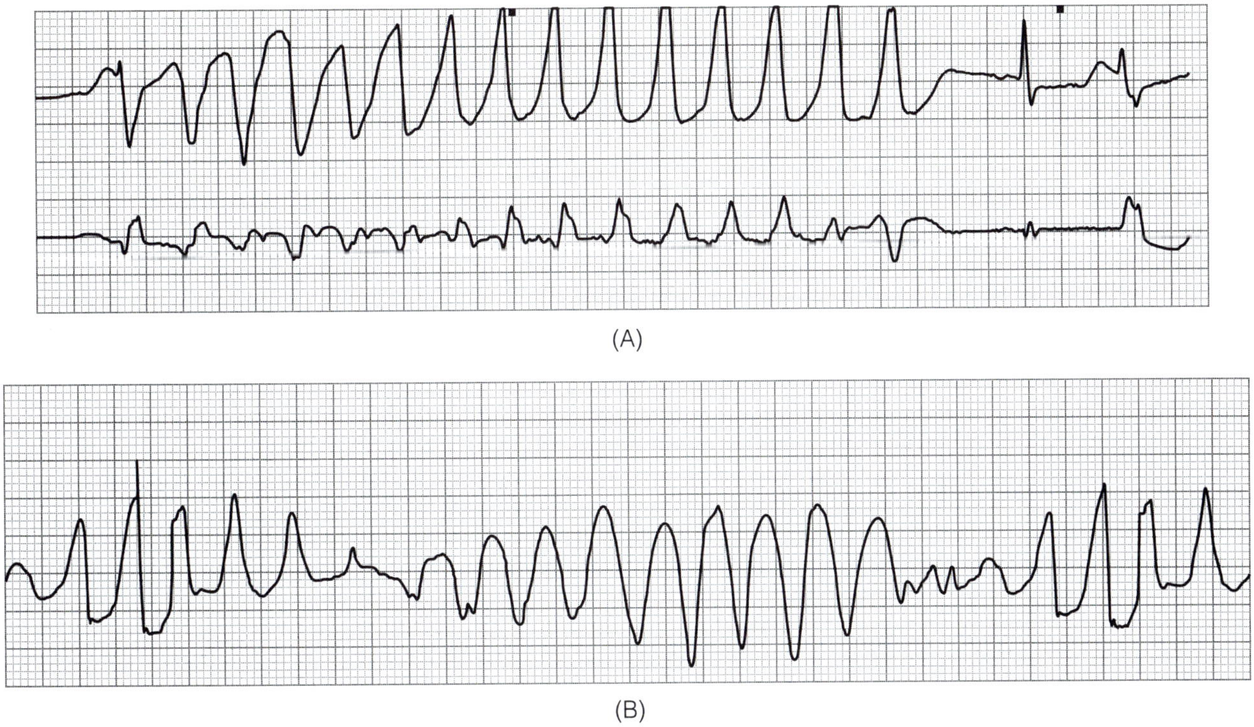

Figure 7-15 Two ECG tracings showing *Torsade de pointes*. (A) The rhythm spontaneously converted after being managed with intravenous (IV) magnesium. The patient was reportedly taking amiodarone. (B) The patient was defibrillated. This patient had alleged tricylic overdose.

in polarity usually occurs gradually and is repeated several times in succession. TdP is frequently initiated by a PVC occurring on a prolonged T or TU wave. The rate range of the tachycardia is usually 250 to 350 per minute. Figure 7-15 are two examples of Torsade.

Torsade de pointes refers to one episode or several points. *Torsades* refers to more than one episode or an episode of sustained duration (Conover 1992; Coumel, Leclercq, & Dessertenue 1984).

The Mechanism of Torsade

A popular explanation for Torsade is the presence of two or more epicardial breakthrough sites vying for control of activation. When the site of activation changes, so does the QRS morphology. The narrower complexes producing the spindlelike effect may be the different shaped QRSs that are really fusion beats resulting from the collision of the two different sites of activation (Conover 1996; Wellens 1992).

Runs of TdP often terminate and recur. Repeated episodes are progressively longer. Left untreated, this arrhythmia may deteriorate into ventricular fibrillation.

TdP can be misinterpreted as ventricular fibrillation. Ventricular fibrillation is chaotic without any characteristic spindle effect, and the QRS rate is immeasurable. Clinically, patients with TdP have pulses, and patients in ventricular fibrillation are pulseless.

Presence of intrinsic cardiac disease, central nervous system (CNS) abnormalities such as subarachnoid hemorrhage, and intracranial trauma can generate TdP.

ECG rhythm disturbances that may deteriorate into TdP include severe bradydysrhythmias such as complete AV block with idioventricular rhythm.

Torsade can also be induced by drugs such as quinidine, procainamide, disopyramide, amniodarone, aprindine. Psychotropic drugs, such as phenothiazines and tricyclic antidepressants, can cause prolonged QT intervals. Organo-phosphate poisoning is another cause of prolonged QT intervals resulting in TdP. Recent studies have highlighted Erhythromycin-related antibiotics with antihistamines contribute to a high incidence of arrhythmias and reported deaths through similar effects on conduction.

Other causes of Torsade are electrolyte disturbances such as hypokalemia and hypomagnesemia. Also, the use of liquid protein and other quick-weight-loss products has been implicated in electrolyte-induced TdP.

Intervention. The use of magnesium IV with an infusion may be indicated because of its effectiveness in stabilizing membrane potential. Where TdP is caused by other than cardiac drugs—the tricylics—treatment includes giving the antidote specific to the offending drug. Correcting this arrhythmia may require multiple defibrillation attempts. When this occurs, and there is a short time where a reasonable rhythm is seen, transcutaneous pacing (TCP) should be initiated at a rapid rate.

This rapid pacing will dominate depolarization and control the rhythm. Transvenous pacing can replace TCP as soon as possible, lessening the patient's discomfort.

Magnesium is the drug of choice. Prolonged QT does not preclude TdP. However, the instances of occurrence are frequent enough to warrant vigilant observation.

Initial treatment for sustained TdP is defibrillation and often requires multiple defibrillation attempts. Torsade frequently persists with increasing duration even after conversion. When this happens, definitive treatment is to initiate transcutaneous pacing at a more rapid rate than the TdP thus preventing its recurrence. This is called *overdrive pacing*. Overdrive pacing can be initiated only between episodes of TdP. Overdrive pacing DOES NOT stop the TdP.

VENTRICULAR FLUTTER

This rhythm is rarely seen because its deteriorates rapidly into ventricular fibrillation. The ECG characteristics of ventricular flutter are:

1. P Wave: P waves may not be distinguishable during ventricular flutter, although atrial activity, dissociated from ventricular activity, may not be affected.
2. PR Interval: Since atrial activity is dissociated from ventricular activity, a PR interval is not measurable.
3. QRS Complex: The QRS complex duration is usually greater than 0.12 second and bizarre in appearance. The T wave may not be separated from the QRS complex.
4. QRS Rate: The ventricular rate is 250 to 350 per minute. Atrial activity often is not determinable.
5. QRS Rhythm: The rhythm is regular or slightly irregular. In ventricular flutter, undulating waves are seen rising and falling.

When the ventricular rate is this fast, the patient is unstable. The rhythm requires immediate unsynchronized cardioversion. Any atrial activity may be un-

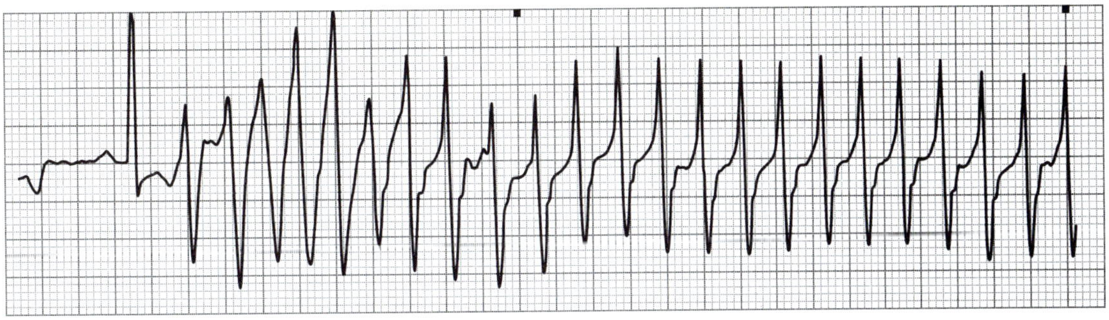

Figure 7-16 An ECG tracing showing a sinus beat followed by an R-on-T PVC, which caused ventricular flutter as confirmed on a 12-lead ECG.

affected. The rhythm is usually short lived, deteriorating into ventricular fibrillation within a very short time. Figure 7-16 is an example of ventricular flutter.

VENTRICULAR FIBRILLATION

Multiple, disorganized complexes characterize ventricular fibrillation and cause cardiac arrest. Ventricular fibrillation may be of sudden onset or may follow PVCs, ventricular tachycardia, and ventricular flutter, or it can occur without any warning ectopic.

Ventricular fibrillation is a terminal rhythm. This means that there is no natural conversion to a normal rhythm. There are no intermittent episodes of ventricular fibrillation.

Clinically, there is no pulse and no cardiac output with ventricular fibrillation. Occasionally, there are erratic movements in the extremities, or agonal breath sounds may accompany this rhythm. The practitioner should not presume that because these movements occur, the rhythm must not be ventricular fibrillation. These are terminal events accompanying the fibrillation.

Ventricular fibrillation may be confused with artifact, for example, when the patient is unresponsive, in a seizure state, or shivering. Assess and confirm pulses and responsiveness. The ECG characteristics of ventricular fibrillation are as follows:

1. P Wave — P waves are unidentifiable.
2. PR Interval: — There is no measurable PR interval.
3. QRS Complex: — There are no discrete QRS complexes.
4. QRS Rate: — Unable to determine
5. QRS Rhythm: — The rhythm is chaotic, with multiple, disorganized contractions of the ventricles.

Figure 7-17 shows three examples of ventricular fibrillation.

Coarse versus Fine Ventricular Fibrillation

Despite the chaos, ventricular fibrillation has a direction to the flow of current. It is easily recognized in a lead parallel to that flow of current and often referred to as *coarse*. If the flow is off in another direction, the amplitude may be diminished.

If the fibrillation is of low amplitude, frequently called *fine* v-fib, it may be confused with asystole. Switch to lead I and lead III to differentiate between ventricular fibrillation and asystole.

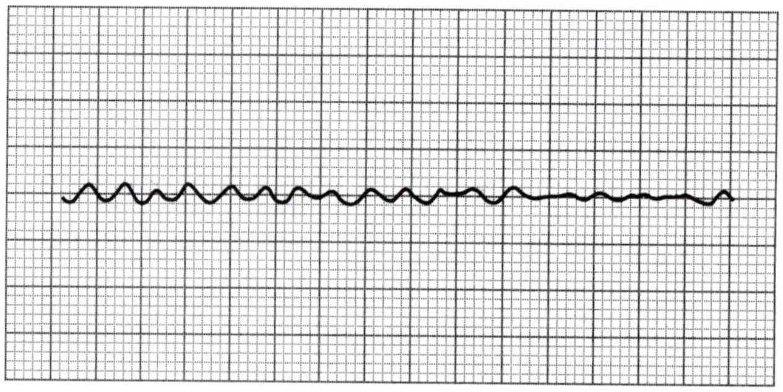

(A)

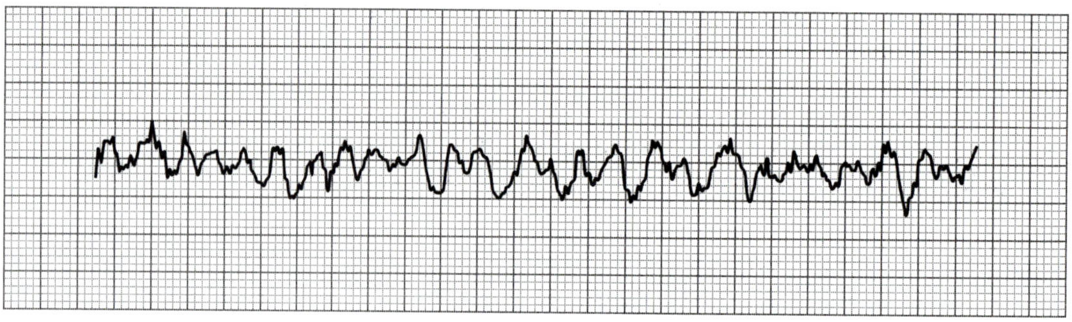

(B)

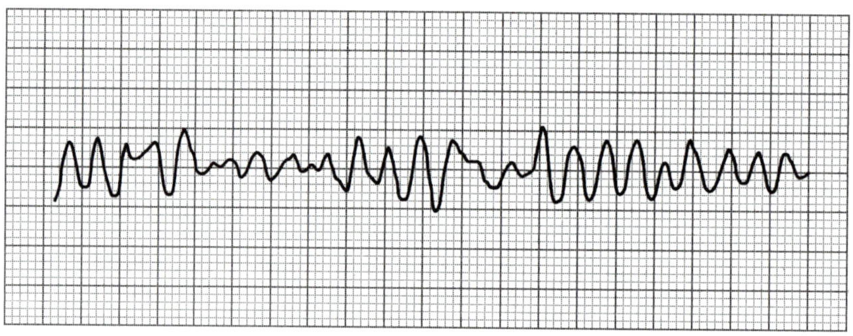

(C)

Figure 7-17 ECG tracings from three patients with ventricular fibrillation.

Once ventricular fibrillation is confirmed, whether fine or coarse, immediate defibrillation is the treatment of choice. There is no clinical difference between fine versus coarse ventricular defibrillation. The term, *coarse* ventricular fibrillation does not imply a more easily converted rhythm; nor does the term, *fine* ventricular fibrillation imply a more lethal situation. Figure 7-18A and B are illustrations of ventricular fibrillation of varying amplitudes.

VENTRICULAR ESCAPE: IDIOVENTRICULAR RHYTHM

With abnormal ventricular depolarization, the ventricular pacemaker is not as efficient as the supraventricular pacemakers. It is the lowest of the series of pacemakers and may become dominant when the higher pacemakers have failed. It may be an "escape" or "safety" rhythm and should never be suppressed.

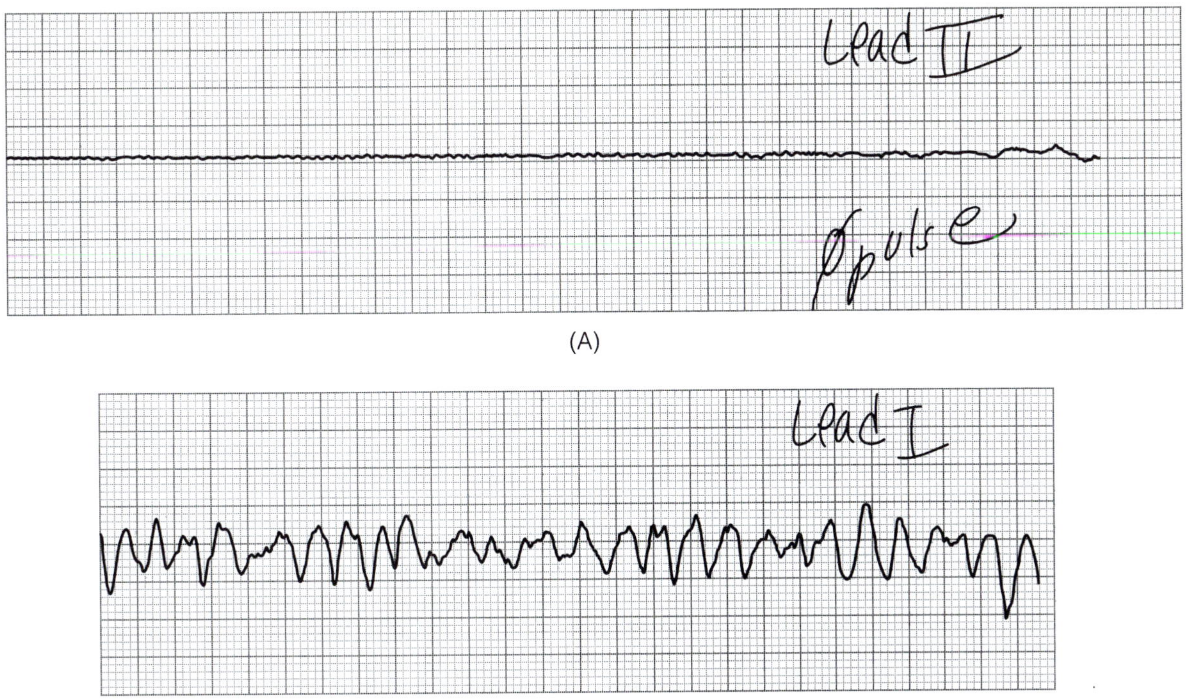

(A)

(B)

Figure 7-18 ECG tracings from the same patient. (A) An apparent asystole or fine ventricular fibrillation. (B) Ventricular fibrillation confirmed on lead I.

Idioventricular rhythm (IVR) appears in the presence of depressed conduction and the ventricles assume the control of the rhythm. The ventricles have the ability to initiate impulses at 20 to 40 beats per minute. The rhythm is usually regular.

Idioventricular rhythm is clinically significant because it is slow and usually does not produce effective perfusion. IVR may accelerate or progress to ventricular tachycardia or fibrillation.

Initial therapies should be directed to *accelerating* the more normal rhythms and subsequently the ventricular rate. For instance, blocking the vagus with atropine may provoke the sinus or junction to generate potential and take control. The ECG characteristics of idioventricular rhythm are as follows:

1. P Wave: P waves may not be present. If they are, they are independent of the IVR.
2. PR Interval: There is no measurable PR interval.
3. QRS Complex: The QRS complex duration is usually greater than 0.10 second, often greater than 0.12 second. However, a ventricular ectopic that occurs within the ventricular fascicles can elicit a narrower than expected QRS.
4. QRS Rate: The inherent rate of the ventricular pacemaker is 20 to 40 beats per minute.
5. QRS Rhythm: The rhythm is usually regular.

Figure 7-19 consists of examples of idioventricular rhythm.

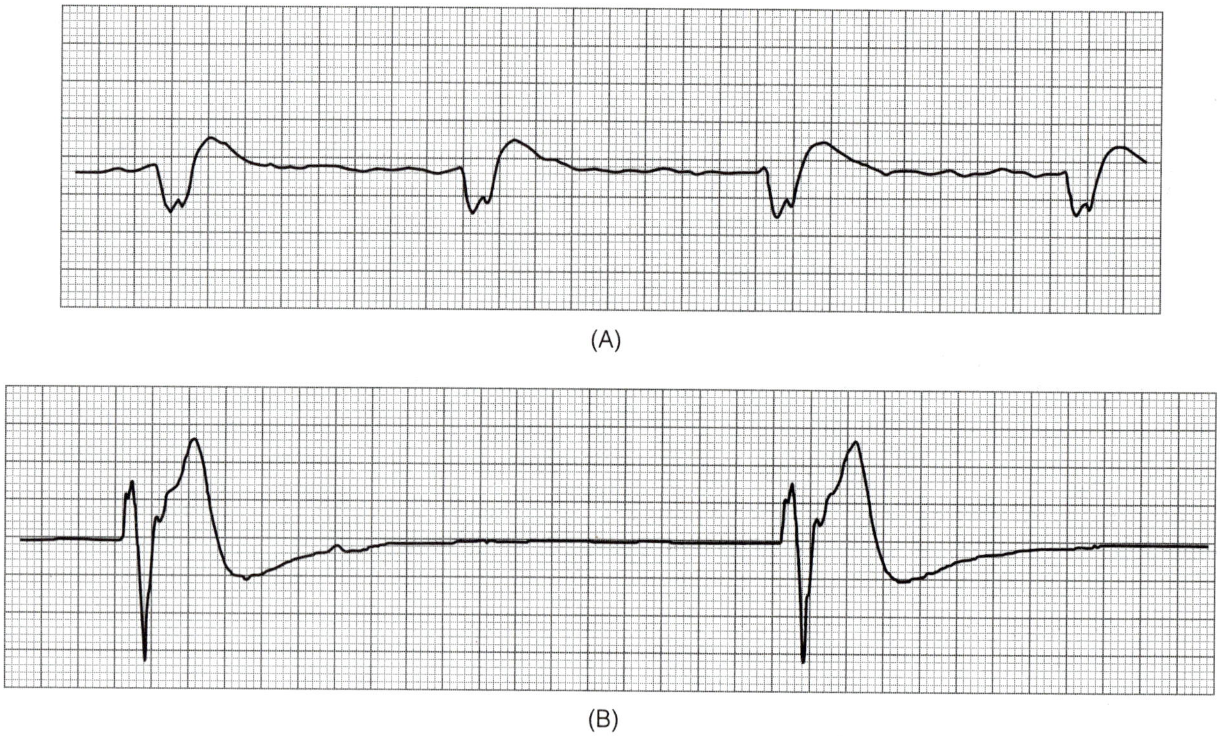

Figure 7-19 (A) An ECG tracings showing idioventricular rhythm at 37 per minute. (B) An idioventricular rhythm at 16 per minute. Both patients were pulseless and did not respond to epinephrine or atropine or to trancutaneous pacing.

ACCELERATED IDIOVENTRICULAR RHYTHM

Accelerated idioventricular rhythm (AIVR) is three or more successive beats in a row, with a rate between 40 and 100 beats per minute. AIVR often begins with a long coupling interval and terminates when the sinus rate emerges at a time when it can conduct through to the ventricles. The ECG characteristics of accelerated idioventricular rhythm are as follows:

1. P Wave: P waves may not be present. If they are, they are independent of the IVR.
2. PR Interval: There is no measurable PR interval.
3. QRS Complex: The QRS complex duration is usually greater than 0.10 second, often greater than 0.12 second. When the origin of a ventricular ectopic is within the ventricular fascicle, the QRS may not exceed 0.12 second.
4. QRS Rate: The accelerated rate of the ventricular pacemaker is 40 to 100 beats per minute.
5. QRS Rhythm: The rhythm is usually regular.

Figure 7-20 is an example of atrial fibrillation progressing to accelerated idioventricular rhythm.

Cause

Accelerated idioventricular rhythm occurs when an area of enhanced automaticity exists within the ventricular conduction system. When the rate is similar to the

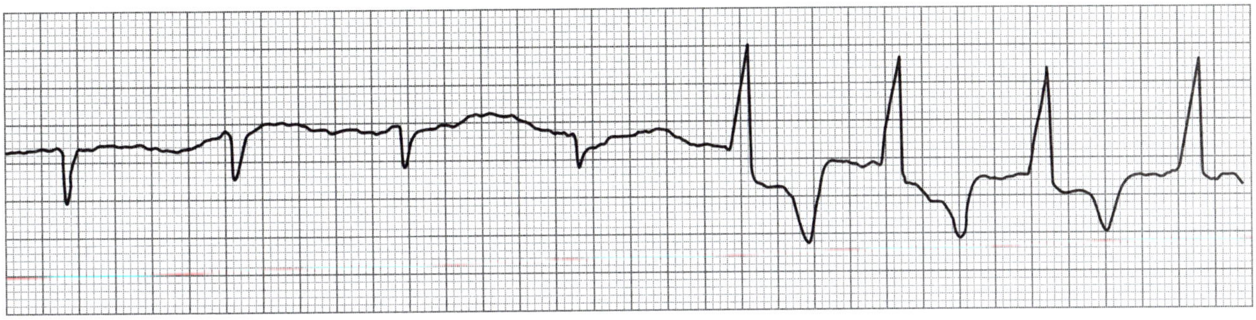

Figure 7-20 An ECG tracing showing atrial fibrillation with an accelerated junctional rhythm at 67 per minute progressing to an accelerated idioventricular rhythm at 75 per minute.

underlying sinus rate, it will begin and end with ventricular fusion beats. Fusion beats are created when ventricular and supraventricular forces collide or fuse and create a different QRS. Fusion beats at the onset show the progressive dominance of the ventricular focus; fusion beats at the end of AIVR show the return to dominance by the supraventricular pacemaker. Figure 7-21 shows AIVR for four beats followed by two fusion beats.

With abnormal ventricular depolarization, the ventricular pacemaker is not as efficient as the supraventricular pacemakers. An idioventricular escape mechanism is the lowest of the series of pacemakers and may become dominant when the higher pacemakers have failed. It may be an "escape" or "safety" rhythm and should not be suppressed. It can be seen post-MI or post-reperfusion procedures.

Intervention

In most cases, intervention for idioventricular rhythm or AIVR with slower rates calls for acceleration of some higher order of rhythm. The use of atropine may block the action of the vagus so that sinus or junctional escape rhythms may surface and take over. The application of the transcutaneous pacemaker is also appropriate.

ABERRANT VENTRICULAR CONDUCTION

Abnormal ventricular activation will occur if one or more of the bundle branches is/are partially refractory at the time of the next electrical stimulation. The term is

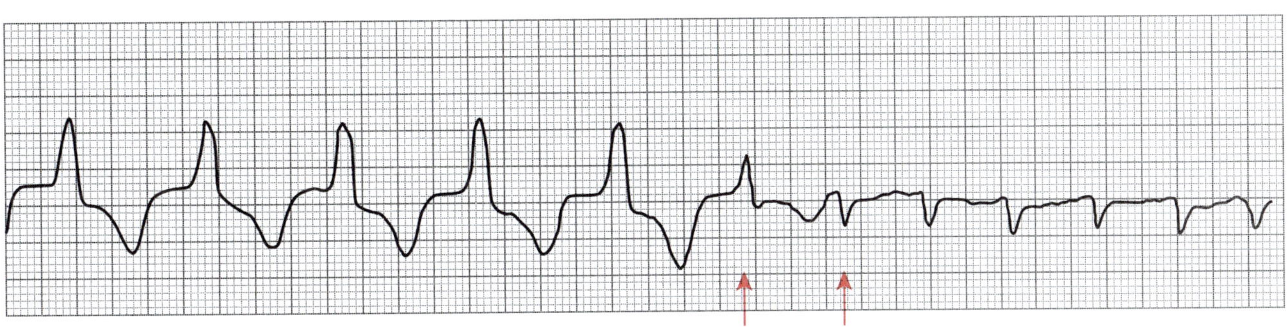

Figure 7-21 An ECG tracing showing AIVR at 84 per minute progressing to atrial fibrillation. Note the two fusion beats commonly seen with AIVR as the dominant supraventricular rhythm resumes control.

usually applied when a PAC occurs and when there is a transient AV conduction defect or, more commonly, a right bundle branch block.

Some PACs have *deviated* from the normal conduction pathways and produce changing QRS complexes that appear ventricular in origin. Therefore, it is important for the examiner to look for the premature P′ that may be hidden in the previous ST segment or T wave.

Another way to recognize the PAC with aberrant ventricular conduction is to carefully plot out the sinus conducted P waves. Remember, in a regularly occurring sinus rhythm, the sinus P′s will plot through, usually undisturbed by a PVC, but be reset by the PAC.

Remember, too, PVCs are different from sinus conducted beats; the QRS is usually opposite from the T wave, and PVCs are usually greater than 0.12 second in duration. However, there are PVCs that are fascicular in origin, and while they are different, they are not broad and bizarre and may be interpreted as PACs. Again, plot out the sinus P waves; they should march through any PVC event without disturbing the cadence of the sinus rhythm.

In most hearts, the right bundle branch has the longest refractory period. Therefore, aberrantly conducted PACs usually find the right bundle still refractory and conduct with a right bundle branch block pattern, that is, rSR′. The PAC with aberrant ventricular conduction may present with its T wave in the same direction. Again, plot out the sinus P waves; they should march through any PVC but be altered if the abnormal beat is atrial in origin.

Although PACs are the source of most aberrantly conducted beats, PJCs can conduct abnormally. These complexes are difficult to differentiate from PVCs. Once again, if these abnormal QRSs occur in a sinus rhythm, the sinus rate will not be disturbed provided there is no retrograde conduction from the His bundle to the atria. QRS complexes that are different from the underlying rhythm should be considered ventricular in origin, until confirmed by 12-lead ECG. Figure 7-22A, B, and C are examples of sinus with PACs and aberrant ventricular conduction.

Intervention. A patient who presents with chest pain and wide complex tachycardia should be treated as though the tachycardia was ventricular in origin until proven otherwise. Intervention in a patient with a slow ventricular rate would be initiated if the patient was symptomatic, hypotensive, and hypoperfusing.

Treatment of a patient with a reasonable ventricular rate would include assessment and intervention for the chest pain and consideration given to the use of lidocaine.

The following is a summary for differentiation of PVC and PAC with aberrancy:

1. Look for the sinus P waves and plot them through the event. Sinus conducted P waves usually plot out independently of the event. The chances of the event being a PVC are better than 12:1 (Conover 1996; Wellens and Conover 1992).
2. If the sinus conducted P waves are disturbed in their cadence and the rhythm is not sinus arrhythmia, look to the left of the event and search for a P′ in the preceding ST segment or T wave.

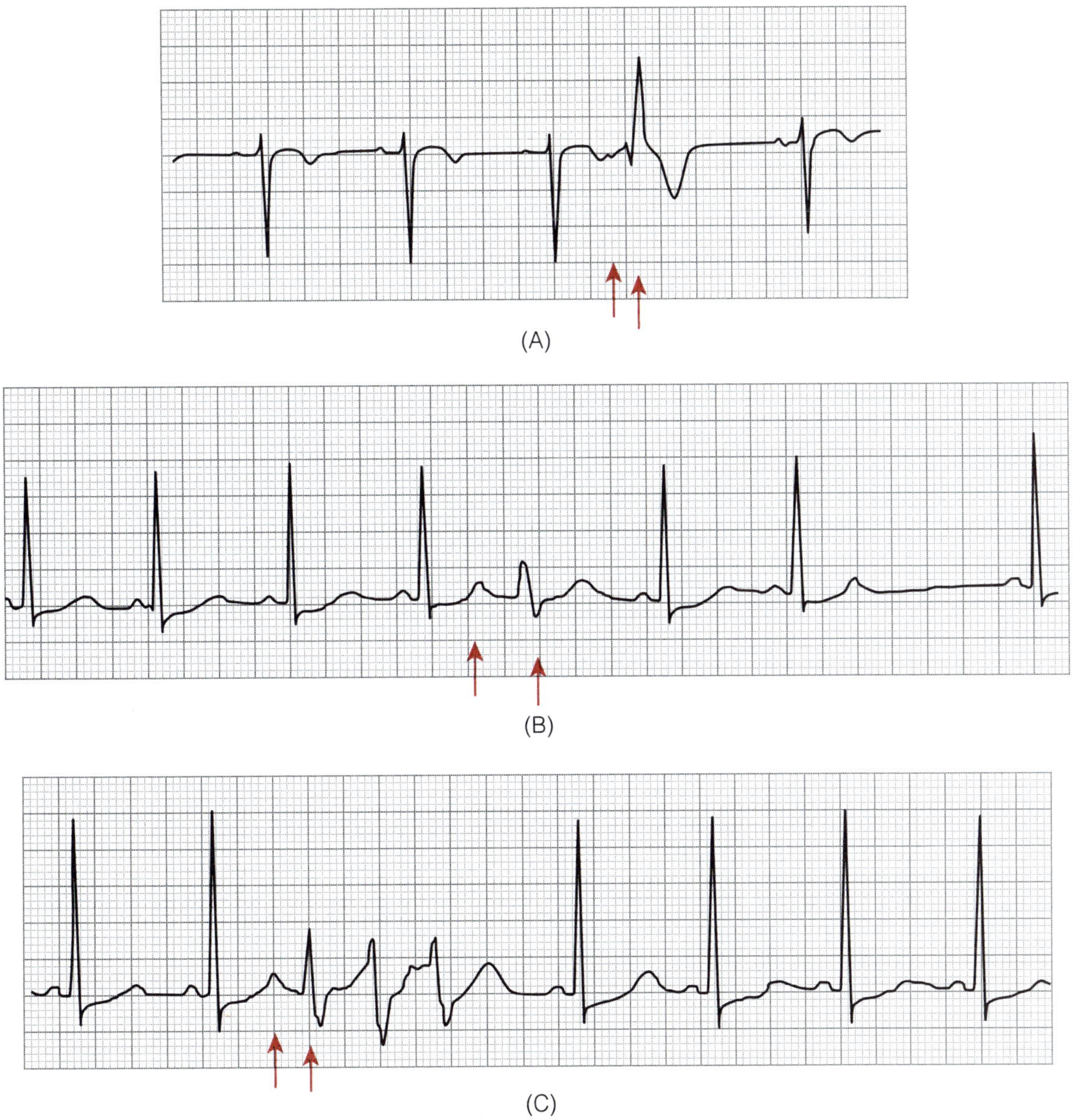

Figure 7-22 Three ECG tracings illustrating aberrant ventricular conduction. Note in (A) there is a PAC in the previous ST segment. The ECG interpretation for (A) would be sinus at 75 per minute with a PAC and aberrant ventricular conduction. Note that the sinus P waves do not plot through the event. In (B) and (C), the T-wave amplitude prior to the aberrant QRSs is increased. The increased amplitude of the T wave is additive, that is, the combined amplitude of the P′ superimposed on the preceding T wave. The ECG interpretation for (B) would be sinus at 75 per minute with a PAC with aberrant ventricular conduction and a nonconducted PAC. Here, too, the sinus P waves do not plot through. (C) would be interpreted as sinus at 75 per minute, 1 to 2 mm ST segment depression, a PAC with aberrant conduction, and a 3-beat run of tachycardia. Note the sinus P waves do not plot through the event. Note that the T wave just prior to the tachycardia is increased in amplitude. That amplitude is ***additive*** and measures as the total of the T wave plus the P wave of complexes prior to the event. PACs that occur this early in the cardiac cycle often find the tissue partially refractory, and thus the impulse conducts abnormally or aberrantly.

3. Look for other PACs and PVCs in the same patient. If you see conducted or blocked PACs, the chance of the event being a PAC with aberrant ventricular conduction is now better than 14:1 (Conover 1996; Wellens and Conover 1992).

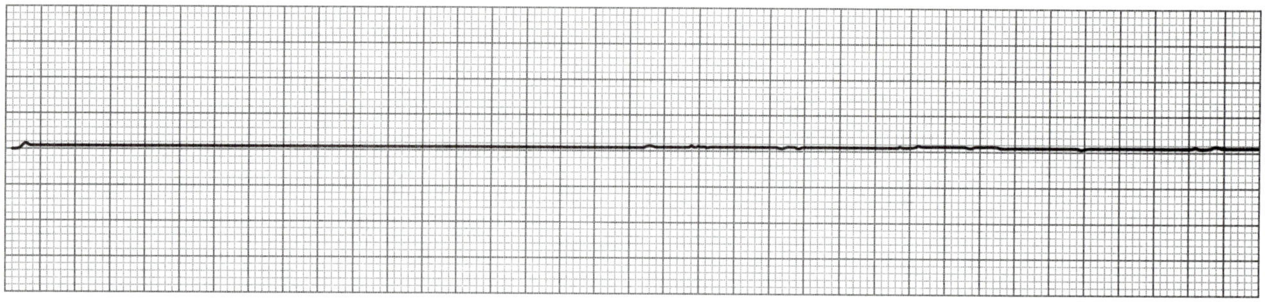

Figure 7-23 ECG tracing illustrating an example of ventricular asystole.

4. If you are dealing with a tachycardia, look at its onset. A PAC will begin the PSVT, and a PVC will begin the tach and/or fib. You also will be able to see the previous QRSs before the event started.
5. Treat the patient clinically. Be aware of drug history if at all possible. If you suspect ventricular tachycardia, then treat the patient accordingly.

ASYSTOLE

Asystole occurs when there are no ventricular complexes, indicating the ventricles are inactive. In some instances, the atria continue to beat in their own time. It is hoped that an escape pacemaker of some kind will take over. Figure 7-23 shows a continuous ECG tracing from a patient with ventricular fibrillation who deteriorated into asystole. Figure 7-24 is a continuous ECG recording of a patient who was defibrillated for ventricular fibrillation and deteriorated into asystole.

Asystole versus Fine Ventricular Fibrillation

Ventricular fibrillation is the result of chaotic activity within the ventricular system. Many fibers are depolarizing, and there is no effective perfusion. When the flow of current is largely parallel to the monitoring lead, the fibrillation is easily recognized. However, when the flow of current is at right angles to the monitoring lead, the EKG may look like asystole. Switch to leads I and III to differentiate asystole from ventricular fibrillation.

Figure 7-25A shows asystole in lead II and confirmed in lead I. Figure 7-25B shows asystole in lead II confirmed as V-fib in lead I.

Intervention

Treatment includes CPR, airway management, and multiple approaches using drugs and devices to initiate and enhance myocardial activity. This includes the use of epinephrine and atropine. Because the cause of asystole is rarely known, pacing should be attempted. The use of transcutaneous pacing is rarely beneficial. However, application and documented lack of response can be comforting to the patient's family, noting that everything possible was attempted.

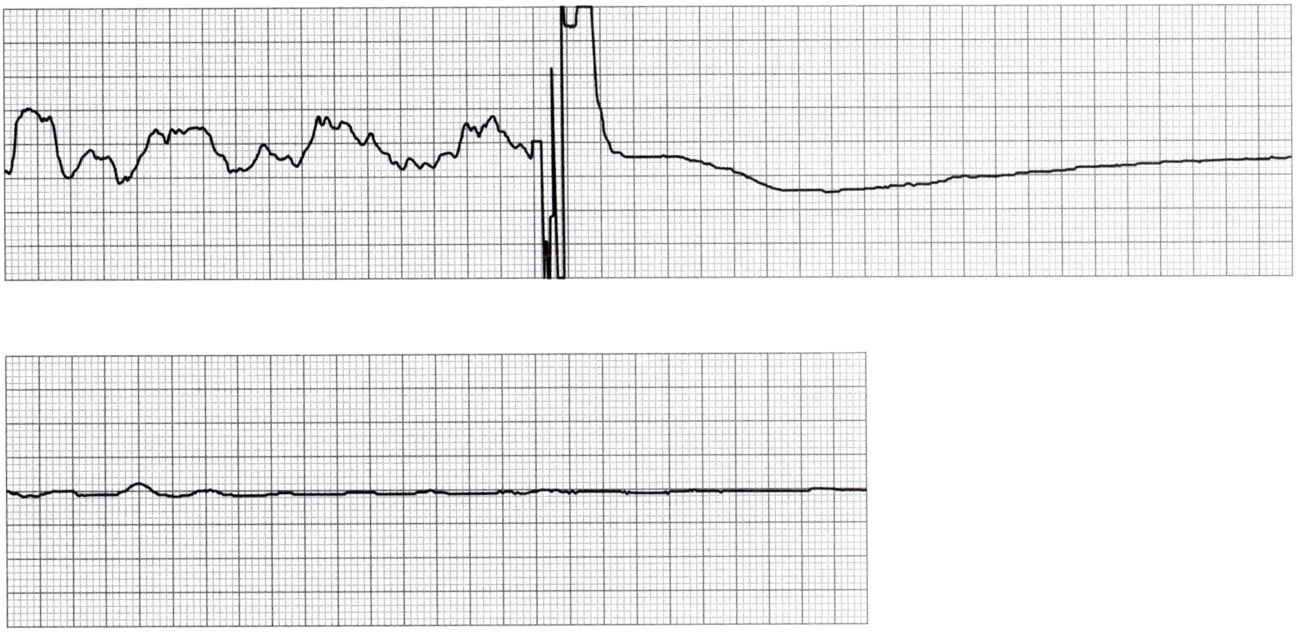

Figure 7-24 A continuous ECG tracing in a patient who was defibrillated. The resulting asystole was confirmed with two leads.

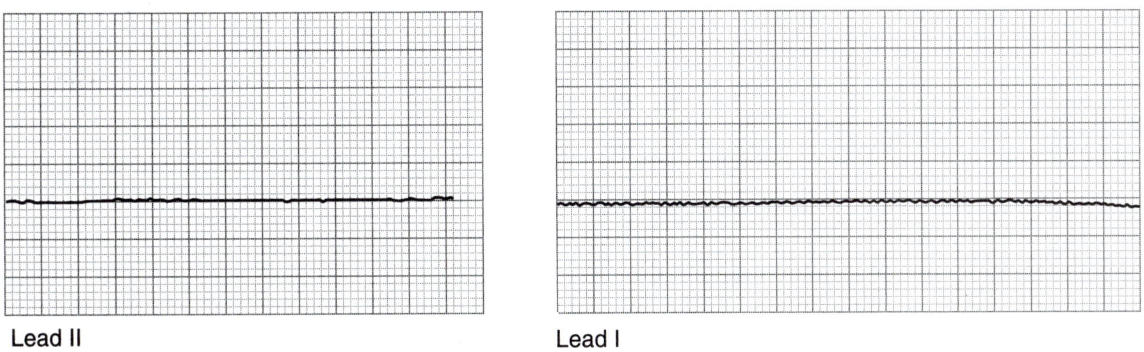

(A)

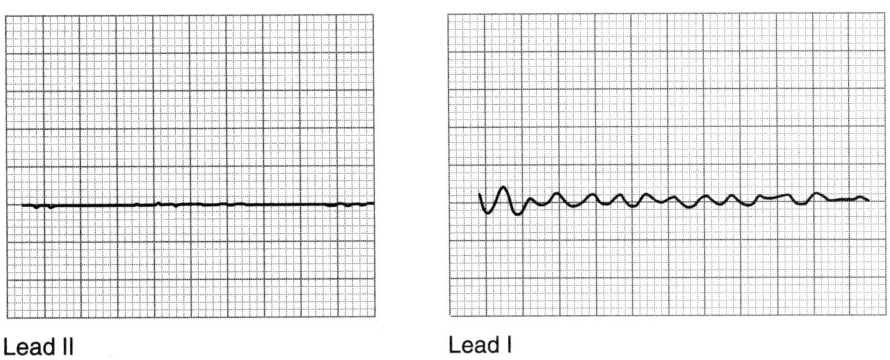

(B)

Figure 7-25 (A) An ECG in a patient where the asystole was confirmed in two leads. (B) The asystole was, in reality, ventricular fibrillation as confirmed in a second lead.

PULSELESS ELECTRICAL ACTIVITY

There are tragic circumstances when the ECG of a patient in cardiac arrest continues to display an identifiable rhythm but the patient is unresponsive and does not have a palpable pulse. The actual ECG rhythm in such cases may present as sinus rhythm, any of the atrial dysrhythmia, AV junctional rhythm, or any of the AV blocks. There may be ectopy of any frequency.

Despite the presence of electrical function (as seen by the ECG), there is no mechanical response, no cardiac output, pulse, or blood pressure, thus the term, *pulseless electrical activity* (PEA).

Electrical mechanical dissociation (EMD), as one explanation, is a catastrophic, physiologic event for which there is little recourse. There are other conditions, termed *mechanical impediments* to cardiac filling and subsequent systole that result in a similar circumstance. These include hypovolemia, tension pneumothorax, severe hypovolemia, and/or hypoxemia, all of which deprive the myocardium of adequate mechanical abilities.

Another cause of PEA is cardiac tamponade. This condition may be reversible, especially when diagnosed quickly and pericardiocentesis is performed. Pericardial effusion may act to mechanically "choke off" the heart by preventing it from adequately filling, therefore, inadequately pumping. The term *tamp* means to plug, and the term *tamponade* is used to describe the situation.

Another case of PEA occurs in cases where the myocardium has sustained injury that may or may not be reversible.

Figure 7-26 is a documented example of a clearly distinct atrial fibrillation in a patient with PEA due to cardiac tamponade confirmed on post mortem examination.

Intervention

Treatment for PEA includes CPR, airway management, and multiple approaches using drugs and devices to initiate and enhance myocardial activity. The treatment also should be directed to identification of the cause of the mechanical impairment to circulation.

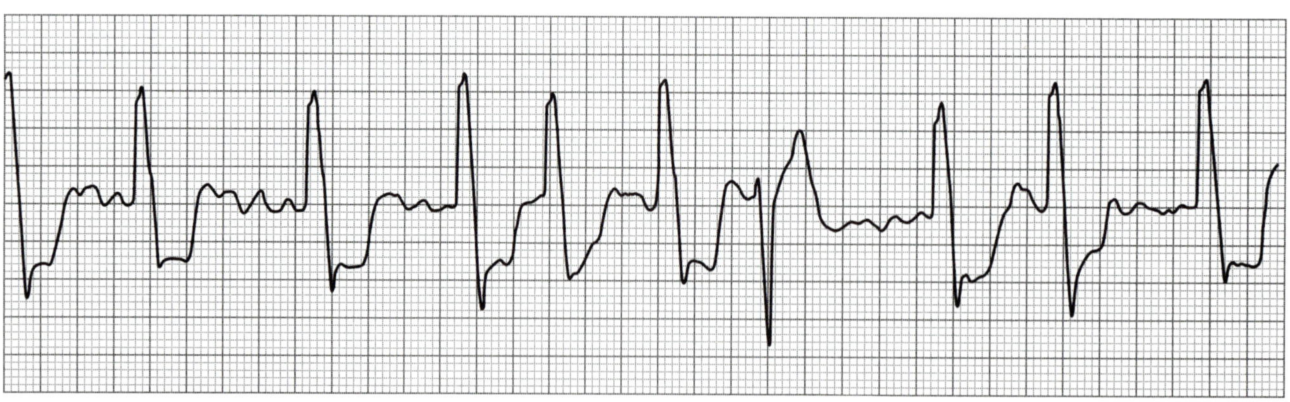

Figure 7-26 An ECG showing atrial fibrillation ventricular rate range of 60 to 100 per minute and a PVC. However, this is a documented example of a patient who was pulseless. Pulmonary embolus and cardiac tamponade were confirmed on autopsy.

SUMMARY

Ventricular ectopy are often signs of myocardial ischemia and hypoxia. They often deteriorate into arrhythmias that are life-threatening. Early recognition and rapid intervention of ventricular ectopics and arrhythmias to protect the patient are some of the critical reasons for the development of CCUs and paramedicine. Table 7-1 is a summary of the characteristics of ECG changes with ventricular mechanisms.

Table 7-1 Guide to ECG analysis of the ventricular mechanisms

	PVC	Idioventricular Rhythm	Accelerated	Tachycardia	Fibrillation	Asystole
P waves	independent or none	independent or none	independent or none	independent or none	unable to see or none	independent or none
P-R Interval						
QRS duration	≥ 0.10 QRS opposite the T wave	≥ 0.10 QRS opposite the T wave	≥ 0.10 QRS opposite the T wave	≥ 0.10 QRS opposite the T wave	≥ 0.10 QRS opposite the T wave	
Rate/minute		20–40	40–100	>100		
Rhythm		regular	regular	regular	irregular	

Table 7-2 Guide to ECG analysis of ectopics

	Atrial	Junctional	Ventricular
P waves	P′ (+) or (-) or none seen; may be lost in previous T or QRS	P′ (-) or none	sinus Ps usually plot through the premature QRS
P-R interval	usually different from the sinus; can be < or > 0 .20	<0.12 sec if the P′ is visible	whatever the sinus is
QRS duration	≤ 0.10	≤ 0.10	>0.10 usually; can be <0.10 if the origin is within the fascicles; QRS is opposite the T wave
Rx	question why; question meds and caffeine/stimulants, medical history; dig; assess for CHF	question why; question meds and medical history; dig	question why; question meds and caffeine/stimulants, medical history; dig

Self-Assessment Exercises

Fill in the Blanks

Complete the statements, and then compare your answers with those in the back of the book.

SINUS RHYTHM	PJC	PAC	PVC
1 (+) P plus QRS	1(-) P′+ QRS or no P	______________	______________
PRI 0.12–0.20	less than 0.12	______________	______________
QRS 0.10 or less	0.10 or less	______________	______________
QRS rate: 60-100/min		______________	______________
QRS rhythm: regular	disturbs sinus cadence	______________	______________

ATRIAL TACH	SINUS TACH	VENTRICULAR TACH
______________	P wave = 1(+)P + QRS	______________
______________	PRI = 0.12– 0.20 second	______________
______________	QRS = 0.10 or less	______________
______________	QRS rate = 100–150	______________
______________	QRS rhythm = regular	______________

ECG Rhythm Identification Practice

For the following rhythms fill in the blanks and then check your answers with those in the back of this book.

Figure 7-27

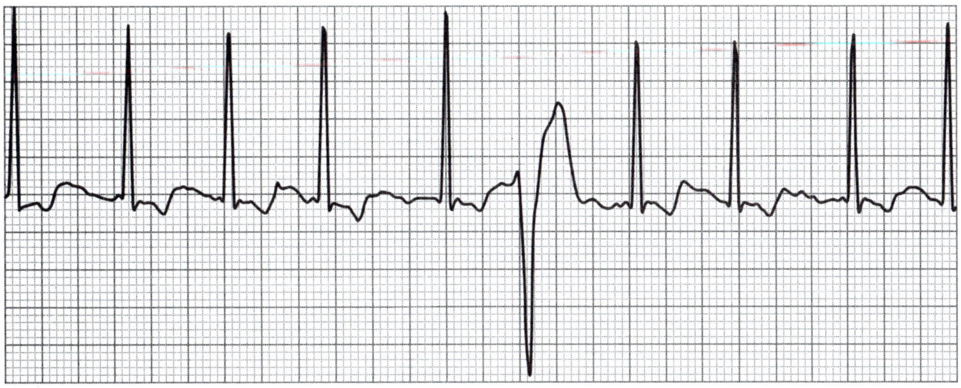

QRS duration ______________ QT ____________
Ventricular rate/rhythm ______________________
Atrial rate/rhythm __________________________
PR interval ________________________________

Identification ______________________________
Symptoms __________________________________
____
Treatment __________________________________

Figure 7-28

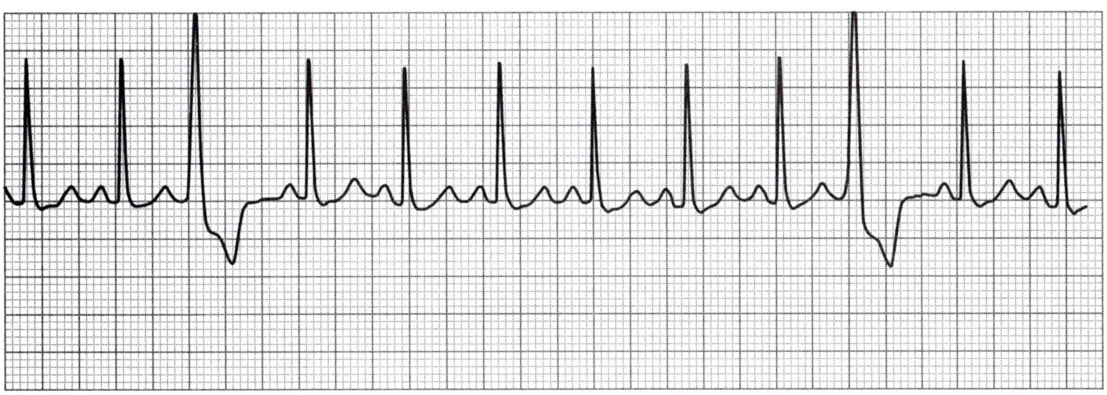

QRS duration ______________ QT ____________
Ventricular rate/rhythm ______________________
Atrial rate/rhythm __________________________
PR interval ________________________________

Identification ______________________________
Symptoms __________________________________
____
Treatment __________________________________

Figure 7-29

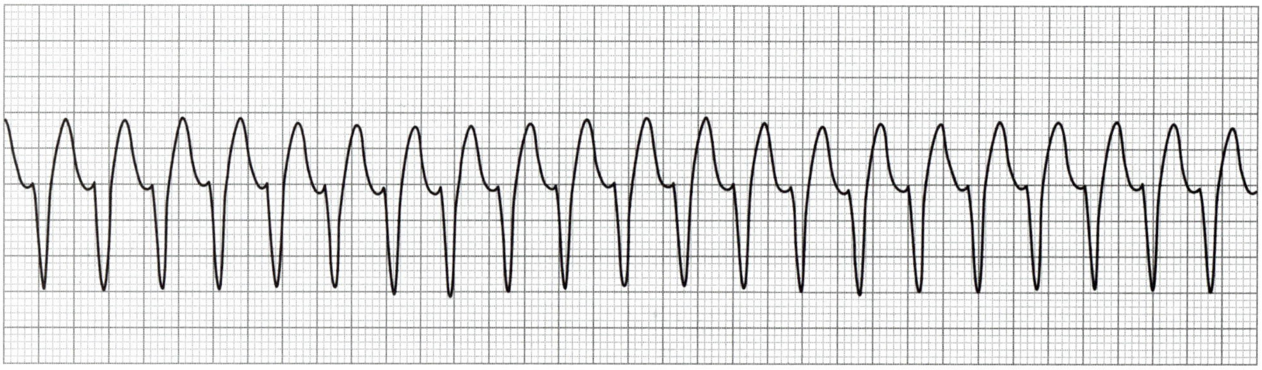

QRS duration ______________ QT ____________

Ventricular rate/rhythm ______________________

Atrial rate/rhythm __________________________

PR interval ________________________________

Identification ______________________________

Symptoms _________________________________

____

Treatment _________________________________

Figure 7-30

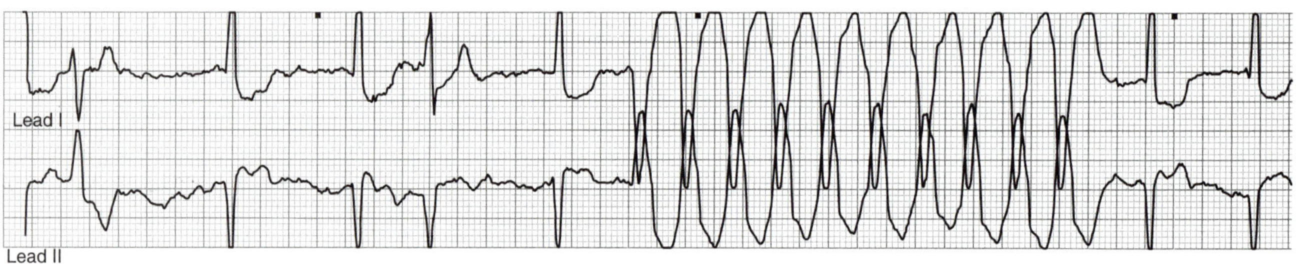

QRS duration ______________ QT ____________

Ventricular rate/rhythm ______________________

Atrial rate/rhythm __________________________

PR interval ________________________________

Identification ______________________________

Symptoms _________________________________

____

Treatment _________________________________

Figure 7-31

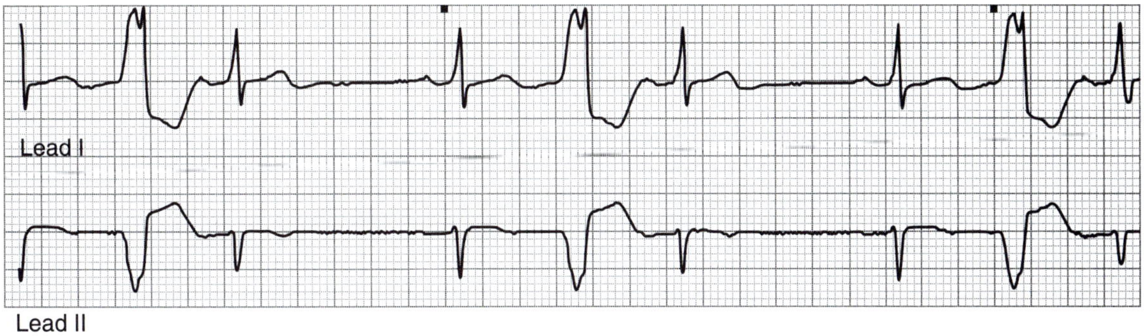

QRS duration ________________ QT ____________

Ventricular rate/rhythm ________________________

Atrial rate/rhythm ____________________________

PR interval __________________________________

Identification ________________________________

Symptoms ____________________________________

____

Treatment ____________________________________

Figure 7-32

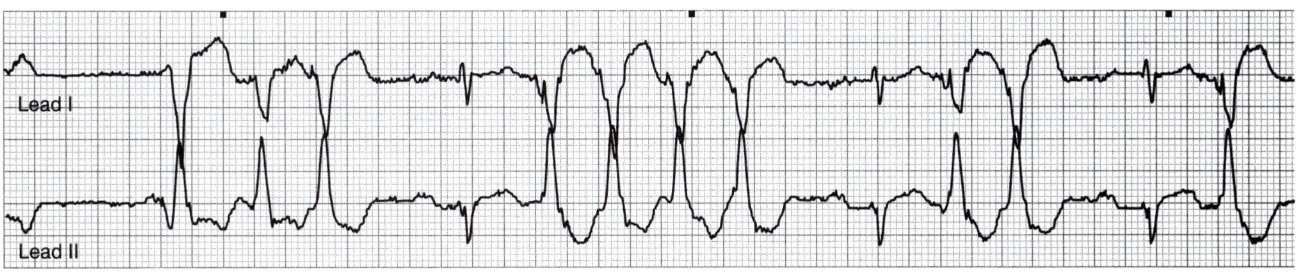

QRS duration ________________ QT ____________

Ventricular rate/rhythm ________________________

Atrial rate/rhythm ____________________________

PR interval __________________________________

Identification ________________________________

Symptoms ____________________________________

____

Treatment ____________________________________

Figure 7-33

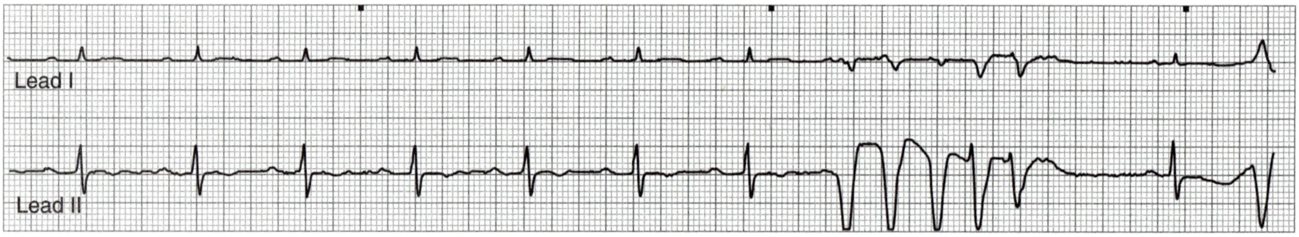

QRS duration ________________ QT ______________

Ventricular rate/rhythm __________________________

Atrial rate/rhythm ______________________________

PR interval ____________________________________

Identification ______________________________________

Symptoms ____

____

Treatment ____

Figure 7-34

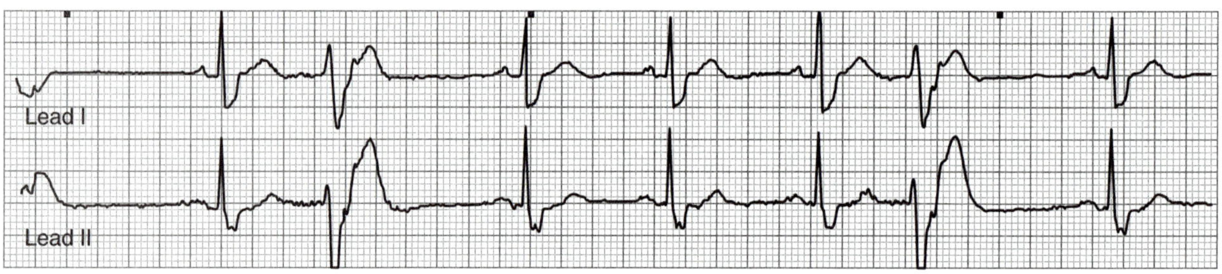

QRS duration ________________ QT ______________

Ventricular rate/rhythm __________________________

Atrial rate/rhythm ______________________________

PR interval ____________________________________

Identification ______________________________________

Symptoms ____

____

Treatment ____

Figure 7-35

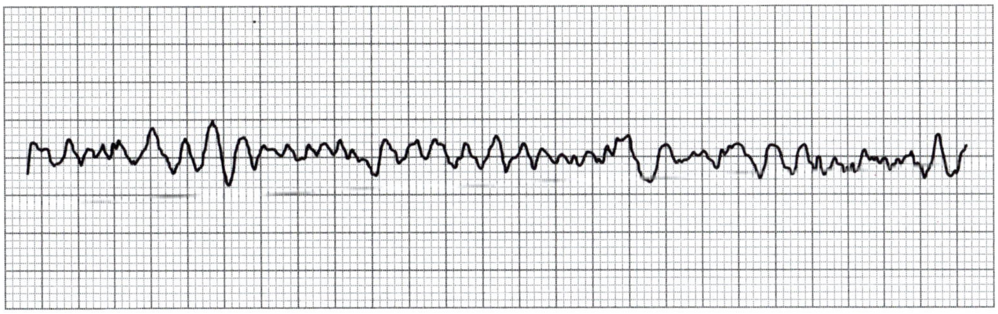

QRS duration ________________ QT ______________
Ventricular rate/rhythm ________________________
Atrial rate/rhythm ____________________________
PR interval ___________________________________

Identification ________________________________
Symptoms _____________________________________
____
Treatment ____________________________________

Figure 7-36

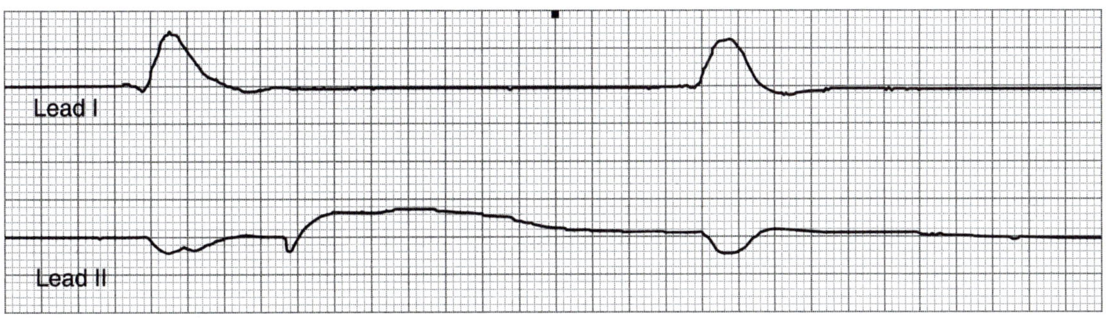

QRS duration ________________ QT ______________
Ventricular rate/rhythm ________________________
Atrial rate/rhythm ____________________________
PR interval ___________________________________

Identification ________________________________
Symptoms _____________________________________
____
Treatment ____________________________________

Figure 7-37

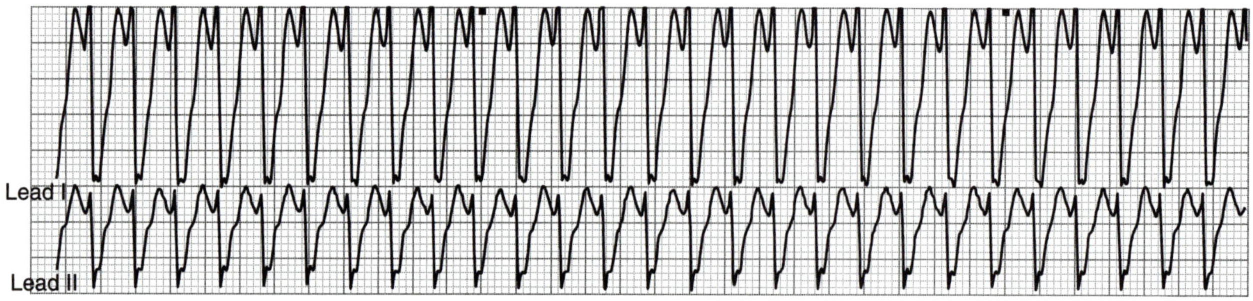

QRS duration ______________ QT ____________

Ventricular rate/rhythm ____________________

Atrial rate/rhythm _________________________

PR interval ________________________________

Identification _____________________________

Symptoms __________________________________

____

Treatment __________________________________

Figure 7-38

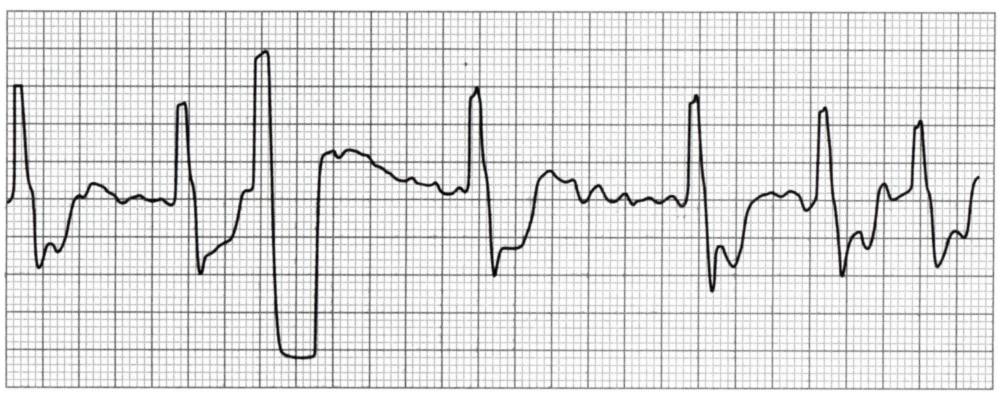

QRS duration ______________ QT ____________

Ventricular rate/rhythm ____________________

Atrial rate/rhythm _________________________

PR interval ________________________________

Identification _____________________________

Symptoms __________________________________

____

Treatment __________________________________

Figure 7-39

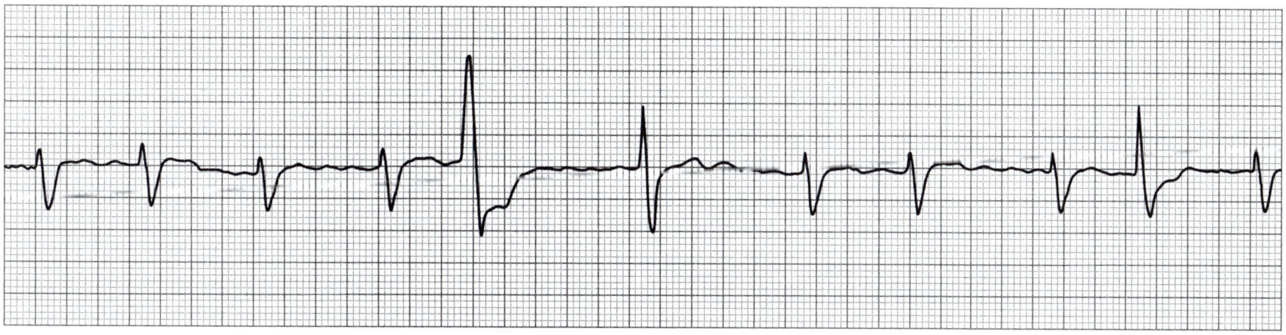

QRS duration ________________ QT ______________

Ventricular rate/rhythm __________________________

Atrial rate/rhythm ______________________________

PR interval ____________________________________

Identification ______________________________

Symptoms ___________________________________

____

Treatment ___________________________________

Figure 7-40

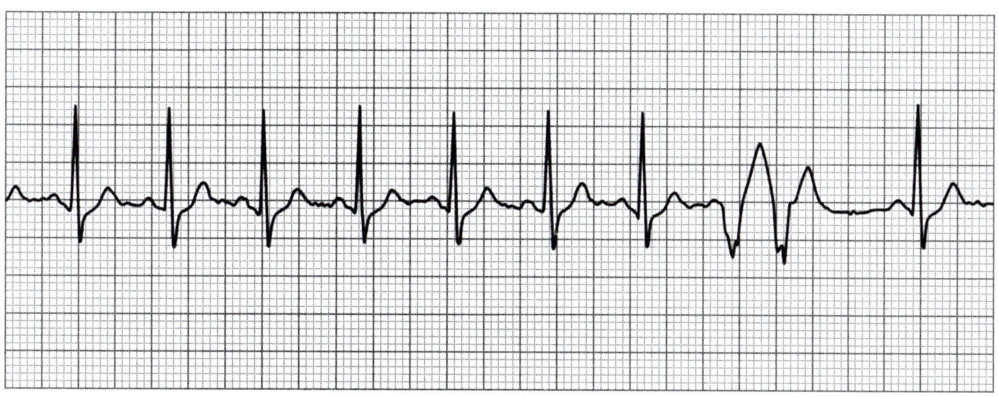

QRS duration ________________ QT ______________

Ventricular rate/rhythm __________________________

Atrial rate/rhythm ______________________________

PR interval ____________________________________

Identification ______________________________

Symptoms ___________________________________

____

Treatment ___________________________________

References

American Heart Association. *Currents in emergency cardiac care.* Vol. 1, No. 1, 1; 1990.

American Heart Association. *Textbook of advanced cardiac life support.* Chapter 4; 1994.

American National Standards Institute (ANSI)/Association for the Advancement of Medical Instrumentation (AAMI). *Cardiac defibrillator devices.* DF-2-1989.

Conover, M. B. *Nurse's pocket guide to electrocardiography* (3rd ed.). St. Louis, MO: C. V. Mosby; 1994.

Conover, M. B. *Understanding electrocardiography: Arrhythmias and the 12-lead ECG* (7th ed.). St. Louis, MO: Mosby-Year Book; 1996.

Conover, M. B. & Wellens, H. J. *The ECG in emergency decision making.* Philadelphia: W. B. Saunders; 1993.

Coumel, P., Leclercq, J. F. & Dessertenne, F. Torsade de pointes. In Josephson, M. E. & Wellens H. J. (Eds.). *Tachycardias: Mechanisms, Diagnosis, Treatment.* Philadelphia: Lea and Febiger; 1984.

Crocket, P. J., Droppert, B. M., Higgins, S. E., & Richards, R. K. *Defibrillation: What you should know.* Redmond, WA; Physio-Control; 1996.

Cummins, R. 0. Automated external defibrillators: Where we've been and where we're going. *Resident and Staff Physician.* Vol. 40, No. 1, 61–67; 1994.

Emergency Cardiac Care Subcommittee and Subcommittees, American Heart Association. Guidelines for cardiopulmonary resuscitation and emergency cardiac care. *JAMA.* 1994.

Ewy, G. A., Hellman, D. A., McClkug, S., et al. Influence of ventilation phase on transthoracic impedance and defibrillation effectiveness. *Critical Care Medicine.* Vol. 8, 164–166; 1980.

Goldberger, E. *Textbook of Clinical Cardiology.* St. Louis, MO: C. V. Mosby; 1982.

Mandel, W. J. (Ed). *Cardiac arrhythmias: Their mechanisms, diagnoses and management* (2nd ed.). Philadelphia: Lippincott; 1987.

Marriott, H. J. *Practical electrocardiography* (8th ed.). Baltimore: Williams and Wilkins; 1988.

Marriott, H. J., & Conover, M. B. *Advanced concepts in arrhythmias,* 2nd ed. St. Louis, MO: C. V. Mosby; 1989.

Schuster, M. & Keller, J. Effect of fire department first-responder automated defibrillation. *Annals of Emergency Medicine,* Vol. 22, No. 4, 106–112; 1993.

Wellens, H.J., & Durrer, D. *Electrical stimulation of the heart in the study and treatment of the tachycardias.* Baltimore, MD: University Park Press, 1987.

CHAPTER 8

AV Conduction Defects: Conduction Problems in the AV Node and His Bundle

Premise

1. In the AV conduction defects, there is a pathology that exists or a medication has been administered that causes an unnatural conduction delay. These problems are simple to analyze if you recall what is normal conduction.
2. The naming of the arrhythmias gives an easy-to-recognize indication as to the source, pacer, or ectopic and the resulting fast or slow heart rate. The titles of the AV conduction defects are less clear and can be mastered if you keep in mind the components of the electrical wiring of the heart.
3. Keep in mind that the various *grades* or *degrees* of second-degree AV block are recognized by the configuration of the QRS complex and sometimes by the frequency and sudden occurrence of the block.

Objectives

After reading the chapter and completing the Self-Assessment Exercises, the student should be able to

1. identify the AV conduction defects
2. realize the implications of the defect

Key Terms

complete AV block
first-degree AV block
infranodal
Mobitz
second-degree AV block
Type I
Type II
Wenckebach

Introduction

Recall that electrical activation normally begins with the SA node, and the wave of depolarization spreads outward through the atrial muscle to the AV junction. In the

AV junction, there is a natural delay in the AV node and then the impulse travels down the His bundle and its branches into the ventricles. This is especially helpful in atrial flutter and fibrillation. In these arrhythmias, the AV node functions in a therapeutic manner, protecting the ventricles from a rapid and chaotic atrial rate.

infranodal
Below or inferior to the AV node/His bundle

In AV conduction defects, the conduction of the normal wave front can be delayed or blocked at any point after atrial depolarization. This can occur within the AV node or below the His bundle or **infranodal** or involving one, two, or all of the bundle branches. Analysis of the ECG must be correlated to patient presentation and within the clinical setting in which it occurs.

In the previous chapters, each of the arrhythmias was identified by two terms; the *pacemaker* or *ectopic*, and the resulting heart rate and rhythm. For example, in sinus tachycardia, the pacemaker is in the sinus node, and the heart rate is greater than 100 beats per minute. In ventricular tachycardia, the pacemaker is in ventricular tissue, and the heart rate is greater than 100 beats per minute.

When identifying the AV conduction defects, the name of the arrhythmia does not identify the pathology. The student must learn by rote, the specific term associated with the conduction defect.

SINUS RHYTHM WITH FIRST-DEGREE AV BLOCK

first-degree block
A delay in AV conduction reflected in a PR interval greater than 0.20 second

The time taken by the spread of depolarization from the SA node to the ventricular muscle is seen on the ECG by the PR interval and does not take more than 0.20 second. Interference with the conduction process within the AV node results in a lengthening of the PR segment and thus the PR interval. When this lengthening of the PR interval is consistently greater than 0.20 second, this is **first-degree AV block**. ECG characteristics of first-degree AV block are

1. P Wave: The P waves are positive and uniform in lead II if the SA node is the pacemaker. Every P wave is followed by a QRS complex.
2. PR Interval: The PR interval is greater than 0.20 second and constant from beat to beat.
3. QRS Complex: The QRS complex duration is 0.10 or less. Every QRS complex is preceded by a P wave.
4. QRS Rate: The rate is dependent on the basic rhythm. If the basic rhythm is sinus, the rate is constant between 60 and 100 per minute.
5. QRS Rhythm: The rhythm is regular as a sinus rhythm is. If sinus arrhythmia is present, the rhythm will vary accordingly.

Table 8-1 shows the comparison in ECG configurations between sinus rhythm and first-degree AV block. Note the only difference is the PR interval.

First-degree atrioventricular (AV) block represents a delay in the transmission of impulses from the atria to the ventricles. This is seen in the ECG by a PR segment greater than 0.12 second. The resulting PR interval will be greater than 0.20 second.

It is vital to differentiate between a prolonged PR segment and a P wave of prolonged duration since both conditions result in a PR interval greater than 0.20 second.

Table 8-1 The comparison in ECG configurations between sinus rhythm and first-degree AV block.

	Sinus	First-degree AV Block
P waves	1 (+) per QRS	1 (+) per QRS
PR interval	0.12–0.20 second	>0.20 second and consistent
QRS duration	≤ 0.10	≤ 0.10
Rate/minute	60–100	60–100
Rhythm	regular	regular

Cause of First-degree AV Block

First-degree AV block is not of itself critical. Clinically, it may be a sign of proximal right coronary artery disease and may be the result of digitalis. First-degree AV block is seen as a congenital anomoly during pregnancy, with endocarditis, myocarditis, electrolyte disturbances, and as a result of advancing age.

Intervention

Typically, the overall heart rate is within normal limits, the patient's symptoms are not related to the rhythm, and no intervention is required.

In patients on digitalis therapy, the concurrent bradycardia should warrant assessment and possible discontinuance of the drug. Figure 8-1 is an ECG rhythm strip showing first-degree AV block.

SINUS WITH SECOND-DEGREE AV BLOCK, THE INTERMITTENT CONDUCTION DEFECTS

In **second-degree AV block**, one or more sinus impulses fail to reach the ventricles. Most sinus beats are conducted, and the PR may be normal or prolonged but always

second-degree AV block

A form of heart block characterized by a missing QRS. A disorder in which one or more of the sinus impulses are not conducted along the AV pathway. One or more sinus impulses are blocked and are unable to stimulate the ventricles.

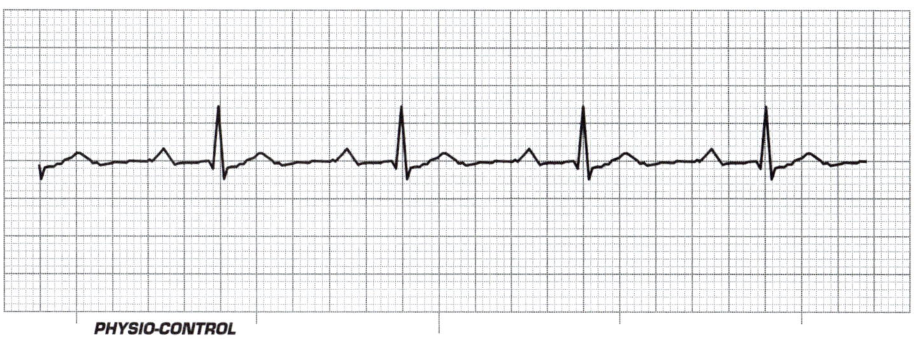

Figure 8-1 An ECG tracing illustrating a sinus rhythm at 60 per minute with a consistently prolonged PR interval, that is greater than 0.20 second. Note the PR segment is greater than 0.12 second. The ECG interpretation would be sinus at 60 per minute with first-degree (1°) AV block.

constant. The hallmark of second-degree block is that there is a predictable P wave and an occasional absent QRS complex. There are several variations of second-degree AV block.

It is critical to plot out the cadence of the P waves to differentiate between a nonconducted PAC and an AV block. In the AV conduction defects, sinus P waves will plot through. Certainly, it is possible to have a sinus arrhythmia with AV block, but the gradual increase and decrease in sinus rate is easy to plot out. The ECG characteristics of second-degree AV block are as follows:

1. P Wave: The P waves are positive and uniform in configuration in lead II. Not every P wave is followed by a QRS complex. Sometimes they conduct, and sometimes they do not; the P wave plots through regularly but may be difficult to identify.
2. PR Interval After the dropped QRS, the PR interval of the conducted beat is constant and may even be greater than the normal 0.20 second.
3. QRS Complex: The QRS complex duration is 0.10 second or less when the disease is within the AV node.
4. QRS Rate: Because of the block in the AV node, the atrial rate is different from the ventricular rate.
5. QRS Rhythm: The rhythm is regular when there is a consistent atrial to ventricular relationship, for example, 2:1. If this relationship varies, the rhythm is irregular.

Figure 8-2 is an ECG tracing showing the missing QRS. Note that the PR after the missed QRS is constant.

Often, atrial rate is once or twice that of the ventricular rate. When the ventricles cannot respond because of the refractoriness of the AV node, the atrial P wave is not followed by a QRS complex. In the following example of second-degree AV block, ventricular activation is normal. However, occasionally, there is no wave front conducting through, resulting in a missing QRS. Figure 8-3 is an ECG rhythm strip showing second-degree AV block with varying ventricular rate.

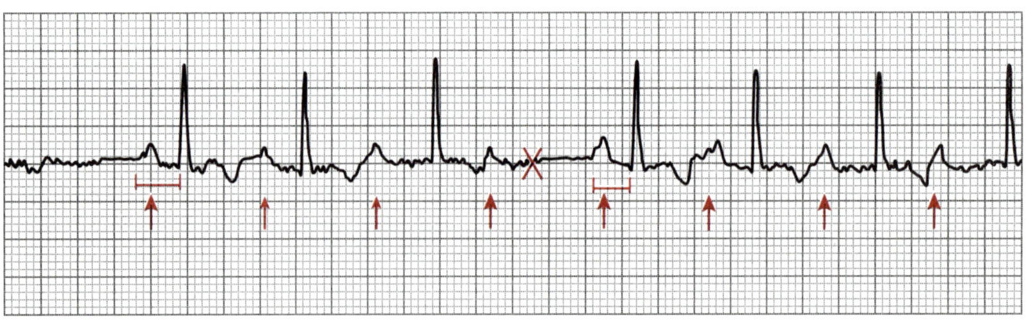

Figure 8-2 An ECG tracing showing sinus rhythm with second-degree (2°) AV block. The P waves plot through, and there is a P wave to the left of each QRS complex. Note the missing QRS. Also, note that the PR after the missed QRS complex is consistent. The QRS duration is within normal limits. There is progressive prolongation of the PR segments of the PR intervals, indicating the Wenckebach phenomenon. The ECG interpretation would be sinus at 86 per minute, with second-degree AV block, probably Type I (QRS = 0.06 to 0.08 second) with Wenckebach.

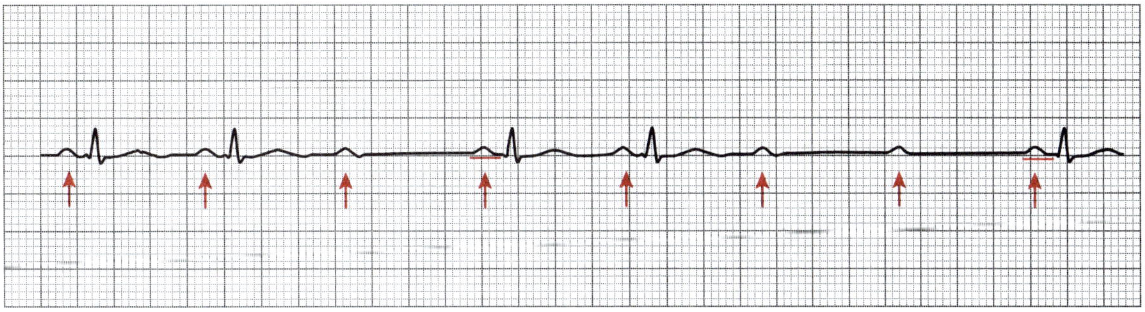

Figure 8-3 An ECG tracing showing the sinus rate at 75. The ventricular response varies at 27–75 per minute. There are P waves to the left of each QRS. However, there are several P waves without QRS complexes. The QRS is within normal limits. The ECG interpretation would be sinus at 75 per minute with high-grade (advanced) second-degree AV block, ventricular rate 27–75 per minute.

SINUS WITH SECOND-DEGREE AV BLOCK, THE WENCKEBACH PHENOMENON, TYPE I, OR MOBITZ TYPE I.

The **Wenckebach** phenomenon occurs when there is a progressive delay in conducting an atrial impulse until, finally, there is no conduction into the ventricles. This phenomenon in conduction delay can occur with sinus rhythm, atrial flutter, or fibrillation. The Wenckebach phenomenon also can occur between sinus depolarization and atrial activation.

Wenckebach
Progressive prolongation of conduction time. Seen in atrial flutter, atrial fibrillation, SA block, and AV conduction defects.

In a sinus rhythm where the disease affects the AV node, there is a progressive lengthening of the PR segment until such time when there is no conduction. The progressive prolongation of the PR interval eventually causes the P wave to fall in the refractory period of the ventricles, resulting in the missed QRS complex. The next sinus beat occurs right on time. The PR interval following the missed QRS is the same as the first PR of the group.

The cycle may repeat itself with variations in the numbers of conducted beats. The progressively prolonged PR segment of the PR interval is a warning of progressive conduction problems and is called the *Wenckebach phenomenon.*

In summary, the Wenckebach phenomenon is characterized by the following:

1. group beating
2. the group begins and ends with a P wave
3. there is one more P wave than QRS within the group
4. the PR after the missed QRS is the same regardless of the numbers of PQRST complexes in the group
5. the greatest PR interval prolongation occurs within the second PR interval of the group.
6. irregular or decreasing R-R intervals

Figure 8-4 is an ECG tracing showing a sinus mechanism with occasional missed QRS complexes. The practitioner must first plot out the P waves to confirm or deny that the missed QRS is because of a nonconducted PAC. In this example, the P waves plot through regularly. Where there is a missed QRS complex, the PR after the missed

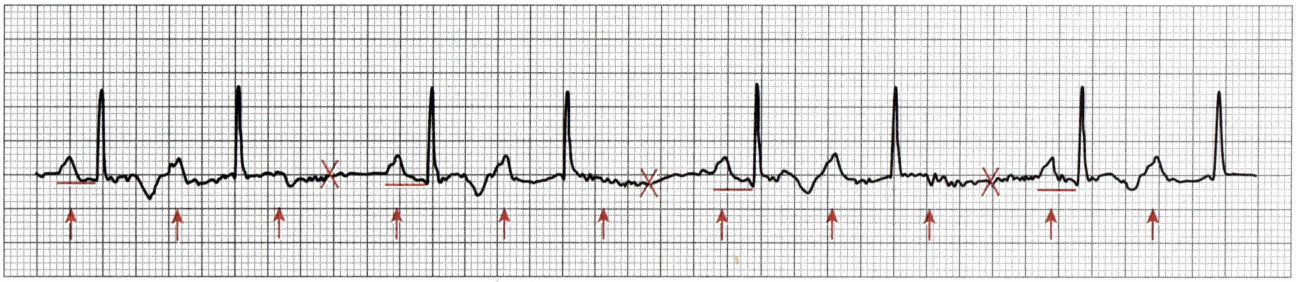

Figure 8-4 An ECG tracing showing progressive prolongation of the PR interval until the sinus P does not conduct into the ventricles. There is no ventricular depolarization, hence the missed QRS. The PR after the dropped beat is consistent with each instance. The ECG interpretation would be sinus at 86 per minute with second-degree (2°) AV block, Wenckebach, probably Type I (QRS 0.08 second) inverted T waves, ventricular rate 57 to 75 per minute.

beat is constant. The PR intervals warn of the difficulty in AV conduction by the progressive prolongation of the PR intervals until, finally, there is no conduction.

Cause of Second-degree AV block

Second-degree AV block, Type I, with or without a Wenckebach phenomenon, occurs above the His bundle, at the level of the AV node, and is associated with right coronary artery disease. Thus, second-degree AV block of Type I or Wenckebach Type is associated with inferior wall myocardial infarction (IWMI). Wenckebach-Type second-degree AV blocks also may occur with digitalis toxicity or chronic lesions of the AV conduction system. In IWMI, the ischemia at the level of the AV node may be reversible.

Electrophysiologic studies have shown that the site of block associated with **Type I** conduction defect is usually within the AV node or at least above the penetrating portions of the bundle branch system. Should a complete AV block occur, there is still the opportunity for a junctional escape rhythm.

Type I
In second-degree AV block, a term that describes a narrow QRS complex

The ECG characteristics of second-degree AV block with the Wenckebach phenomenon are as follows:

1. P Wave: The P waves are positive and uniform in lead II. Not every P wave is followed by a QRS complex.
2. PR Interval: After the dropped QRS, the PR interval of the conducted beat is constant and may even be greater than the normal 0.20 second. With a Wenckebach phenomenon, the PR intervals become progressively longer until an atrial depolarization no longer initiates a ventricular response; the cycle is then resumed. The PR after the dropped QRS is constant each time this occurs.
3. QRS Complex: The QRS complex duration is 0.10 second or less when the disease is within the AV node.
4. QRS Rate: The atrial rate is constant between 60 and 100 per minute. The ventricular rate is slower than the atrial rate due to the nonconducted beats.

5. QRS Rhythm: The rhythm is irregular with "group" beating, that is, more Ps than QRSs. There is a pause after each group. The phenomenon may be 3:1, 5:4, 11:10, or 2:1 conduction, referring to the length of the phenomenon.

In AV block with the Wenckebach phenomenon, ventricular beats are dropped in a cyclic manner. The second PR interval in the group usually demonstrates the greatest amount of prolongation; its PR segment is sometimes dramatically longer than the first in the group.

After that, there is a series of prolonged PRs, and, although they do get longer, the amount of increase is less each time. The last event in the group is a P wave without a subsequent QRS.

Intervention

Quick interpretations of the AV block can lead to incorrect diagnosis and treatment. True differentiation of types is critical. Interpretation should not be done on a single ECG monitoring lead. Assessment using a 12-lead ECG, correlated with patient presentation, medication and past medical history is critical. Prematurely treating with agents that will increase the sinus rate will not increase AV conduction when the underlying pathology is in the AV junction.

Note: In the presence of AV block, agents that increase the sinus rate will not invariably increase AV conduction and thus ventricular rate. In fact, the use of such agents can result in rapid sinus rates with complete AV block or use of accessory pathways and abnormal ventricular conduction and possibly ventricular tachycardia.

Figure 8-5A and B are ECG tracings showing second-degree AV block Type I, one with and one without an obvious Wenckebach phenomenon.

SECOND-DEGREE AV BLOCK WITH WIDE QRS COMPLEX (TYPE II)

Conduction defects that occur below the His bundle and within one or more of the bundle branches are usually associated with left coronary artery disease. The left coronary artery supplies most of the right bundle branch as well as the left anterior fascicle, and partially, the left posterior fascicle. Left coronary artery occlusion produces anterior-wall myocardial infarction (AWMI). When intraventricular conduction defects occur, the QRS duration is prolonged and takes on specific morphology reflecting the affected fascicle.

Second-degree AV block **Type II** occurs as a result of chronic lesions within the conduction system and also occurs in AWMI as a result of the necrotic process. Second-degree AV block Type II is diagnosed when a dropped QRS complex is *not* preceded by progressive prolongation of the PR interval. The PR interval may be normal or prolonged but remains fixed and constant.

Type II

In second-degree AV block, a term used to describe a wide QRS complex, i.e., greater than 0.12 second. It indicates disease within one or more of the ventricular fascicles.

The QRS duration and morphology are critical in making the diagnosis of second-degree AV block Type II. ECG diagnosis requires that there be evidence of bundle branch pathology. Figure 8-6 is an ECG tracing showing second-degree AV block and the Wenckebach phenomenon. The QRS is 0.08 second. The PR after the

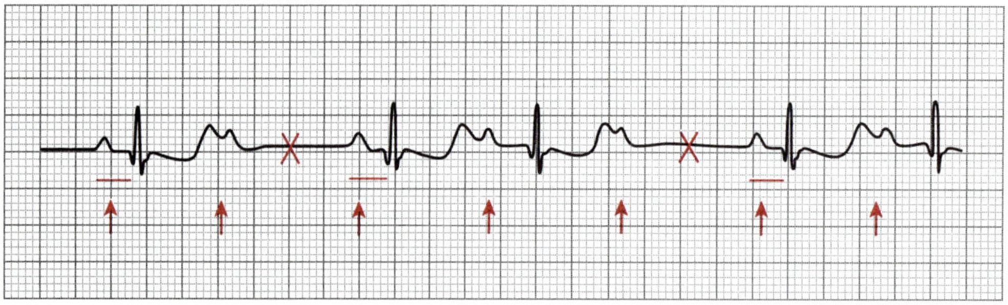

(A)

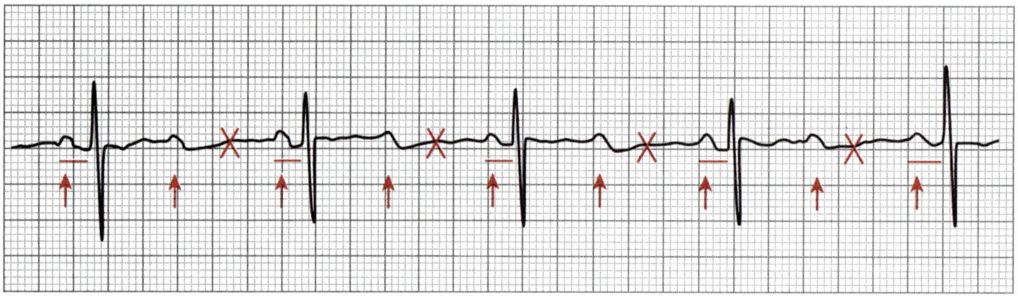

(B)

Figure 8-5 In each ECG tracing, plot out the P waves and determine that there are no PACs. Note that after the missed QRS, the PR interval is the same. The QRS in each example is within normal limits. The PR segment of the PR interval is progressively longer until the sinus P does not conduct into the ventricles. The ECG interpretations would be: (A) sinus at 86, ventricular rate 43 to 86 per minute, second-degree AV block, probably Type I (QRS 0.10 second), with Wenckebach; (B) sinus at 100 per minute with ventricular response at 50 per minute, second-degree AV block, probably Type I (QRS 0.08 second).

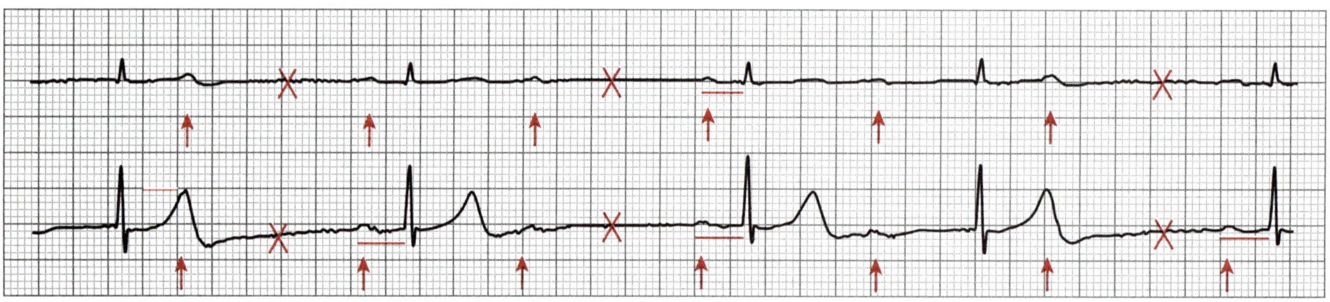

Figure 8-6 An ECG tracing showing second degree AV block. The P waves plot through. The PR lengthens progressively, but the PR is constant after the missed beat. The QRS is within normal limits at 0.08 second, probably Type I. The ECG interpretation would be sinus at 67 per minute with second-degree AV block, probably Type I (QRS= 0.04–0.06), ventricular rate 30–57 per minute, with Wenckebach.

missed QRS is constant. Figure 8-7, in contrast, shows the Wenckebach phenomenon with QRS that is an rS configuration and 0.12 second. The QRS in this patient was confirmed on 12-lead ECG to be indicative of left anterior fascicular block; that is, the disease affected the penetrating portions of the bundle branch system.

Figure 8-8 is an ECG tracing from a patient who had a confirmed myocardial infarction. Note the difference between atrial and ventricular rates—the fixed PR interval and the QRS that is 0.16 second in duration.

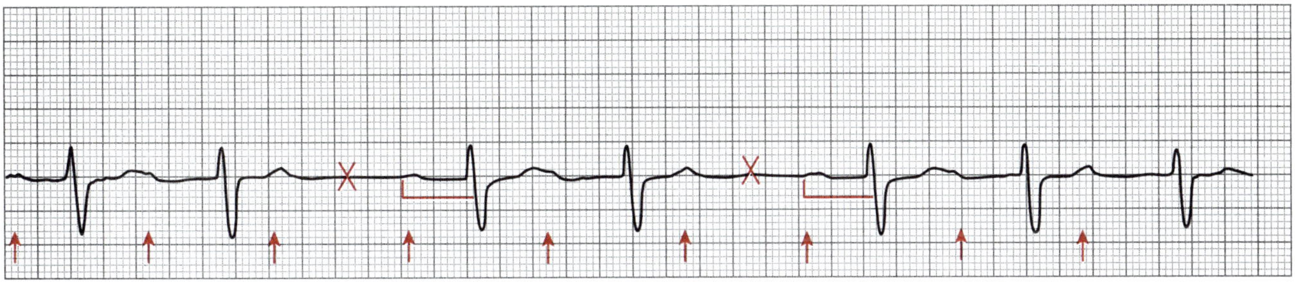

Figure 8-7 An ECG tracing showing second-degree AV block. The P waves plot through, and the PR lengthens progressively, but the PR is constant after the missed beat. The QRS is broader than normal at 0.12 second and is an rS configuration, which may indicate an intraventricular conduction defect. The ECG interpretation would be sinus at 75 per minute with second-degree AV block, probably Type II (QRS = 0.12 an rS configuration), ventricular rate 37 to 75 per minute, with Wenckebach.

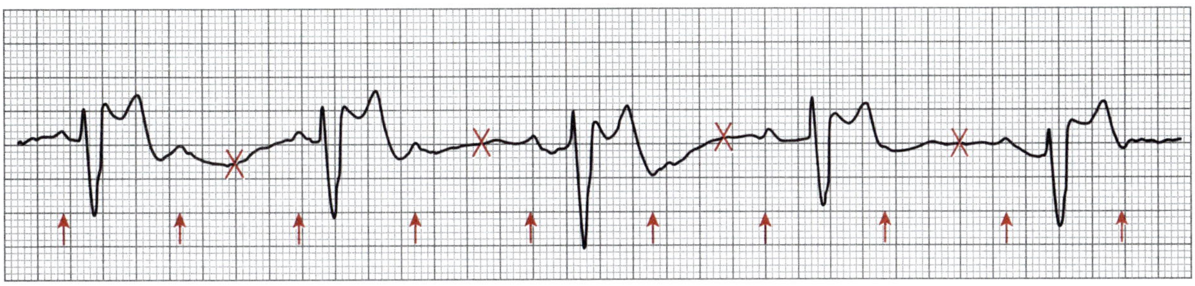

Figure 8-8 An ECG tracing from a patient with confirmed anteroseptal wall myocardial infarction. Plot out each of the P waves as they occur within the ST segment and T waves. The PR interval is constant after the missed QRS. The QRS is 0.16 second and an rS configuration. Every other sinus P does not conduct. The ventricular rhythm is regular. This is an example of AV block with 2:1 conduction. The ECG interpretation would be sinus at 75 per minute, second-degree AV block, probably Type II (QRS = 0.12 an rS configuration), ventricular rate 43 per minute.

Type II AV block is clinically significant because

1. it may be associated with fall in cardiac output
2. it can be a precursor of complete AV block dependent on the potential for a ventricular escape pacemaker.

Intervention

Initial therapy may be directed toward accelerating SA/AV conduction and thus ventricular rate. Because of disease in the bundle branch, the response is poor and may even result in chaotic ventricular arrhythmias. Hypoperfusion with this arrhythmia is the rule rather than the exception. Hence, rapid intervention with electronic pacing is usually necessary to manage these patients. Figure 8-9 is an ECG tracing allegedly from a patient who received atropine because of bradycardia with second-degree AV block. Note that in this rhythm the sinus rate is 150 per minute, and the ventricular response is 37. The PR interval is constant and the QRS 0.12. The patient was reported to become hypotensive with altered levels of consciousness.

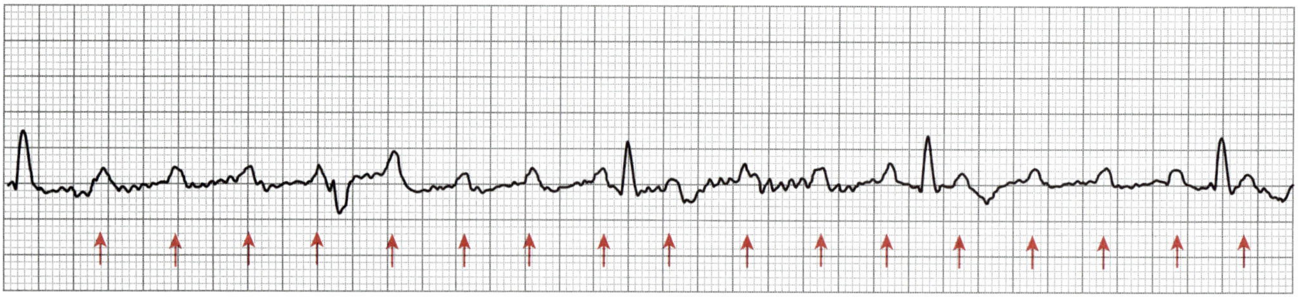

Figure 8-9 An ECG tracing showing an atrial rate of 150 and ventricular response of 37 per minute in a patient who allegedly received atropine for a bradycardia. The ECG interpretation would be complete AV block, sinus rate is 150 per minute, and the ventricular rate is 37 per minute. It is critical to report atrial and ventricular rates.

Second-degree AV block, AV Block with 2:1 Conduction or Fixed-rate Second-degree AV Block

Second-degree AV block may be a result of Type I or Type II conduction defects, that is, associated with right or left coronary artery disease. In second-degree AV block that occurs as a result of Type I disease, the QRS complexes are narrow, 0.10 second or less.

In fixed-ratio second-degree AV block that occurs as a result of Type II disease, the QRS complexes are altered, and the duration is greater than 0.10, often 0.12 to 0.16 second. Table 8-2 is a summary of ECG configuration in Type I and Type II second-degree AV blocks.

Table 8-3 is a summary of the differences in pathology, the ECG characteristics, and proposed interventions in Types I and II second-degree AV block.

SINUS WITH HIGH-GRADE (ADVANCED) AV BLOCK

Second-degree high-grade AV block can be interpreted when the atrial rate is reasonable, two or more consecutive atrial impulses are not conducted, and the conducted beats have consistent PR intervals. There is no competition from a subsidiary pacer, as with accelerated junctional rhythm, for example. The ratio of atrial to ventricular conducted beats may vary from 3:1, 4:1, and so on, and the ratio may vary. Figure 8-10 is an ECG tracing of high-grade second-degree AV block.

SINUS WITH COMPLETE AV BLOCK

Pathology involved in AV block can progress in severity until all the sinus impulses are completely blocked. Regardless of the site of the lesion, there is *no* conduction through to the ventricles.

complete AV block
Progression of an AV block so severe that all the sinus impulses have become completely blocked

When **complete AV block** occurs at the level of the AV node, the His bundle will control the ventricular rhythm at 40 to 60 beats per minute. The ventricular rhythm will be regular. Figure 8-11 is an example of complete AV block. The QRS rhythm is regular at 37 beats per minute. The atrial rate is faster at about 60 per minute. The QRS and P waves are independent of each other.

Table 8-2 Summary of ECG configuration in Type I and Type II second-degree AV blocks.

AV BLOCKS	Second-degree* Wenckebach	Second-degree* 2:1 Type I	Second-degree* 2:1 Type II
P waves	independent and regular	independent and regular	independent and regular
PR Interval	progressively longer, but the PR after the missed QRS is the same	can be < or > than 0.20 second The PR after the missed QRS is the same.	can be < or > than 0.20 second The PR after the missed QRS is the same.
QRS duration	<0.10**	<0.10 probably Type I **may present as 2:1 conduction	>0.10 probably Type II **may present as 2:1 conduction
Rate	varies	atrial rate is twice ventricular rate	atrial rate is twice ventricular rate
Rhythm	varies	regular	regular

Misses a QRS. PR after dropped PR after dropped QRS is consistent
**in the absence of preexisting bundle branch block

When complete AV block occurs below the His bundle, the ventricular rhythm is controlled by a ventricular escape mechanism between 20 to 40 beats per minute. The ventricular rhythm will be regular. Figure 8-12 is an example of complete AV block. The atrial and ventricular rates are independent, and each is regular. The QRS is 0.18 to 0.20 second.

Table 8-3 Summary of differences in pathology, ECG characteristics and interventions in Types I and II second-degree AV block.

Type I QRS 0.10 or less with or without Wenckebach Phenomenon	Type II QRS greater than 0.10
AV lesion: above the bundle of His	Lesion in the bundle branch system
Associated with IWMI, digitalis, chronic AV lesions	Associated with AWMI or chronic lesions within the bundle branch system
Nature: ischemic, reversible, transient	Lesion is usually chronic in nature
ECG: Ps plot through; PR interval may prolong prior to missing QRS; PR after the dropped QRS is consistent	P waves plot through; dropped QRS preceded by a fixed PR interval
Ventricular rhythm can be regular or irregular	Ventricular rhythm can be regular or irregular
In the presence of sinus bradycardia, usually responds well to pharmacologic intervention	Usually does not respond well to pharmacologic intervention
Rarely requires electronic pacing	Usually requires electronic pacing

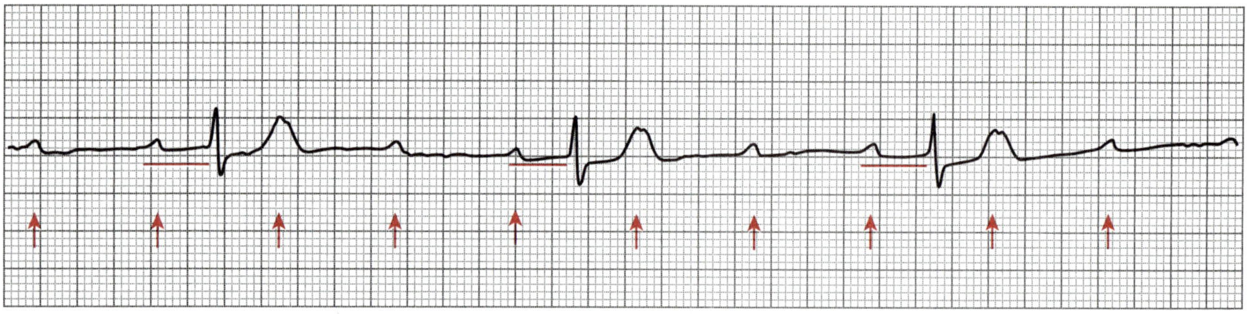

Figure 8-10 An ECG tracing illustrating high-grade, second-degree (advanced) AV block. The atrial rate is 86 per minute, the ventricular rate is 30 per minute. The conducted beats have consistent PR intervals. The ECG interpretation would be sinus rate at 86 per minute with advanced second-degree AV block, ventricular rate 30 per minute.

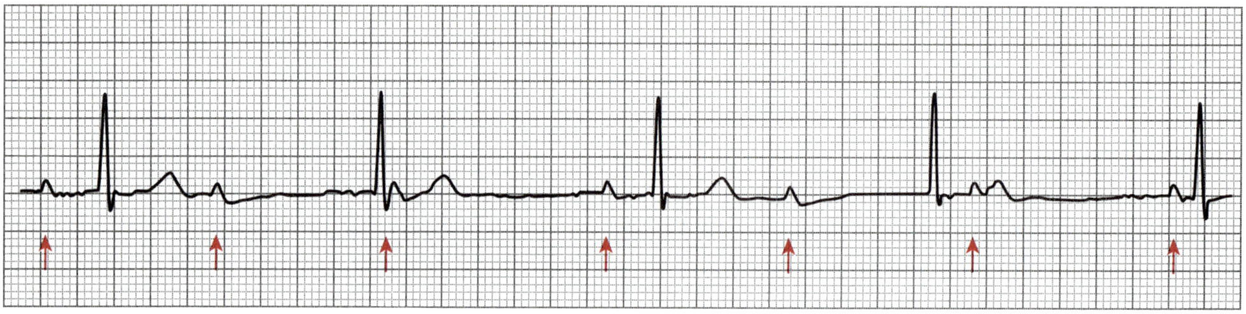

Figure 8-11 An ECG illustrating complete AV block, probably at the level of the AV node since the QRS is 0.06 second. The atrial rate is faster than the QRS rate, and the P waves and QRS complexes are independent of each other. There are no consistent PR intervals. The ECG interpretation would be sinus at 50 per minute with complete AV block, a junctional rhythm with a ventricular rate at 40 per minute.

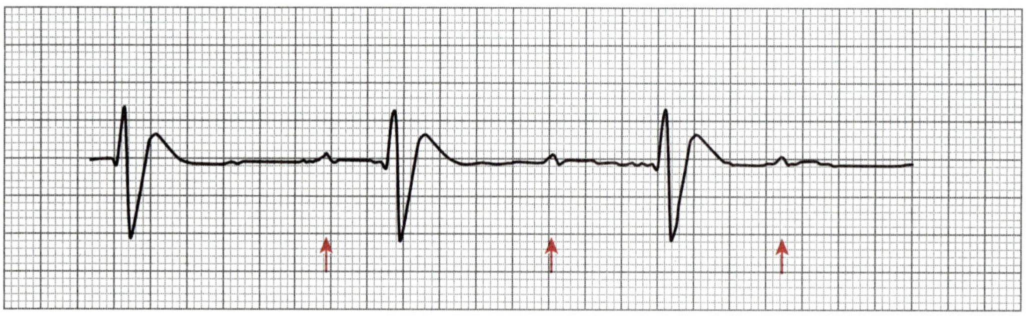

Figure 8-12 An ECG illustrating complete AV block that is probably infranodal since the QRS is 0.16 second. The sinus rate is faster than the QRS rate, and the P waves and QRS complexes are independent of each other. There are no consistent PR intervals. The ECG interpretation would be sinus at 50 per minute with complete AV block, possibly an idioventricular rhythm (or a QRS showing bundle branch conduction defect) and a ventricular rate at 40 per minute.

In complete AV block, the atrial rate is different, faster and independent of the ventricular rate. There is no relationship between P and QRS; thus there is *NO* PR interval. The atria, remaining under the control of the SA node, or in atrial flutter or fibrillation, are beating at their own intrinsic rate and are completely dissociated from the ventricles. The ECG characteristics of complete AV block are as follows:

1. P Wave: The P waves are positive and uniform in lead II and are not associated with the QRS complexes. The atrial rate is independent and faster than the escape ventricular rate.
2. PR Interval: Since there is no relationship between the P waves and the QRS complexes, there is no measurable PR interval.
3. QRS Complex: The QRS complex duration, depending on the site of impulse formation, may be normal, with the pacemaker in the AV junction, or greater than 0.12 with the QRS opposite in direction from the T wave, when the pacemaker is from the ventricle.
4. QRS Rate: While the atrial rate often is controlled by the SA node, the ventricles are controlled by either an escape junctional pacemaker with a normally narrow (0.10 or less) QRS complex or a ventricular escape pacemaker with a QRS greater than 0.12 second.
5. QRS Rhythm: The ventricular rhythm is regular since the escape pacemaker is from the AV junction or an escape ventricular focus.

AV DISSOCIATION

In various arrhythmias, the atria and ventricles beat independently for a number of reasons. *AV dissociation* is a generic term that describes this independent function. The term describes an ECG sign and does not provide the diagnosis of the problem. After all, jaundice does not always indicate liver failure, dizziness does not always imply a cerebral vascular accident, adventitious lung sounds do not imply only pneumonia.

In ventricular tachycardia, the atria and ventricles beat independently. In most instances, the P waves may not be visible in all leads. Occasionally, a condition exists where the sinus node slows and the AV junctional tissue accelerates and takes control of the ventricular rate. Analysis of the ECG will see the slowing of the sinus node, acceleration of the junction (usually only a few beats faster), and then acceleration of the sinus, taking control once again. Thus, there is a time when the atria and ventricles are dissociated and under control of different pacemakers. When the atrial and ventricular rates are the same, but independent, the arrhythmia is *isorhythmic AV dissociation.*

Cause of Isorhythmic AV Dissociation

AV dissociation can be medication induced, the most common cause being digitalis therapy. AV dissociation can occur with enhanced automaticity in the AV junction due to physiologic stretching secondary to mitral or aortic valve disease. AV disso-

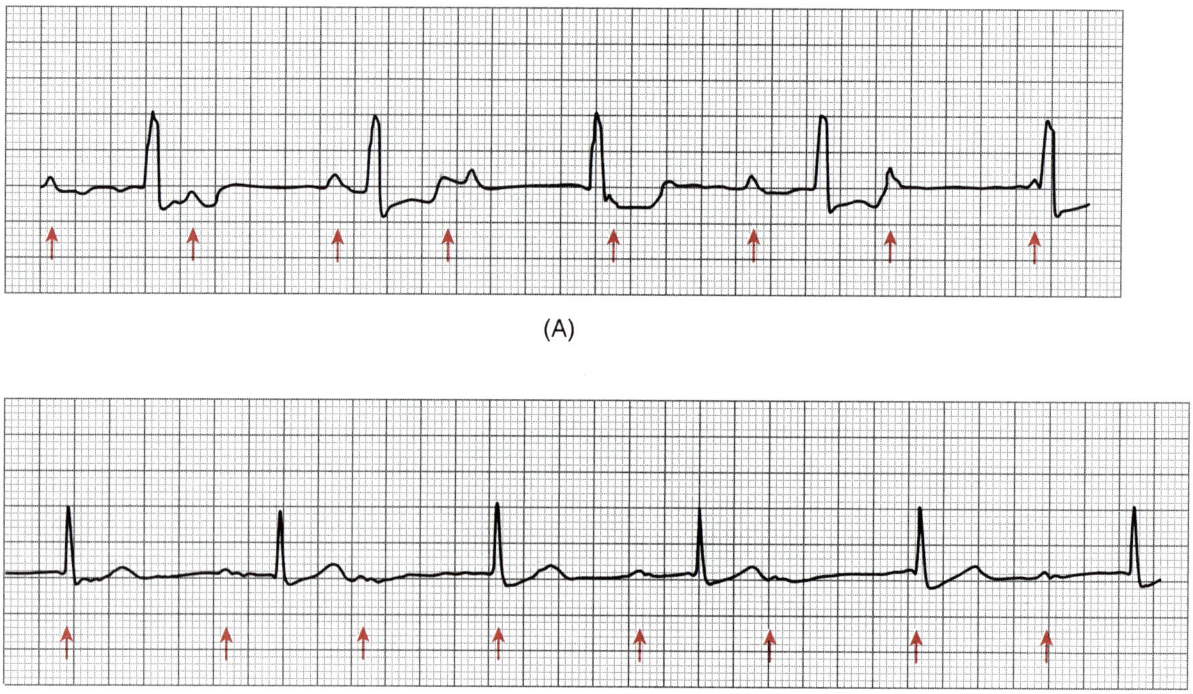

Figure 8-13 ECG tracings showing AV dissociation. In (A), atrial rate is 75 per minute, and the independent ventricular rate is 50 per minute. In (B), the atrial rate is 75 per minute and ventricular rate is 50 per minute. Both are examples of complete AV block, that is, the atrial and ventricular rates are independent.

ciation also is seen immediately after cardiac surgery. Figure 8-13A and B are examples of AV dissociation.

Intervention

AV dissociation is a sign. Treatment should be directed to identifying the cause of the dissociation. Is it complete AV block due to pathology in the AV node? Is it accelerated junctional rhythm as seen in cases of digitalis toxicity? Is it ventricular tachycardia? Recall in ventricular tachycardia that the ventricular ectopic controls ventricular response, while the sinus node is still in control of the atria.

Communication between medical personnel concerning this tracing should include atrial rate, ventricular rate, patient presentation, medical and medication history.

Summary

We have just discussed AV dissociation as a result of complete AV block and AV dissociation that can occur with ventricular tachycardia, atrial flutter, or fibrillation with a junctional rhythm. Even in ventricular fibrillation, the atria still may be under the control of the sinus node and simply not seen. Each of these arrhythmias has obvious clinical implications, and the ECG pattern must be described in its entirety. Table 8-4 provides a summary of AV block configurations.

Table 8-4 Summary of ECG configurations of first, second, and complete AV blocks

	First Degree	Second-Degree Wenckebach	Second-Degree* 2:1 Type I	Second-Degree* 2:1 Type II	Complete
	every P has a QRS	*misses a QRS; *PR after dropped; QRS is consistent	misses a QRS; *PR after dropped; QRS is consistent	misses a QRS; *PR after dropped; QRS is consistent	AV dissociation
P waves	(+)/QRS	independent and regular	independent and regular	independent and regular	independent and regular
PR Interval	>0.20 but consistent	progressively longer, but the PR associated with the missed QRS is the same	can be < or >0.20 second; the PR after the missed beat is the same	can be < or >0.20 second; the PR after the missed beat is the same	there is no PR interval
QRS duration	<0.10	<0.10	<0.10 probably Type I *may present as 2:1 conduction	>0.10 probably Type II may present as 2:1 conduction	<0.10 if from a junctional pacer; >0.10 and slow if from a ventricular pacing site
Rate/minute	60–100	varies	atrial rate is twice ventricular	atrial rate is twice ventricular	atrial rate is faster than the ventricular
Rhythm	regular	varies	regular	regular	regular
Rx	symptomatic: question rate question meds question chest pain	symptomatic: consider Atropine, fluids, Dopamine, pacemaker	symptomatic: consider Atropine, fluids, Dopamine, pacemaker	symptomatic: consider fluids, Dopamine, pacemaker	symptomatic: consider fluids, Dopamine, pacemaker

Self-Assessment Exercises

Fill in the Blanks

Complete the statements, and then compare your answers with those in the back of the book.

SINUS RHYTHM	FIRST-DEGREE AV BLOCK	SECOND-DEGREE AV BLOCK TYPE I
1 (+) P plus QRS	1 (+) P plus a QRS	________
PRI 0.12–0.20	greater than 0.20	________
QRS.10 or less	0.10 or less	________
QRS rate: 60-100/min	________	________
QRS rhythm: regular	________	________

SINUS RHYTHM	COMPLETE AV BLOCK	SECOND-DEGREE AV BLOCK TYPE II
1 (+) P plus QRS	sinus Ps plot through	________
PRI 0.12–0.20	no PRI	________
QRS 0.10 or less	0.10 or less	________
QRS rate: 60-100/min	________	________
QRS rhythm: regular	________	________

ECG Rhythm Identification Practice

For the following rhythms fill in the blanks and then check your answers with those in the back of this book.

Figure 8-14

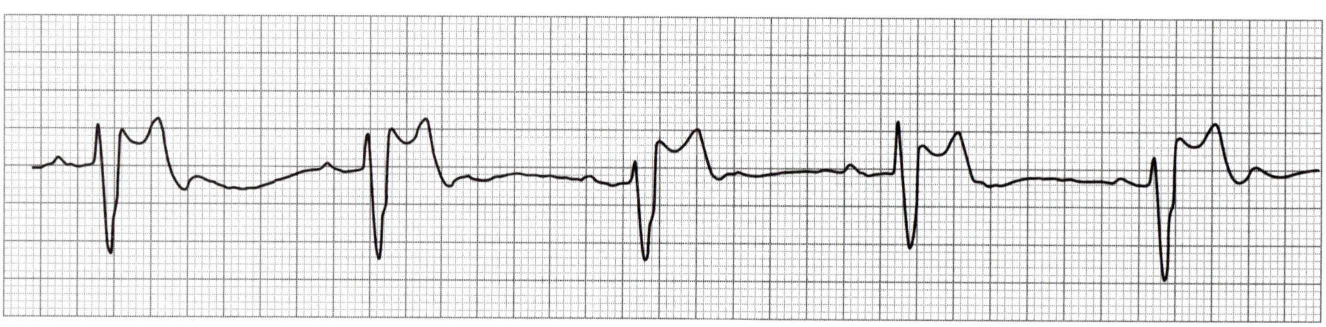

QRS duration ________ **QT** ________
Ventricular rate/rhythm ________
Atrial rate/rhythm ________
PR interval ________

Identification ________
Symptoms ________
____
Treatment ________

Figure 8-15

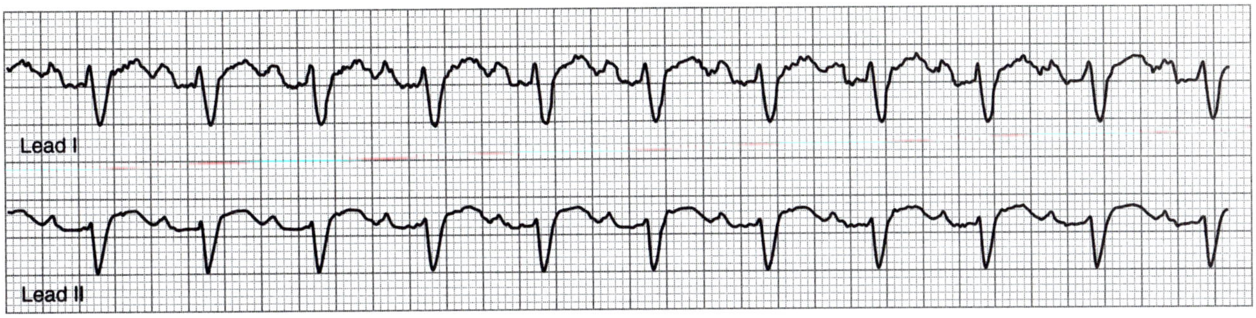

QRS duration ______________ QT ____________

Ventricular rate/rhythm ____________________

Atrial rate/rhythm ________________________

PR interval ______________________________

Identification ______________________________

Symptoms ________________________________

____

Treatment ________________________________

Figure 8-16

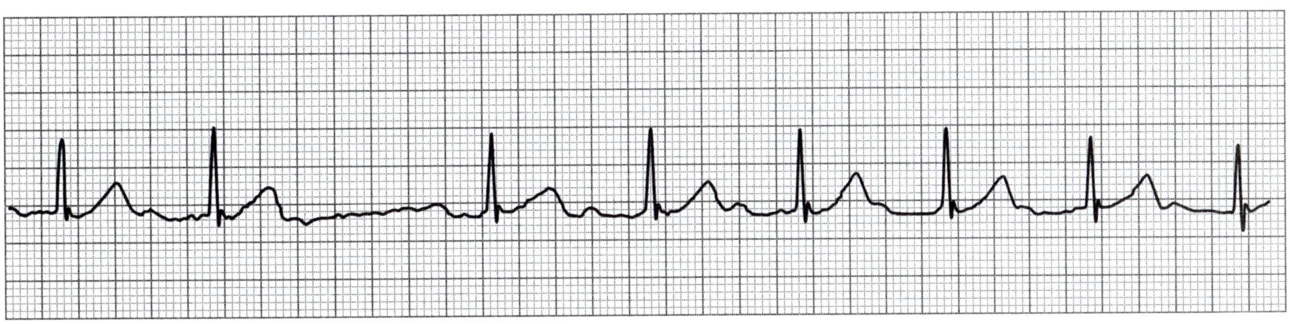

QRS duration ______________ QT ____________

Ventricular rate/rhythm ____________________

Atrial rate/rhythm ________________________

PR interval ______________________________

Identification ______________________________

Symptoms ________________________________

____

Treatment ________________________________

Figure 8-17

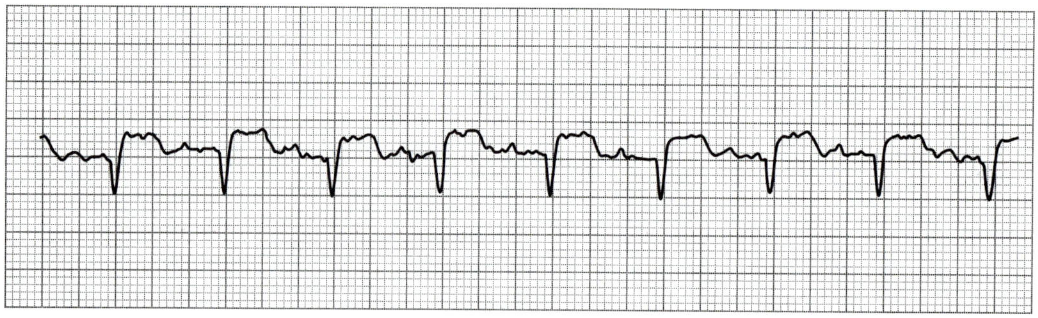

QRS duration ______________ QT __________

Ventricular rate/rhythm ____________________

Atrial rate/rhythm ________________________

PR interval ______________________________

Identification ____________________________

Symptoms ________________________________

____

Treatment ________________________________

Figure 8-18

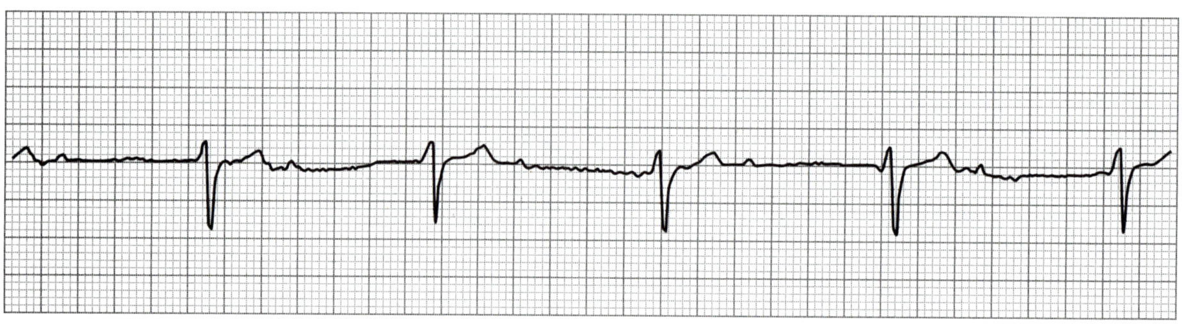

QRS duration ______________ QT __________

Ventricular rate/rhythm ____________________

Atrial rate/rhythm ________________________

PR interval ______________________________

Identification ____________________________

Symptoms ________________________________

____

Treatment ________________________________

Figure 8-19

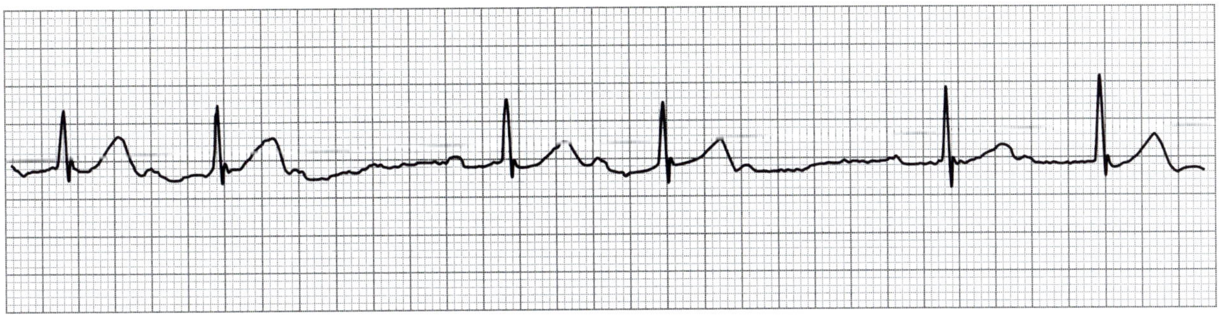

QRS duration ________________ QT ____________
Ventricular rate/rhythm ____________________
Atrial rate/rhythm ________________________
PR interval ______________________________

Identification ______________________________
Symptoms ________________________________
____
Treatment ________________________________

Figure 8-20

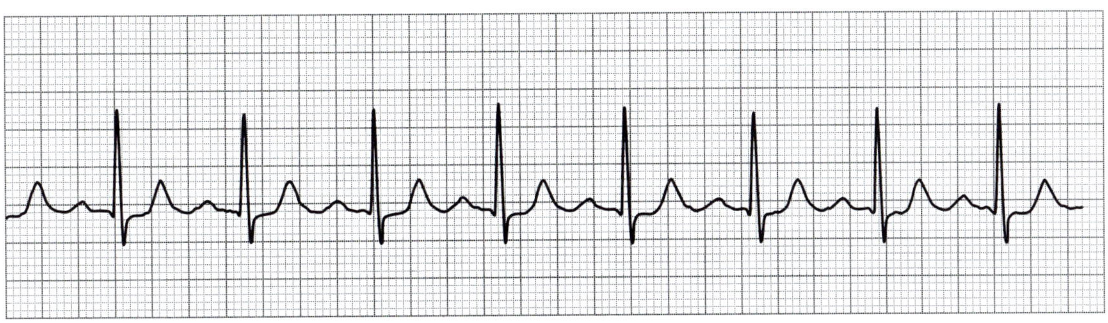

QRS duration ________________ QT ____________
Ventricular rate/rhythm ____________________
Atrial rate/rhythm ________________________
PR interval ______________________________

Identification ______________________________
Symptoms ________________________________
____
Treatment ________________________________

Figure 8-21

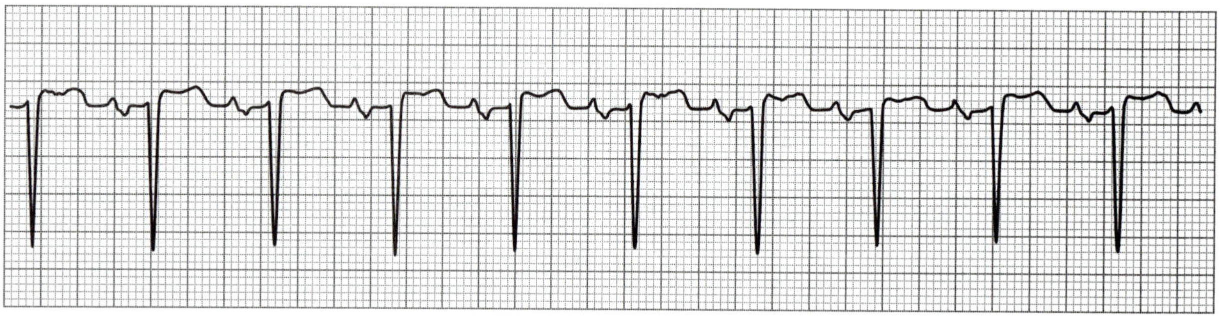

QRS duration ______________ QT ___________

Ventricular rate/rhythm ______________________

Atrial rate/rhythm ________________________

PR interval ______________________________

Identification ______________________________

Symptoms ________________________________

____

Treatment ________________________________

Figure 8-22

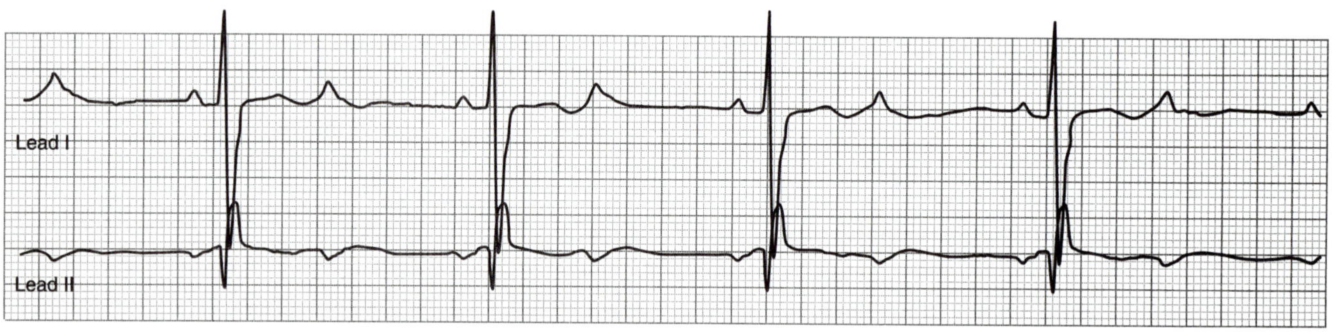

QRS duration ______________ QT ___________

Ventricular rate/rhythm ______________________

Atrial rate/rhythm ________________________

PR interval ______________________________

Identification ______________________________

Symptoms ________________________________

____

Treatment ________________________________

Figure 8-23

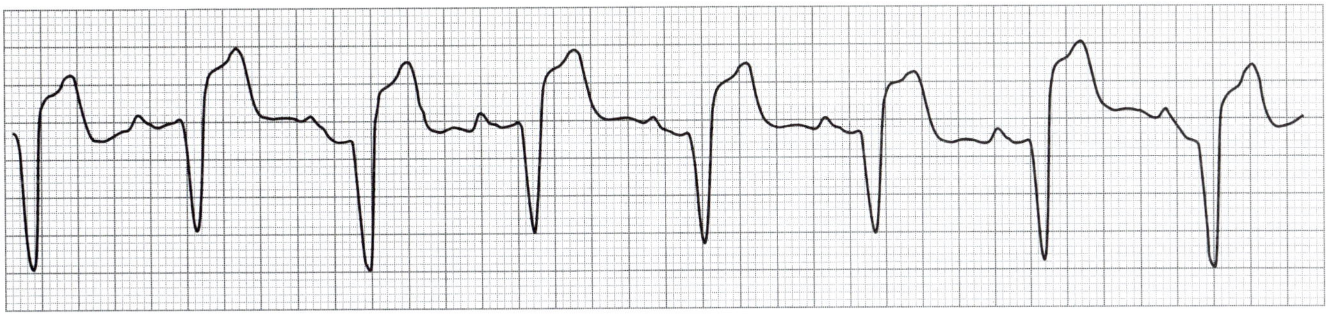

QRS duration ________________ **QT** ____________

Ventricular rate/rhythm ________________________

Atrial rate/rhythm ___________________________

PR interval ________________________________

Identification ______________________________

Symptoms ________________________________

____

Treatment ________________________________

References

Conover, M. B. *Nurse's pocket guide to electrocardiography* (3rd ed.). St. Louis, MO: C. V. Mosby; 1994.

Conover, M. B. *Understanding electrocardiography: Arrhythmias and the 12-lead ECG* (7th ed.). St. Louis, MO: Mosby-Year Book; 1996.

Conover, M. B. & Wellens, H. J. *The ECG in emergency decision making*. Philadelphia: W. B. Saunders; 1993.

Emergency Cardiac Care Subcommittee and Subcommittees, American Heart Association. Guidelines for cardiopulmonary resuscitation and emergency cardiac care, *JAMA*. 1994.

Mandel, W. J. (Ed). *Cardiac arrhythmias: Their mechanisms, diagnoses and management* (2nd ed.). Philadelphia: Lippincott; 1987.

Marriott, H. J. & Conover, M. B. *Advanced concepts in arrhythmias* (2nd ed.). St. Louis, MO: C. V. Mosby; 1989.

CHAPTER 9

Electrical Interventions

Premise To defibrillate is to halt the death process. Rapid recognition of the need for defibrillation will save lives.

Objectives

After reading the chapter and completing the Self-Assessment Exercises, the student should be able to

1. identify the purpose and mechanisms of defibrillation and synchronized cardioversion
2. describe the difference between defibrillation and synchronized cardioversion
3. identify and describe the indications, factors favoring, complications, and contraindications for defibrillation, and synchronized cardioversion.
4. identify and describe indications and use of the automated external defibrillator.

Key Terms

automated external defibrillation
available energy
cardioversion
defibrillation
delivered energy
impedance
joules
precordial thump
resistance
stored energy
synchronized
unsynchronized

Introduction

Over 600,000 patients die each year from cardiovascular diseases; half of those occur outside the hospital, with sudden death (collapse) being the first sign of cardiac disease in 50 percent of the population. Ventricular fibrillation is not self-terminating and will persist unless defibrillation is performed as soon as possible. The longer the time from onset to defibrillation, the less likely ventricular fibrillation will terminate with treatment. Rapid defibrillation is the major determinant of survival in cardiac arrest caused by ventricular fibrillation.

Synchronized cardioversion is another type of electrical intervention that will be discussed in this chapter. While this is usually an elective procedure, it is used successfully when medications cannot otherwise control arrhythmias other than ventricular fibrillation.

KEY CONCEPTS

defibrillation
Termination of ventricular fibrillation by electrical shock

joules
Unit of energy equal to approximately 0.7375 foot-pounds

stored energy
Amount of joules available in the defibrillator's capacitor

delivered energy
Amount of joules administered to a patient

impedance
Interference to the flow of energy (resistance)

resistance
Opposition to the flow of energy (impedance)

available energy
Amount of actual energy that is delivered to a patient with an impedance of 50 ohms

Defibrillation is the delivery of a high intensity charge to the heart that results in complete depolarization of the myocardium. This charge of electricity has the potential for interrupting some arrhythmias and allow for a normal pacemaker to resume control of heart rate and rhythm.

Defibrillation energy is measured in **joules**. **Stored energy** is the amount of joules actually available in the defibrillator's capacitor. **Delivered energy** is the amount of joules actually administered.

The amount of patient **impedance** or **resistance** to the flow of energy causes a variation in the flow of energy. An *ohm* is the unit of measurement of impedance. Typically, an adult is considered to have 50 ohms of resistance. A joule is the amount of electrical energy expended by a current of one ampere flowing for one second through one ohm of resistance.

The amount of impedance varies depending on many factors, including but not limited to the size of the patient, the heart, metabolic status, medications and electrolyte balance. **Available energy** is the amount of actual energy that will be delivered to a patient with an impedance of 50 ohms.

EQUIPMENT

Defibrillators deliver energy from the energy source through electrodes. Some electrodes are in the form of hand-held paddles, others are disposable electrodes that are pregelled with a conductive medium. Internal paddles are also available for direct application to the heart. This requires opening of the chest cavity.

Traditional hand-held paddles require application of a conductive medium designed to reduce skin resistance. Placement of the hand-held paddles is along the long axis of the heart, anterior-lateral (lead II, sternum-apex) position. That is, one to the right of the sternum at the third and fourth intercostal space. The other hand-held paddle is placed over the apex of the heart, to the left of the midclavicular line. The use of hand-held paddles requires that firm pressure be applied equivalent to 25 pounds of pressure.

The disposable, pregelled electrodes minimize the amount of time taken for set up and delivery of current, and reduce the variation in electrode placement and application of pressure between operators as well as applications by the same operator. The disposable electrodes also reduce safety hazards since the operator will not be reaching across the patient, or handling the electrodes. Placement of these disposable electrodes is the same as with hand-held paddles. The operator will discharge the energy from the source. This procedure is also called *hands-free* or *remote* defibrillation.

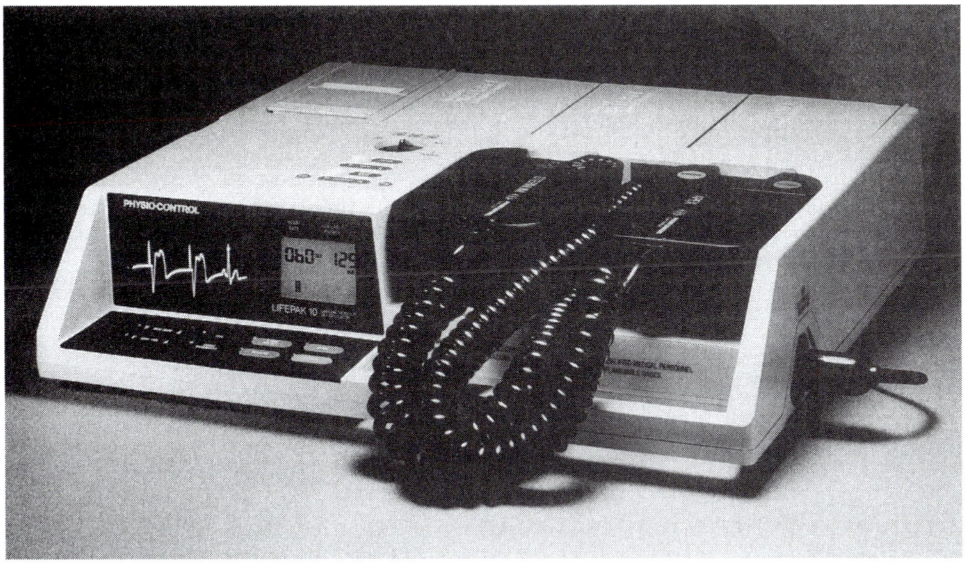

Figure 9-1
A defibrillator/monitor (Courtesy of Medtronic Physio-Control.)

The basic controls are standard and include an on/off switch; energy selection, charge, and discharge buttons; and a synchronized control button. Some defibrillators have the capability of discharge control or internal and external applications (see Figure 9-1).

DEFIBRILLATION

Defibrillation is the **unsynchronized** delivery of a high-intensity charge to the heart that results in complete depolarization of the myocardium. The term *unsynchronized* implies that there is no sensing mechanism. The current is delivered regardless of the ECG rhythm. Figure 9-2 is a continuous ECG tracing illustrating ventricular fibrillation and the deflections recorded during the delivery of shock current.

unsynchronized
No use of a sensing mechanism to deliver shock current

After conversion, the resulting rhythm depends on the capability of the first, fastest, and strongest pacemaker repolarized. The probability of conversion to a higher order of rhythm is directly related to the duration of ventricular fibrillation. The status of the heart's muscle, oxygenation, and overall metabolic condition are critical factors in successful conversion to a natural pacemaker.

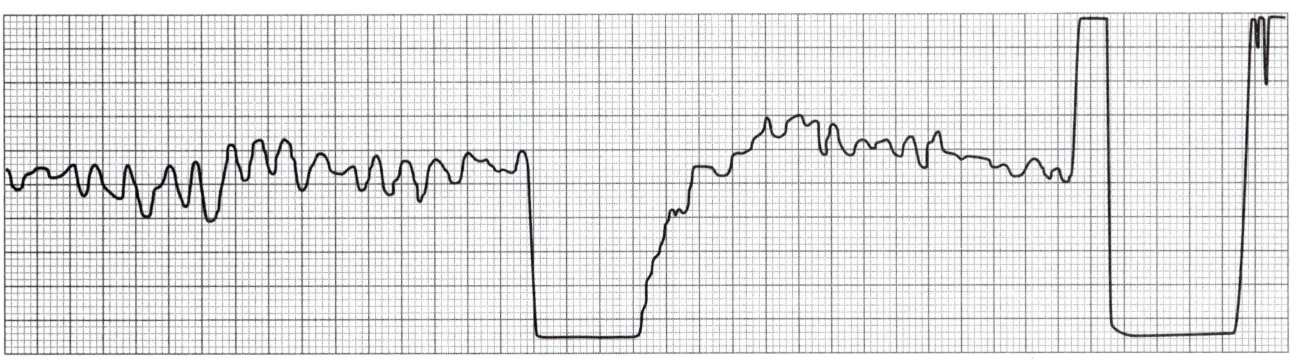

Figure 9-2 An ECG tracing showing ventricular fibrillation and the point of defibrillation. Note the prominent deflections at the time of shock.

Defibrillation does not guarantee conversion. Following delivery of the electrical charge to the myocardium, there is a period of myocardial instability that may result in arrhythmias. Therefore, any factors that enhance instability should be managed as soon as possible. These include hypoxia, extremes in acidosis or alkalosis, digitalization and electrolyte imbalance.

Another form of unsychronized shock may be delivered by a forceful blow to precordium, a **precordial thump**. This mechanical shock can result in depolarization of the myocardium and can terminate some arrhythmias. Precordial thump should be done only with a standby defibrillator since the mechanisms cause deterioriation to ventricular fibrillation. Complications from a precordial thump can include damage to the sternum and rib cage or even damage to the liver, spleen, myocardium, and lungs.

precordial thump
An unsynchronized, mechanical shock delivered by a forceful blow to the precordium

Indications for Defibrillation

The delivery of an unsynchronized charge is indicated where there is no QRS complex present, as in ventricular fibrillation or when ventricular tachycardia is present and the patient has no palpable pulse. When the rhythm does not convert, subsequent shocks are rapidly delivered and the amount of voltage increases. Repeated discharge of energy over short periods of time may decrease the resistance and improve the chance for conversion.

SYNCHRONIZED CARDIOVERSION

Cardioversion has several definitions and interpretations. The generic definition is any method used to terminate an arrhythmia. Another is any method of electrical termination of any arrhythmia. A third definition is the delivery of shock to terminate atrial fibrillation and flutter with rapid ventricular rates, and supraventricular tachycardia. Since confusion with terminology still exists, the clinician is best advised to define the method of delivery, that is synchronized or unsychronized.

cardioversion
Delivery of an electrical discharge used to terminate dysrhythmias that are refractory to drugs; or when an immediate conversion to sinus rhythm is needed

Synchronized cardioversion means the machine is programmed to deliver the charge *in synch with* or simultaneous to the patient's QRS complex. Synchronized cardioversion is used to treat arrhythmias other than ventricular fibrillation and polymorphic ventricular tachycardia. The term *synchronized* implies that there is a sensing mechanism so that the charge will only be released when the unit recognizes the QRS complex (often and more simply referred to as the *R wave*), therefore preventing the charge from falling during the relative refractory period.

synchronized
Delivery of an electrical discharge programmed simultaneously to the patient's QRS complex

A QRS complex of at least 10 mm may not be visible in lead II, the common monitoring lead. It may be necessary to switch leads to visualize the QRS complex and then synchronize.

When the synchronize control, or synch-mode, is activated, the monitor searches for certain criteria, such as amplitude and slope of the wave form, in an effort to differentiate from the P, T, or U waves. Most units will easily detect an R wave that is tall and narrow. The monitor will *mark* the R wave and indicate this on the ECG paper and the LED display. Figure 9-3 shows the markings indicating the QRS complex sensed and recognized by the monitor/defibrillator.

When the monitor/defibrillator is charged in the synch mode, it will discharge only energy when the monitor detects the R wave. This seek-and-find mechanism

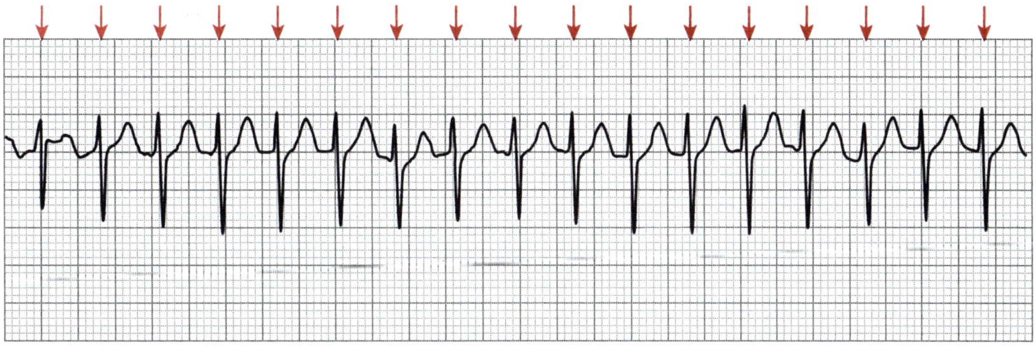

Figure 9-3 A continuous ECG tracing from a patient with a narrow-QRS tachycardia. Note the arrows over each QRS indicating that the unit is in the synchronized mode.

causes a short delay while the machine confirms the R wave. Figure 9-4 is a continuous ECG recording of synchronized cardioversion showing the preshock markings of the QRS complex, the time of discharge, and the postshock ECG.

Figure 9-5 is an example of cardioversion in a patient with atrial flutter showing the time of shock and the resulting rhythm.

Indications

Synchronized cardioversion is used in the management of patients with narrow QRS-complex tachycardia, such as PSVT, atrial fibrillation, or atrial flutter with a rapid ventricular response and certain junctional and ventricular tachycardias.

In wide-complex, ventricular tachycardia, when the rate is very rapid or the QRS complex is wide and bizarre, it may be difficult for the monitor/defibrillator to discriminate between QRS and T waves, and the chance for discharge during the time seen as the T wave is a risk. If the patient is in jeopardy, the operator should not take the time to synchronize; defibrillation should be applied immediately.

Synchronized cardioversion is usually an elective procedure. Administration of medication to sedate the concious patient and relax skeletal muscles is indicated.

AUTOMATED EXTERNAL DEFIBRILLATION

Automated external defibrillation (AED) is indicated for patients who are apneic and pulseless. AEDs are designed to analyze cardiac electrical activity and deliver a series of shocks through electrodes attached to the patient's chest. The technology for automated external defibrillation has advanced to a point where lay persons can be trained in the delivery of shock. Successful resuscitation of out-of-hospital arrest depends on a series of critical interventions known as the *chain of survival.* This chain includes early recognition, early access, early application of CPR, early defibrillation, and early access to advanced life support (ALS).

automated external defibrillation
The use of a computer voice synthesizer to guide the operator through the steps of defibrillation

Many EMS systems have demonstrated increased survival outcomes of cardiac arrest patients experiencing ventricular fibrillation. The increase in survival rates occured after early defibrillation programs were implemented and when all of the links in the chain of survival were present.

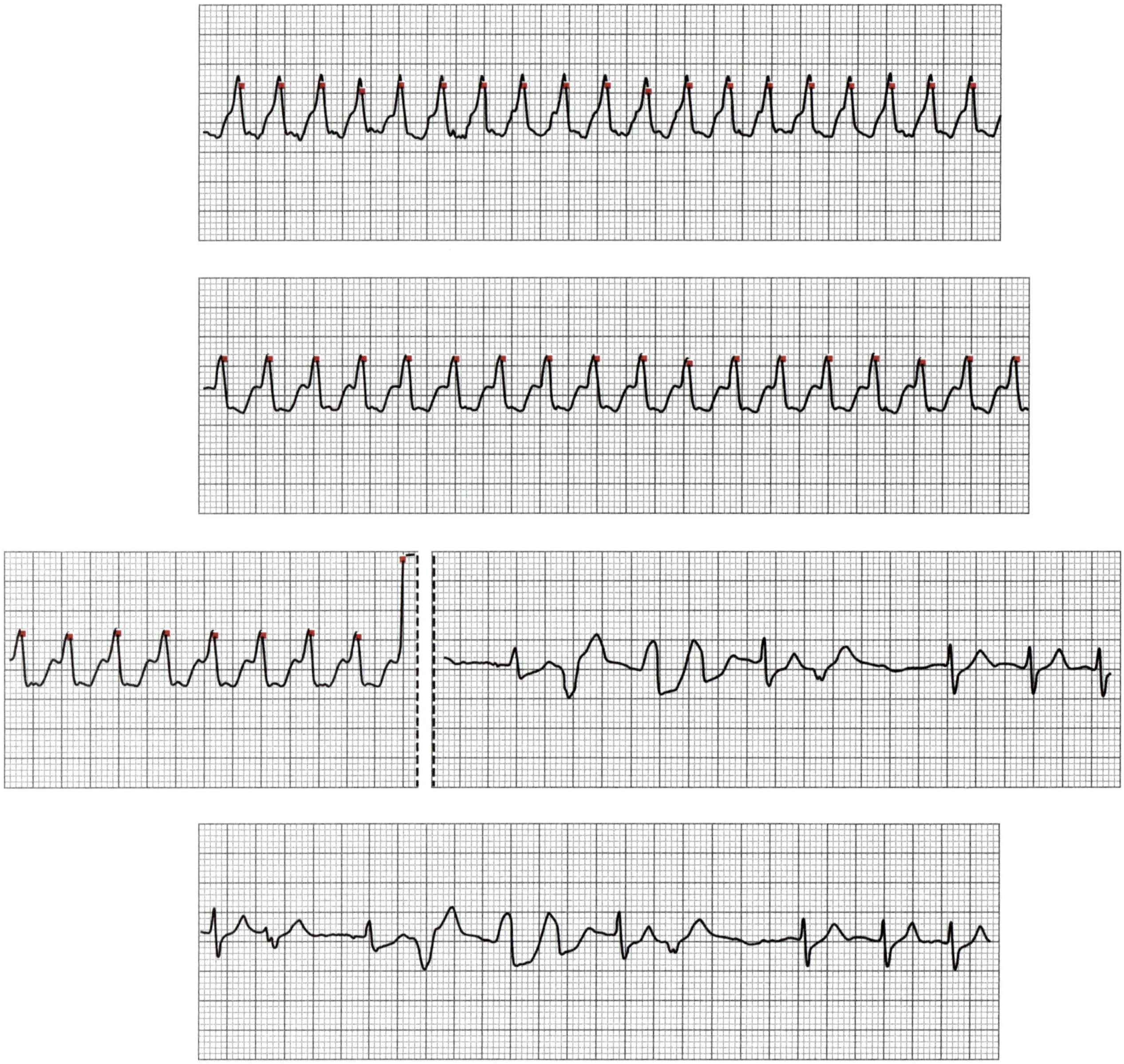

Figure 9-4 A continuous ECG tracing from a patient with supraventricular tachycardia. Note the deflections superimposed on the R wave indicating that the unit is in the synchronized mode. The deflection at the time of shock in the third tracing is followed by a conversion. Note in the fourth tracing that ectopy is still present. Finally, in the last tracing, allegedly after 47 minutes, sinus rhythm begins to prevail without ectopy.

Currently, AEDs are used in medical patients over the age of 12. Rescuers authorized to use AEDs must also learn the following:

1. Use of bag-valve-mask devices with supplemental oxygen attached.
2. Use of flow restricted, oxygen-powered ventilatory devices.
3. Techniques of lifting and moving patients.
4. Suctioning of airways.
5. Use of airway adjuncts.

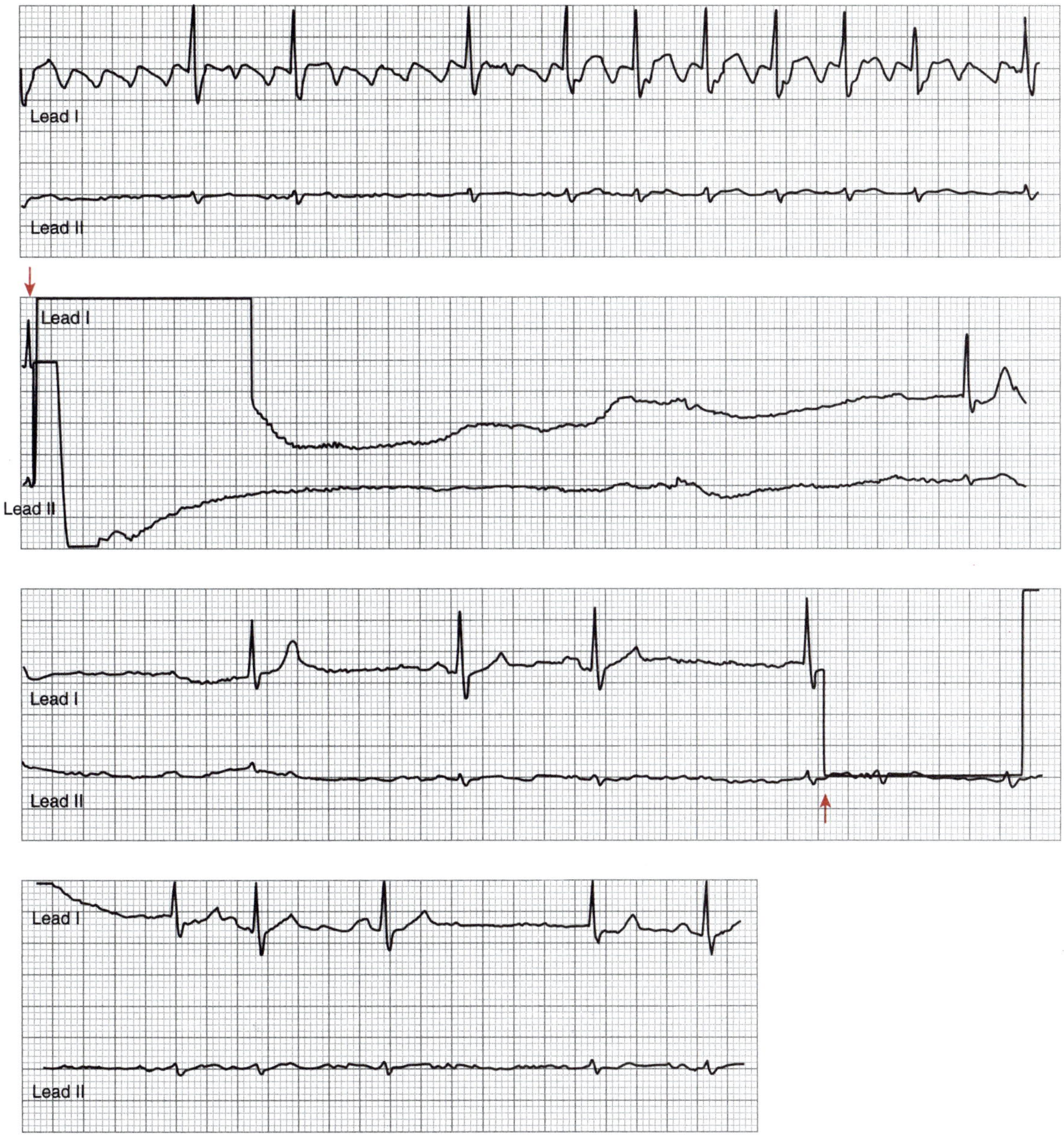

Figure 9-5 A continuous ECG tracing from a patient with atrial flutter. This tracing has two leads, lead I and lead II. Note that the atrial flutter is better visible in this patient in lead I. The patient underwent synchronized cardioversion at 25 joules. The deflection at the time of shock is visible as well as the subsequent conversion to a sinus rhythm with PACs.

6. Use of body substance isolation for infections when necessary.
7. How to interview bystanders and family members to obtain facts related to arrest events.

Semi-automatic versus Fully Automated External Defibrillation

Fully automated external defibrillation works without action by the operator, except to turn on power. The semi-automatic defibrillator uses a computer voice synthesizer to advise the operator of the steps to take based upon its analysis of the patient's cardiac rhythm.

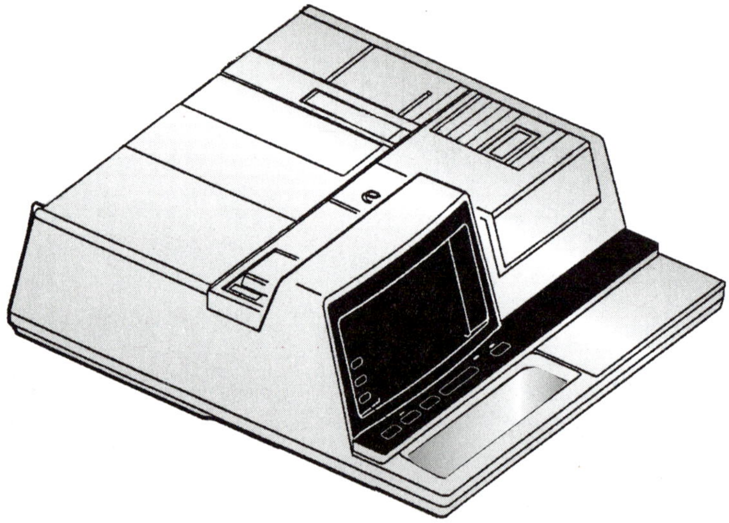

Figure 9-6 An AED device (Adapted with permission from Medtronic Physio-Control.)

Analysis of cardiac rhythms is done by the defibrillator computer microprocessor, which evaluates the patient's rhythm and confirms the presence of a rhythm for which a shock is indicated.

Accuracy of devices in rhythm analysis has been high in detecting both rhythms needing shocks and rhythms that do not need shocks. The analysis is dependent on properly charged defibrillator batteries.

Application must be interruped for any movement, even during transportation of the patient. Some AEDs cannot differentiate patient movement of any kind from ventricular fibrillation. Therefore, no CPR is performed during the time the machine is analyzing the rhythm, as well as at times shocks are delivered. No person should be touching the patient when rhythm is being analyzed and when shocks are delivered. Chest compressions and artificial ventilation are stopped when the rhythm is being analyzed and when shocks are delivered. Defibrillation is more effective than CPR, so stopping CPR during the process is more beneficial to patient outcome. CPR may be stopped up to 90 seconds if three shocks are necessary, and CPR is resumed only after the first three shocks are delivered.

Some models of SAED have an override feature so that if motion is detected, the operator can move to manual mode and assume full responsibility for rhythm recognition, choice of energy strength, and the ultimate delivery of the charge. These operators function under strict protocols and have physician oversight. Refer to Figure 9-6 for an example of an AED device.

Advantages of Semi-automated External Defibrillation

The operator completes initial training and validates CPR knowledge and skills and must memorize treatment sequence. The speed of operation is very quick; the first shock can be delivered within 1 minute of arrival at the patient's side.

Another advantage is that remote defibrillation occurs through adhesive pads. Remote defibrillation is a safer "hands-off" method. In addition, the electrodes are large, so they cover a larger area. Rhythm monitoring is an option on some defibrillator models, but this is not required. Documentation of preshock and postshock

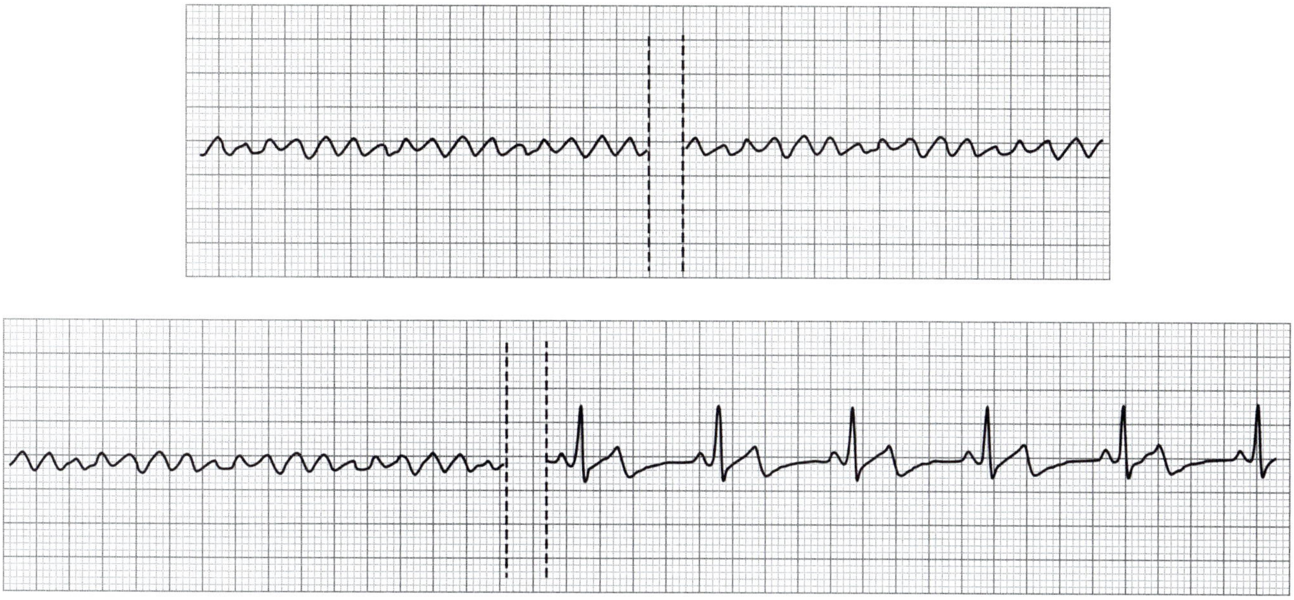

Figure 9-7 A continuous ECG recording showing the documentation from an SAED. A log of activity showing date and time, joules selected, and the pre- and postshock rhythms is available in this model SAED. The option for a continuous recording of rhythm and data is available on most models.

events, the date, time, and joule strength are options on various models. Figure 9-7 is a continuous ECG tracing documenting the activity of this model defibrillator.

Automatic Implantable Cardioverter Defibrillator (AICD)

Patient-activated antitachycardia implanted devices were made available as early as the 1960s. The patient was instructed to activate the device by delivering a burst of pacing, suppressing the arrhythmia, and allowing the sinus node to regain control.

In the 1970s, advanced technology made it possible to implant a device that monitors heart rate, and when a tachycardia is sensed, the device provides a defibrillating current. There were two monitoring electrodes attached to the ventricular epicardium, and two large electrodes similarly attached to deliver the shock. Figure 9-8 is a graphic of the application of epicardial pacing and sensing patches.

Beginning in 1990, transvenous application of the electrodes was made possible. Advanced technology also has developed a single, multifunctional device that can be programmed specific to patient needs, providing high-energy shock, synchronized cardioversion, automated antitachycardia burst pacing, and conventional ventricular pacing. Figure 9-9 shows the position of the transvenous sensing catheter and the position of the implanted defibrillator.

While the electrical termination of recurrent supraventricular tachycardias can be achieved, ablation may be the treatment of choice in cases where the arrhythmia reccurs frequently or the AICD therapy is insufficient to patient needs. Physiologic testing is usually done to determine the cause, and surgical ablation may be recommended as a more successful cure.

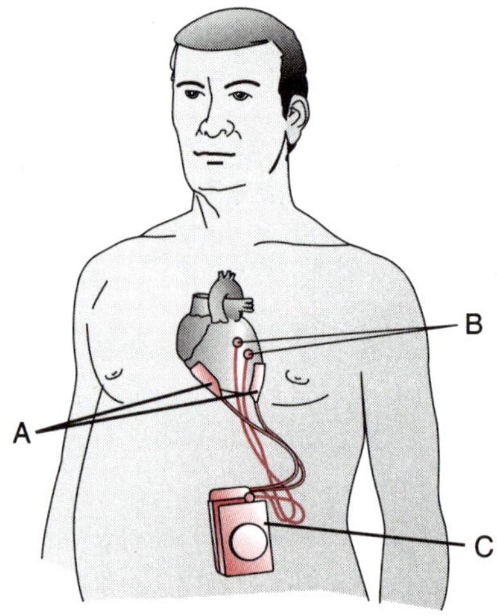

Figure 9-8 (A) Application of the epicardial pacing, (B) sensing electrodes, and (C) the position of the implanted defibrillator.

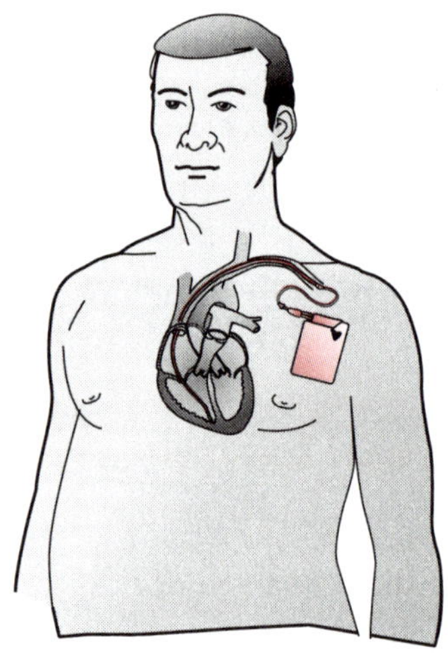

Figure 9-9 A transvenous catheter and an implanted defibrillator device.

Summary

Defibrillation, cardioversion, and AEDs provide a mechanism by which an operator can halt the death process associated with ventricular fibrillation. The successful resuscitation of the patient requiring defibrillation or synchronized cardioversion depends on the duration of ventricular fibrillation or pulseless ventricular tachycardia, as well as the condition of the myocardium, heart size, and body weight.

AEDs are designed for simple operation and application for use on medical patients who are apneic and pulseless. The accurate assessment of the patient is essential to provide the most appropriate technology. Education, practice, medical oversight, and continuing education also are critical links in the survival of the patient and safety of the operator.

Self-Assessment Exercises

Matching

Find the phrase in the right column that matches the numbered word or phrase in the left column, and compare your answers to those in the back of the book.

____ 1. Available energy
____ 2. Defibrillation
____ 3. Delivered energy
____ 4. Fully automated
____ 5. Impedance or resistance
____ 6. Joule
____ 7. Ohm
____ 8. Semi-automatic
____ 9. Stored energy
____ 10. Synchronized

A. Device that advises the operator to deliver a shock
B. Amount of energy actually accessible in the defibrillator's capacitor
C. Amount of energy actually administered
D. Amount of actual energy that will be delivered to a patient with an impedance of 50 ohms
E. Automatic delivery of shock
F. Measurement of defibrillation energy
G. Opposition to the flow of current
H. Process where a sensing mechanism provides delivery of current during the QRS complex
I. Unit of measurement of impedance
J. Unsensed delivery of electrical current

References

Conover, M. B. *Nurse's pocket guide to electrocardiography* (3rd ed.). St. Louis, MO: C. V. Mosby; 1994.

Conover, M. B. *Understanding electrocardiography: Arrhythmias and the 12-lead ECG* (7th ed).. St. Louis, MO: Mosby-Year Book; 1996.

Conover, M. B. & Wellens, H. J. *The ECG in emergency decision making*. Philadelphia: W. B. Saunders; 1993.

Marriott, H. J. & Conover, M. B. *Advanced concepts in arrhythmias* (2nd ed.). St. Louis, MO: C. V. Mosby; 1989.

CHAPTER 10

Electronic Pacemakers

Premise The purpose for electronic pacing is to provide an energy source that will guarantee a minimum ventricular rate when the heart's conduction system cannot. Electronic pacing does not guarantee myocardial tissue response.

Objectives

After reading the chapter and completing the Self-Assessment Exercises, the student should be able to

1. identify pacemaker artifact, and calculate its rate and the escape interval
2. identify the chambers of the heart that are being paced
3. identify the mechanism by which the pacemaker is being activated or inhibited
4. recognize ECG signs of pacemaker malfunction

Key Terms

A-V interval
asynchronous
demand
electronic capture
escape interval
failure to capture
failure to sense
fusion
hysteresis
inhibited
milliampere (mA)
millisecond (ms)
millivolt (mV)
mode of pacemaker response
overdrive suppression
oversensing
pacemaker
pacemaker identification code
programmed upper rate limit (PURL)
rate-adaptive or physiologic
sensitivity
threshold
undersensing

Introduction

The heart has an intrinsic system that provides for the source and conduction system of electrical energy in an organized fashion. Disturbances in the source or within the conduction system can cause life-threatening arrhythmias. These may be drug-induced or due to intrinsic conduction defects.

Electronic pacemakers are used primarily in the management of bradycardia resulting from the heart's inability to stimulate or conduct electrical impulses. They are also used to suppress ectopics and the onset of certain tachycardias.

PACEMAKER CODES

To better understand, more easily evaluate, and document ECG characteristics of **pacemakers**, additional language should be added to the ECG vocabulary, to clarify intrinsic function from pacemaker function. The five-letter **pacemaker identification code** of the Intersociety Committee on Heart Disease (ICHD) was designed in an effort to explain how a pacemaker operates.

pacemaker
The site that controls the heart rate because it has the fastest rate of automaticity

pacemaker identification code
A five-letter code designed to explain the operation of a pacemaker

mode of pacemaker response
The vibration pattern of the pacemaker's shock wave

The first letter of the code does not mean right and left; it indicates the chamber being paced: Atrial (A), Ventricular (V), or Dual (D), indicating both chambers are being paced.

The second letter indicates which chamber's activity is being sensed: Atrial (A), Ventricular (V), or Dual (D), indicating both chambers' activities are being sensed, or O, meaning neither.

The third letter indicates the **mode of pacemaker response**, Inhibited (I), Triggered (T), or Dual (D), indicating the pacer is capable of both functions, or O, meaning not applicable.

The fourth letter stands for the type of changes or the programmability that can be made by noninvasive means, that is, P-programmability of rate and/or output; R-rate modulation; C-communicating; or M-multiprogrammable. These include rate, energy output, ability to sense, refractory period, and other variables as technology increases.

The fifth letter stands for the response of the pulse generator to sensing tachycardias and reflects the antitachycardia function.

Commonly, the first three letters of the code are used to describe pacemaker activity. For example, in a demand, single chamber (ventricular) pacer, both sensing and pacing circuits are in use. Thus, this pacer would be called a VVI pacer; V for the ventricular chamber being paced, V for the intrinsic ventricular activity being sensed, and I for the ventricular function inhibited by the sensed intrinsic QRS.

Another example would be the DDD pacemaker. The first D means dual pacing activity; both atrial and ventricular chambers are paced. The second D means dual sensing activity; both atrial and ventricular intrinsic activity is being sensed. The third D identifies what the pacer will do (pace or not) based on sensed event.

A-V interval
In pacemaking, the distance between the paced atrial wave form and the paced ventricular wave form.

For example, a sensed event in the atrium inhibits atrial pacing and triggers a ventricular pacing stimulus after the programmed **A-V interval**. A sensed beat in the ventricle inhibits the pacer's output in the ventricle.

THE LANGUAGE OF PACEMAKER FUNCTION

In addition, the names given to pacemaker-generated wave forms and intervals differentiate them from the patient's intrinsic wave forms and intervals.

A refers to pacer-induced atrial depolarization.

Committed is a term used in dual-chambered pacing, when ventricular stimulation will occur after atrial stimulation at a preset interval. If ventricular stimulation is programmed to occur *always* after atrial stimulation, this is termed *fully committed.* When normal or paced atrial excitation occurs and normal (intrinsic) AV conduction results, ventricular pacing will be inhibited.

Partially Committed refers to pacemakers that have *safety pacing.* For example, after the atrial spike occurs, the pacemaker looks for any sensed event within 110 **milliseconds (ms)**. If a ventricular event is sensed during that time, the pacemaker forces a ventricular spike at the end of 110 ms. If nothing is sensed during the first 110 ms following the atrial spike, the pacer will inhibit on any ventricular sensed event after 110 ms or it will pace at the end of the A-V interval.

millisecond
One thousandth of a second

V-A Interval is the time between paced ventricular and paced atrial activity.

V-V Interval is the distance measured between two paced ventricular events.

R-V Interval: The distance from the intrinsic ventricular event and the paced ventricular event that follows, the pacemaker's escape interval.

Notation is a set of numbers indicating pacer mode and programmed timing parameters, seen on patient identification cards. For example, a notation may be 60/160/150. The 60 is the lower rate limit. The pacemaker is programmed to track spontaneous rate, and if this intrinsic rate falls below 60 per minute, the pacer is programmed to provide the stimulus. The 160 is because in dual-chambered pacing, the A-V interval is measured in milliseconds; for example, 160 milliseconds equals 0.16 second. The 150 is the pacemaker's programmed maximum rate of delivery. In this example, the paced rate should never exceed 150 per minute.

Table 10-1 is a summary of the intrinsic ECG terms and correlating pacemaker terminology.

When referring to the intervals between intrinsic function and pacing function, the terminology will afford an easy explanation. For example, in atrial pacing, the interval between the intrinsic P wave and the paced atrial beat would be the P-A interval. Similarly, the interval between the intrinsic QRS and the paced QRS, would be the R-V interval. Figure 10-1 is an ECG tracing indicating the R-V and V-V intervals.

PACEMAKER COMPONENTS

Pulse Generator

An electronic pacemaker consists of two primary components: the pulse generator, which is the energy source, and the pacing electrode, which delivers the electrical

Table 10-1 Analogous terminology for intrinsic and pacemaker wave forms and measurements.

Intrinsic Wave Forms	Pacemaker Term
P wave	A wave
P-R interval	A-V interval
P-P interval	A-A interval
QRS complex	V wave
R-R interval	V-V interval

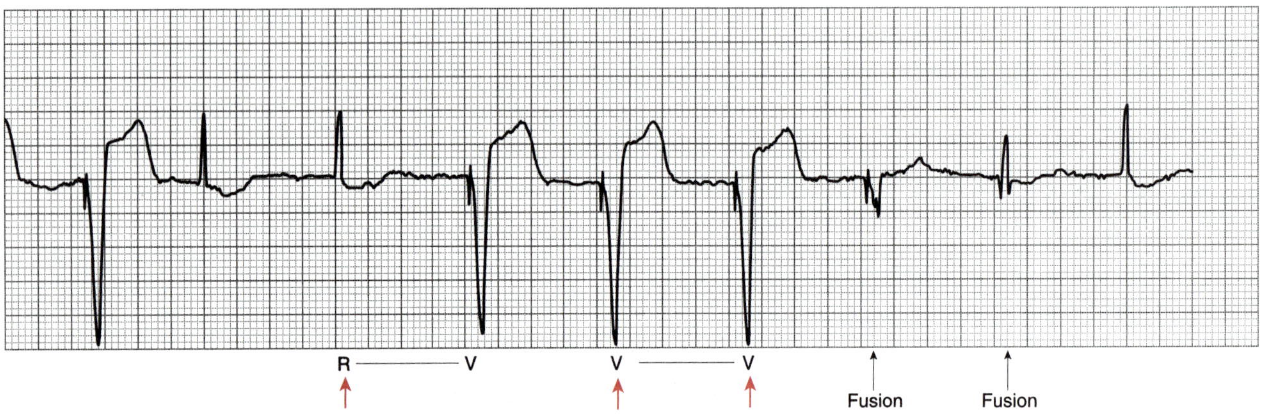

Figure 10-1 An ECG tracing indicating the R-V and V-V intervals. Note the distance between the second, intrinsic QRS (R) and the first paced QRS (V), the distance between two paced QRS complexes (R-R). The R-V = the V-V interval. There are two paced QRS complexes that are a merging of paced and normal forces depolarizing the ventricles. The V-V interval remains constant as the supraventricular source had not yet accelerated beyond the pacer's preset rate. Note the combination or fusion of the pacer spike and the intrinsic QRS complex. The pacer fires on time, and there is a combination of paced and intrinsic forces.

stimulus. External pacemakers that deliver a current through the skin from one electrode to another are called *transcutaneous* (*trans*–through, *cutaneous*–the skin). The pulse generator of the transvenous pacemaker can be external or implanted. A transvenous pacemaker (*trans*–through, *venous*–the vein) uses a pacing catheter that is connected to the pacemaker and threaded into the right ventricle so that it comes in contact with the right ventricular endocardial tissue.

Pacemaker generators are frequently of the built-in cardiac monitor/defibrillator type or hand-held devices. Implanted pacemaker generators are encased in titanium or stainless steel housing that is hermetically sealed to protect the circuitry.

Pacemaker circuitry changes constantly. It has evolved from transistorized circuits, and their sizes have decreased appreciably. Newer pacemakers are very small and programmable, sometimes using telephone transmission. Figure 10-2 is a drawing of the torso with anterior and posterior (AP) transcutaneous pads superimposed.

Transcutaneous pacemakers (TCPs) are external devices manufactured separately or incorporated into defibrillator/monitors. Some are designed with a pacing cassette to be inserted into the defibrillator console, and others have pacing controls integrated into the system. In a transcutaneous pacemaker, the electrodes are attached to the patient and to the pacemaker by a special pacing cable. ECG leads also are attached to the patient as the intrinsic ECG signal must be monitored constantly.

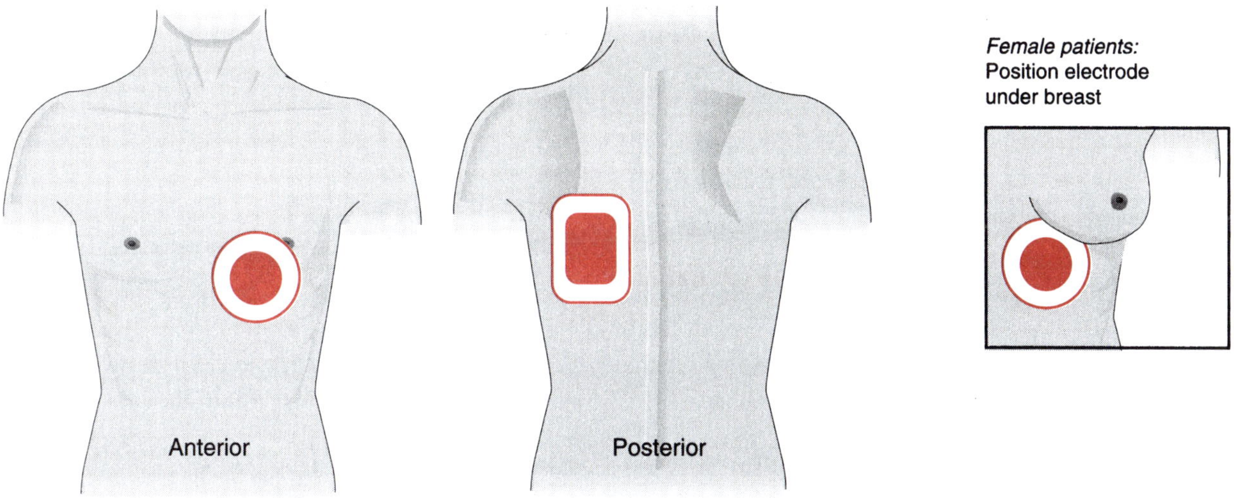

Figure 10-2 A torso with anterior and posterior (AP) transcutaneous pads, indicating their placement. The insert shows the position of the anterior pad for female patients.

Pacemaker Catheters and Electrodes

Transvenous pacing is relatively new, beginning in the 1959. A pacemaker catheter is inserted using a venous approach so that the distal tip is in the right ventricle. The pacemaker catheter is attached to a pulse generator.

Pacemaker catheters, often referred to as the *lead* or the *electrode*, are the link between the pacemaker and the heart. These catheters transmit an impulse to the heart, and in some pacemakers, transmit the heart's intrinsic electrical activity back to the pacemaker.

Pacemaker catheters are either bipolar or unipolar. Bipolar catheters have positive and negative electrodes, which come in contact with heart tissue. The distal, negative electrode is the stimulating electrode.

Unipolar electrodes have only the negative electrode at the distal tip of the catheter. The positive or indifferent electrode is part of the pulse generator. Unipolar systems are very sensitive to intracardiac as well as extracardiac signals.

Noninvasive, transcutaneous pacing electrodes are large, pregelled patches that can be anterior-posterior (AP) or anterior-left lateral (AL). The AP placement is most common and does not interfere with defibrillation if needed. The landmarks for placement of the TCP pacing electrodes are well defined by the manufacturer, and the polarity should not be reversed. If the electrodes are reversed, failure to capture may occur.

External pacing electrodes may be multifunctional (ECG monitoring, defibrillation/synchronized cardioversion, and pacing) or single function (pacing only). Whatever the manufacture capabilities, during demand pacing the patient's ECG must be monitored through ECG electrodes. Current technology does not permit multifunction electrodes to pace and monitor the patient at the same time. The repetitive pacing current is usually large in comparison to the intrinsic ECG and would be disruptive to the ECG display.

The proximity of pacing electrodes with TCP to the ECG electrodes may cause artifact and distortion on the ECG. The ECG electrodes should be placed far enough away from the site of the pacemaker electrodes so that the ECG tracing is clear and distinct. For instance, the left leg electrode usually placed under the rib cage can be placed on the left side of the abdomen, away from any bony prominence or even on the left thigh.

Pacemaker Energy

milliampere
One thousandth of an ampere

threshold
The least amount of energy needed to generate a response

sensitivity
The ability of a pacemaker to process the heart's intrinsic signals

millivolt
One thousandth of a volt

undersensing
The inability of a normally operating pacemaker to sense depolarization

oversensing
The pacemaker's sensing of interference as if it were a depolarization wave form

The current output from the pacemaker is measured in terms of **milliamperes**. The amount of mAs, or signal, must be of such an amplitude to cause capture but not so strong as to cause diaphragmatic pacing. The minimum amount of current required to elicit electronic and mechanical capture is **threshold**.

Sensitivity is the ability of the pacemaker to process the heart's intrinsic signals and is programmed in **millivolts** (mVs). When the sensitivity is set at its smallest number, the pacemaker senses all intrinsic signals. As the sensitivity is set at larger numbers, the pacemaker progressively ignores intrinsic signals.

For example, pacemakers set at zero or low numbers are sensitive to the heart's function as with demand pacing. Conversely, if the pacemaker sensitivity is set at a large number, the pacemaker would function at a fixed-rate mode or synchronously.

When depolarization is not sensed, the pacemaker is said to be **undersensing**. Some ectopic intrinsic activity may vary in amplitude, and the pacemaker may not be sensed by a normally operating pacemaker. When interference is sensed as if it were a depolarization wave form, the pacemaker is said to be **oversensing**.

In a transcutaneous system, a higher current of output is required to overcome chest wall resistance. The result is a painful procedure to the patient. The possibility of skin burn is minimized by the large surface area of the pregelled pacing pads.

Pacemaker Artifact and Pacer-induced QRS Complexes

When a pacemaker stimulus is delivered, a sharp, perfectly vertical artifact is seen on the ECG. This is the pacer *artifact*, or *spike*. On the ECG, the pacemaker spike of a unipolar system usually generates a signal (the pacer spike) that is larger than the stimulus from a bipolar signal. Sometimes bipolar spikes are difficult to see, and some may not be seen at all.

electronic capture
A pacer spike directly associated with the ECG complex

failure to capture
A pacer spike with *no* associated ECG complex

Each pacer spike will be seen on the ECG in direct association with the wave form of the chamber being paced. This association is called **electronic capture**. When a pacer spike occurs at the appropriate time, and there is no QRS complex associated with it, this is called **failure to capture**.

The QRS from a unipolar system is usually seen as a large QS complex with the T wave in the opposite direction. The QRS from a bipolar system is primarily negative but may not be greater than 0.12 second. Regardless of the amplitude and direction of every pacer-induced QRS, every captured QRS should result in mechanical capture, that is, a palpable carotid pulse. Figure 10-3 is an ECG tracing showing a rhythm with a paced QRS.

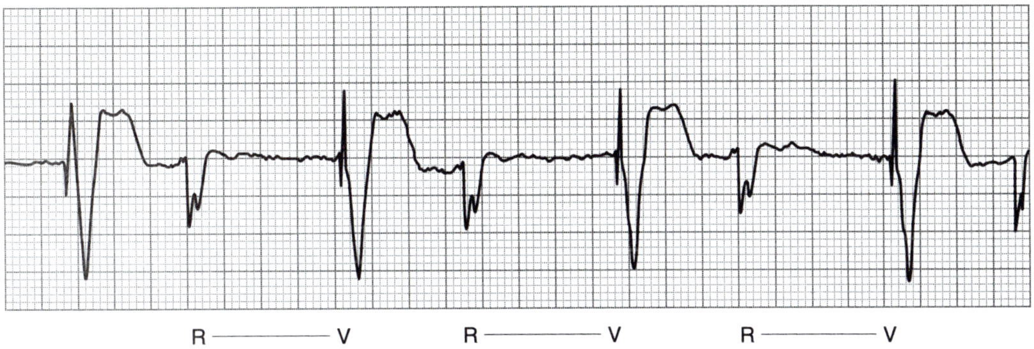

Figure 10-3 An ECG tracing showing the intrinsic QRS (0.12 second) followed by a paced QRS. The rhythm takes on a bigeminal pattern; the R-V intervals are consistent.

Pacemaker Fusion

Occasionally, the pacemaker fires at the same time a supraventricular impulse reaches the ventricles, and the two forces will collide or fuse and simultaneously depolarize the ventricles. This collision of forces, **fusion**, will cause a change in the pacer-induced QRS. The pacer-induced fusion beat will take on the characteristics of both energy sources, causing a decreased amplitude and duration. Figure 10-4 is an ECG tracing showing evidence of pacemaker fusion. Note the decreased amplitude of the QRS.

fusion

A complex produced by the simultaneous discharge of two pacemakers as with an atrial and ventricular focus. As a result of the two waves colliding within the ventricles or atria, the two forces somewhat blend or cancel each other, producing a smaller or narrower complex than normal. The resulting complex shows some characteristics of the ectopic and the sinus beat.

TEMPORARY AND PERMANENT PACING

The word *temporary* in electronic pacing varies in interpretation and is relative to the purpose and goal desired for the patient. For instance, temporary pacing can be noninvasive (transcutaneous) for a short period of time, minutes for an example, or transvenous, yet externally controlled, and used for only a few days. If the problem is corrected, the pacing electrode is easily removed.

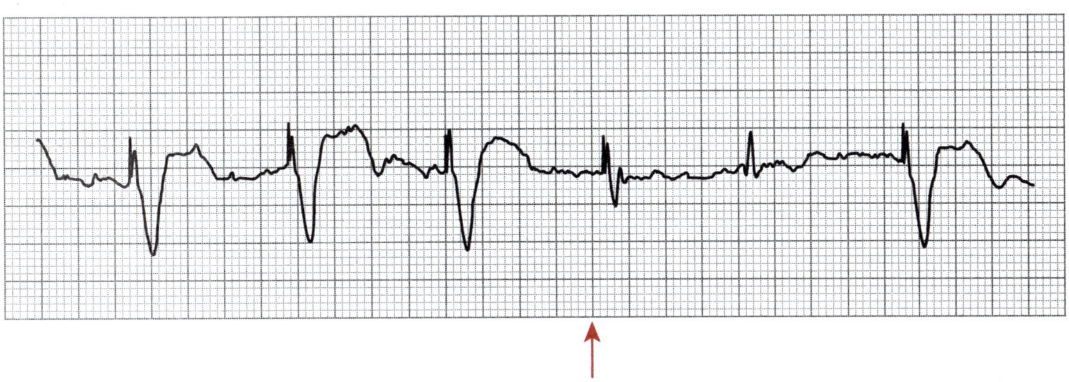

Figure 10-4 An ECG tracing showing four paced QRS complexes. The fourth (↑) complex is a combination of pacer and normal QRS activation. This is pacemaker fusion. The R-V and V-V intervals are consistent.

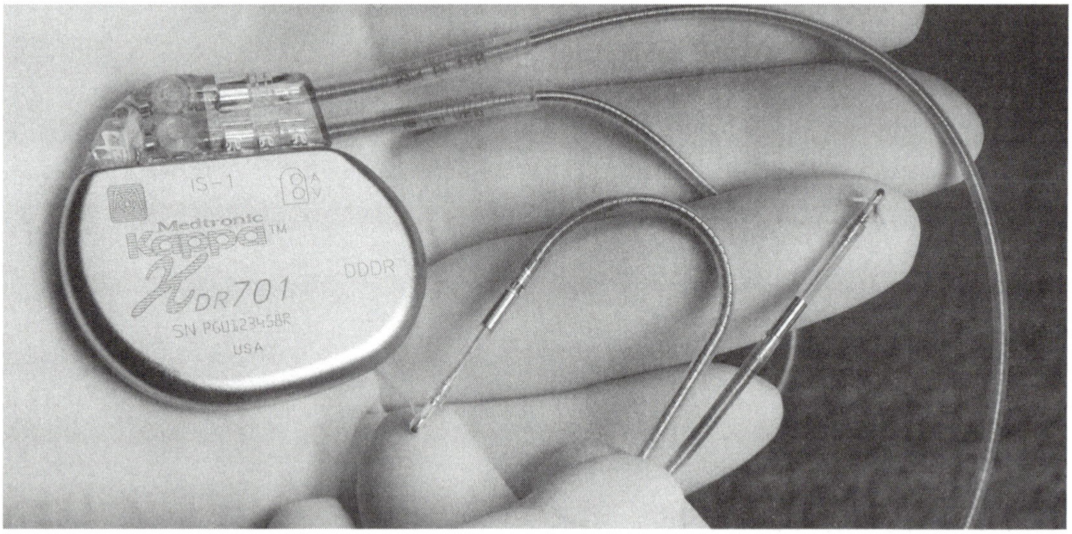

Figure 10-5 An implantable pulse generator (pacemaker) and the platinized pacemaker electrodes. Note the relative size of the pacemaker. It generates the electrical impulse that is transmitted through the electrodes to the endocardium. These implantable, flexible electrodes have soft plastic tines or phlanges that are compressed during implantation. Once inserted, these tines deploy to hold the pacemaker in place and limit the chance of dislodgement. (Courtesy of Medtronic, Inc.).

Implanted pacemaker generators can be a temporary solution for a patient and can be utilized for months or even years. The pacemaker is designed to manage the heart rate until a definitive operative procedure can be performed. For instance, in a child whose weight is slight, and in whom pulmonary function would improve with age, the use of temporary transvenous implanted pacing would provide a satisfactory ventricular rate until such time as the corrective procedure could be accomplished. Figure 10-5 shows a a transcutaneous, a hand-held, and an implanted pacemaker generator.

Classification

Pacemakers are classified according to their activity as either asynchronous or demand pacemakers.

asynchronous
A pacemaker current generated at a fixed, preset rate

Asynchronous Pacemakers (VOO). **Asynchronous** pacemakers are also called *fixed-rate* or *continuous* pacemakers and generate a current at a fixed, preset rate. These pacemakers may be used in cases of congenital AV block or other conditions where there is no functional (natural) intrinsic rhythm. A fixed-rate or continuous pacemaker fires continuously, regardless of the patient's intrinsic rhythm. The possibility of a pacing stimulus firing during the heart's vulnerable period is great, and the patient could suffer pacer-induced ventricular tachycardia or fibrillation. There is no sensing mechanism in a fixed-rate pacemaker.

demand
When an artificial pacemaker senses intrinsic cardiac activity and does not discharge. This prevents competition between the artificial pacemaker and sinus activity.

Demand Pacemakers (VVI/AAI). Demand or inhibited pacemakers fire only when needed, or on **demand**. Demand or synchronous pacemakers have a sensing device and a timer that is preset for a specific rate, or escape interval. The sensing mechanism interprets the signal received from the patient's rhythm, allowing for intrinsic function. If an impulse is sensed within the pacemaker's preset rate, the pacemaker is inhibited, does not pace, and the timer is reset. If an impulse is not generated after the appropriate interval, the pacer fires, and the timer is again reset. Usually, the distance between the intrinsic QRS and the first paced QRS (R-V interval) is the same as the distance between two consecutive paced beats (V-V interval).

The **escape interval** is the time from the last sensed beat to the first pacer spike. The duration of the escape interval is preset according to the desired rate. For example, if the preset rate is 60 per minute, the escape interval is one second, or five large blocks on ECG paper. A pacer-induced QRS should occur within one second of the previously sensed QRS complex.

escape interval
The preset amount of time from the last sensed beat to the first pacer spike

Similarly, if the preset rate is 75 per minute, the escape interval is 0.8 seconds, or 4 large blocks on the ECG paper. If the patient rate drops below the preset rate, the pacemaker will guarantee the minimal preset rate. In most demand pacemakers, the escape interval is programmed to be constant.

If the sensing electrodes are located in the atrium, the pacemaker senses the patient's intrinsic atrial depolarization. If the sensing electrodes are located in the ventricle, the pacemaker senses the patient's intrinsic ventricular depolarization.

If a demand pacemaker fires prematurely, this is **failure to sense**. This is dangerous to the patient since the premature pacer energy can occur during the vulnerable phase of the intrinsic T wave, and pacemaker-induced tachycardia or fibrillation may result.

failure to sense
The premature firing of a demand pacemaker that can be dangerous to the patient

Sensing failure can be oversensing or undersensing. Undersensing would cause the pacemaker to behave like an asynchronous device. Oversensing could cause long pauses beyond the escape interval.

Hysteresis

Hysteresis is a feature of some permanent pacemakers that allows for programming of a longer escape interval between the intrinsic complex and the first paced event. It is a delay mechanism that allows a little more time for the intrinsic pacemaker to generate a natural impulse. This prolonged interval should be the same every time it occurs and should occur only between the intrinsic and first paced event.

hysteresis
A delay mechanism on some permanent pacemakers to allow programming of prolonged intervals used to promote normal intrinsic function as long as possible

The advantage to hysteresis is to allow for intrinsic function within a safe and reasonable rate range, thus promoting normal function as long as possible. The problem is that some pacemakers are programmed with long periods of hysteresis, and on the ECG, this feature may be mistaken for pacemaker malfunction. Differences in escape and pacing intervals should cause concern for pacer malfunction until proven otherwise. Figure 10-6 shows examples of hysteresis. Note the difference in the measurements between the R-V and V-V intervals. This is a documented ECG from a patient with hysteresis programmed into the pacemaker function. The observer would interpret this as pacemaker malfunction, and without documentation about this patient's pacemaker specifications, the operator would be correct.

Atrial Pacemakers

Atrial pacemakers are often used in conditions of sinus (SA) arrest and when conduction through the AV node is intact. The pacing catheter is threaded transvenously so that the electrode is located in the right atrium and acts as an artificial SA node and senses the patient's intrinsic P wave.

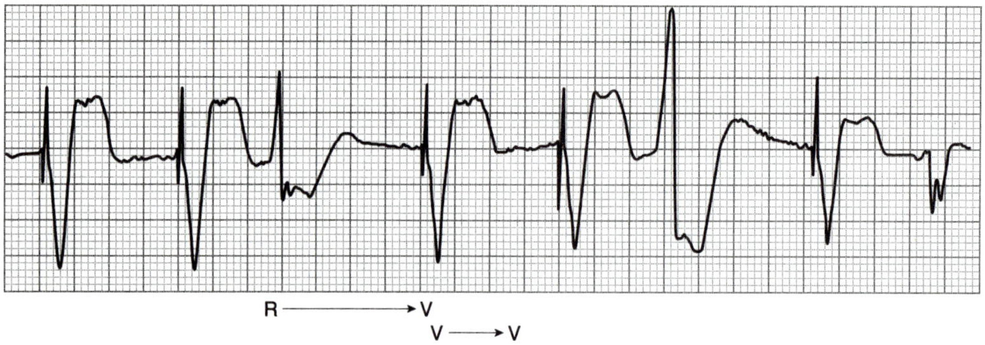

(A)

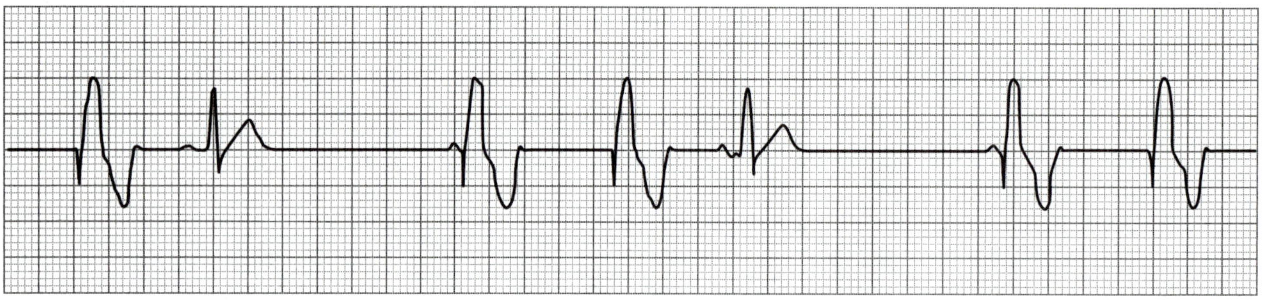

(B)

Figure 10-6 Examples of hysteresis. In (A), note the difference in the measurements between the R-V and V-V intervals; the first R-V interval is 0.12 second longer than the V-V interval. This is consistent, even when the next intrinsic QRS is a PVC. In (B), note the long R-V which is clearly longer than the V-V interval. This would be interpreted as pacemaker malfunction unless the clinician knew the patient was programmed with hysteresis. (ECG courtesy of John Stasic, MEDTRONIC Corp.)

Atrial pacemakers also are used in bradycardia; they drive the heart at a rate faster than the intrinsic rate. When a pacemaker is stimulating the atrium, each pacing spike should produce a P wave. Atrial pacemakers are not used in patients with atrial arrhythmias.

VENTRICULAR PACEMAKERS

The earliest and most common mode of pacing is ventricular. Ventricular pacing can be external (transcutaneous or transvenous) or implanted. In ventricular pacing, the impulse stimulates the ventricles. The paced QRS will be preceded by a pacing spike and the pacer-induced QRS should result in a palpable carotid pulse (mechanical capture).

Fixed-rate ventricular pacing is seldom used. Recall that fixed-rate pacing is not sensitive to the intrinsic QRS and fires continuously without regard for the patient's own heart rhythm. The fixed-rate pacing current could fall during the vulnerable phase of the cardiac cycle and cause repetitive firing, pacer-induced ventricular tachycardia, or fibrillation.

When an ECG tracing shows only ventricular pacing, the observer will be unable to determine if the pacemaker is an asynchronous pacer or a demand pacer functioning 100 percent of the time. Sometimes the patient knows the type of pacemaker, and sometimes the patient will carry an identification card explaining the

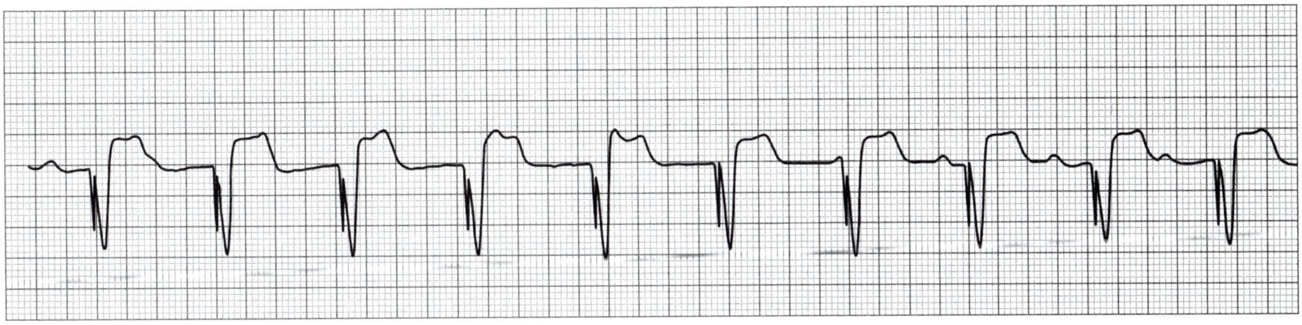

Figure 10-7 An ECG tracing of a ventricular pacer. There are no intrinsic QRS complexes. It is not vital that the clinician determine the underlying rhythm. It is not possible to determine if this is a demand or an asynchronous pacemaker as there are no intrinsic beats. The ECG is interpreted as a ventricular pacer at 75 per minute.

name and type of pacer implanted. Figure 10-7 is an ECG tracing of a ventricular pacer. There are no intrinsic QRS complexes.

Ventricular Demand Pacemakers

Ventricular demand or QRS-inhibited pacemakers are used frequently and are the only type used for transcutaneous pacing at this time. This pacemaker has both sensing and pacing mechanisms. Both mechanisms are situated in the ventricle and thus sensitive to the patient's intrinsic QRS complex. The pacemaker is programmed not to fire; thus, the pacemaker is **inhibited** by the patient's own QRS complex. The demand ventricular pacemaker is ideal in the use of any bradycardia because of these two unique features:

inhibited
Restrained from firing

1. sensing the patient's intrinsic QRS
2. ability to fire only when needed

Figure 10-8 is an ECG tracing showing the escape intervals with a demand ventricular pacemaker.

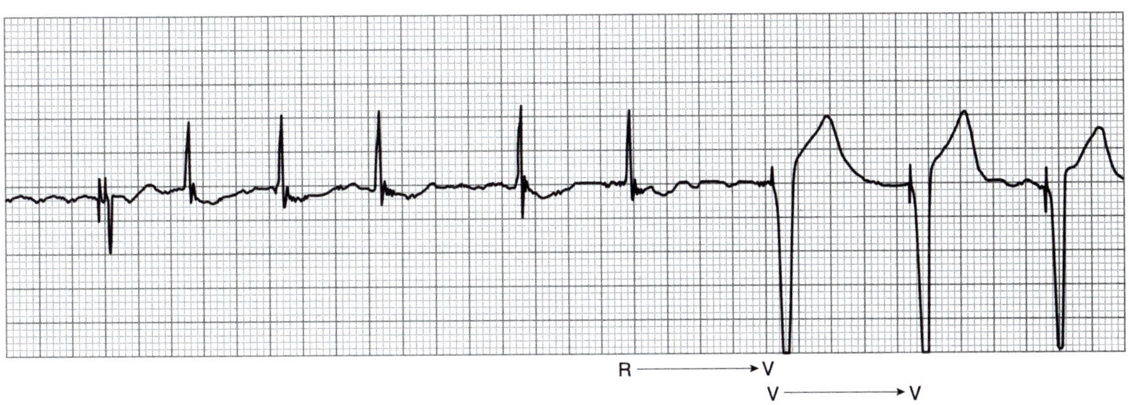

Figure 10-8 An ECG tracing of atrial fibrillation with an ventricular demand pacemaker. Note that the R-V and V-V intervals are similar.

Noninvasive *transcutaneous* pacemakers (TCPs) are ventricular demand pacemakers and are a temporary solution to a bradycardia. A transcutaneous pacemaker provides quick and safe, although uncomfortable, application of a pacing device. With TCP, the external electrodes and lead wires are attached to the monitor/defib/pacer apparatus. The advantages are that the application is very quickly done and the operator can control the rate and amplitude of impulses. The major disadvantage is that it is uncomfortable for the patient. As soon as possible, a transvenous catheter is inserted and attached to the external pacemaker during the definitive stage of patient care.

Triggered Ventricular Pacemakers

Like a ventricular-inhibited pacemaker, the triggered ventricular pacemaker has both sensing and pacing capabilities. This pacemaker fires when the patient's intrinsic rate falls below a preset limit but differs from a QRS-inhibited pacer in the manner in which it is programmed to respond. A demand ventricular pacemaker will be inhibited by the QRS and not issue a stimulus; the triggered pacemaker *does* issue a stimulus. In fact, the pacemaker spike is seen in the middle of the QRS. The spike does alter the QRS morphology, making it difficult to assess for pacemaker malfunction.

Dual-chamber Pacemakers. Dual-chamber pacing is when transvenous catheters are implanted into the right atrium and the right ventricle. The advantage to this mode of pacing is that the atria and ventricles are paced in sequence, allowing for atrial contribution to cardiac output. Dual-chamber pacemakers depend on a stable atrial rhythm for proper function.

The dual-chambered pacemaker can be preset with variations:

1. atrial inhibited
2. ventricular inhibited
3. atrial synchronous ventricular inhibited

In each of these settings, the pacer A-V interval is programmed to a specific duration. The dual-chamber pacemaker can be used for problems with sinus node function, firing in the atria and allowing normal progress through the AV conduction system, and ultimately causing ventricular depolarization. If AV block occurs, the ventricular pacer will fire at the end of the programmed A-V interval, thus guaranteeing a minimum ventricular rate.

Regardless of the mode of pacing, if all the components are functioning, the pacing stimulus will be released as designed, each pacemaker stimulus will result in myocardial response or capture, and the escape interval will be constant. Finally, for every captured QRS complex, there should be a mechanical capture, that is, a palpable carotid pulse. Figure 10-9A is a drawing of an implanted dual-chamber pacemaker. Figure 10-9B is an ECG tracing of a dual-chamber pacer. Note the pacer spike before A and V wave forms.

If the intrinsic arrhythmia is atrial fibrillation or flutter, or frequent episodes of atrial tachycardia occur, this pacemaker may not be suitable. In patients whose atrial arrhythmias may preclude them from the use of the DDD or VDD pacemakers, but would benefit from an increase in paced atrial and ventricular function, the physician might consider the use of a biosensor to reflect physiologic needs and alter pacing function accordingly. These are the **rate-adaptive** or **physiologic** pacers.

rate-adaptive or physiologic
A pacemaker that has physiologic sensors and alters pacing functions according to the changes noted

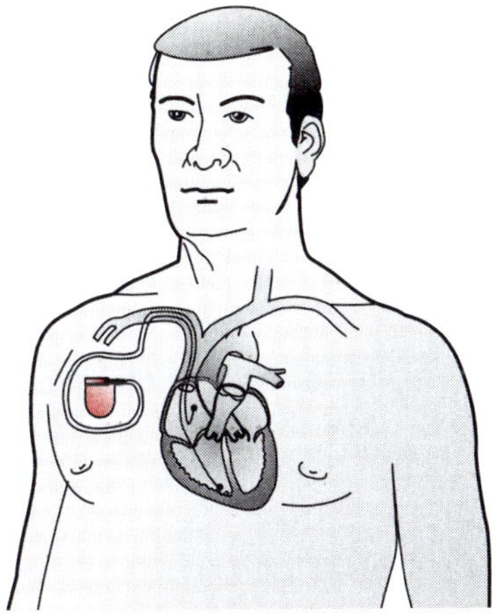

(A)

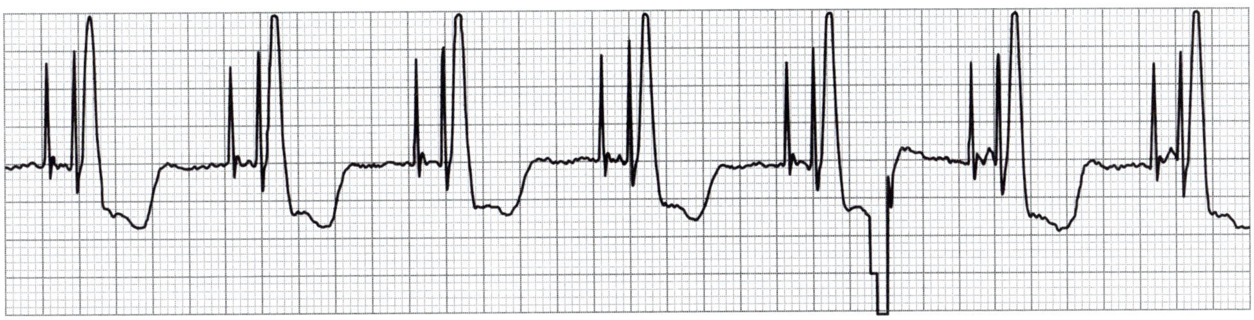

(B)

Figure 10-9 (A) An implanted dual-chamber pacemaker. Note the position of the atrial and ventricular pacemaker catheters. (B) is an ECG tracing of a dual-chamber pacemaker. Note the fixed A-V intervals.

There are pacemakers with a feature that will give a **programmed upper rate limit (PURL)** at which the pacemaker can pace the ventricle. In instances where the atrial rate exceeds the ventricular rate, each ventricular pace is delayed until the PURL is reached. In other words, if the PURL is 100 per minute, the ventricular pacer will not fire at an interval less than 600 ms.

programmed upper rate limit (PURL)

The fastest rate the pacer is programmed to function. The pacer cannot exceed a programmed number of pacing impulses.

Rate-responsive Pacemakers

As technology accelerates, pacemakers are being designed that support the patient's quality of life and respond to the body's demands. For instance, there are demand pacemakers that can be programmed to respond to a change in physiologic demand. These pacemakers are sensitive to the patient's activity and respiratory rate and blood temperature. There are other parameters under investigation, such as metabolic status and blood pH. Once the sensing mechanism processes the information, the pacemaker determines what the desired rate should be and increases or decreases accordingly.

Since these pacemakers are sensor-controlled, rate determination changes to match patient activity moment-to-moment. These pacemakers are *rate-responsive*, *rate-adaptive*, or *rate-modulating* pacemakers.

overdrive suppression
Pacing at very rapid rates to overcome an ectopic

Overdrive Suppression

Overly excitable myocardial tissue can result in unwelcome tachycardias that recur and may render the patient unstable. For example, in the case of Torsade de Pointes, this arrhythmia may be suppressed with defibrillation, but it recurs, requiring the patient to be defibrillated frequently. Despite the good intention, the frequent shocks cause damage to the myocardium.

Another example is refractory bouts of atrial tachycardia. In either of these situations, the application of transvenous or transcutaneous pacing at an R-V interval less than the intrinsic normal QRS-to-ectopic interval may prevent recurrence of the tachycardia until such time as other therapies can be invoked.

During the temporary pacing at high rates, the voltage and rate can be lowered slowly until a reasonable rate range is reached. If the ectopic recurs, the rate and voltage can be increased to regain control.

PACEMAKER MALFUNCTION

Demand pacers should never be late, nor should they ever be premature.

Failure to Function

Problems with pacemaker function are related to timing and the ability to fire, sense, and capture. If the patient's implanted pacemaker fails to function or fire the stimulus, there will be no pacer spike, and the ECG will show what remains of the patient's intrinsic rhythm. In cases of suspected pacemaker malfunction, a transvenous or transcutaneous pacer can be applied as soon as possible and set to a reasonable rate. There is no danger of competition to the suspected defunct implanted pacemaker. Figure 10-10 is an ECG showing failure to function. There is a paced rhythm and suddenly, no pacing artifact; the patient is in complete AV block.

A timing problem exists when the escape interval alters or takes too long. This could be a problem with the timing mechanism or indicate end of life (EOL) for the pacemaker. It should be noted that the least likely problem is timing mechanism failure. Interval changes are usually due to oversensing. An *abrupt* change in an interval, but consistent over time, would indicate EOL. The danger here is the resulting inappropriate bradycardia.

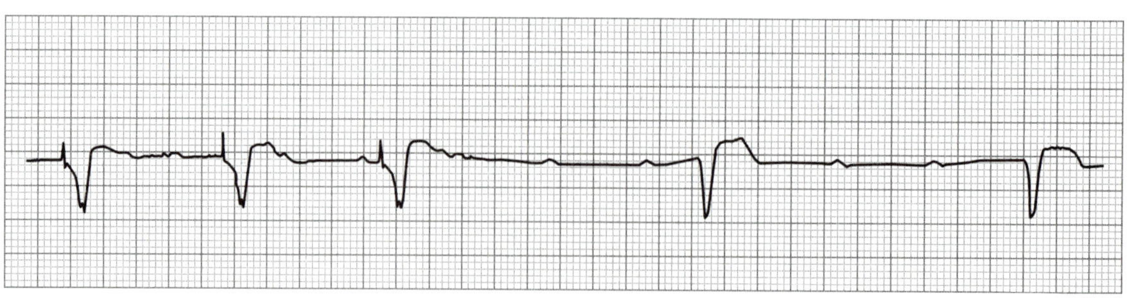

Figure 10-10 ECG showing failure to function. The first four complexes are paced beats. Following is a visible sinus at 100 per minute with complete AV block with a ventricular rhythm at 30 per minute.

Failure to Sense

Failure to sense is the occurrence of premature pacing. The chamber involved may respond to the pacing stimulus or not, depending on the state of refractoriness of the tissue involved. The pacemaker fires without regard to the patient's intrinsic function and competes with the patient for control of heart rate. The danger here is that the pacing spike may fall during the vulnerable period of the cardiac cycle, causing repetitive firing, ventricular tachycardia, or fibrillation.

Occasionally, the patient rate and the pacemaker rate are so similar that it appears that there is failure to sense. Plot out the V-V intervals and then the R-V intervals. If they are the same, the pacemaker is said to be *isorhythmic* (the same rhythm).

Failure to Capture

When a pacemaker is stimulating adequately, each pacer spike would produce a wave form indicating electronic capture. An atrial pacer should produce a pacer-induced P wave; a ventricular pacer should produce a pacer-induced QRS. When a pacer spike fails to produce the paced complex or the pacer-induced QRS fails to produce a pulse, the problem is a failure to capture. This may be a problem with the position of the catheter or inadequate voltage. Failure to capture also may reflect the inability of the heart to respond to the stimulus.

If failure to capture persists, occurs frequently, or results in a bradycardia, application of a transcutaneous or transvenous pacer is in order. Figure 10-11 is an ECG tracing showing failure to capture.

ASSESSING THE PACEMAKER ECG

Approach the ECG in a stepwise fashion:

1. Whenever possible, identify the patient's underlying rhythm
2. Identify the mode of pacing; demand versus asynchronous
3. Evaluate the pacer. To identify a pacer in the demand mode, you must see the patient's own intrinsic QRS.
    a. Measure the distance between two paced beats (the pacing interval).

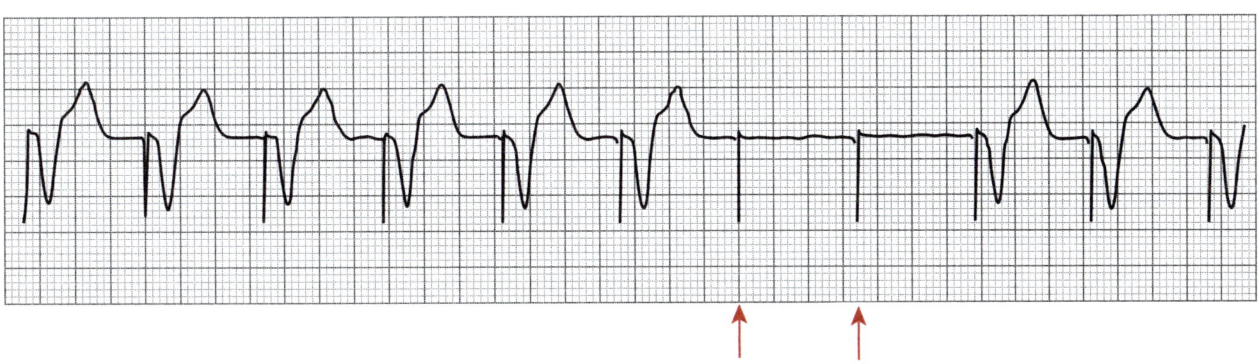

Figure 10-11 An ECG tracing of a ventricular paced rhythm with two episodes of failure to capture (arrows).

b. Compare the distance between the patient's last normal beat and the first paced beat (the escape interval—sometimes called the *demand interval*) These measurements should be the same. In other words, the paced interval equals the escape interval. The documentation will include identification of the patient's rhythm and rate and an assessment of the pacer. For example, "atrial fib at 70 to 85 per minute, a ventricular demand pacer at 72 per minute. The escape and paced intervals are constant." Recall that the demand pacer is set or timed to function within the escape interval. That interval should not change. If the interval is measured to be longer or shorter than what is expected, this is reportable as the pacer may not be functioning properly.

4. Assess the patient's pulse and perfusion. Assess for dizziness, episodes of fainting, edema, dyspnea, chest pain, and hiccough.

Assessing Dual-chamber Pacemaker on ECG

The dual-chambered pacer is programmed to provide both atrial and ventricular function in sequence. This is to provide as near normal perfusion as possible. It is important to determine how the pacer functions in terms of its sensing capabilities.

1. Identify the patient's underlying rhythm.
2. Evaluate the escape interval.
   a. Measure the distance between the first of the pacer artifacts for two paced beats.
   b. Plot back in time and determine which wave forms match this interval, that is, the patient's P wave or the QRS complex. This will give an indication of which complex is being sensed by the pacer.
3. Assess the patient's pulse and perfusion. Assess for dizziness, episodes of fainting, edema, dyspnea, chest pain, and hiccough.

COMPLICATIONS OF PACING

Catheter Dislodgement

Dislodgement of the catheter electrode is a problem that occurs one percent of the time. Dislodgement of the transvenous catheter can result in failure to capture or in inappropriate stimulation. If there is a change in the position of the catheter, the paced ECG pattern will change. One complication is perforation of the ventricular septum. In this instance, the catheter electrode may penetrate the ventricular septum and pace from the left ventricle. While the pacer stimulus (spike) may be seen on the ECG, there may not be a captured QRS complex. An indication of perforated septum is a positive pacer-induced QRS.

Perforation

The pacemaker catheter can perforate the right ventricular septum or the right ventricular wall. If the catheter perforates the right ventricular wall and stimulates the

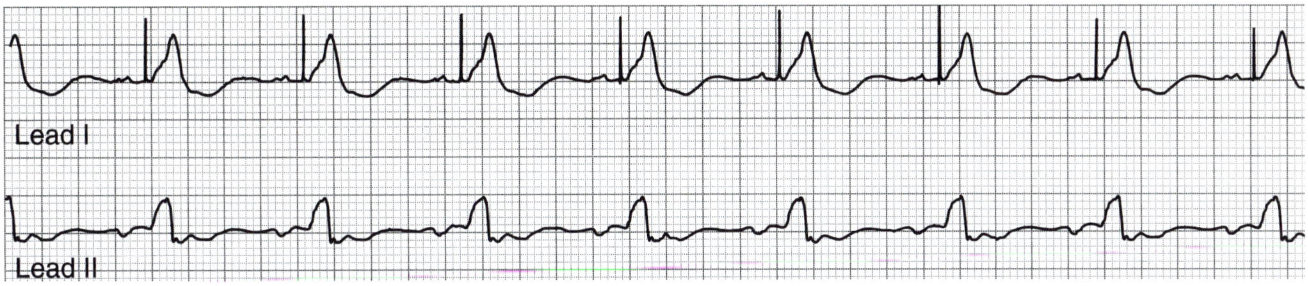

Figure 10-12 An example of positive (+) paced QRSs in a patient with documented perforated septum. Note the (+) paced complexes.

diaphragm, the patient will hiccough to the ventricular paced rate. If a pacemaker catheter perforates the myocardium, pacemaker capture will stop. In addition, a perforated myocardium can lead to cardiac tamponade.

When an electrode perforates the septum, this will cause a sudden change in the polarity of the paced QRS complex. Recall that the paced right ventricle elicits a broad negative (QS) deflection on leads II and V_1. If the left ventricle is stimulated by the pacer, the pacing spike will be followed by a broad positive (QS) deflection on leads II and V_1. In addition, the pacer catheter may not come in contact with ventricular tissue, which will result in failure to capture. Figure 10-12 is an example of positive (+) paced QRSs in a patient with documented perforated septum.

Skeletal Muscle Inhibition

Newer pacemakers have better filtering devices and are less susceptible to interference. Some pacemakers are more interactive and sensitive to intrinsic cardiac activity and may be more susceptible to interference. Unipolar pacemakers are more susceptible to interference than bipolar pacemakers. In either of these situations, the pacemaker may sense the activity, and being unable to discriminate the source, become inhibited from its programmed function. On ECG, this will be interpreted as failure to function.

This should not be confused with skeletal muscle movement seen with transcutaneous pacing. As the pacing current passes through skin and skeletal muscle, a predictable twitching will occur. As current is increased until electronic capture is achieved, the intensity of muscle twitching also will increase. This does not interfere with transcutaneous pacing function.

Interference. Depending on the type and amplitude of an external source of energy, a demand pacer may be unable to discriminate between intrinsic electrical forces and the unknown source. The pacer may be inhibited from functioning near a microwave or cellular telephone, and the patient may be in jeopardy.

Summary

The function of the electronic pacemaker is to provide an artificial stimulus when the heart's own electrical system is failing. The wide range of technology has provided an increase in the pacemaker options for a variety of problems. With the increase in variability of application comes an increase in complexity.

Assessing pacemaker function to determine problems with failure to function, sense, and capture are consistent with all pacing devices. The use of a consistent approach to ECG rhythm analysis will help detect problems with any of these functions.

Self-Assessment Exercises

Matching

Find the phrase in the right column that matches the numbered word or phrase in the left column, and compare your answers to those in the back of the book.

____ 1. A-A interval
____ 2. A-V interval
____ 3. asynchronous
____ 4. capture
____ 5. committed
____ 6. demand pacer
____ 7. failure to capture
____ 8. failure to sense
____ 9. hysteresis
____ 10. inhibited
____ 11. milliamp (mA)
____ 12. millivolt (mV)
____ 13. overdrive suppression
____ 14. pacemaker code
____ 15. pacer spike plus a (+) broad QRS
____ 16. programmed upper rate limit (PURL)
____ 17. rate-adaptive
____ 18. R-V interval
____ 19. sensing
____ 20. threshold
____ 21. V-V interval

A. Ability of the pacemaker to process the heart's intrinsic signals
B. Ability to allow a longer escape interval for the first paced event
C. A pacer spike and no paced QRS or P wave
D. A pacer functions prematurely
E. A pacer that recognizes intrinsic function and paces only when necessary
F. A series of letters to describe pacemaker function
G. Distance between the intrinsic beat and the first paced event. Also known as the pacer escape interval.
H. Distance between two paced atrial events
I. Distance between two paced ventricular events
J. Fixed-rate pacing; no sensing mechanism
K. In dual-chamber pacing, when the A-V interval is preset
L. May indicate septal perforation on the ECG
M. Minimum amount of current required to elicit electronic capture
N. Pacer spike plus a P or broad, negative QRS
O. Pacemaker ability to increase or decrease pacing rates in response to biosensor
P. Preset time between paced atrial and paced ventricular activity
Q. Rapid rate pacing to deter tachycardias
R. Rate limit for pacemakers
S. Sensitivity
T. The ability for the pacer to sense a P and/or QRS and *not* fire
U. Unit of measurement for electrical sensitivity
V. Unit of current in pacemakers

ECG Rhythm Identification Practice

For the following rhythms fill in the blanks and then check your answers with those in the back of this book.

Figure 10-13

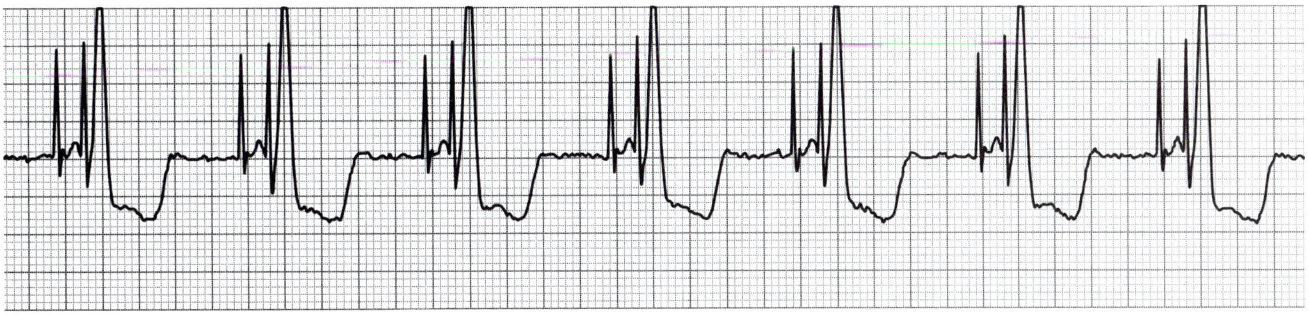

QRS duration ______________ QT ____________

Ventricular rate/rhythm ______________________

Atrial rate/rhythm __________________________

PR interval ________________________________

Identification ________________________________

Symptoms ___________________________________

____

Treatment ___________________________________

Figure 10-14

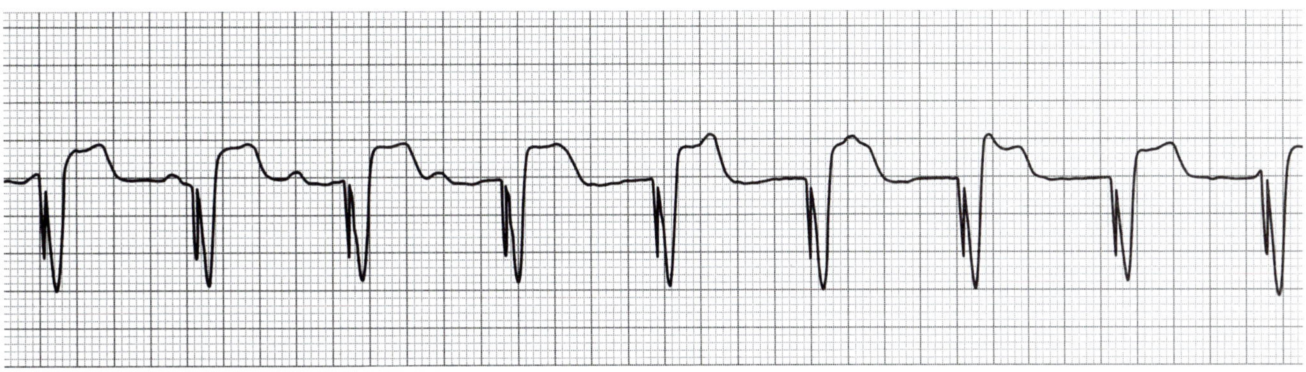

QRS duration ______________ QT ____________

Ventricular rate/rhythm ______________________

Atrial rate/rhythm __________________________

PR interval ________________________________

Identification ________________________________

Symptoms ___________________________________

____

Treatment ___________________________________

Figure 10-15

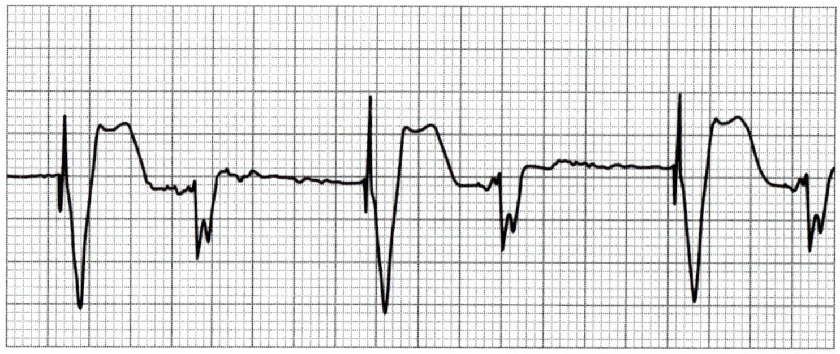

QRS duration ________________ QT _____________
Ventricular rate/rhythm _________________________
Atrial rate/rhythm ______________________________
PR interval ____________________________________

Identification ____
Symptoms ____
____
Treatment ____

Figure 10-16

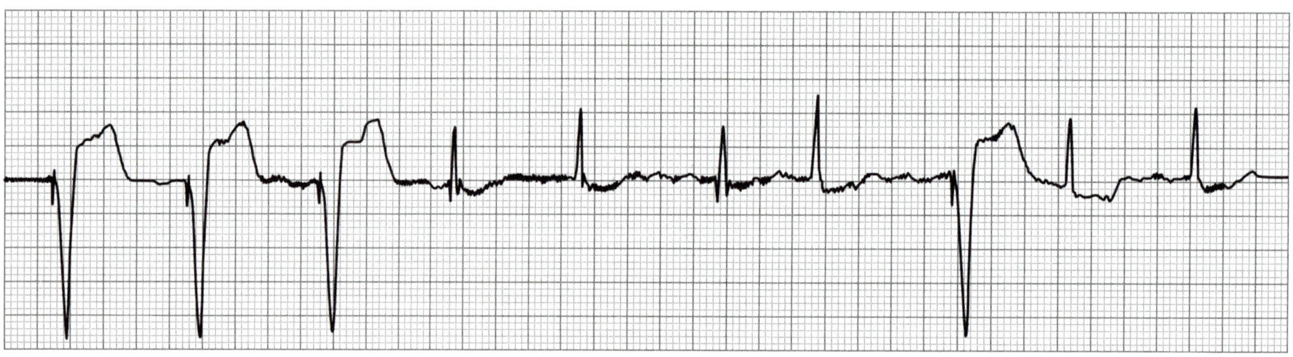

QRS duration ________________ QT _____________
Ventricular rate/rhythm _________________________
Atrial rate/rhythm ______________________________
PR interval ____________________________________

Identification ____
Symptoms ____
____
Treatment ____

Figure 10-17

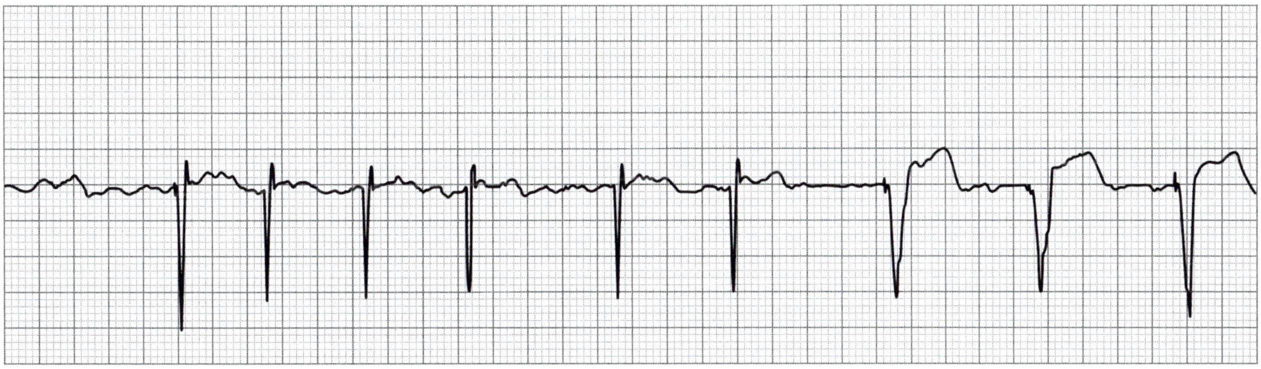

QRS duration ______________ QT ____________

Ventricular rate/rhythm ______________________

Atrial rate/rhythm __________________________

PR interval _______________________________

Identification _______________________________

Symptoms ___________________________________

____

Treatment __________________________________

Figure 10-18

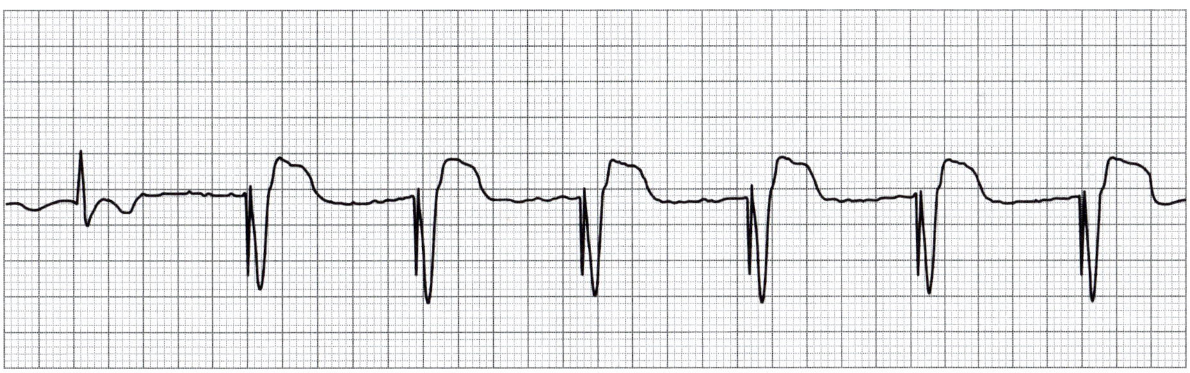

QRS duration ______________ QT ____________

Ventricular rate/rhythm ______________________

Atrial rate/rhythm __________________________

PR interval _______________________________

Identification _______________________________

Symptoms ___________________________________

____

Treatment __________________________________

Figure 10-19

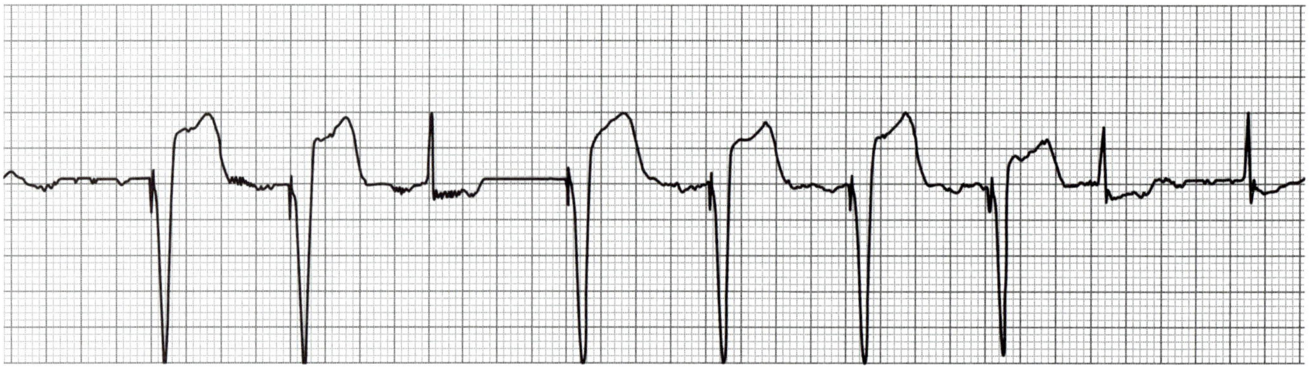

QRS duration ________ QT ________

Ventricular rate/rhythm ________

Atrial rate/rhythm ________

PR interval ________

Identification ________

Symptoms ________

Treatment ________

Figure 10-20

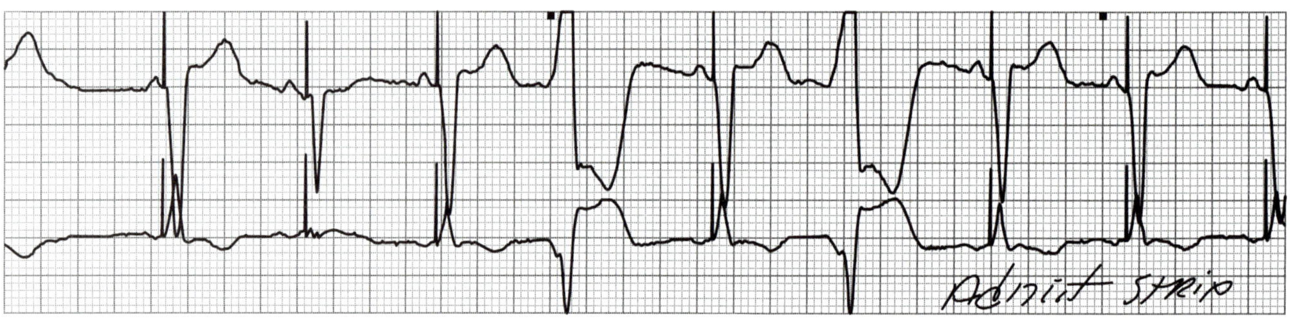

QRS duration ________ QT ________

Ventricular rate/rhythm ________

Atrial rate/rhythm ________

PR interval ________

Identification ________

Symptoms ________

Treatment ________

Figure 10-21

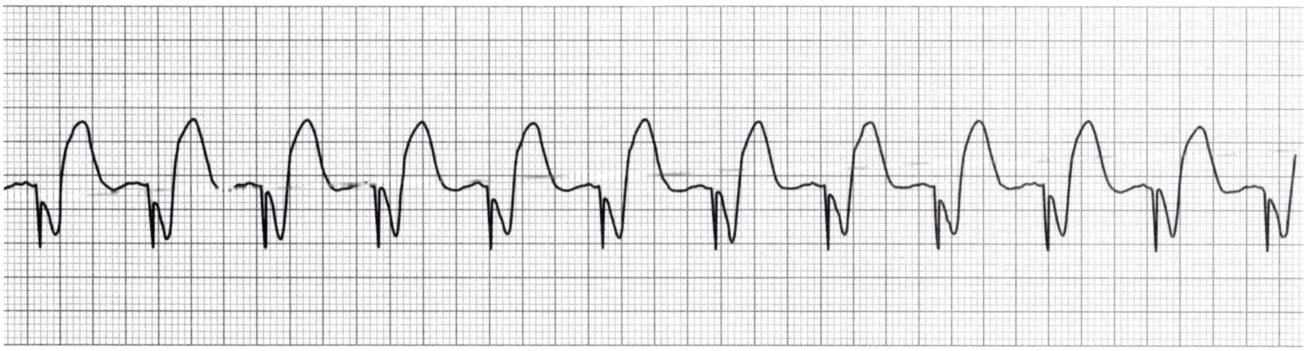

QRS duration ______________ QT ____________

Ventricular rate/rhythm ______________________

Atrial rate/rhythm __________________________

PR interval ________________________________

Identification ________________________________

Symptoms ____________________________________

____

Treatment ____________________________________

Figure 10-22

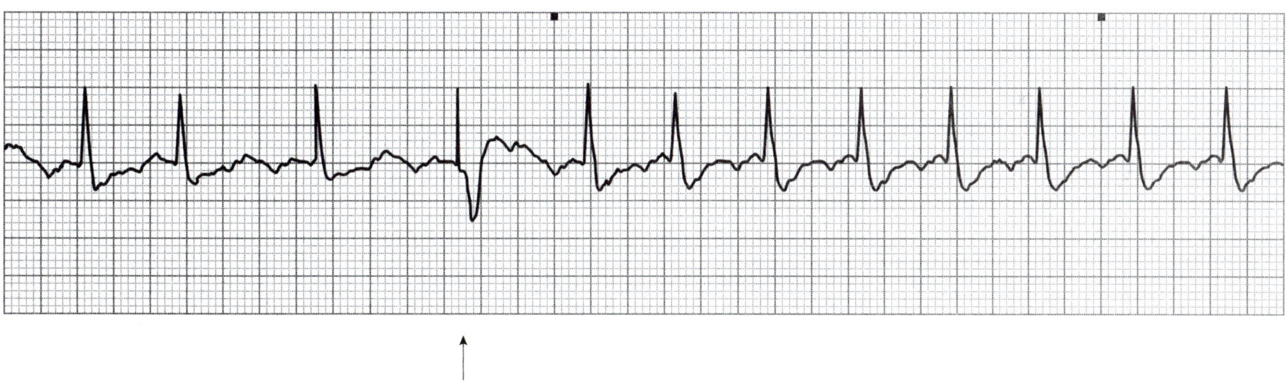

QRS duration ______________ QT ____________

Ventricular rate/rhythm ______________________

Atrial rate/rhythm __________________________

PR interval ________________________________

Identification ________________________________

Symptoms ____________________________________

____

Treatment ____________________________________

References

Conover, M. B. *Nurse's pocket guide to electrocardiography* (3rd ed.). St. Louis, MO: C. V. Mosby; 1994.

Conover, M. B. *Understanding electrocardiography: Arrhythmias and the 12-lead ECG* (7th ed.). St. Louis, MO: Mosby-Year Book, Inc.; 1996.

Conover, M. B. & Wellens, H. J. *The ECG in emergency decision making*. Philadelphia: W. B. Saunders; 1993.

Del Monte, L. & Gamrath, B. *Noninvasive pacing: What you should know.* Redmond, WA. Physio-Control; 1996.

Emergency Cardiac Care Subcommittee and Subcommittees, American Heart Association. Guidelines for cardiopulmonary resuscitation and emergency cardiac care, *JAMA*. 1994.

Marriott, H. J. & Conover, M. B. *Advanced concepts in arrhythmias* (2nd ed.). St. Louis, MO: C. V. Mosby; 1989.

CHAPTER 11

The 12-Lead ECG

Premise Interpretation using 12-lead ECGs is not difficult if you

1. know the normal configurations of the wave forms
2. remember the direction from which the various leads "look" at the heart
3. practice

Objectives

After reading the chapter and completing the Self-Assessment Exercises, the reader should be able to

1. identify the surfaces of the heart visualized by the 12 leads
2. identify the components of the wave forms that signify myocardial ischemia and/or infarction by using the 12-lead ECG
3. identify the site of infarction and select the appropriate monitoring lead system
4. relate the site of infarction to the anticipated fascicular complications
5. identify the ECG changes specific to fascicular block
6. describe methods to calculate axis and the significant abnormal axis

Key Terms

akinesis
axis deviation
current of injury pattern
dyskinesis
fascicular block
nontransmural
precordial
transmural
ventricular aneurysm

Introduction

In ECG rhythm identification, almost all ECG tracings studied are lead II. There are many monitoring devices that are configured to observe a combination of leads. The visualization of the surfaces of the heart, differentiation of the tachycardias, identification of sites of ischemia, injury, and infarction as well as the complications of bundle branch block are best studied using multiple leads.

Interpretation of ECGs using lead II and sometimes MCL_1 is considered "basic." The clinician learns and practices identification of normal wave forms, measurement, durations, and associated calculations to determine normal versus abnormal. This mastery requires organization, practice, and application of basic rules and principles.

The use of 12-lead ECG requires the same diligence, effort, and an equally-organized approach, only with nine more leads. The newer cardiac monitors offer a choice of one, three, and 12 leads in portable devices easily applied to the patient.

MYOCARDIAL INFARCTION

Ischemia, injury, and necrosis may be obvious in some leads and not in others. The patient with chest pain deserves the best visualization of all of the surfaces of the heart. Since time is muscle, it is becoming increasingly common to have 12-lead ECG application and transmission from the prehospital scene to a receiving hospital. Confirmation of myocardial changes within the short window of opportunity provides the patient with the best possible opportunity for re-perfusion.

This chapter is a brief overview of 12-lead ECG analysis. It is meant to help the clinician realize the hazards of relying on one or two leads for insight and to help with interpretation. This chapter is not meant to be all inclusive of the fine points associated with this topic.

Application of 12-lead ECG rhythm analysis is available in some prehospital settings and is not meant to delay patient care, delay on-scene time, or replace clinical assessment of the patient. The 12-lead system is invaluable in the clinical setting for further confirmation and trending the changes at frequent intervals.

The use of the 12-lead ECG system in a prehospital setting should improve patient care by providing evidence of patient status to medical direction so that steps for reperfusion can be rapidly available to the patient on arrival to an emergency facility. Again, time is muscle, and whatever can be done to minimize the delay from recognition to reperfusion should be appreciated.

The Surfaces of the Heart and the 12 ECG Leads

As noted in Chapter 3, the electrocardiographic leads that best explore a particular area of left ventricular myocardium are those that face the specific surface in question. Exploring leads that are perpendicular to a specific aspect of left ventricular muscle will record loss of tissue there, although leads that are parallel or tangential to that particular area may show little if any change.

Each area of left ventricular muscle, with its distinct blood supply, has specific electrocardiographic leads that explore it. The inferior (diaphragmatic) surface is visualized in limb leads II, III, and AVF; the septal surface is best seen in V_1 and V_2 and the anterior wall in V_2 to V_4. Lateral left ventricular muscle is reflected in I, AVL, V_5 and V_6 and the true posterior surface by subtle changes in leads V_1 and V_2. Figure 11-1 is a graphic representation of the limb leads, superimposed on the heart.

The inferior surface of the left ventricle (also termed "diaphragmatic surface") lies close to a horizontal plane. Standard leads I, AVR, and AVL, as well as the **precordial** leads, all explore forces of depolarization nearly parallel to the inferior sur-

precordial
The area of the anterior surface of the chest, overlying the heart.

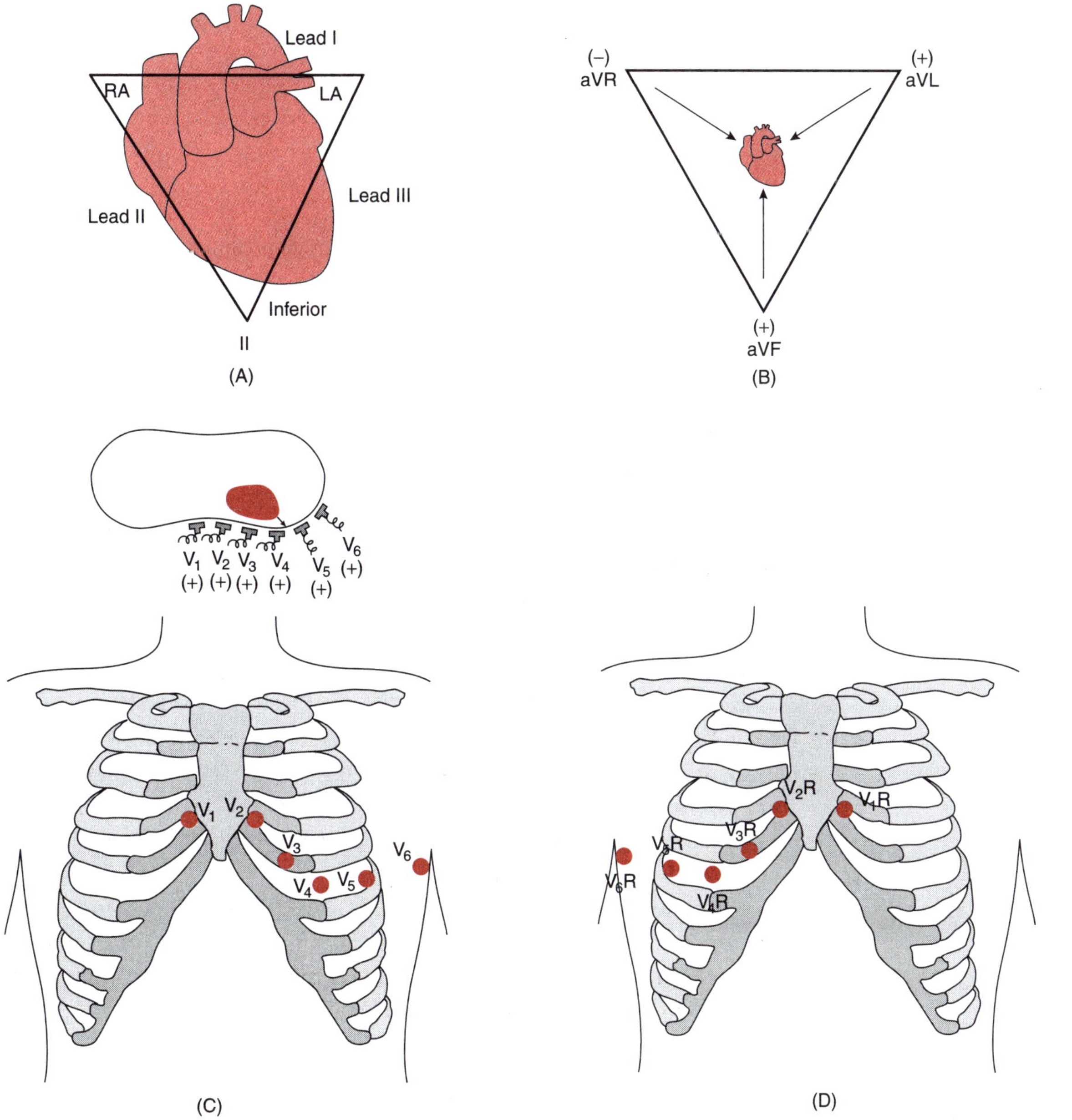

Figure 11-1 (A) Limb leads I, II, and III superimposed on the heart, (B) the augmented leads in relationship to the heart, (C) placement of the precordial leads in relationship to the heart, (D) placement of the right precordial leads on the chest.

face and thus may not record damage there. However, limb leads II, III, and AVF are perpendicular of near perpendicular to the inferior surface and will thus reflect problems in the heart muscle in that area. These are also termed the "inferior leads." Figure 11-2 shows the position of limb leads II, III, and AVF in relationship to the inferior surface of the heart.

All abnormal ECG tracings indicating inferior wall changes require the use of right precordial lead analysis. The right chest leads are V_{3R}, V_{4R}, V_{5R}, V_{6R}. The positive electrodes of each lead are in the same position as the left, but to the right of the sternum. V_{1R} is in the same position as traditional left precordial leads.

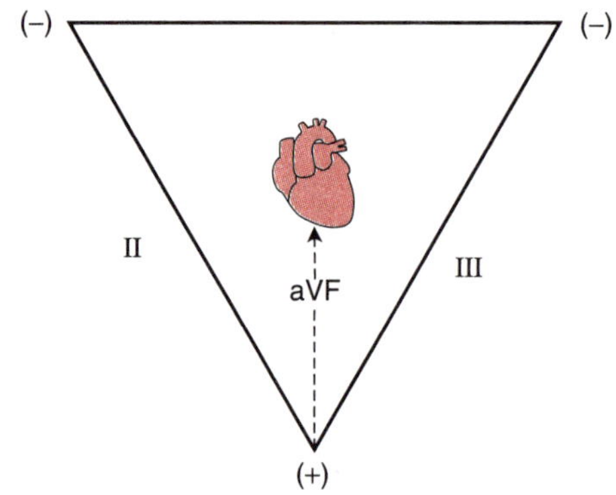

Figure 11-2 The proximity of leads II, III, and AVF to the inferior surface of the heart.

The positive electrode for V_{4R} is at the midclavicular line, fifth intercostal space, right chest. V_{3R} is halfway between V_{4R} and V_1. The electrodes for V_{5R} and V_{6R} are on the same level as V_{4R} in the anterior and midaxillary lines, respectively.

The septal surface and anterior wall of the left ventricle will be best visualized in the precordial leads V_1 to V_4, for these leads are approximately perpendicular to that surface. Lead V_1 is particularly important because the initial small R wave represents septal depolarization in a left to right direction. Leads V_2 to V_4 explore most of the anterior surface. Thus, loss of septal and anterior wall muscle, by occlusion of the proximal left anterior descending coronary artery before the first septal perforation, will be reflected as changes in V_1 to V_4 (the anteroseptal leads). Figure 11-3 shows the position of the precordial leads in relationship to the inferior anterior surface of the heart.

A more distal obstruction of the left anterior descending coronary artery, with preservation of the first septal branch, will cause primary damage over the anterior wall and will be reflected as changes in V_1 through V_4, the anterior leads.

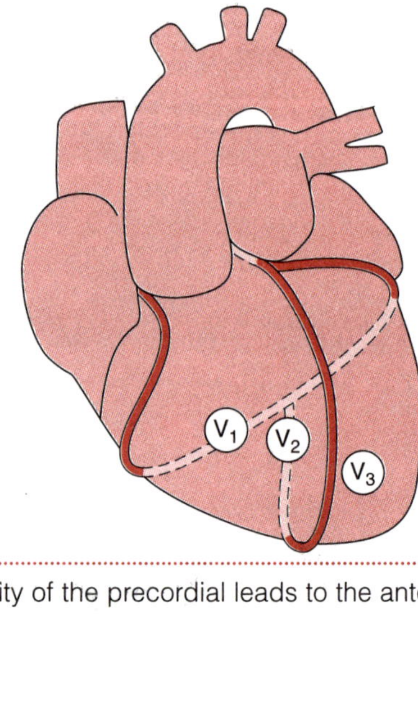

Figure 11-3 The proximity of the precordial leads to the anterior surface of the heart.

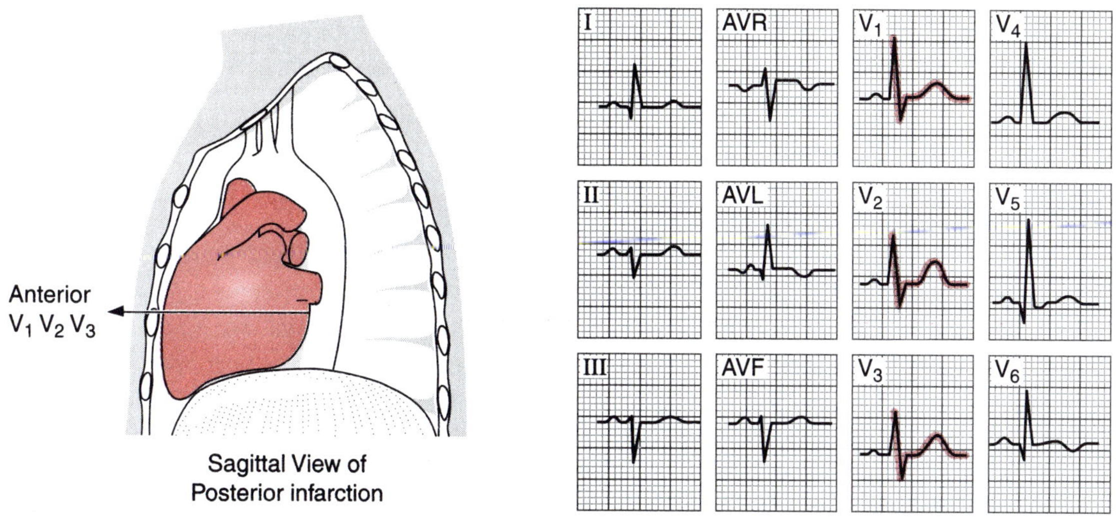

Figure 11-4 The position of the anterior precordial leads as they mirror the posterior surface of the heart.

The lateral surface of the left ventricle, primarily supplied by the left circumflex marginal arteries with potential contribution from the diagonal branches of the left anterior descending coronary artery, will be best explored by leads V_5 and V_6. In addition, lead I is perpendicular to this surface, and AVL is nearly perpendicular. Thus, I, AVL, V_5, and V_6 are considered the anterolateral leads. Obviously, if damage is extensive over the anterior and lateral wall, changes will be seen in leads through V_4 as well as in I, AVL, V_5, and V_6.

The posterior surface of the left ventricle lies in a plane parallel to the frontal plane and is hidden from the precordial exploring electrodes by the anterior and septal surfaces. Infarctions of the posterior surface, usually by occlusion of the posterior descending coronary artery, thus may produce subtle electrocardiographic changes. Such damage will be reflected primarily in accentuation of depolarization forces over the anteroseptal surface, in V_1 to V_3, as a mirror image of the posterior surface. Figure 11-4 shows the position of anterior precordial leads as they reflect the changes in the posterior surface of the heart.

PATHOPHYSIOLOGY OF MYOCARDIAL INFARCTION

While myocardial infarction is an acute process, it may occur because of a chronic accumulation of atheromatous plaque in the coronary arteries. The bulging of the plaque may significantly obstruct blood flow. In most cases, without total occlusion, a stenosis of a coronary artery can lead to myocardial infarction. The fibrous cap of the atheromatous plaque can fracture or rupture. Subsequent ulceration of the plaque frequently results in the creation of an obstructive thrombus or spasm of the artery. This can cause acute, total occlusion and subsequent mycardial infarction. Thrombus formation, resulting from ulceration of the atherosclerotic plaque, is stimulated by the exposure of underlying collagen and other thrombogenic substances to blood flow, leading to the release of thromboplastic elements from the plaque's necrotic core. This exposure is followed by:

- platelet adhesion and aggregation
- release of thromboplastin which initiates the coagulation cascade
- formation of the platelet plugs
- incorporation of fibrins, red blood cells, and plasminogen into the final clot

In 1998, the PURSUIT trial in multiple centers began testing inhibition of platelet factor therapy added to aspirin and heparin. This remains an area of research.

DeWood reported the causative role of intracoronary thrombus in acute myocardial infarction. In this study, patients with 24 hours of symptoms underwent coronary angiography to detect the presence or absence of thrombus in the occluded artery. In 87 percent of patients who were evaluated within 24 hours after symptom onset, total coronary occlusion was observed. This was confirmed in 88 percent of those patients who subsequently underwent coronary artery bypass surgery.

The incidence of observed thromboembolic occlusion decreases with time after onset of symptoms. DeWood suggests that spontaneous reperfusion may be an important feature in the evolution of anterior wall myocardial infarction.

Coronary artery spasm can occur in nonoccluded coronary arteries. Coronary artery spasm can result in myocardial infarction because of restricted blood flow distal to the spasm. Coronary artery spasm can also occur in *fixed atherosclerotic obstruction.* Fixed atherosclerotic obstruction is a lesion in a vessel with an atheromatous plaque. Coronary artery spasm also occurs in the grafts used in coronary bypass surgery.

The process of myocardial injury in an acute MI is time dependent. Necrosis develops over several hours in the presence of coronary occlusion. The evolution of MI follows the wave front phenomenon of myocardial necrosis. Injury in necrosis originates in the ischemic subendocardium and progresses outward toward the epicardium to involve an entire area of myocardium perfused by the coronary artery involved. This phenomenon was first described by Reimer and his colleagues in 1977.

Initially, the injury is said to be reversible and salvage of myocardial muscle mass is possible if blood flow is restored, but this must occur early. With increased duration of occlusion, the area of necrosis will enlarge and myocardial damage becomes irreversible. Thromboembolic occlusion is the precipitating cause in most infarctions. The best results with percutaneous transluminal coronary angioplasty (PCTA) occur when PCTA is done within one hour after onset. If there is unavoidable delay, thrombolysis should be considered.

Rapid intervention reduces mortality and improves left ventricular function. Reperfusion increases as time-to-treatment decreases. Various studies (GUSTO and ISIS) are evaluating other therapies for use in the acute situation.

ECG Changes in Myocardial Infarction

Myocardial infarction leads to loss of depolarizing cardiac muscle. Specific areas of necrosis, injury, and ischemia are reflected by changes in the electrocardiogram (ECG) that explore those specific surfaces of the left ventricle.

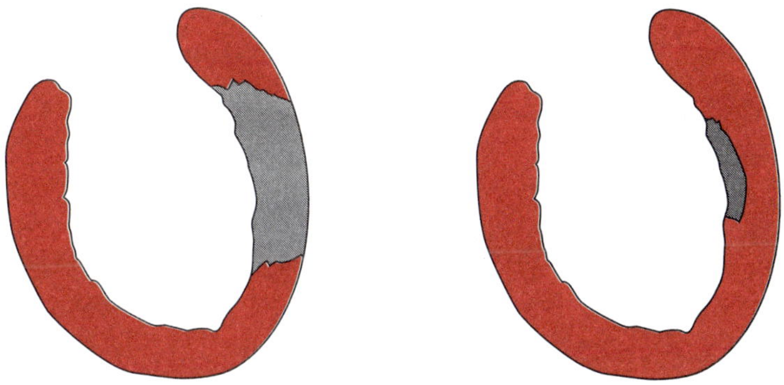

Figure 11-5 (A) Transmural myocardial infarction, (B) Nontransmural myocardial infarction. Note the differences in penetration of the infarcted tissue.

With acute myocardial necrosis, the forces of depolarization are no longer generated in the damaged areas, thus, the remaining forces of ventricular depolarization are accentuated, displacing the mean QRS vector in each lead system away from the zone of necrosis. This generates the abnormal, pathologic Q waves of myocardial infarction. The necrotic area no longer will be capable of depolarization, contraction, or repolarization, but it is always surrounded by an area of ischemic myocardium, incompletely depolarized with each ventricular activation.

Such incomplete depolarization generates ST segment elevation in the area of ischemia surrounding the acute myocardial infarction. ST segment depression may be seen in those leads that explore a portion of ischemic ventricular tissue opposite the necrotic area. Because the sequence of ventricular repolarization is altered by acute myocardial ischemia and necrosis, the T waves become inverted or occasionally accentuated.

There are two major types of myocardial infarction. An infarction may be **transmural**, for example, with necrosis there is fibrosis of the full thickness of the myocardial wall, or it may be **nontransmural**, confined to the subendocardium or inner aspects of the myocardium. Figure 11-5 is a graphic representation of transmural and nontransmural infarction.

transmural
A myocardial infarction with necrosis, where there is fibrosis of the full thickness of the myocardial wall

nontransmural
A myocardial infarction confined to the subendocardium or inner aspects of the myocardium

Transmural Infarction Pattern

The QRS morphology, the ST segment, and the T wave will be altered with a transmural myocardial infarction. The QRS change is more important than ST-segment or T-wave changes and thus will be considered first.

QRS Changes. The foremost change is in the QRS complex with the development of Q waves. The new Q waves will be seen in those leads that explore the particular area of infarction. With transmural necrosis, the specific area of damaged ventricular tissue will cease to be depolarized. Those leads that explore this specific area no longer will record forces of depolarization directed toward them; rather, some forces of depolarization will be seen moving away, and a Q wave, or negative deflection, will be recorded.

The normal precordial leads are generated by depolarization forces moving toward the exploring electrode. Following infarction, these forces will be lost and the exploring electrodes will record depolarization moving away from the positive electrode in the lead facing the infarction. This will be recorded as a Q wave. The time is takes for the Q wave to develop can be as little as four hours.

A word of caution is indicated. A normal ECG may exhibit deep Q waves, especially in I and V_5 to V_6, which represent septal depolarization in a left-to-right direction. Q waves, to be considered diagnostic of myocardial infarction, should meet one of the following criteria:

1. Duration of 0.04 second (one small box) or greater.
2. The depth of the Q wave is 25 percent or more of the height of the R wave.
3. The Q waves are "new" to the patient.
4. Once formed, the Q wave usually becomes the permanent electrocardiographic evidence of myocardial infarction.

In a prehospital setting, it is difficult to determine if Q waves are "new" or "old" for the patient. Thus, detailed clinical history and accurate reporting of the QRS configuration are necessary. Application of the 12-lead ECG on any patient with chest pain becomes necessary so that transmission of data and accurate reporting can be instrumental in providing rapid intervention at the receiving facility.

ST-Segment Changes

current of injury pattern

The ST-segment elevation that occurs immediately following the insult

ST-segment elevation is also known as the **current of injury pattern**. ST-segment elevation occurs soon after the insult and is seen in the leads that explore the damaged area. The ST-segment elevation associated with infarction usually encompasses the T wave in its contour. This is to be contrasted with other minor causes for alterations in ST-segment contour. One such change, *early repolarization*, is a normal variant to the ST segment often seen in younger patients and is easily confused with the ST-segment changes of ischemia. It is critical to assess clinical presentation-as the ECG is only one tool in making the diagnosis. Figure 11-6 is a graphic representation of the injured myocardium and the accompanying ECG changes in the lead facing the injury.

Following acute infarction, or when resolution of ischemia has taken place, the ST segment usually returns toward baseline; this usually occurs in the first 72 to 96 hours after damage. Persistent ST-segment elevation is electrocardiographic evidence for the development of left **ventricular aneurysm**.

ventricular aneurysm

A condition where a portion of the infarcted myocardial tissue does not contract or expand normally causing the myocardium to bulge outward

Ventricular aneurysm is a condition where a portion of infarcted myocardial tissue does not contract or expand normally. During ventricular systole, that portion of the myocardium bulges outward instead of contracting. This major wall motion disorder is usually seen on the ECG as the persistent ST-segment elevation well after the infarction is resolved and lasts months or even years afterward. However, it should be noted that wall motion disorders can be present without ECG changes. Left ventricular aneurysm following extensive infarction may show persistent ST-segment

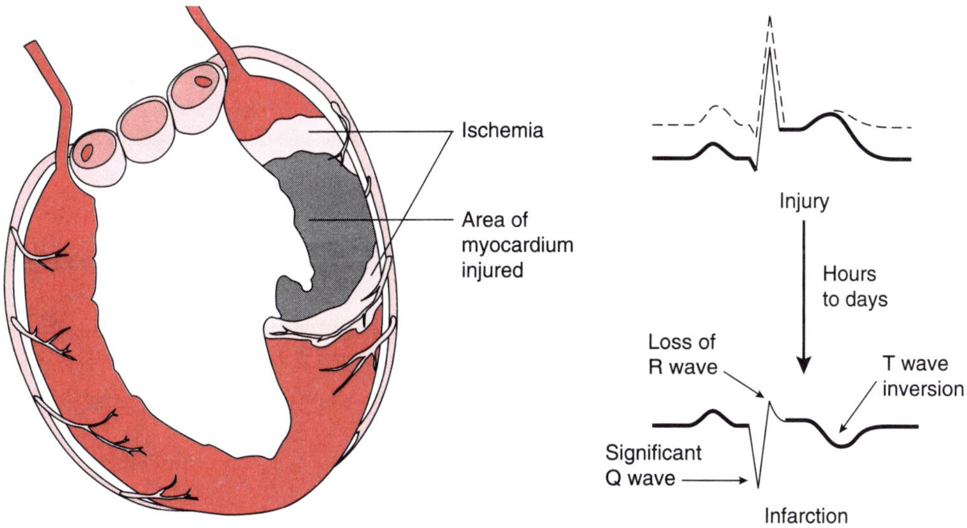

Figure 11-6 The injured myocardium and the accompanying acute changes in the Q wave, ST segment, and T wave initially and after time passed.

inversion over the damaged muscle. This ST-segment elevation may be present for years and may be confused with acute necrosis. Such ST-segment elevation and aneurysm formation may mask future ischemic episodes. Figure 11-7 is a graphic representation of ventricular wall aneurysm.

Akinesis is the lack of motion, and **dyskinesis** is the paradoxical bulging during ventricular systole. Patients with suspected wall motion disorders are described as chronically fatigued due to low cardiac output.

akinesis
Lack of motion

dyskinesis
The paradoxical bulging during ventricular systole

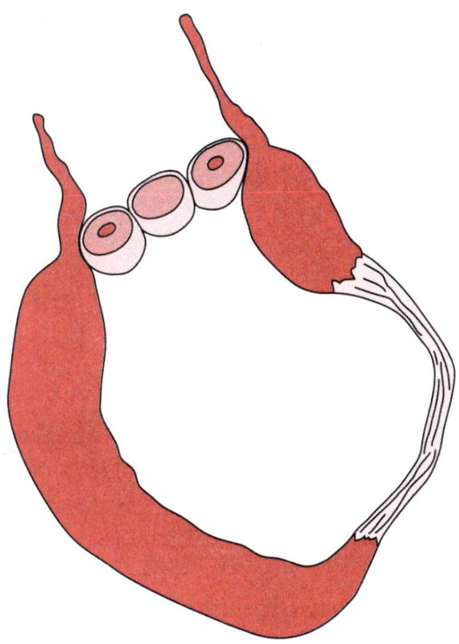

Figure 11-7 A ventricular wall aneurysm.

T-Wave Changes. During the acute phase of myocardial necrosis, the T wave is incorporated into ST-segment elevation. As the ST segment returns to baseline, the T wave becomes inverted and may not return to normal for weeks or months. T-wave inversion, like ST-segment changes, has multiple etiologies and must be interpreted in light of the patient's clinical presentation.

U-Wave Changes. An abnormal U wave is a frequent sign of ischemic heart disease. It is most often recorded in lead I, II, and precordial leads V_4 toV_6. A negative U wave is seen in 10 to 60 percent of patients with anterior myocardal infarction, and in up to 30 percent of patients with inferior myocardial infarction. Appearance of a negative U wave may precede other ECG changes of infarction by up to several hours (Lepeschkin, 1992).

Nontransmural (Non-Q Wave) Myocardial Infarction

The nontransmural myocardial infarction, also known as non-Q wave subendocardial infarction, will not produce significant alteration in the QRS complex because there has been no transmural damage. Rather, the ST segment will be depressed, and the T wave will be inverted in those leads that explore the damaged area. These changes will resolve slowly over 48 to 96 hours. In light of the fact that digitalis and ventricular hypertrophy with systolic overload will produce similar alterations to the ST segment and T wave, such electrocardiographic changes always must be placed in context with the clinical setting and supporting laboratory data to be considered diagnostic of a nontransmural myocardial infarction.

Inferior Wall (Diaphragmatic) Myocardial Infarction

In inferior wall myocardial infarction (IWMI), there are Q waves and ST elevation in leads II, III, and AVF. With further evolution, the ST depression resolves, the T wave is less inverted, but the Q waves persist. Eventually, the T waves return to normal, and the fibrotic scar on the inferior wall is represented by Q waves. There are two aspects of inferior wall MI that deserve emphasis at this point:

1. With Q waves in II, III, and AVF, the mean axis of depolarization may be shifted to the left, more negative than -30 degrees. In the setting of inferior wall infarction with leftward shift of axis, left anterior hemiblock cannot be diagnosed.
2. A Q wave in standard lead III may be entirely normal and thus must always be interpreted in light of electrocardiographic changes seen in standard leads II and AVF. The Q wave in these two leads must be 0.04 second in duration and 25 percent of the amplitude of the R wave to be considered diagnostic for myocardial damage.

Figure 11-8 is an illustration of the inferior surfaces of the heart affected by disease. The accompanying ECG patterns reflect the Q waves and ST elevation in limb leads II, III, and AVF. Note the reciprocal changes in lead I.

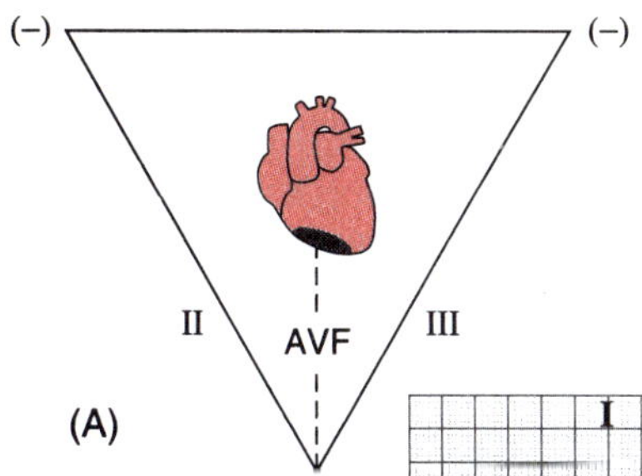

(A)

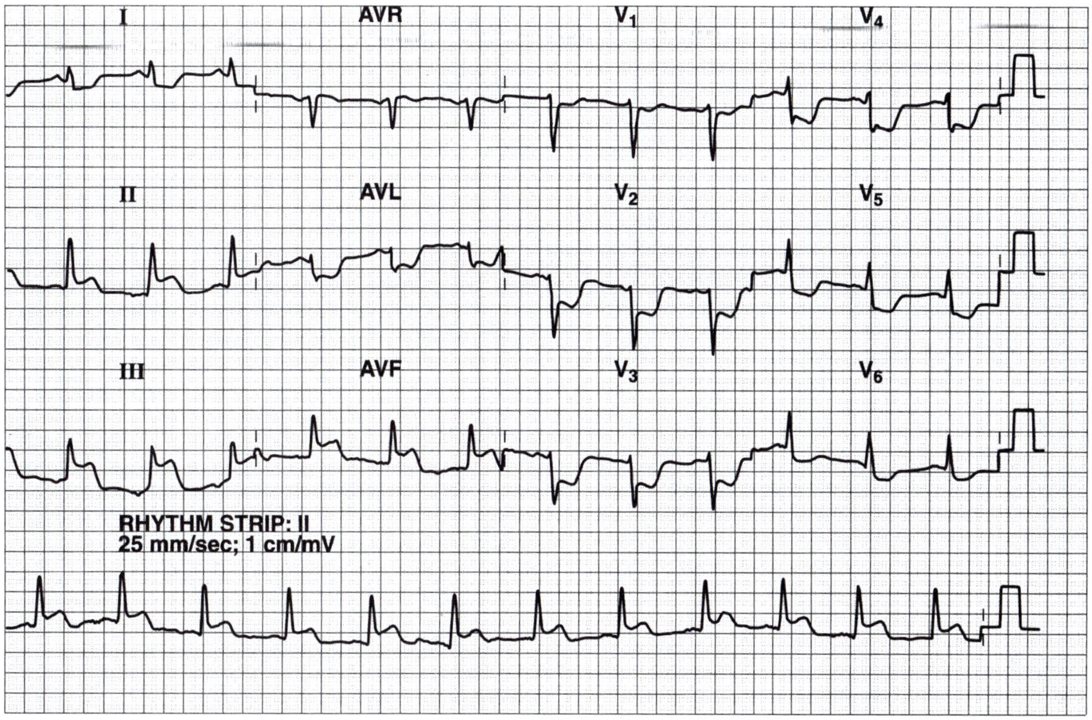

(B)

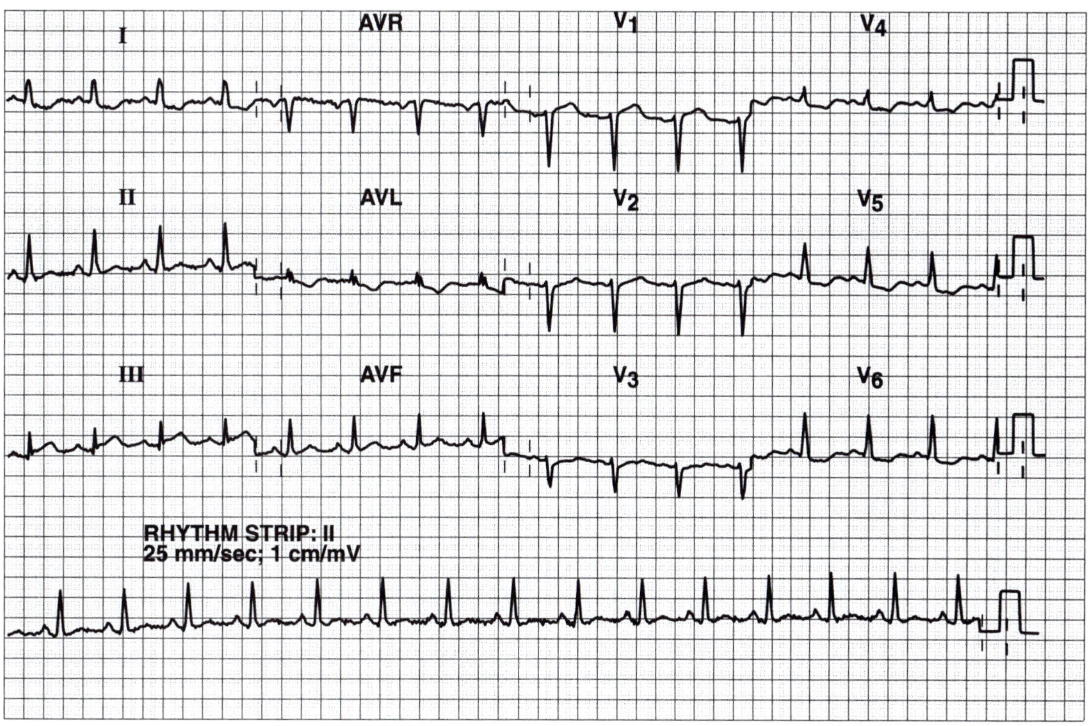

(C)

Figure 11-8 (A) A schematic of the leads that face the inferior surface of the heart; (B) a 12-lead ECG showing the changes reflecting the injury pattern in the limb leads, II, III and AVF; note reciprocal ST-segment depression in lead I; (C) the return of the ST segment to baseline is evident six minutes after successful reperfusion.

Approximately half of all inferior myocardial infarctions may lose criteria for significant Q waves about 6 months following necrosis. Therefore, small Q waves in the inferior leads that do not fulfill criteria for significant Q waves still must be interpreted with caution and should alert the observer that an acute inferior myocardial infarction pattern might once have been present.

An infarction of the inferior (diaphragmatic) surface will be recorded by a Q-wave formation in leads II, III, and AVF, the inferior leads. An anterolateral wall infarction will logically be seen as Q waves in leads I, AVL, V_5, and V_6. Figure 11-9 is a 12-lead documentation of inferior wall myocardial infarction.

All abnormal ECG tracings indicating inferior wall changes require the analysis of right precordial lead. Of critical importance is the analysis of lead V_{4R} which identifies:

1. the affected coronary artery
2. presence of right ventricular wall infarction
3. presence of AV nodal conduction defect

ECG changes include ST elevation with proximal right coronary disease, elevated T wave in distal right coronary disease, and inverted T wave with distal left circumflex disease.

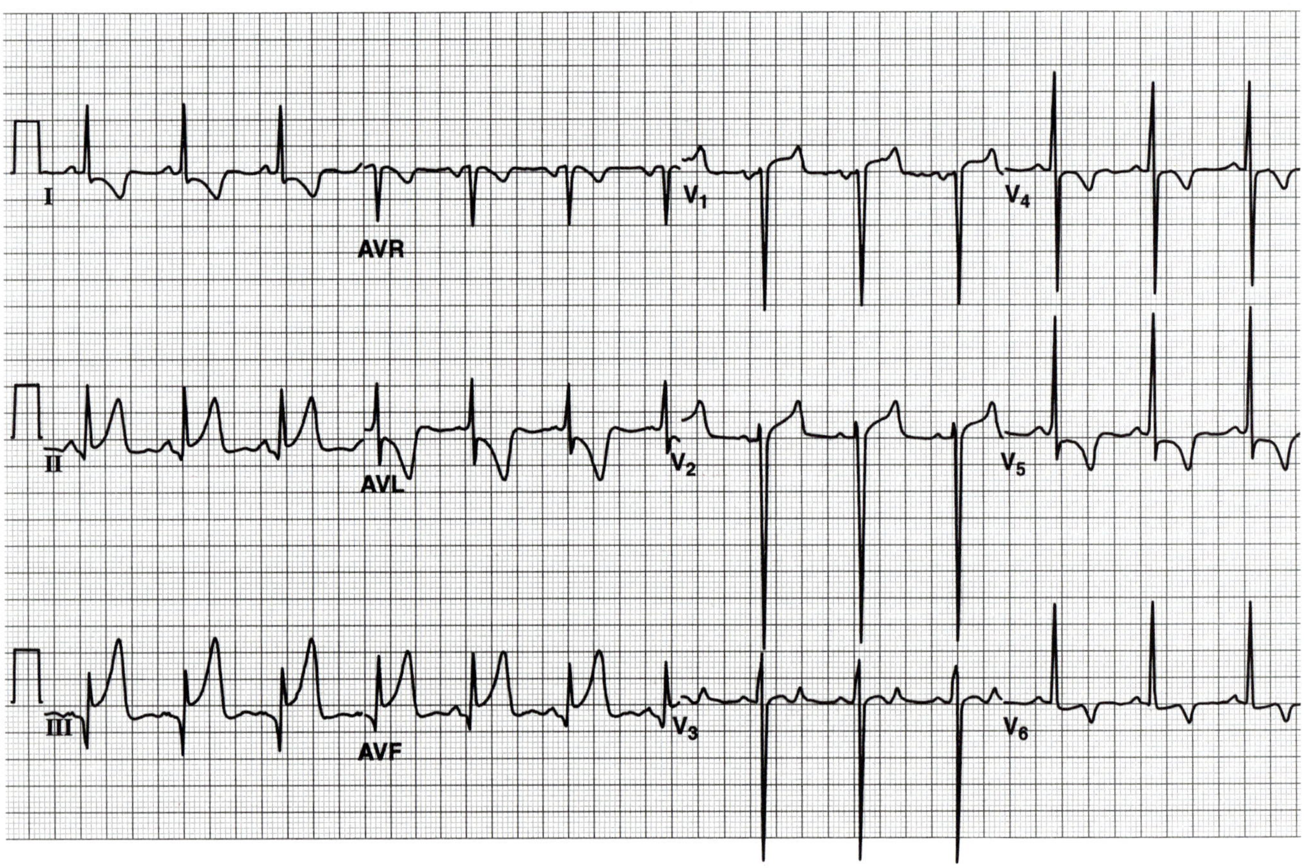

Figure 11-9 12-lead evidence of inferior myocardial infarction. Note the appearance of Q waves, ST elevation in leads II, III, and AVF. There are reciprocal changes in the ST segment and T wave in leads I and AVL.

Anteroseptal and Anterior Myocardial Infarctions

A QS or QR complex in V_1 to V_4 is diagnostic of an acute anterior wall MI. A decrease in the R-wave height (excursion) over the anterior precordial leads also is consistent with acute anterior necrosis. Reversed R-wave progression, the R wave diminishing from V_1 to V_4, often is overlooked as a criterion for anterior wall damage. In addition, absent or poor R wave progression over the anterior precordial leads may be seen in left ventricular hypertrophy or type C right ventricular hypertrophy. It should be reemphasized that T-wave inversion over the anterior precordial leads may be a normal variant, most often seen in female patients under 30 years of age. Figure 11-10 is a 12-lead documentation of anterior wall myocardial infarction.

In non-Q wave anterior wall myocardial infarction, there is ST depression with

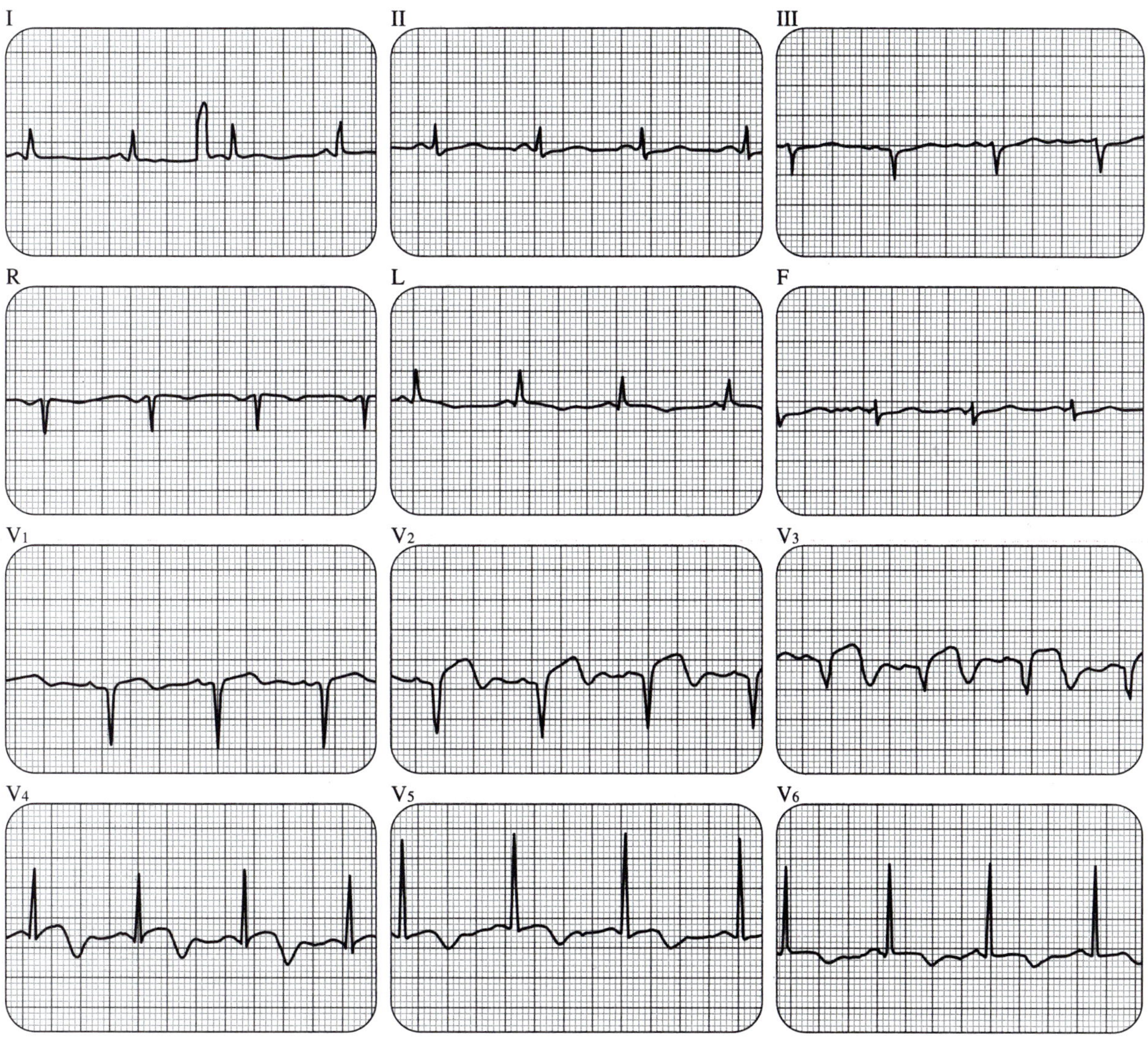

Figure 11-10 12-lead evidence of myocardial infarction. There are no significant changes in lead II; however, the 12-lead ECG demonstrates acute changes: Q waves, ST elevation, and inverted T waves in the precordial leads in V_2 and V_3; ST coving persists in V_4; with a horizontal ST segment and T wave inversion in V_5. This ECG contributed to the diagnosis of an anterolateral wall maycardial infarction.

T-wave inversion in I, AVL, and V_6, but no significant alteration of the QRS configuration. These changes will slowly return to the baseline as acute necrosis resolves.

In summary, the magnitude of anteroseptal or anterior myocardial infarction may be judged by the extent of the precordial leads involved. Sequential ECGs should be scrutinized carefully for evidence of a damaged and unstable conduction system.

Anterolateral Myocardial Infarction

There may be instances where electrocardiographic evidence for acutė necrosis is evident in I and AVL, but absent in V_5 or V_6. This represents an infarction on the high lateral wall of the left ventricle (high lateral infarction), not seen in conventional leads V_5 and V_6, for the explore ventricular tissue in a horizontal plane below the damaged area. In such instances, all precordial leads should be moved up one intercostal space (high lateral leads). Such a simple manipulation may unmask acute infarction changes in V_5 and V_6 that otherwise would be missed. These criteria are important since small, insignificant Q waves may be generated in the normal lateral precordial leads, representing septal depolarization in a left-to-right direction.

Figure 11-11 is an illustration of the surface of the heart affected by anterolateral wall MI. The accompanying ECG patterns reflect the Q waves and ST elevation in precordial leads V_5 and V_6.

Significant Q waves in the lateral precordial leads, V_2 to V_5, and are at least 25 percent of the total amplitude of the QRS complex.

Posterior Myocardial Infarction

As previously mentioned, infarction of the posterior wall of the left ventricle will not generate Q-wave formation or ST-segment elevation in the conventional 12-lead ECG. Rather, there will be changes in the magnitude of the R waves in V_1 and V_2.

Configuration is generated by forces moving both toward and away from the exploring electrode. The posterior wall of the left ventricle generates many of the latter forces moving away from V_1. With infarction of the posterior wall, these forces are lost, thus the forces moving toward V_1 become accentuated. In such an instance, the usually small R waves seen in V_1 and V_2 are magnified, and the R wave may become taller than the S wave. There is electrocardiographic evidence for a posterior myocardial infarction when the R/S ratio in V_1 becomes equal to or greater than one. This may be confusing in patients with right ventricular hypertrophy, because right **axis deviation** is not present with posterior wall infarctions. The posterior infarction pattern often is seen in patients with acute inferior infarction because both areas of left ventricular myocardium are usually supplied by the same coronary artery.

axis deviation
The direction of the mean flow of electrical current outside the normal limits.

Figure 11-12 is an illustration of the surface of the heart affected by inferior-posterior wall MI. The accompanying ECG patterns reflect the tall R waves and ST depression in leads V_2, V_3, and V_4 as these leads are reciprocal to the surface affected.

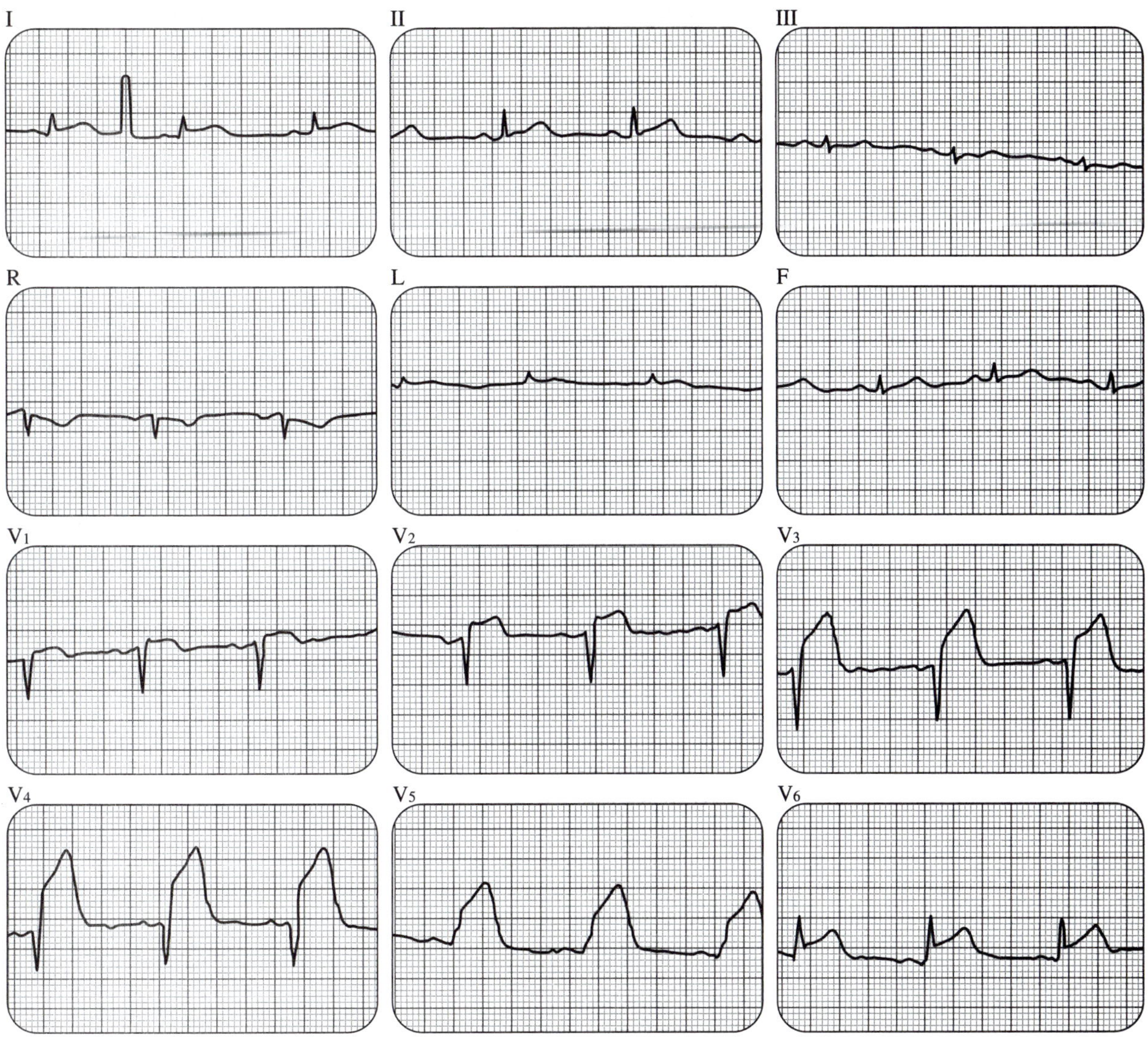

Figure 11-11 12-lead ECG from a patient with diagnosed anterolateral wall infarction. Note the 1 mm ST-segment elevation in lead II which might be discounted as irrelevant. Lead I shows 1 mm ST elevation. If only limb leads are available for initial monitoring of the patient with chest pain, the acute signs seen in leads I and II are significant enough to warrant 12-lead analysis.

Pseudo Infarction Patterns

Left ventricular hypertrophy may generate poor R-wave progression over the anterior precordial leads, suggesting an anterior wall myocardial infarction. Such poor R-wave progression is due to enhanced forces of ventricular depolarization over the lateral wall of the left ventricle. This pseudo infarction pattern is of particular importance in patients with aortic valve disease, whose initial clinical presentation may include significant anginal pain.

Pulmonary embolus, emphysema, and chronic obstructive pulmonary disease with right ventricular hypertrophy also may present with poor R-wave progression. In this instance, the right axis deviation is adequate to differentiate anterior wall myocardial infarction and right ventricular hypertrophy.

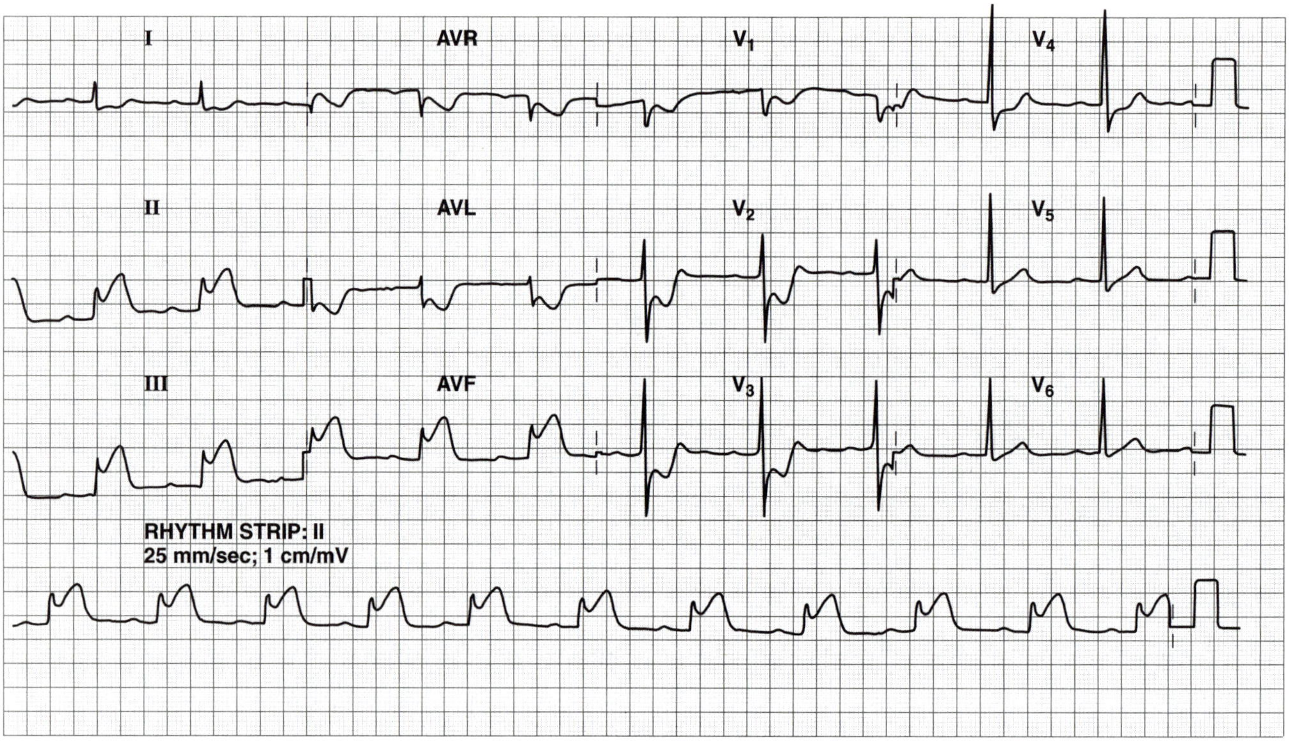

(A)

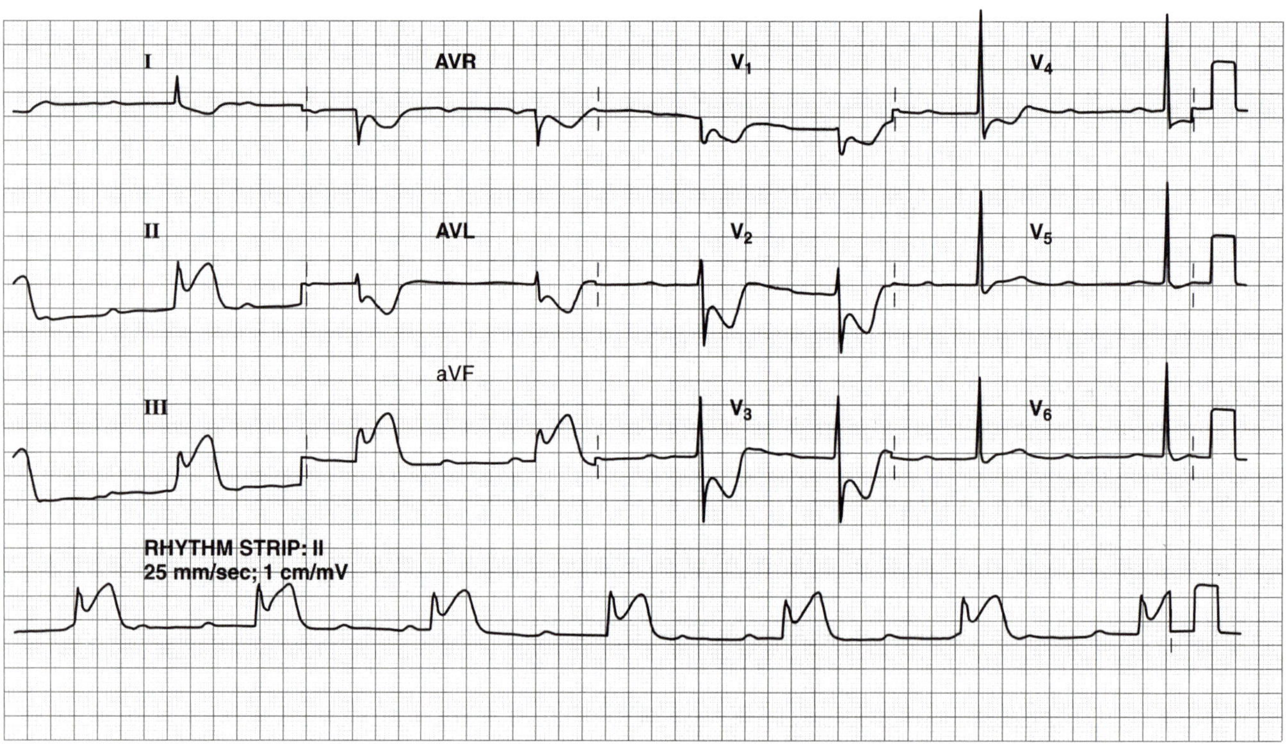

(B)

Figure 11-12A and B Two 12-lead ECGs from a patient with acute inferior-posterior MI. Note the acute changes in limb leads II, III, and AVF indicating inferior involvement. Note the acute changes in $V_1 - V_3$ reflecting the posterior involvement.

Pneumothorax is another common etiology of a pseudo infarction pattern on ECG. Because of displacement of the heart and mediastinum, the QRS voltage may be reduced and the QRS axis significantly shifted, generating what is interpreted as pathologic Q waves.

Hyperkalemia classically causes peaked T waves, which may incorporate some ST-segment elevation. This can be easily confused with the acute current of injury of myocardial necrosis.

Wolff-Parkinson-White (preexcitation) syndrome can cause what may appear to be pathologic Q waves in both the inferior and anterior leads due to initial aberrant forces of depolarization through the accessory bypass tract. In patients with this condition, conduction down the accessory tract often creates a delta wave on many of the ECG leads. This makes further conclusions regarding the QRS morphology (infarction and the like) difficult and, at times, impossible.

Pericarditis of any etiology may show localized ST-segment elevations and subsequent T-wave inversion and is easily mistaken for acute myocardial damage. However, there is never Q-wave formation with pericarditis, and the resolution of the ST segment and T-wave changes takes place over a much longer time.

Patients with idiopathic hypertrophic subaortic stenosis (IHSS) may often have significant Q waves on their ECG. Rather than infarction, these Q waves represent hypertrophied asymmetric ventricular muscle with distortion of the normal patterns of depolarization. A pseudo infarction pattern should always be suspected when the clinical setting and laboratory data do not correlate with electrocardiographic findings.

There may also be dramatic alterations to the T waves and ST segments with sudden increases in the intracranial pressure. These changes do not reflect a primary myocardial problem, but rather changes in repolarization due to enhanced sympathetic nervous system activity.

Early Repolarization

Early repolarization with ST-segment elevation in the anterior leads is also a normal variant. There is usually a 1 to 2 mm ST-segment elevation, but it can also be more pronounced in some individuals, leading to the erroneous diagnosis of either pericarditis or acute myocardial necrosis. In such instances of early repolarization, there is usually a notch at the end of the R wave with an upward concavity to the ST segment. In addition, the T-wave morphology remains distinct and separated from the ST segment. This latter figure is of some help in differentiating the ST segments of acute myocardial necrosis from those of early repolarization.

DIFFUSE ST-SEGMENT AND T-WAVE ABNORMALITIES

ST-Segment Abnormalities

ST-segment depression is nonspecific. While it may be an index of myocardial ischemia or injury, identical ST-segment alteration in the lateral as well as inferior leads can be produced by digitalis, left ventricular hypertrophy, hyperkalemia, hypokalemia, or hypomagnesemia. Such changes over the right precordial leads are slightly more reliable for specific pathologic conditions, present with right ventricular hypertrophy and infarction of the true posterior wall.

T-Wave Abnormalities

The T-wave contour is susceptible to many extra cardiac factors. T-wave inversion or flattening is nonspecific for ischemic heart disease, but the presence of deep, symmetric T-wave inversion is somewhat more suggestive of the diagnosis of ischemia. T-wave contour not only is affected by many pathologic cardiac conditions but may also be altered by exercise, hyperventilation, food ingestion, smoking, or significant electrolyte disturbance.

The normal amplitude for T-wave excursion has never been firmly established. In precordial T waves that are greater than 10 mm in deflection, however, hyperkalemia should be highly suspected. They may also be seen in the right precordial leads in patients with left ventricular hypertrophy. It is because of these considerations that the ST segment and T wave should be interpreted only after the QRS has been carefully analyzed.

FASCICULAR CONDUCTION DEFECTS

One of the purposes of rapid identification of the site of an infarction is to identify any further complication, such as a disturbance to the ventricular conduction system. An anterior, anteroseptal wall MI can cause deterioration of the left bundle branch fascicles. Often in a monitoring lead II, the clinician may observe a change in QRS polarity. In previous chapters, the measurement of the QRS complex was always stressed. In Chapter 8, the implications of second-degree AV block Type II was a great concern and had several implications for interventions. This section will provide insight into the background for that concern.

The anatomy of the penetrating portions of the bundle branch system is such that the right bundle branch and the left anterior fascicles are closely associated at the point of bifurcation. The left posterior fascicle is thicker and situated quite apart from the rest of the bundle branch system. Many of the ventricular conduction defects occur as a result of poor or occluded coronary artery circulation. Figure 11-13 is a graphic representation of the ventricular conduction system and its coronary artery perfusion.

Recall that the flow of current toward the positive electrode creates a positive deflection in that lead. For example, if the greater flow of current moves toward leads II and III, the QRS in leads II and III will be positive in those leads and negative in leads I and AVL.

If the flow of current is directed away from the positive electrode in a lead system, the QRS will be a predominantly negative QRS complex. For example, if the greatest flow of current moves toward lead I and AVL, the QRS in I and AVL will be positive and predominantly negative in leads II and III.

Finally, if the flow of current is perpendicular to the positive electrode in a lead, the complex will be equiphasic, just as positive as negative.

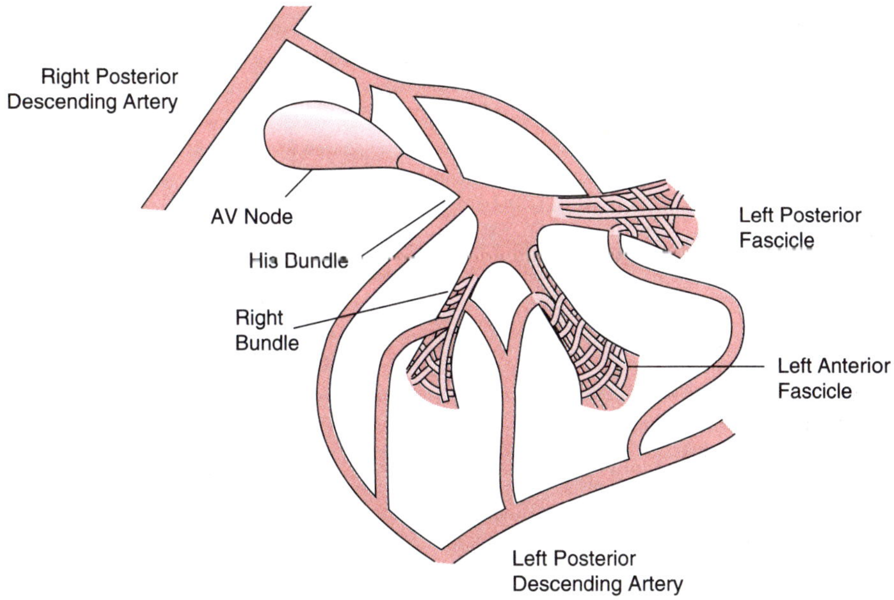

Figure 11-13 The AV and ventricular conduction system with relation to coronary artery perfusion.

Left Anterior Fascicular Block

Interruptions in left anterior conduction will delay activation of the anterior ventricular septum on the anterior wall of the left ventricle. Initial forces of depolarization will occur on the interior and to the right, due to normal activation of a healthy septum but then be driven to the left, along the left posterior fascicle. As a result, the ECG will display a small R wave (initial septal depolarization) and a deep S wave (leftward flow away from lead II). What is most important is that the duration of the QRS will be prolonged greater than 0.10 second, indicating a conduction delay.

Recall that the wave forms are written in uppercase letters. With the fascicular blocks, the morphologic description of the QRS will reflect the discrepancy in the flow of current. So, instead of saying the QRS in leads II and III are predominantly negative, the clinician will report an rS configuration in leads II and III. Figure 11-14 is an ECG tracing showing the characteristic shift in the QRS pattern reflecting left anterior **fascicular block**.

fascicular block
Interruptions in conduction delaying activation of the ventricular septum on the wall of the ventricle

Left Posterior Fascicular Block

Interruptions in left posterior fascicular conduction will delay activation of the left free wall and of the superior wall of the left ventricle. Initial forces of depolarization will first occur superior and to the left, and the later activation will then be driven to the right and inferior, along the left anterior fascicle. The ECG will display a small R wave, the initial depolarization, and a deep S wave, indicating the rightward flow away from leads I and AVL. Again, and most important, the QRS will measure greater than 0.10 second. Figure 11-15 is an ECG tracing showing the characteristic shift in the QRS pattern reflecting left posterior fascicular block.

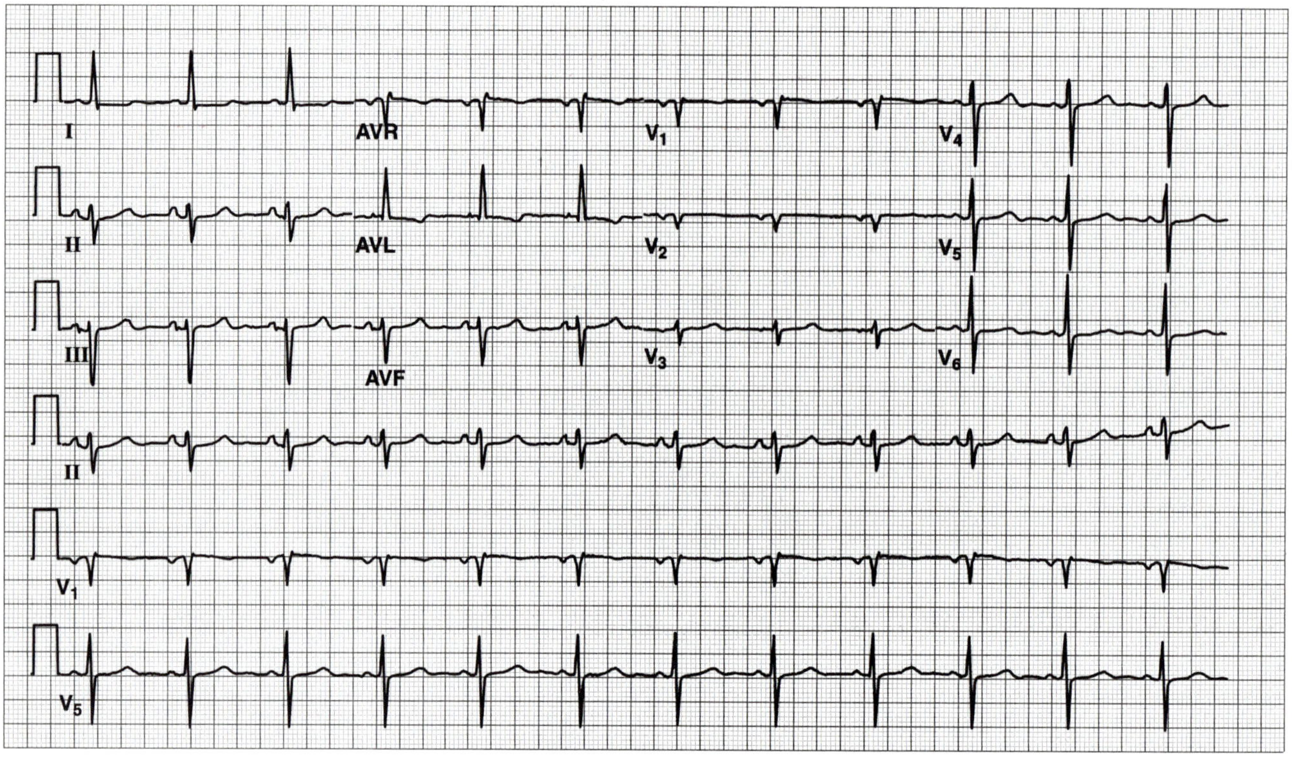

Figure 11-14 In the ECG tracing, leads II, III, and AVF reflect rS configurations greater than 0.10 second while leads I and AVL reflect positive QRS deflections. Note the Q wave in V_2. In a 3-lead monitoring system, the changes in QRS polarity can be easily documented as suspicious of LAFB.

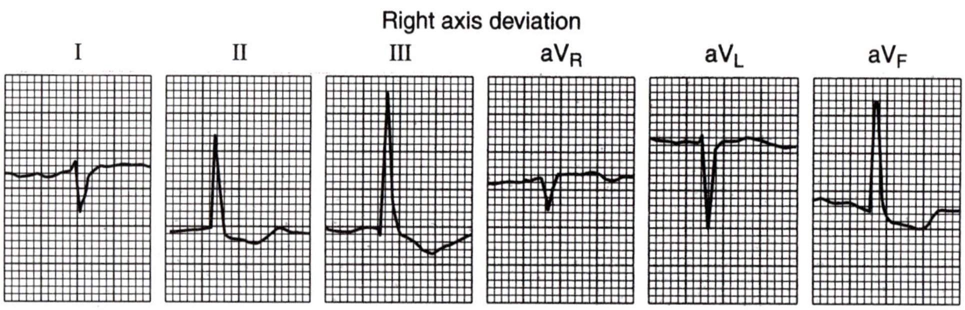

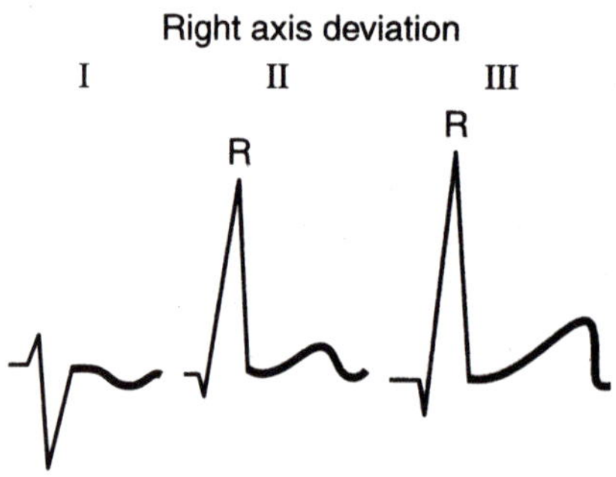

Figure 11-15 In the ECG tracing, leads II, III, and AVF reflect positive QRS configurations greater than 0.10 second while leads I and AVL reflect rS QRS deflections. In a three lead monitoring system, the changes in QRS polarity can be easily documented as suspicious of LPFB.

Right Bundle Branch Block

Interruptions in right bundle branch conduction will delay activation of the right ventricle. Initial forces of depolarization will occur first inferior and then superior and to the left, and the later activation will be driven to the right. The ECG will display a QRS with a broad, terminal S wave in the limb leads, often without any change in axis. The QRS in V_1 will have a characteristic RSR′ as it reflects the RBBB. Again, and what is most important, the QRS will measure greater than 0.10 second. Figure 11-16 is an ECG tracing showing the characteristic right bundle branch block patterns in the limb leads and in V_1 and V_2.

CALCULATING AXIS

The calculation of the mean axis determines the predominant direction of the flow of electrical current in the heart. This is usually measured during ventricular depolarization (QRS) and utilizes the morphology of the QRS complexes in the limb leads. Calculation of axis is one more tool used in determining fascicular block.

The hexaxial reference system refers to an intersecting pattern of 6 limb leads. The hexaxial reference system is used to determine the axis of the heart in the frontal plane. In other words, this will reference the flow of current as it occurs within the heart's conduction sytem. Clinically, this is important because deviation from normal can aid in a differential diagnosis of many cardiac conditions and pathology within the heart's conduction system.

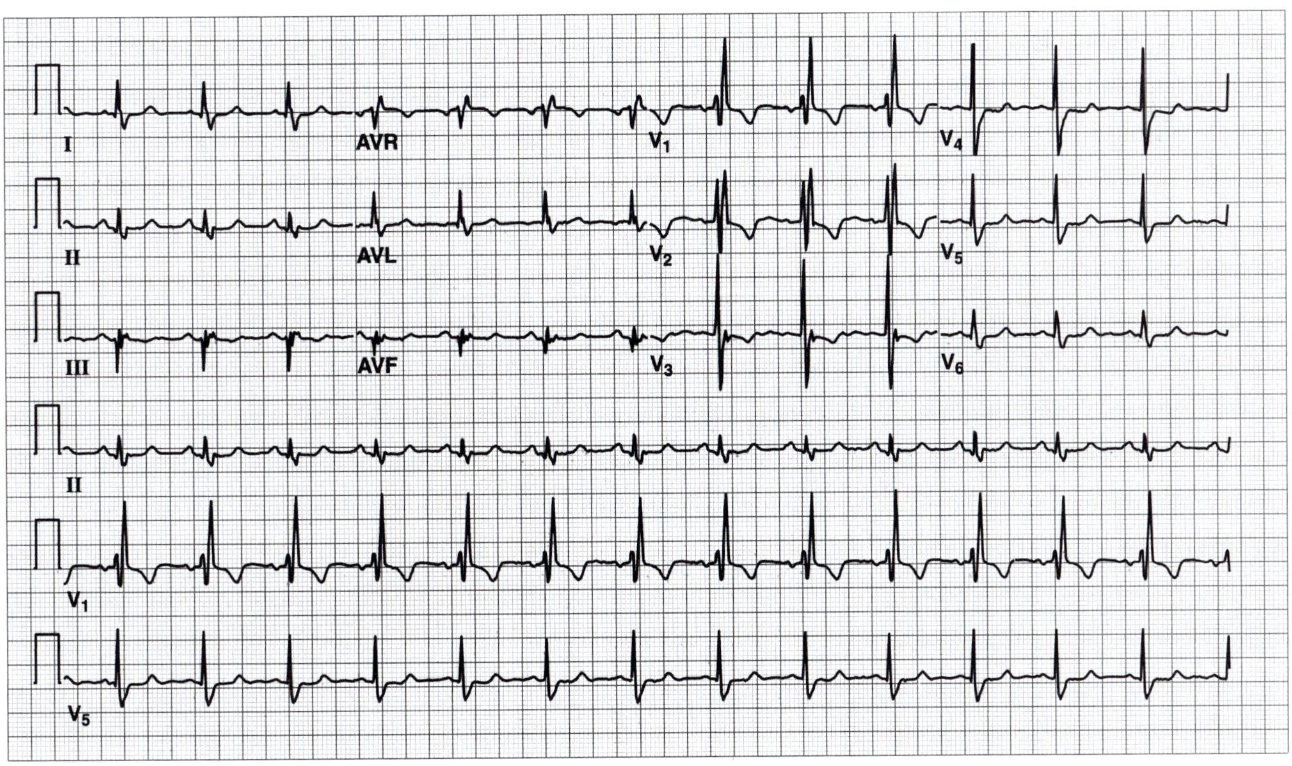

Figure 11-16 In the ECG tracing, leads II and III reflect the positive QRS configurations greater than 0.10 second with broad, terminal S waves. The rSR' in V_1 and RSR' in V_2 reflect RBBB.

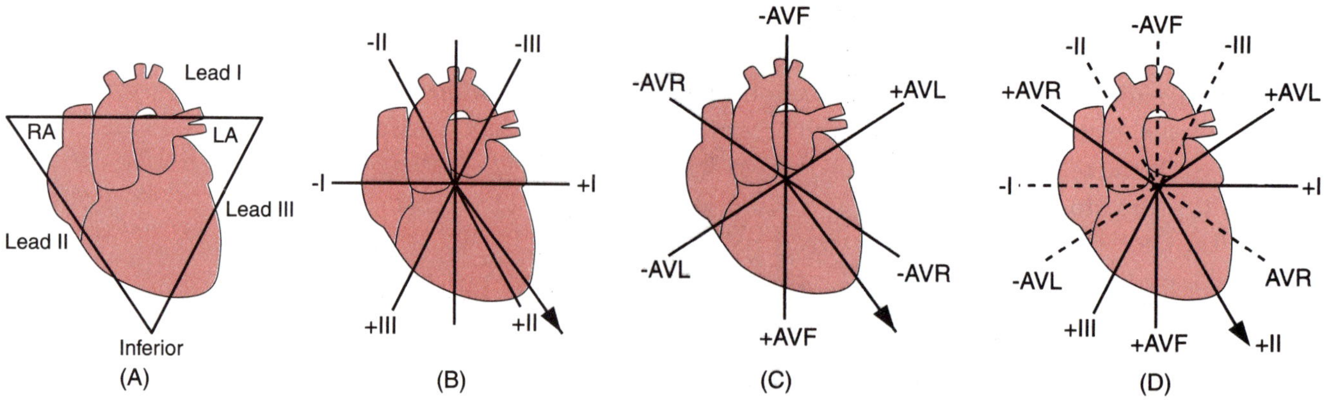

Figure 11-17 (A) The triangle formed by leads I, II, and III. (B) The intersection of the lines of I, II, and III as they form the skeleton of the hexaxial figure. (C) The addition of AVR, AVL, and AVF, and the completed hexaxial system.

To understand and apply the hexaxial system, the clinician must first understand the concept of vectors. A *vector* is the direction of force of electrical energy within the heart. The mean cardiac vector is a representation of the flow of electrical current during a cardiac cycle. In order to understand the hexaxial system, first imagine the triangle formed by leads I, II, and III. As those lines intersect, they create the skeleton for the hexaxial system. Next, add the position for AVR, AVL, and AVF, which also intersect, producting three additional lines of reference. You would now see 12 lines as they visualize the heart's electrical system. Figure 11-17 is an illustration of the building of the hexaxial reference system.

Recall in the normal heart, the flow of electrical current usually travels downward from right to left. This is called the *normal axis* of the heart. Figure 11-18 illustrates the mean flow of current in a heart with normal conduction.

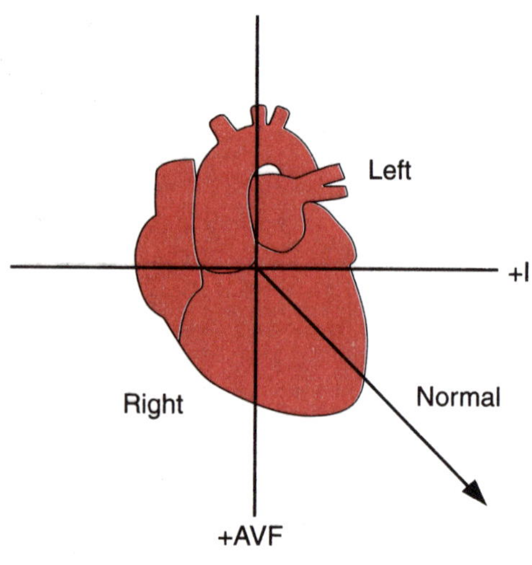

Figure 11-18 The arrow illustrates the direction of the mean flow of current in a heart with normal ventricular conduction.

Calculation of Axis

Calculating the mean flow of current (axis) can be done in several ways. The common and successful two-step method is as follows:

1. Identify the equiphasic QRS.
2. Identify the lead that is perpendicular and positive to this lead. (Remember, lead I is at right angle to AVF, lead II is at right angle to AVL, and lead III is at right angle to AVR.) The flow of current, or axis, will be parallel to that lead.

Figures 11-19A and B illustrate the two-step method.

Another method is the quadrant method. This is successful when there are no equiphasic complexes or when there is more than one lead with equiphasic deflection.

1. Look at lead I and determine if the flow of current is to the right or the left; draw an arrow in that direction:
   a. a positive (+) QRS indicates the flow is to the left
   b. a negative (-) QRS indicates the flow is to the right
2. Look at lead AVF and determine if the flow is superior or inferior; draw an arrow in that direction:
   a. a positive (+) QRS indicates the flow is inferior, towards AVF
   b. a negative (-) QRS indicates the flow is superior, away from AVF

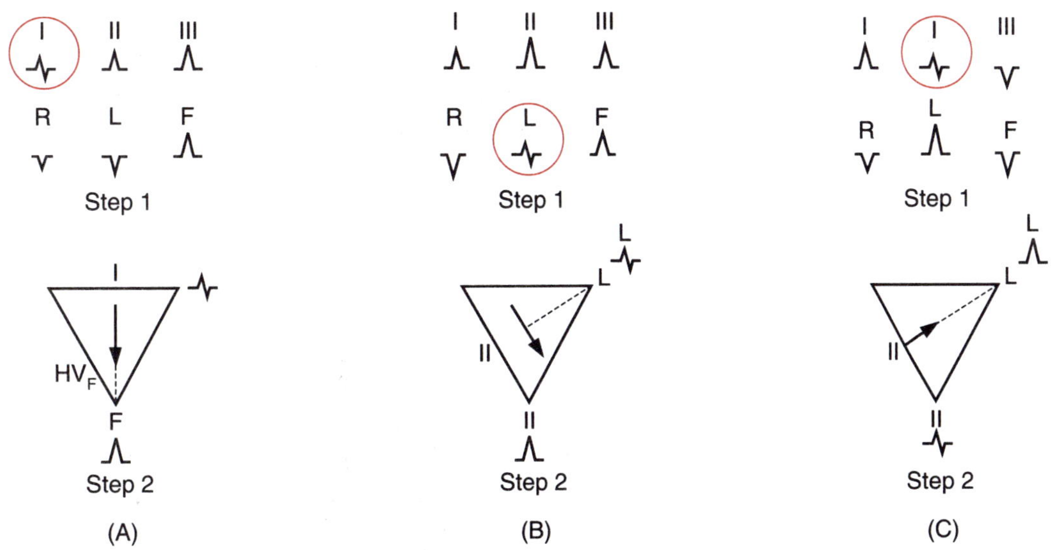

Figure 11-19 (A) Step 1: Look for the equiphasic deflection. In this fiugre, it is lead I, therefore, the current flow must be perpendicular (ar right angle) to lead I. In this example, it is lead AVF. Conclusion: the current is flowing inferior toward the positive electrode of AVF. (B) Step 1: Look for the equiphasic deflection. In this figure, it is lead AVL, therefore, the current flow must be perpendicular to that lead. Step 2: Look for the lead that is perpendicular to lead AVL. It is lead II. Conclusion: The flow of current is flowing inferior toward the positive electrode of lead II. (C) Step 1: Look for the equiphasic deflection. In this figure, it is lead II, therfore, the current flow must be perpendicular to that lead. Step 2: Look at the lead that is perpendicular to lead II. In this example, it is lead AVL. Conclusion: The current is flowing superior toward the positive electrode of lead AVL. (Adapted with permission from Conover, M.B. *Understanding Electrocardiography*, 6th ed. C. V. Mosby, 19–22; 1992.)

3. This creates a quadrant—look for the lead that is positive in that quadrant. This will tell you the direction (axis) of current flow for that patient's QRS.

Figures 11-20A and B illustrate the step-by-step use of the quadrant method.

POINTS TO REMEMBER

1. If the QRS in leads I and II are both positive, there is no deviation. If the QRS in either lead I or II is negative, there is a deviation and further calculation is required.
2. A flow of current far to the left (superior) is considered a deviation from the normal flow, i.e., left axis deviation. The QRS will be more positive in leads I and AVL than in lead II; leads II and III will be predominantly negative.
3. A flow of current far to the right (inferior) is considered a deviation from the normal flow, i.e., right axis deviation (RAD). The QRS will be more negative in leads I and AVL than in lead II; leads II and III will be predominantly positive—III being most positive.

Another quick method is the Handal-Lewis method:

1. Look at lead I—if the current flow is toward the right, lead I will be negative.
2. Look at lead III—if the current flow is too far right (inferior), lead III will be very positive and show the greatest positive deflection of all the limb leads. This is right axis deviation.

Once more:

1. Look at lead I—if the current flow is toward the left, lead I will be positive.
2. Look at lead III—if the current flow is too far left (superior), lead III will be very negative and show the greatest negative deflection of all the limb leads. This is left axis deviation.

Figures 11-21A and B are ECG tracings highlighting the QRS complexes in leads I and III.

Normal and Abnormal Values

We have learned that deviation of current far to the left is considered abnormal. This may be caused by a problem with conduction in the left anterior fascicle of the bundle branch system, driving the current upward and to the left.

Deviation beyond far to the right is considered abnormal. This may be caused by a problem with conduction in the left posterior fascicle of the bundle branch system, driving the current far to the right.

Identify the axis by degrees so that each lead has a landmark:

lead I	=	0 degrees
lead II	=	(+) 60 degrees
lead III	=	(+) at 120 degrees (right) or
		(-) at (-) 60 degrees (left)
lead AVF	=	(+) at (+) 90 degrees or
		(-) at (-) 90 degrees

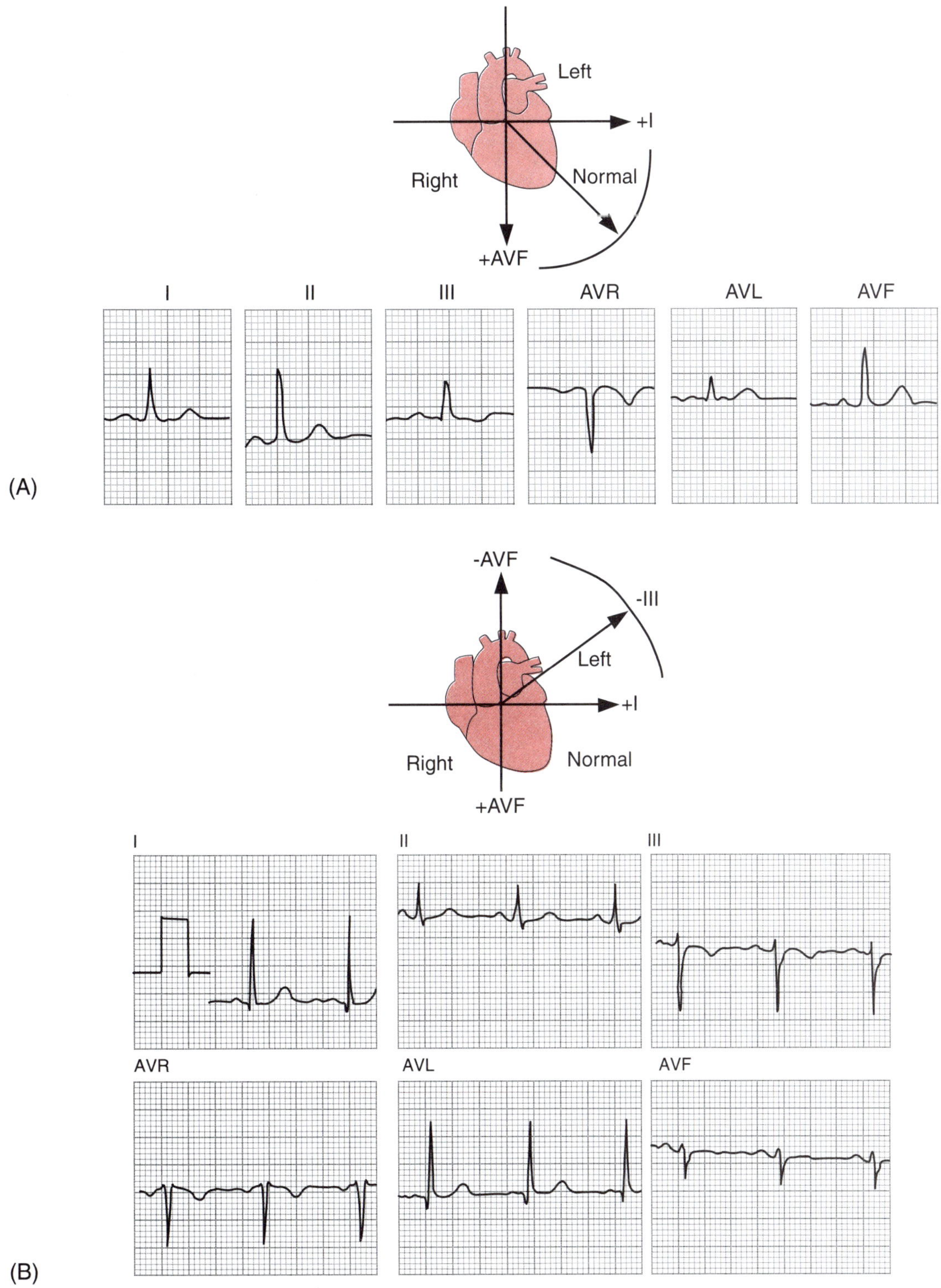

Figure 11-20 (A) Lead I is positive , the first arrow is toward the positive electrode in the lead. Next, lead AVF is perpendicular to lead I and the QRS in lead AVF is positive, so draw an imaginary arrow toward AVF. You have now localized the flow of current between leads I and AVF. The QRS in lead II is most positive so that the current of flow is directed inferior and to the left, within the normal limits. (B) Lead I is positive, the first arrow is from the positive electrode in the lead. Next, lead AVF is perpendicular to lead I and the QRS in lead AVF is negative, so draw an imaginary arrow away from the positive of AVF. You have now localized the flow of current between the positive electrode in lead I and the negative electrode in lead AVF. The QRS in lead III is most negative so the current of flow is directed superior and to the left, outside the normal limits. This deviation from normal is called *left axis deviation*. (Adapted with permission from Conover, M.B. *Understanding Electrocardiography*, 6th ed. C. V. Mosby; 1992.)

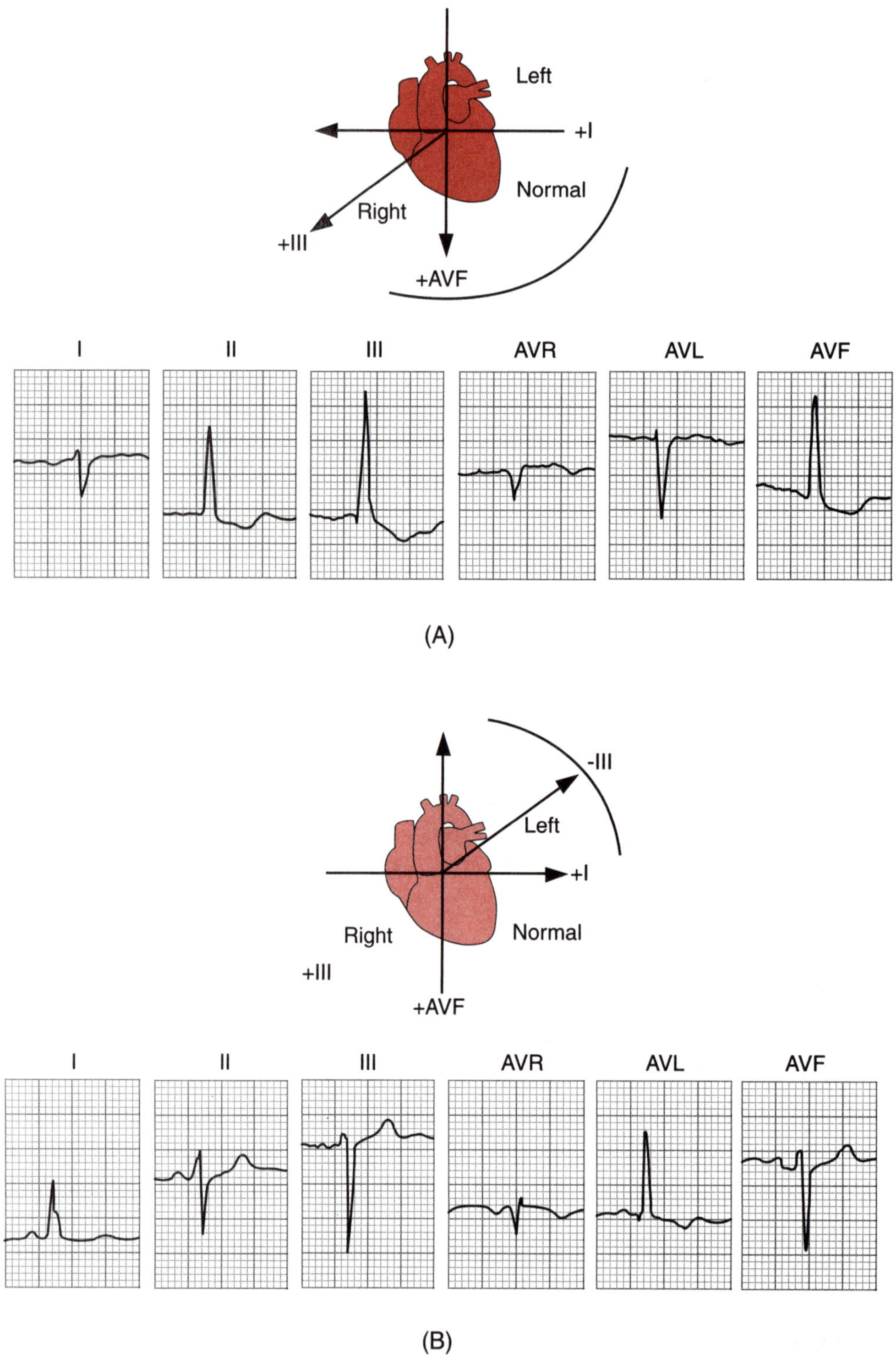

Figure 11-21 (A) An ECG tracing of leads I, II, and III highlighting the QRS complex in leads I and III. Note that in lead I, the QRS is negative, and in lead III, the QRS is positive. Note also the QRS in lead III is the most positive QRS seen in the limb leads. (B) An ECG tracing of leads I, II, and III highlighting the QRS complex in lead I and III. Note that in lead I, the QRS is positive, and in lead III, the QRS is negative. Note also the QRS in lead III is the most negative QRS seen in the limb leads. (Adapted with permission from Conover, M.B. *Understanding Electrocardiography*, 6th ed. C. V. Mosby; 1992.)

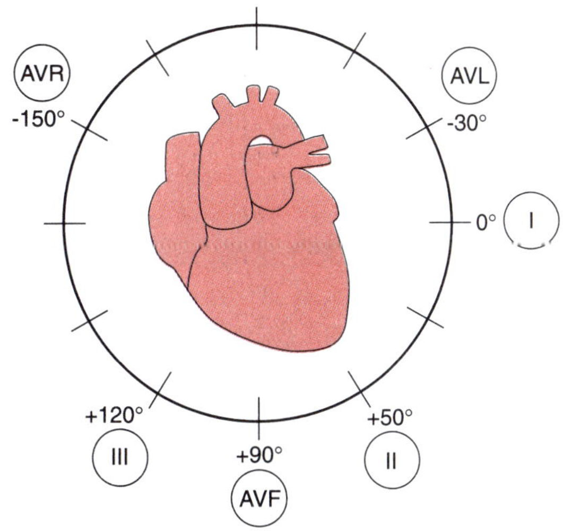

Figure 11-22 The Lewis circle, designed for quick reference, has degree values assigned to the limb and augmented leads as they reflect the heart's surface.

Figure 11-22 is the Lewis circle, designed with degree values assigned to the limb and augmented leads as they reflect the heart's surface.

HOW TO LOOK AT A MONITOR PATTERN USING THE 12-LEAD ECG

1. What is the standard? This is the measurement against which we compare the amplitude of the wave forms.
2. What is the underlying rhythm?
3. Look for the acute changes, according to the surfaces of the heart: Qs, ST segment changes, T-wave inversion
   a. Leads II, III, AVF: the inferior wall
   b. Leads I, AVL, V_6: left lateral wall
   c. $V_1 \rightarrow V_4$: anterior walls
   d. V3R → right anterior wall
4. Look for ventricular conduction disturbances:
   a. Leads II, III, AVF: left anterior fascicle
   b. Leads I, AVL, V_6: left posterior fascicle
   c. Lead VI for RBBB
5. What is the axis?
6. What can happen next? Which lead to observe?

Summary

The ECG is a sensitive tool. The changes in ST segments and PQRST morphology can provide insight into ischemia, injury and necrosis. Unfortunately, the changes are not always present on the ECG, and the patient may present with all the other signs and symptoms. Once present on the ECG, the changes cannot be ignored and must be describe accurately and in detail to minimize the time delay between recognition and reperfusion. Table 11-1 is a summary of ECG changes as seen with myocardial infarction.

The conduction system must always be considered when infarction in this area is suspected. Extensive septal and anterior wall damage may lead to damage of both bundle branches. With evolution of an anteroseptal infarction, there may be development of significant life-threatening intraventricular conduction defects. Table 11-2 is a summary of normal ECG ranges and variations seen on the 12-lead ECG.

This chapter was designed to acquaint the clinician with the concepts of 12-lead ECG analysis and focused on the patient with myocardial ischemia, injury, and infarction. The impact of infarction on the electrical conduction system was also introduced. This is not an all-inclusive chapter for the study of 12-lead analysis requires much more in-depth material. The purpose was to remind the clinician that changes in the heart's perfusion may not always be visible in the ECG, and limb leads may not reflect acute changes in monitoring leads. Finally, the clinician should have an appreciation that in a patient with chest pain, limb leads are insufficient. The 12-lead ECG and rapid clinical assessment are vital for perfusion of heart muscle.

Table 11-1 A quick reference to the surfaces of the heart as seen on the 12-lead ECG

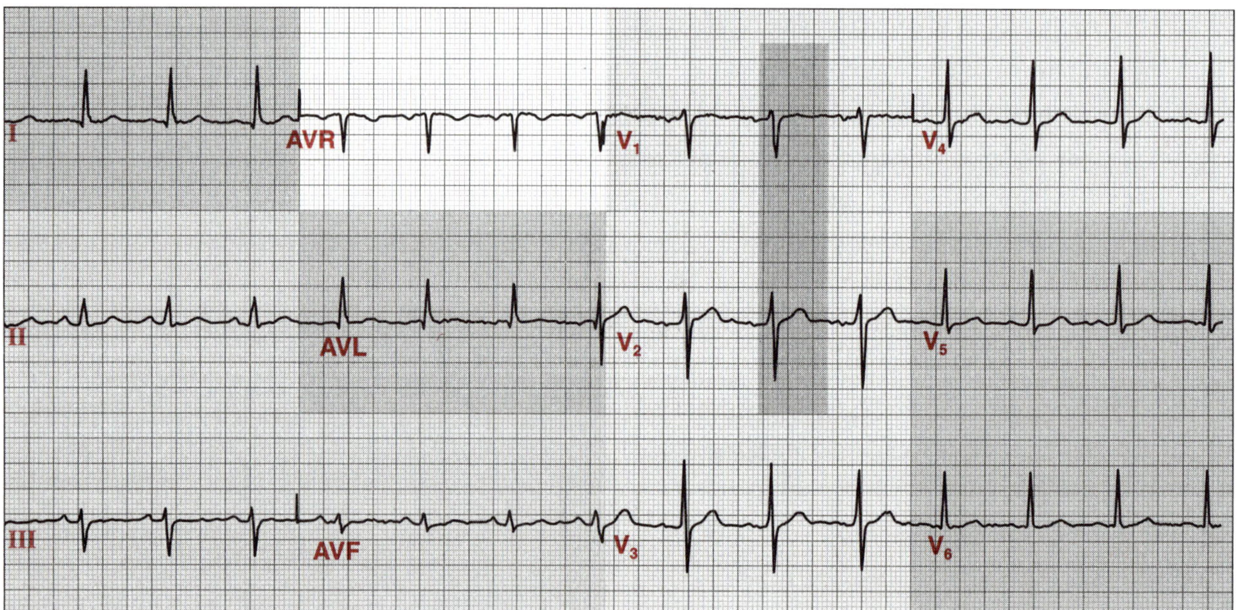

Infarction	Wave Abnormality	ECG Segments	Occlusion
Anterior	ST Elevation	V_1, V_2, V_3, V_4	Left Anterior Descending Artery
Inferior	ST Elevation	II, III, AVF	Right Coronary Artery (RCA)
Lateral	ST Elevation	I, AVL, V_5, V_6	Left Circumflex (LCX) Atery
Posterior	ST Depression, Tall R Wave	V_1, V_2	RCA and/or LCX Artery
Subendo	Diffuse or Localized Changes, Non-Q Wave		

Table 11-2 Normal ranges and variations in adults in a 12-lead electrocardiogram

The configurations in the following grid can provide a guide to the patient's condition but must be interpreted as only a tool. The ECG like any other sign must be judged in the context of patient history and presentation.

LEAD	P	Q	R	S	ST	T
I	upright	<.04 seconds <25% of the R wave	largest deflection of the QRS complex	< R or none	isoelectric; may vary 1 mm (+) or (-)	upright
II	upright	small or none	dominant	< R or none	isoelectric; may vary 1 mm (+) or (-)	upright
III	(+) or (-) flat, or diphasic. (depends on frontal plane axis)	small or none 0.04–0.05 seconds or >25% of the R wave (depends on frontal plane axis)	none to dominant depending on frontal plane axis	none to dominant depending on frontal plane axis	isoelectric; may vary 1 mm (+) or (-)	upright, flat diphasic or inverted depending on frontal plane axis
AVR	inverted	small, none, or large	small or none depending on frontal plane axis	dominant; may appear as a QS configuration	isoelectric; may vary 1 mm (+) or (-)	inverted
AVL	upright, flat or diphasic; inverted depending on frontal plane axis	small, none, or large	small, none or dominant depending on frontal plane axis	none to dominant, depending on the frontal plane axis	usually isoelectric; may vary from +1 -0.5 mm	upright, flat or diphasic; may be inverted depending on frontal plane axis
AVF	upright	small or none	small, none or dominant depending on frontal plane axis	none to dominant, depending on the frontal plane axis	usually isoelectric; may vary from +1 -0.5 mm	upright, flat or diphasic; may be inverted depending on frontal plane axis
V_1	inverted, flat, upright or diphasic	none, may be a QS	less than S_1 or none, (QS) small R' may be present	dominant, may be a QS	0 to (+) 3 mm	upright, flat, diphasic, or inverted
V_2	upright, less commonly diphasic or inverted	none, may be a QS	less than S_1 or none, (QS) small R' may be present	dominant, may be a QS	0 to (+) 3 mm	upright, less commonly flat; diphasic or inverted
V_3	upright	small or none	R<S or R>S or R=S	S>R or S<R or R=S	0 to (+) 3 mm	upright
V_4	upright	small or none	R>S	S<R	usually isoelectric; (+)1 to (-)0.5 mm	upright
V_5	upright	small	dominant, less than 26 mm	S less than SV_4	usually isoelectric; (+) 1 to (-) 0.5 mm	upright
V_6	upright	small	dominant, less than 26mm	S less than SV_4	usually isoelectric; (+) 1 to (-) 0.5 mm	upright

Self-Assessment Exercises

Matching

Match the term in the left column with the definitions in the right column and compare your answers to those in the back of the book.

	Term	Definition
____	1. anterior wall MI	A. ST elevation 3 to 4 week post-MI
____	2. current of injury	B. ST elevation
____	3. inferior wall MI	C. Q wave, ST elevation II, III, and AVF
____	4. transmural MI	D. Q wave, ST elevation V_3,V_4,V_5, V_6
____	5. ventricular aneurysm	E. Q, ST elevation, hyperacute T wave

ECG Rhythm Identification Practice

Identify the ECG criterion listed below each 12-lead ECG and check your answers with those in the back of the book.

Figure 11-23

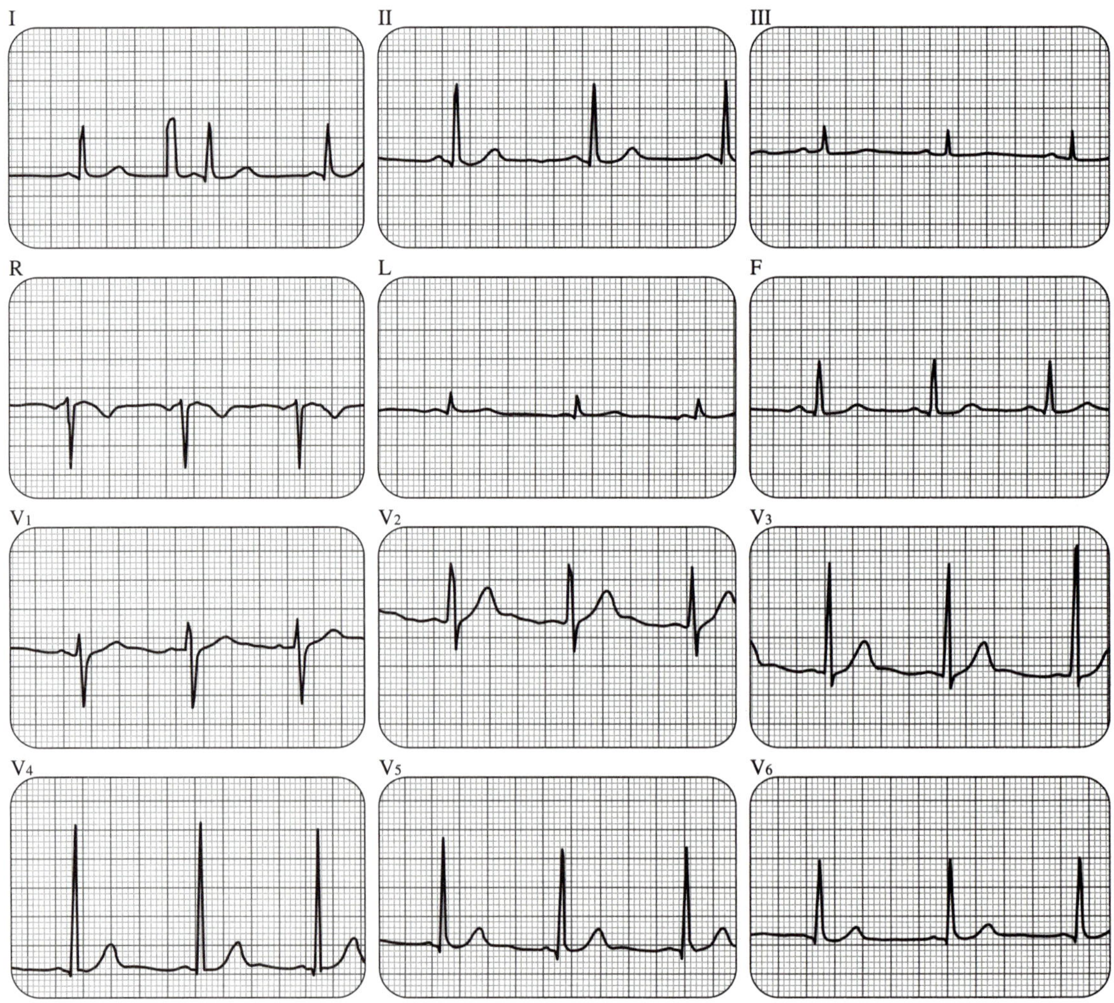

1. What is the underlying rhythm?
2. What are the acute changes?
3. What is your interpretation?
4. What can happen next?

Figure 11-24

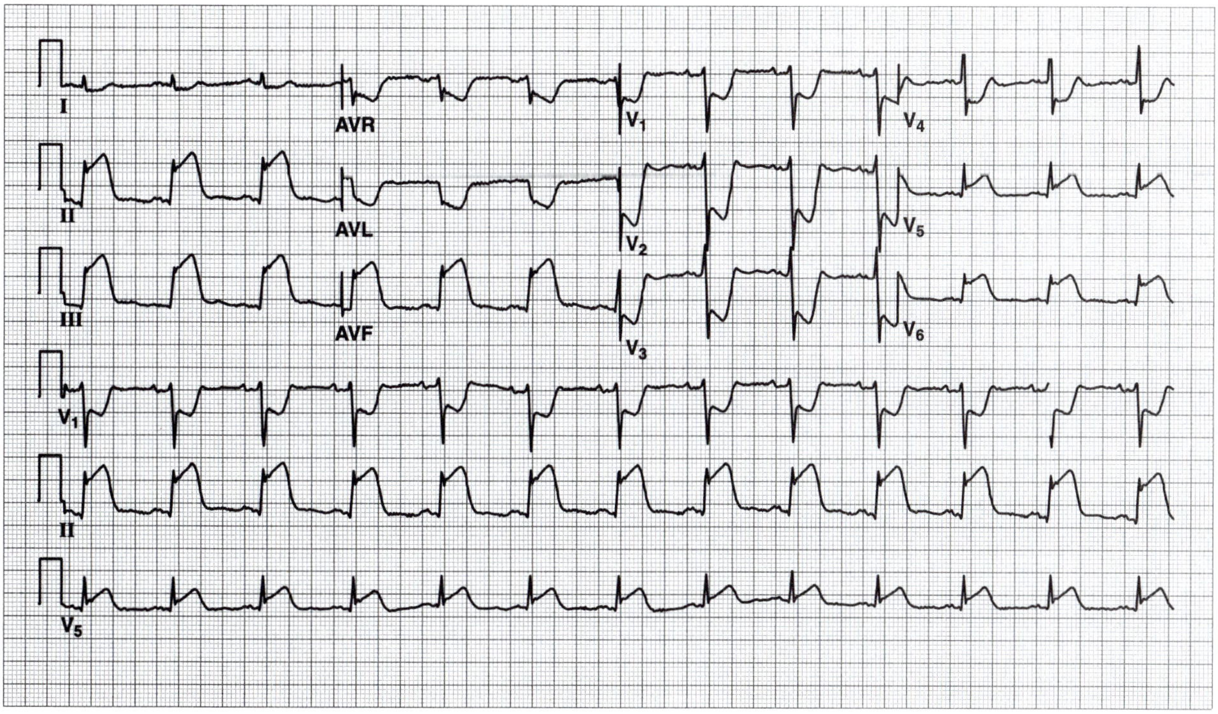

1. What is the underlying rhythm?
2. What are the acute changes?
3. What is your interpretation?
4. What can happen next?

Figure 11-25

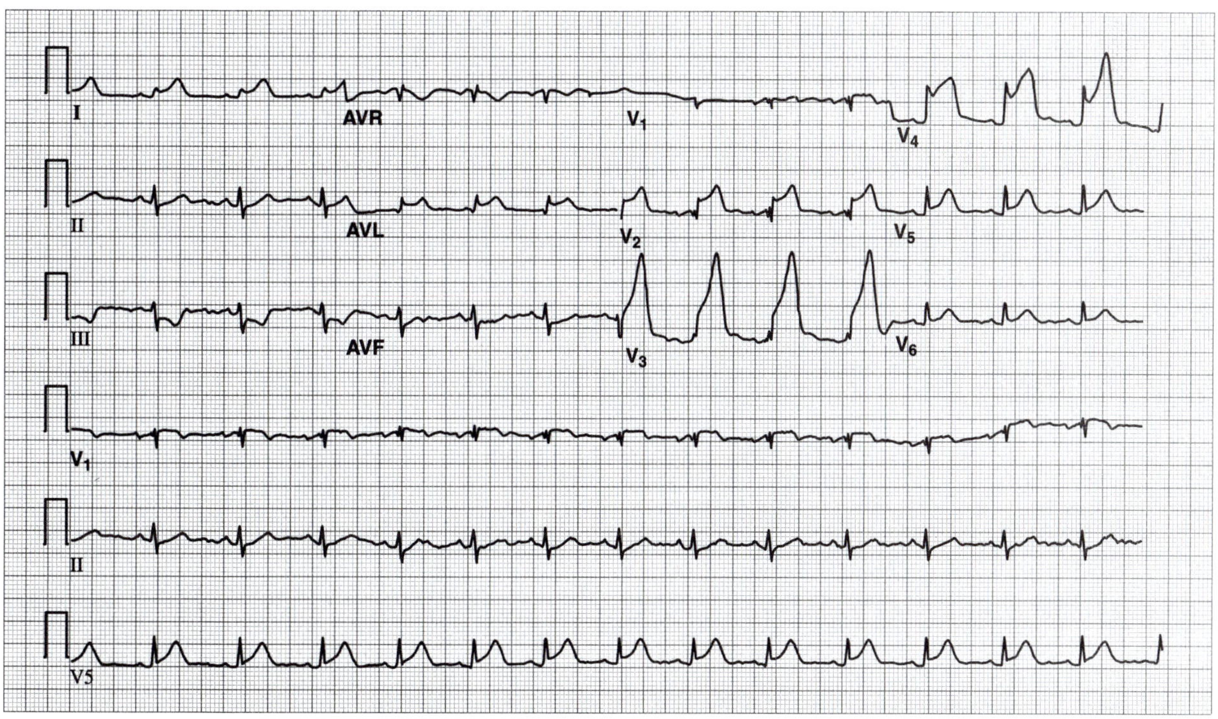

1. What is the underlying rhythm?
2. What are the acute changes?
3. What is your interpretation?
4. What can happen next?

Figure 11-26

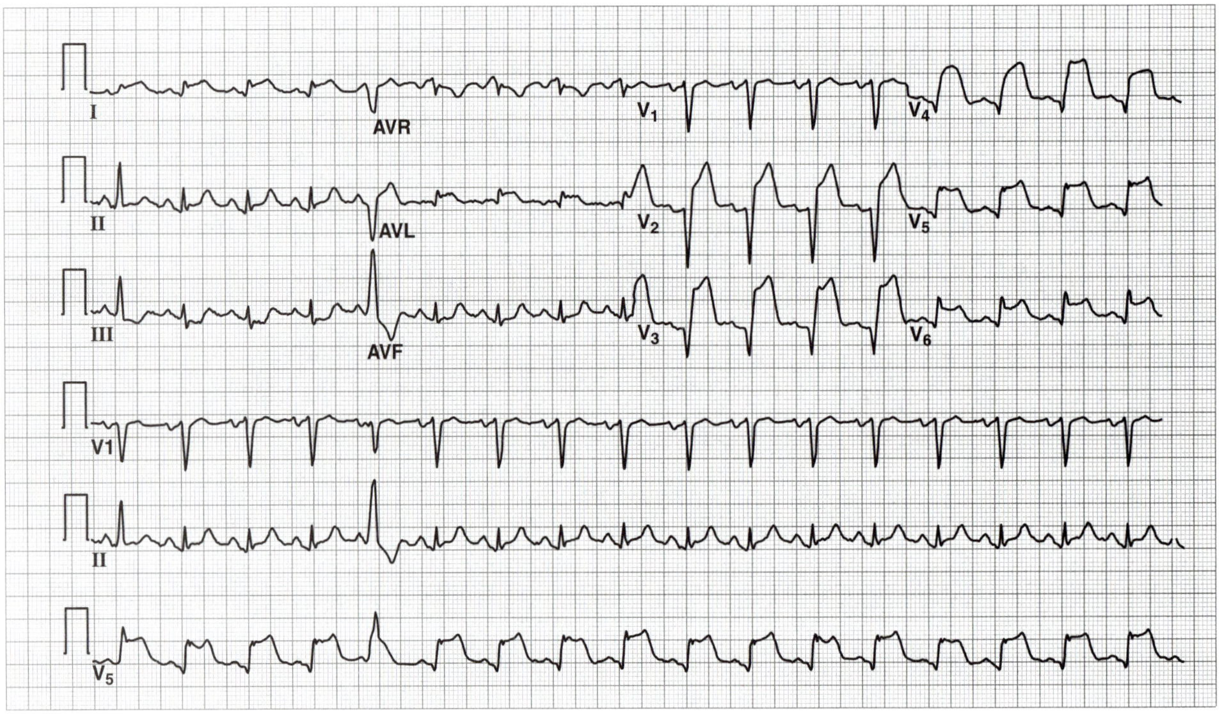

1. What is the underlying rhythm?
2. What are the acute changes?
3. What is your interpretation?
4. What can happen next?

Figure 11-27

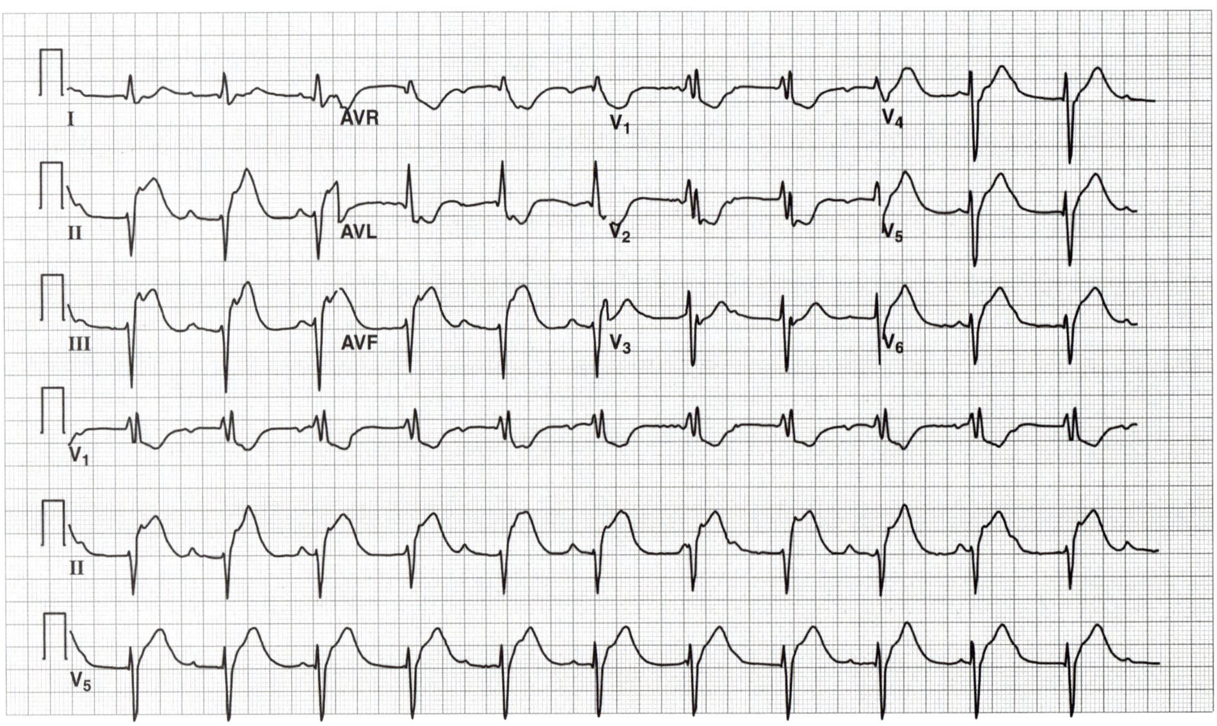

1. What is the underlying rhythm?
2. What are the acute changes?
3. What is your interpretation?
4. What can happen next?

Figure 11-28

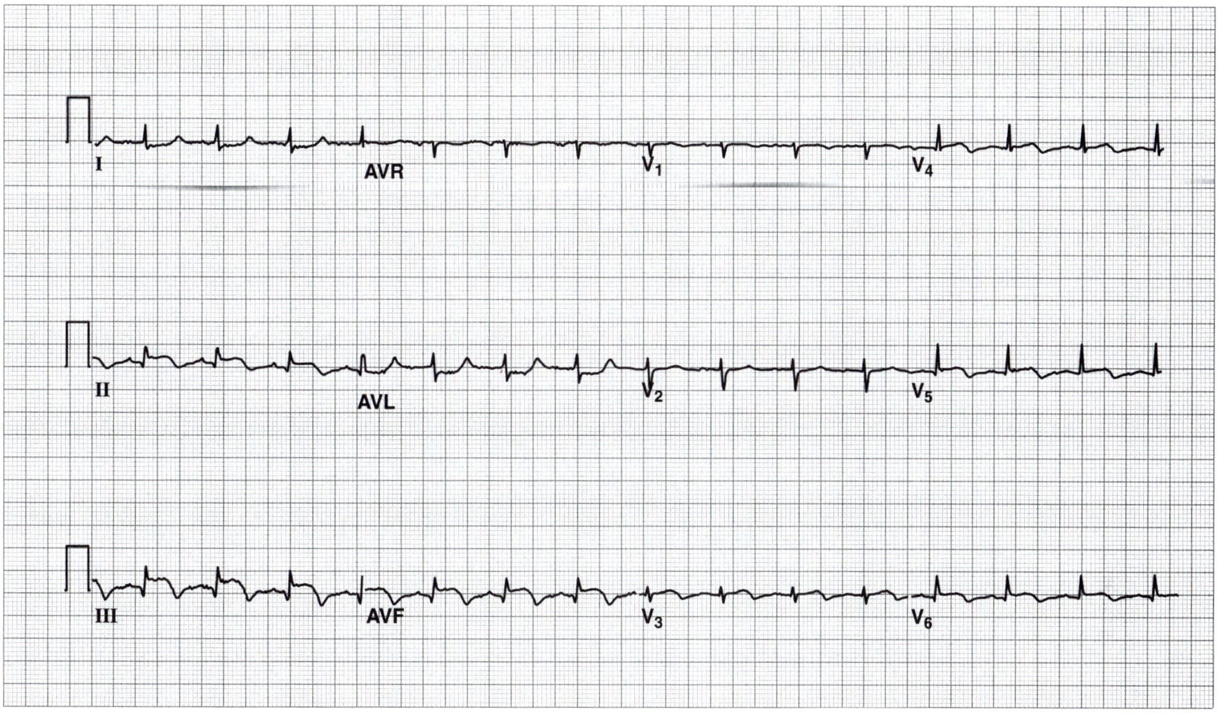

1. What is the underlying rhythm?
2. What are the acute changes?
3. What is your interpretation?
4. What can happen next?

Figure 11-29

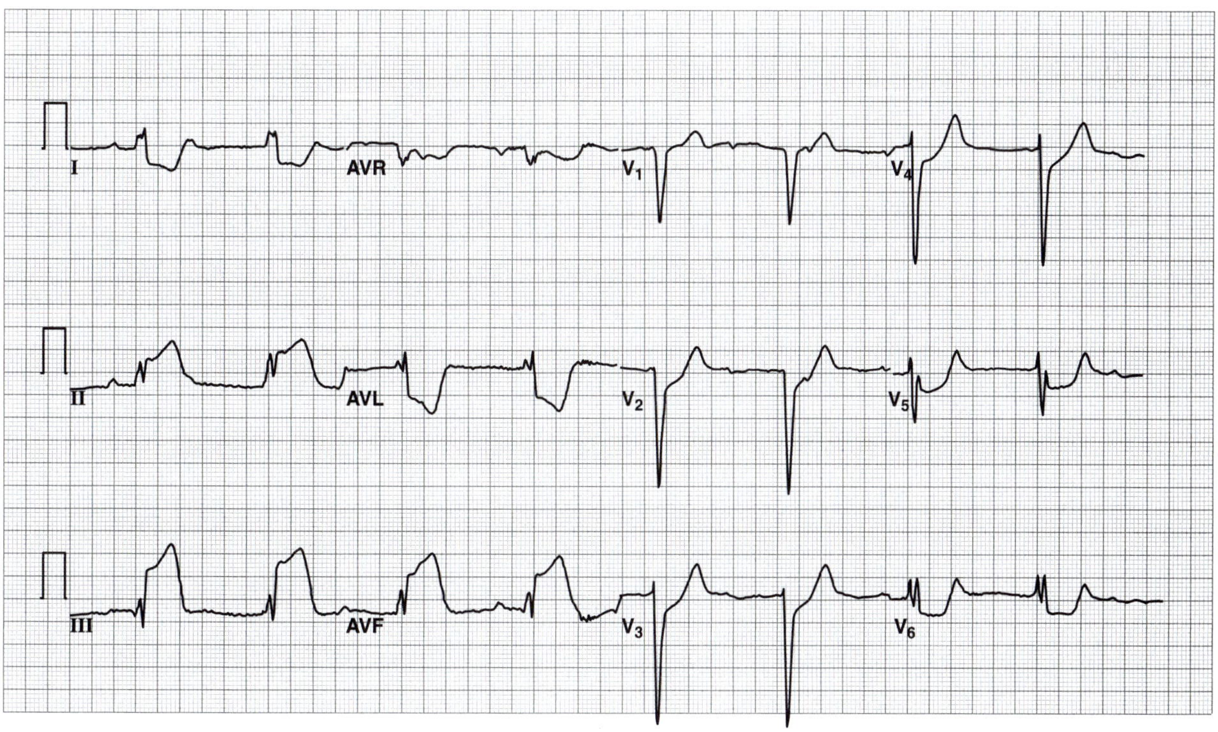

1. What is the underlying rhythm?
2. What are the acute changes?
3. What is your interpretation?
4. What can happen next?

Figure 11-30

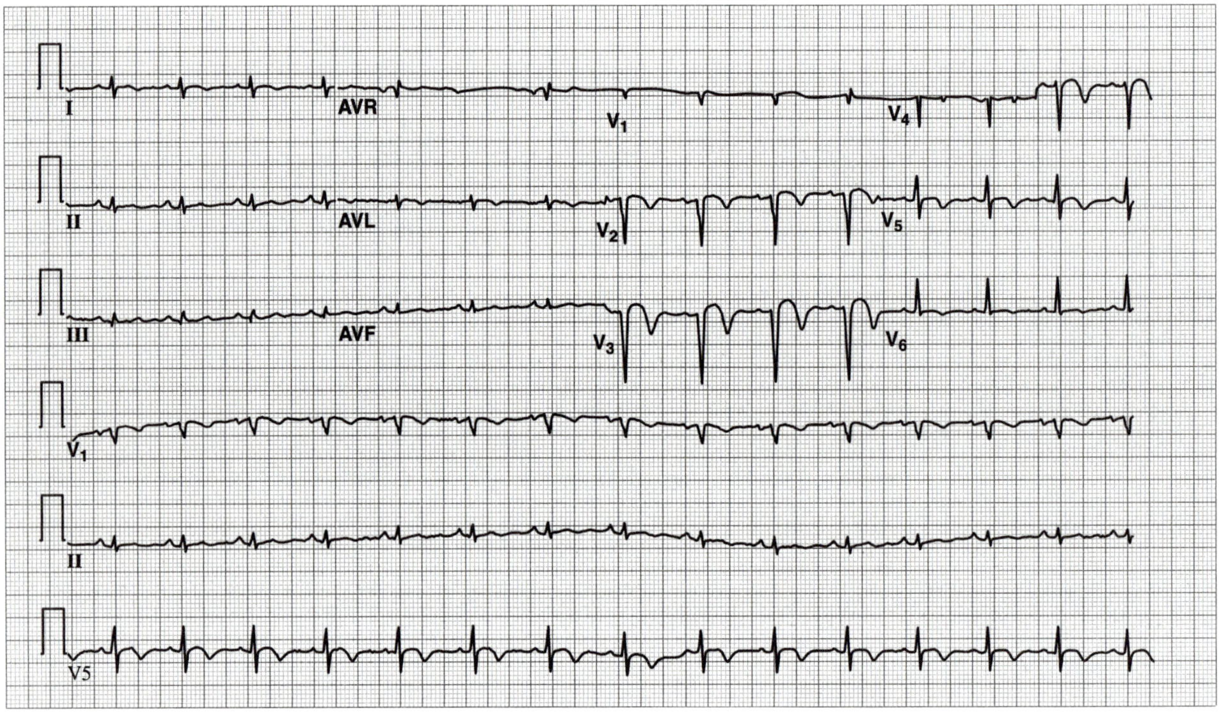

1. What is the underlying rhythm?
2. What are the acute changes?
3. What is your interpretation?
4. What can happen next?

Figure 11-31

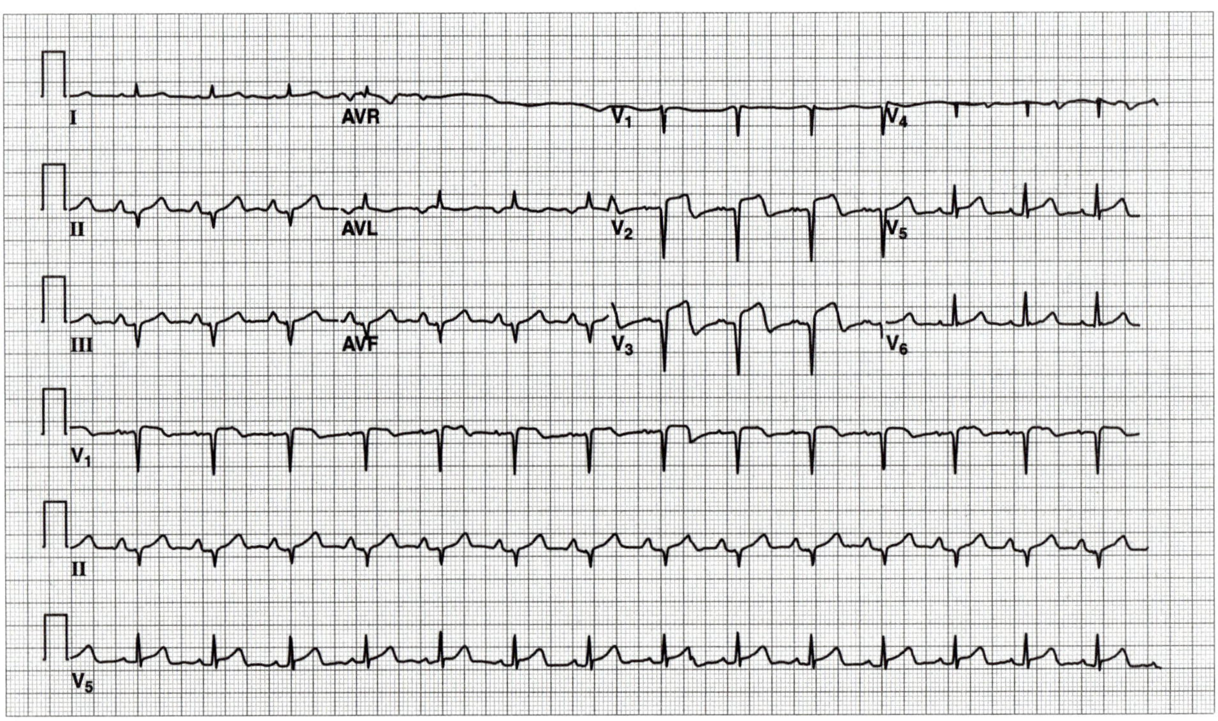

1. What is the underlying rhythm?
2. What are the acute changes?
3. What is your interpretation?
4. What can happen next?

Figure 11-32

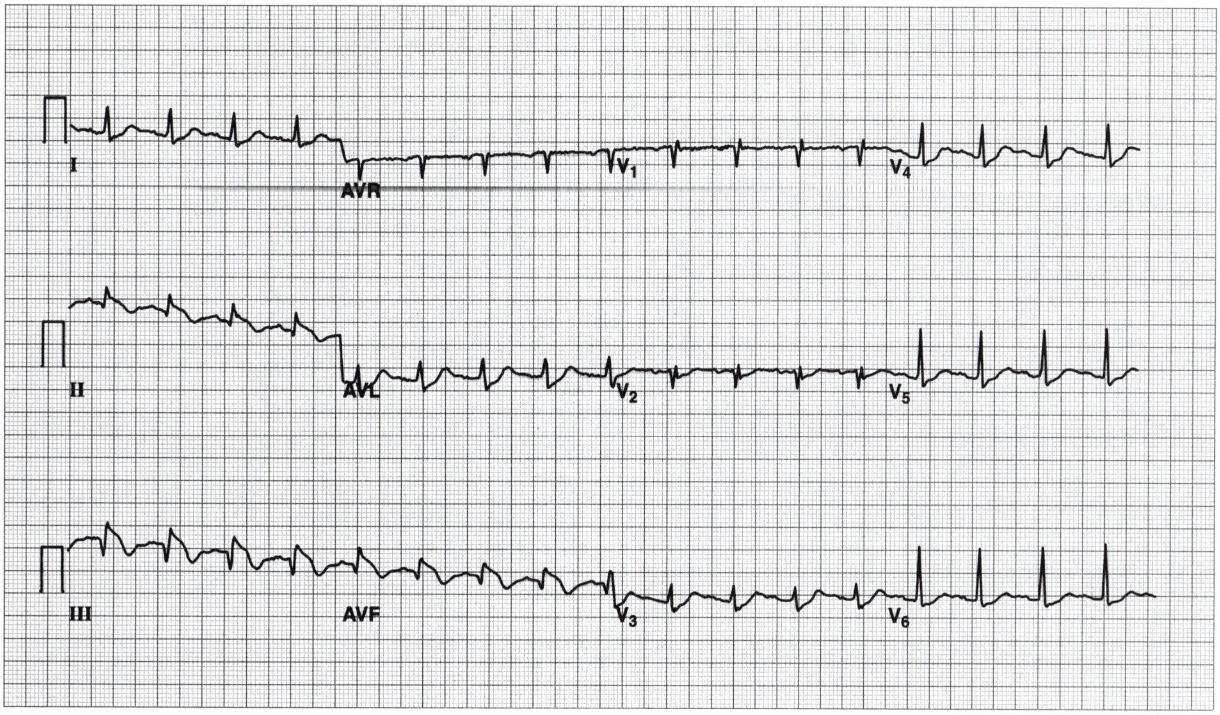

1. What is the underlying rhythm?
2. What are the acute changes?
3. What is your interpretation?
4. What can happen next?

Figure 11-33

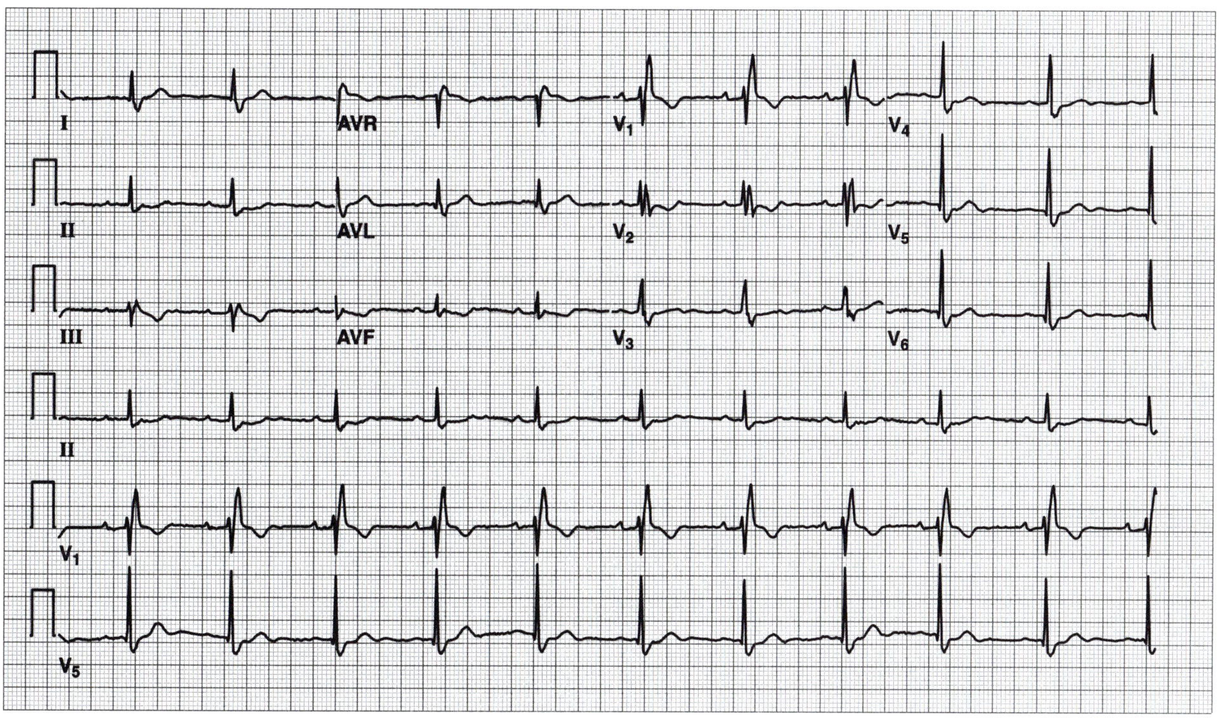

1. What is the underlying rhythm?
2. What are the acute changes?
3. What is your interpretation?
4. What can happen next?

REFERENCES

Conover, M. B. *Nurse's pocket guide to electrocardiography* (3rd ed.). St. Louis, MO: C. V. Mosby; 1994.

Conover, M. B. *Understanding electrocardiography: Arrhythmias and the 12 lead ECG* (7th ed.). St. Louis, MO: Mosby-Year Book, Inc.; 1996.

Conover, M. B. & Wellens, H. J. *The ECG in emergency decision making*. Philadelphia: W. B. Saunders; 1993.

Emergency Cardiac Care Subcommittee and Subcommittees, American Heart Association. Guidelines for cardiopulmonary resuscitation and emergency cardiac care, *JAMA*. 1994.

Lepeschkin, E. Physiological basis of the U wave. In Schlant, R.C. & Hurst, J. W. (Eds.). *Advances in electrocardiography*. New York: Grune and Stratton. 431–477; 1992.

Marriott, H. J. & Conover, M. B. *Advanced concepts in arrhythmias* (2nd ed.). St. Louis, MO: C. V. Mosby Company; 1989.

CHAPTER 12

Arrythmias Due to Abnormal Conduction Pathways

Premise Widening of the QRS does not always imply bundle branch block.

Objectives

After reading the chapter and completing the Self-Assessment Exercises, the reader should be able to

1. define accessory pathway
2. identify the ECG characteristics of presence of an accessory pathway
3. identify the consequences of arrhythmias that are the result of an accessory pathway (AP)

Key Terms

accessory AV pathway
antidromic
bypass tracts
delta wave
intranodal bypass tract
James fibers
Kent bundles
Lown-Ganong-Levine (LGL) syndrome
Mahaim's fibers
orthodromic
Wolff-Parkinson-White (WPW) syndrome

Introduction

Depolarization from the sinus node travels through atrial tissue and terminates at the crest of the AV node. The PR interval is comprised of the time taken for atrial depolarization, forming the P wave, and depolarization of the AV node, bundle of His and both bundle branches, and the PR segment. Slow conduction through the AV node accounts for most of the PR segment. If the wave of depolarization can bypass the AV node, then the normal delay that would have been encountered is circumvented, and the PR segment and thus the PR interval will be shortened.

Most patients with AP are not affected nor diagnosed until adulthood. Males are affected more than females. There is evidence to support that there is genetic predisposition to AP and the resulting tachycardias.

Kent Bundles
Accessory AV pathways that connect the atrium to the ventricles

accessory AV pathway
Muscular connection between the atria and ventricles that bypasses the AV node

intranodal bypass tract
An AP that connects atrial fibers to the upper part of the AV node

Mahaim's fibers
AP that connect the AV node and the ventricle, or the bundle of His and the bundle branch nodofascicular, or the bundle branch and the fascicular ventricle.

bypass tracts
An abnormal bundle of muscle connecting the atria and ventricles but bypassing the AV node. The AV node no longer controls the rate of ventricular stimulation because the atrial impulses follow an alternate pathway.

PREEXCITATION DEFINED

Preexcitation describes early ventricular depolarization, using an *accessory pathway* rather than the normal AV conduction system. An accessory pathway is an extra muscle bundle composed of ventricular tissue that exists outside the normal, specialized conduction tissue. This bundle forms a connection between the atria and ventricles. *Preexcitation syndrome* describes clinical situations where preexcitation causes tachycardias.

Preexcitation is of concern since there is a potential for supraventricular tachyarrhythmias. In addition, paroxysmal supraventricular tachycardia (PSVT) and atrial fibrillation that result from an unrecognized preexcitation syndrome, can deteriorate into ventricular fibrillation. In some cases of preexcitation, the resulting QRS complex is widened and may be confused with bundle branch block. Also wide-QRS complex arrhythmias occurring with preexcitation may be confused with ventricular tachycardia.

PHYSIOLOGY OF ACCESSORY PATHWAY (AP)

There are several accessory pathways (AP) connecting the atria to the ventricles. **Kent Bundles** are accessory AV pathways that connect the atrium to the ventricles. **Accessory AV pathways** are a common type of preexcitation.

- James' bundle is an AP that connects atrial fibers to the upper part of the AV node. This is also termed an **intranodal bypass tract**.
- **Mahaim's fibers** are AP that connect the AV node and the ventricle (nodoventricular), or those that connect the bundle of His and the bundle branch nodofascicular or from the bundle branch to the ventricles (fascicular ventricular).
- Atriofascicular **bypass tracts** are fibers that connect the atrium to the bundle of His.

Figure 12-1 is an illustration of accessory pathways connecting atrial and ventricular tissue.

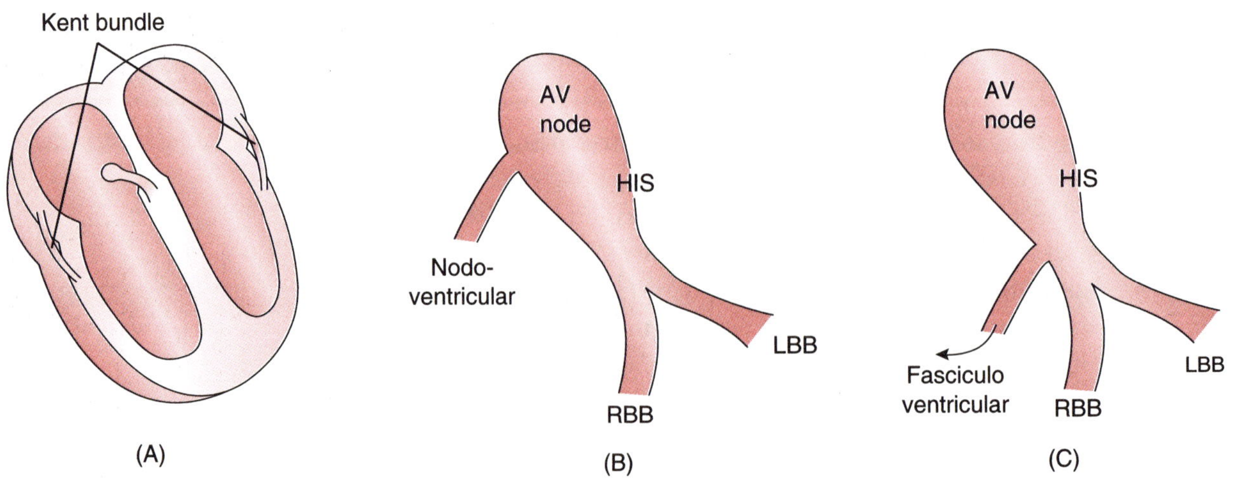

Figure 12-1 (A) The site of the Kent bundles, (B) the James bundle, (C) the Mahaim's fibers. (Adapted from Conover, M.B. *Understanding Electrocardiography: Arrhythmias and the 12 lead ECG* (7th ed.). St. Louis, MO: Mosby-Year Book, Inc.; 1996.)

THE ECG WAVE FORMS AFFECTED BY PREEXCITATION

The ECG pattern of preexcitation consists primarily of a short PR interval because the descending impulse bypasses the normal AV conduction delay. Often, this is the source of AV nodal reentrant tachycardias. During the tachycardia, the QRS can be narrow, wide, and aberrant. If atrial fibrillation occurs with an accessory pathway, the ventricular response is usually very rapid, irregular and with aberrant ventricular conduction. Figure 12-2 is the ECG tracing of a patient with atrial fibrillation complicated by the accessory pathway.

In addition, the early depolarization of the ventricles will cause a widened QRS complex called a **delta wave**, with characteristic slurring in the initial wave forms of the QRS. The delta wave is caused by slow intramyocardial conduction rather than normal intraventricular conduction pathways. The widened QRS is a result of the asynchronous depolarization of the ventricles.

delta wave
Initial slurring of the QRS complex; seen in preexcitation states such as Wolff-Parkinson-White syndrome. As a result, the P-R interval is shortened. It does not have to be seen in all leads.

The polarity of the delta wave may be positive or negative depending on the direction of conduction as viewed by a particular lead. If the forces of excitation are toward the positive electrode in a lead, the polarity of the delta wave will be positive. Similarly, if the forces of excitation are away from the positive electrode in a lead, the polarity of the delta wave will be negative and produce an abnormal Q wave in leads

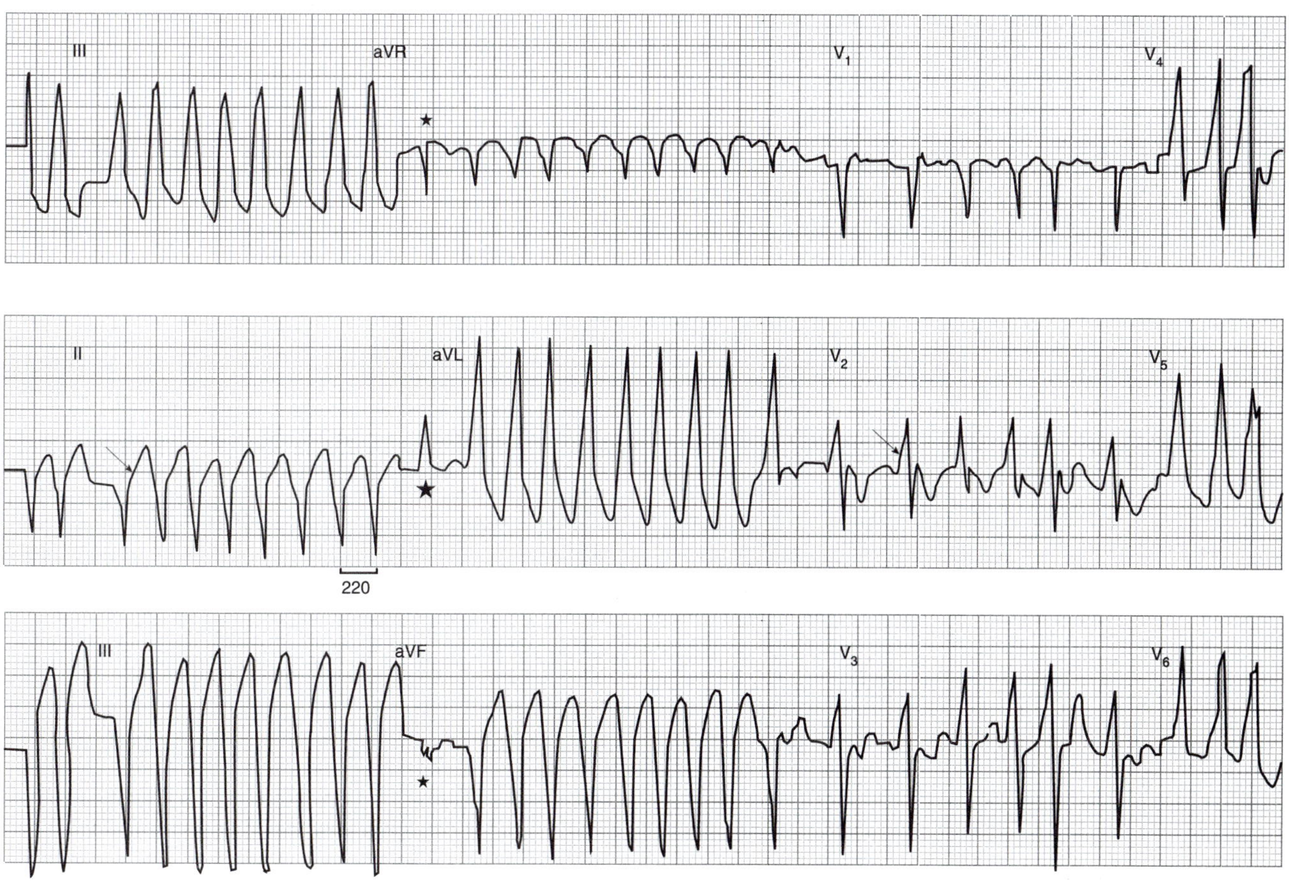

Figure 12-2 An ECG tracing of a patient with atrial fibrillation compounded by the use of an accessory pathway. The delta waves are seen in some of the QRS complexes. Note the irregular rhythm, which differentiates this ECG from ventricular tachycardia. The short R-R interval reflects the use of the accessory pathway rather than conventional AV node delay.

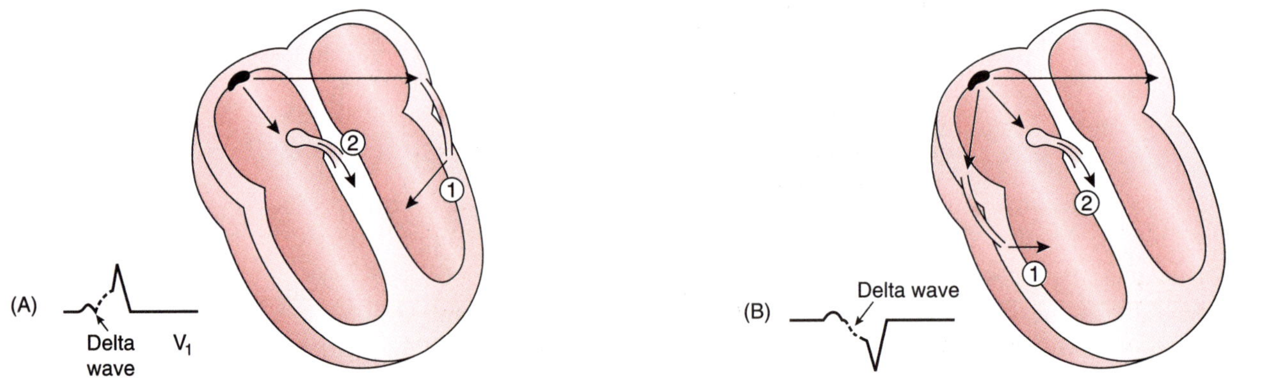

Figure 12-3 The presence of delta waves. Note the distortion on the ascending arm in (A) and on the descending arm in (B) of the QRS complexes as they reflect early activation of ventricular conduction system. (Adapted from Conover, M.B. *Understanding Electrocardiography: Arrhythmias and the 12 lead ECG* (7th ed.). St. Louis, MO: Mosby-Year Book, Inc.; 1996.)

III and V_1. Finally, if the forces of excitation are perpendicular to the positive electrode in a lead, the polarity will be isoelectric. Figure 12-3 is a diagram of the conduction from the atria to the ventricles using an accessory pathway and the resulting changes in the QRS complex.

The amplitude of the delta wave depends on several factors, but primarily how quickly the accessory pathway conducts the current ahead of the normal wave of depolarization. If normal and accessory wave fronts arrive simultaneously, there may be no delta wave and the PR interval would be unchanged. However, since there will be sources depolarizing the ventricles, the resulting QRS will be a fusion of both wave fronts.

In summary, the width of the QRS depends on several factors:

1. the length of time it takes for conduction through the accessory pathway
2. the location of the accessory pathway
3. conduction time between the sinus and AV nodes

Since ventricular depolarization does not follow a normal conduction pathway, repolarization will be out of sequence. The extent of ST-segment and T-wave abnormalities occurring with altered ventricular repolarization depends on the source and degree of preexcitation.

Degrees of Preexcitation

There are four degrees of preexcitation:

1. *None.* The patient has a latent accessory pathway and the PR interval and QRS duration are normal. The anatomical source of the pathway is on the lateral side of the left ventricle. This pathway may become active with atrial fibrillation and is capable of antegrade conduction which can result in a life-threatening arrhythmia.
2. *Minimal*, where the size of the delta wave is very small and not seen in all leads.

3. *Less than maximum*, where the impulse arrives in the ventricle, first using the accessory pathway (short PR interval) and then using the AV node, causing a fusion beat. The resulting QRS may not have the classic delta wave, but may exhibit an abnormal Q wave, or distortion of the ascending arm of the R wave, or increased QRS voltage. In less than maximum preexcitation, it is difficult to differentiate between ventricular hypertrophy, bundle branch block, and acute myocardial infarction. Clinical presentation, serial ECG, and enzyme studies will facilitate diagnosis.
4. *Maximum preexcitation* is the term used when both ventricles are activated by the accessory pathway. There is almost no PR interval and the fusing of P to the QRS complex results in the widened QRS.

When preexcitation is suspected, the clinician must assess the PR interval and a delta wave in all leads. The PR may not be obviously shortened and a delta wave may not be visible in all leads taken simultaneously. A 12-lead ECG must be taken during the tachycardia episode and compared with the resting, or normal, ECG to rule out preexcitation. Figure 12-4 is a diagram with corresponding ECG tracings for the four degrees of preexcitation.

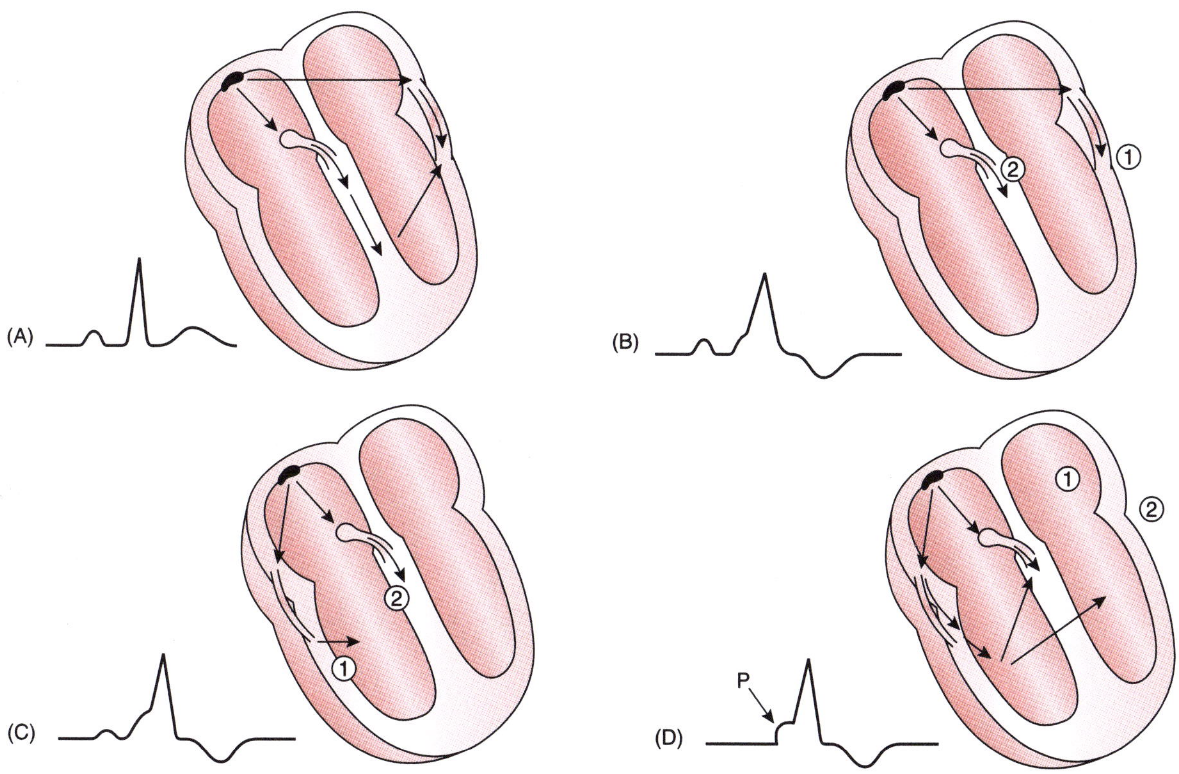

Figure 12-4 (A) Normal activation. QRS complex showing no visible delta wave, no visible change in the QRS to identify the presence of an accessory pathway. (B) Minimal activation. QRS complex showing (+) wave on the ascending arm of the QRS. (C) Less than maximal activation. QRS complex showing (+) delta wave in ascending arm of the QRS. Note the short PR interval. Diagram shows the fusion of normal and early forces arriving in the ventricle. The QRS will be a *fusion* of early and normal depolarizing forces. (D) Maximum activation using an accessory pathway. The PR interval is so minimal as to be nonexistent. The delta wave is obvious as it fuses into the ascending arm of the QRS. (Adapted from Conover, M.B. *Understanding Electrocardiography: Arrhythmias and the 12 lead ECG* (7th ed.). St. Louis, MO: Mosby-Year Book, Inc.; 1996.)

Concealed Accessory Pathway

When an accessory pathway conducts only in a retrograde direction it is *concealed*. This is because during sinus rhythm, conduction down the AV junction, through, to, and within the ventricles is normal. The PR interval and QRS duration are within normal limits and there is no delta wave.

ARRHYTHMIAS WITH PREEXCITATION

orthodromic

Reciprocating tachycardia that conducts down the normal AV conduction system, but reenters the atria through the accessory pathway.

Reciprocating tachycardia occurs when a premature atrial focus conducts down the normal AV conduction system, but uses the accessory pathway to reenter the atria. This is also called circus-movement or reentry tachycardia or **orthodromic** (narrow QRS) reciprocating tachycardia.

The P′ polarity may be (-) or (+) in lead I and may be seen after the QRS complex. There will be a short PR interval. *QRS alternans* may be seen. QRS alternans is the alteration of the amplitude of the R and S waves of the QRS complex. Figure 12-5 is an ECG tracing showing QRS alternans.

A PVC can cause a tachycardia by accessing the atria via the accessory pathway, then traveling down the AV node, His bundle, and into the ventricles. This will result in a narrow QRS tachycardia.

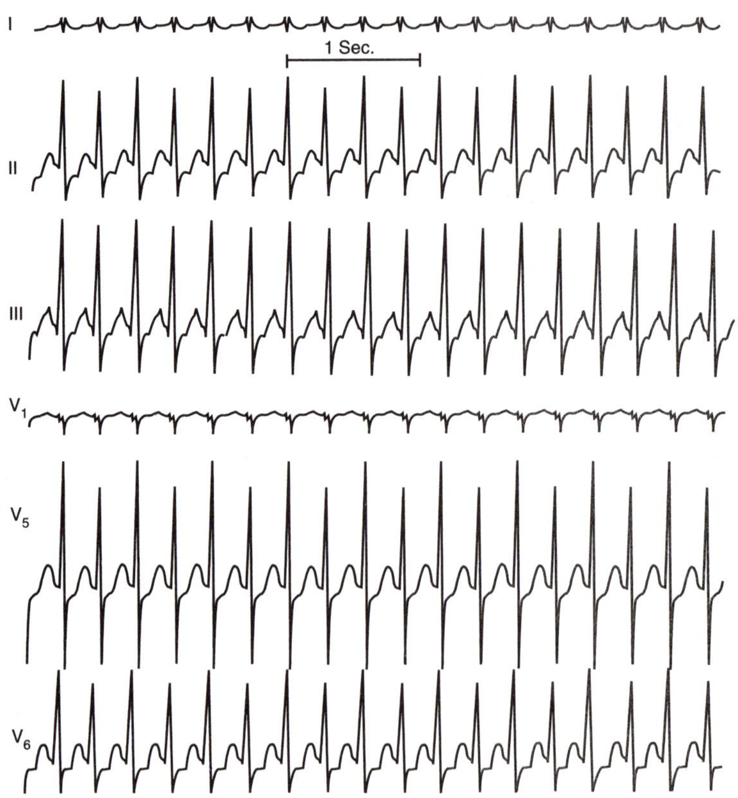

Figure 12-5 QRS alternans. Note the alternating amplitude of the QRS complex in several of the ECG leads in a patient with circus movement tachycardia. Alternans is not always visible in all the ECG leads. (Adapted from Conover, M.B. *Understanding Electrocardiography: Arrhythmias and the 12 lead ECG* (7th ed.). St. Louis, MO: Mosby-Year Book, Inc.; 1996.)

During sinus tachycardia, when a critical rate is reached, the accessory pathway is blocked in an antegrade fashion. The impulse may conduct normally, and reenter the atria using the accessory pathway in a retrograde fashion, thus establishing the reentry circuit.

Orthodromic tachycardia can occur using a slower conducting accessory pathway. The reentry circuit uses the AV node in an antegrade direction and a slower conducting accessory pathway in the retrograde direction. The slower conduction time from ventricle to atria over the slow accessory pathway will produce an RP interval that is long. In fact the P′ will be closer to the QRS that follows it rather than the one that precedes it. The rhythm appears as a junctional tachycardia but the ventricular rate is 130 to 200 per minute. Figure 12-6 is a 12-lead ECG tracing from a patient with orthodromic reciprocating tachycardia. The QRS complexes are narrow and delta waves are present in leads III, AVF, and V_2.

antidromic
Reentry tachycardia that uses the accessory pathway in an antegrade fashion and the AV node in a retrograde direction

Antidromic (wide QRS) tachycardia is a reentry tachycardia that uses the accessory pathway in an antegrade fashion and the AV node in a retrograde direction. The resulting QRS will be wide and the ventricular rhythm may be irregular because retrograde conduction though the ventricular pathways may differ. In some cases, a P′ because of the retrograde stimulation of the atria. This P′ may be seen after the QRS, but not in all leads, since the QRS is so broad. Figure 12-7 is a 12-lead ECG showing a patient with antidromic reciprocating tachycardia.

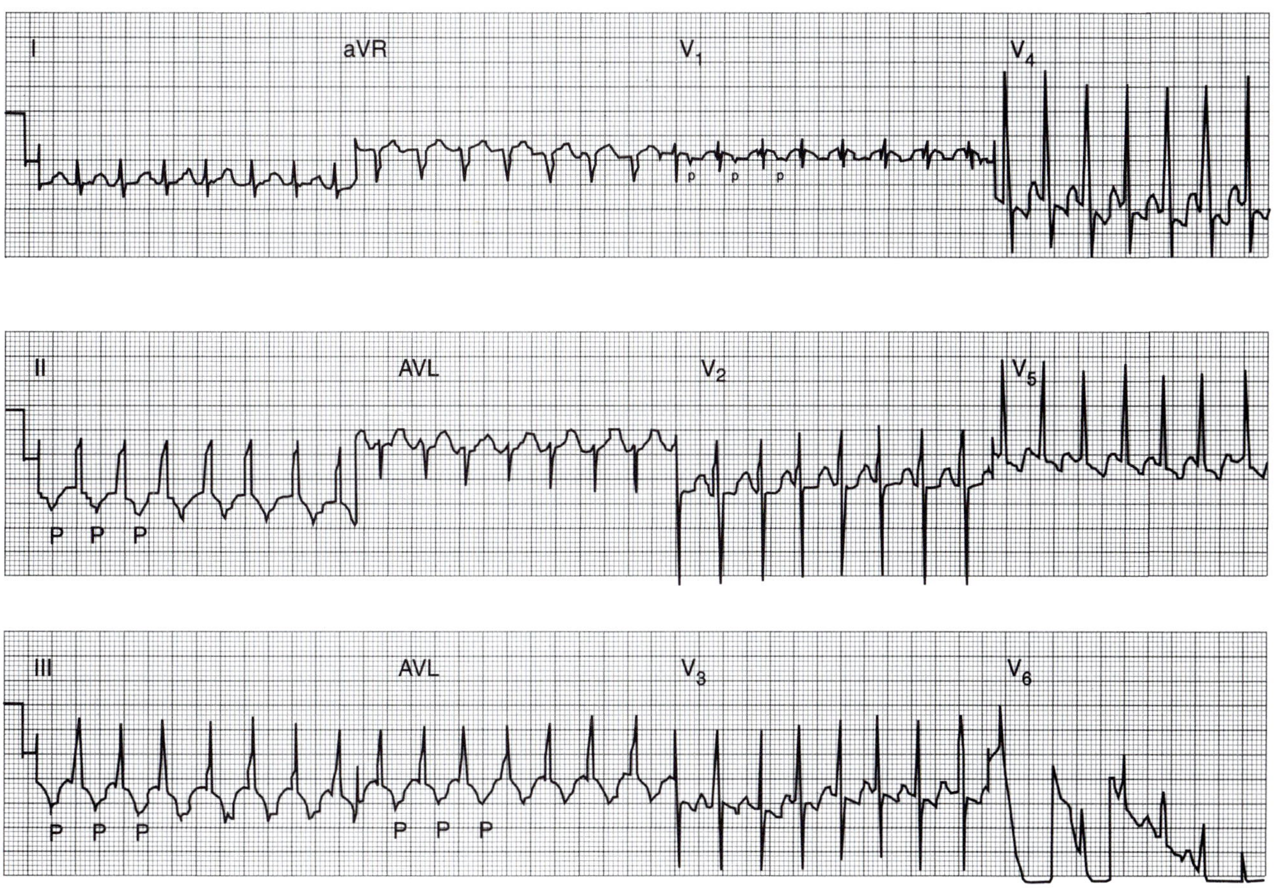

Figure 12-6 A 12-lead ECG from a patient with orthodromic reciprocating tachycardia. Note that the QRS complexes are narrow, PR intervals are short, and delta waves are present in leads III, AVF, and V_2.

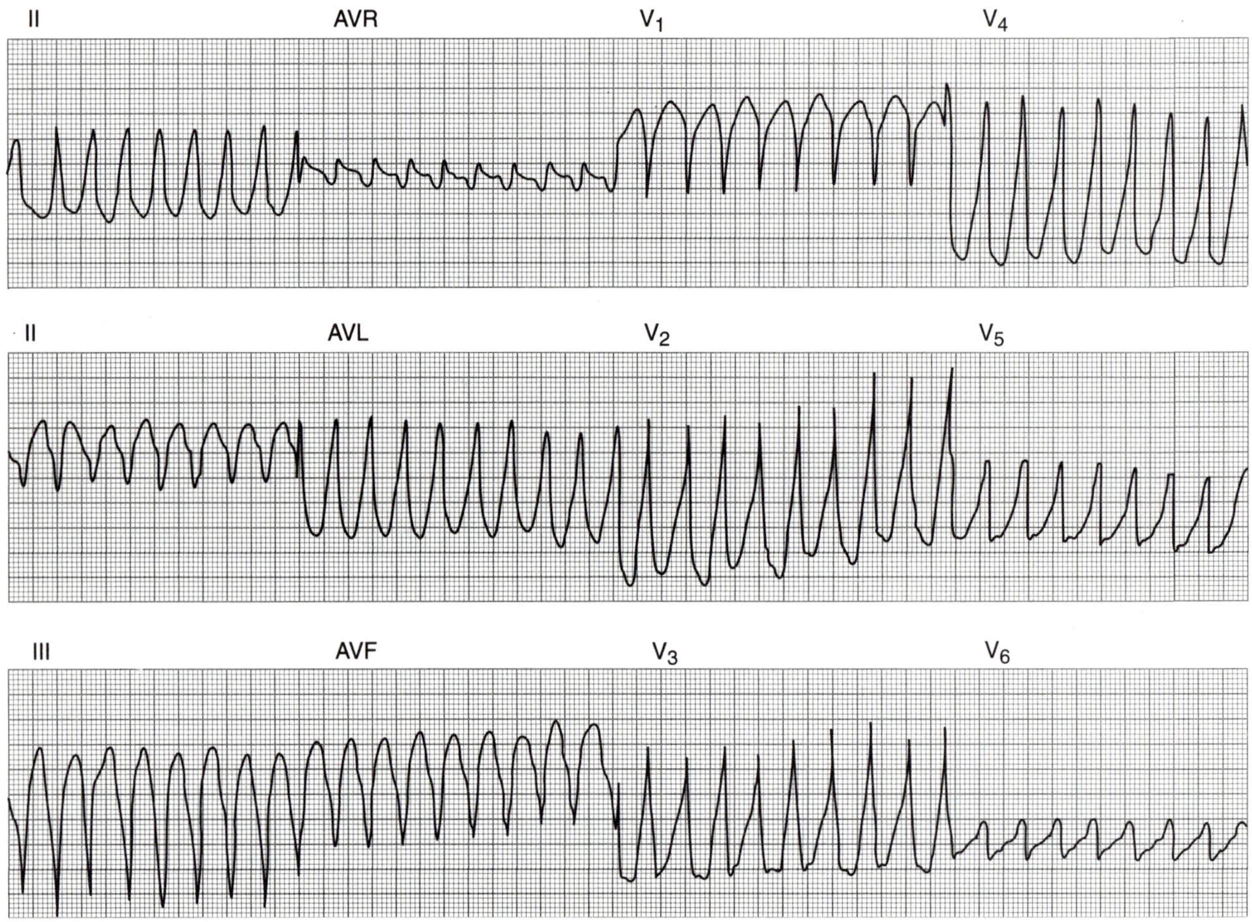

Figure 12-7 A 12-lead ECG showing a patient with antidromic reciprocating tachycardia. Note the broad QRS with opposite T-wave polarity, similar to ventricular tachycardia. Note the delta waves on the ascending and descending arms of the QRS which, in fact, have broadened the QRS complex. Concordant negativity is not present in the precordial leads; a differential for a tachycardia that is supraventricular in origin.

Tachycardia can be caused by the use of two APs. There can be antegrade conduction down one accessory pathway and retrograde conduction using another accessory pathway. In this instance, the QRS will be wide and very difficult to differentiate from ventricular tachycardia.

Atrial fibrillation conducts to the ventricles over an accessory pathway in an antegrade fashion. This result is a ventricular rate sometimes greater than 200 per minute, but with irregularity that is characteristic of the atrial fibrillation. Conduction through a rapidly conducting accessory pathway can result in an irregular ventricular rate that rapidly deteriorates into ventricular fibrillation. Figure 12-8 is a lead II ECG tracing from a patient with diagnosed digitalis toxicity. The ECG is showing atrial fibrillation using an accessory pathway.

Lown-Ganong-Levine (LGL) syndrome

A combination of a short PR interval, normal QRS configuration, and recurrent supraventricular tachycardias. With this condition, the intranodal fibers bypass the crest of the AV node and one of the intranodal fibers terminates near the bundle of His.

LOWN-GANONG-LEVINE SYNDROME

The Lown-Ganong-Levine (LGL) syndrome also known as intranodal bypass tract syndrome was initially described as a combination of a short PR interval, normal QRS configuration, and recurrent supraventricular tachycardias. It was subsequently shown that in patients who exhibit LGL, intranodal fibers bypass the crest of the AV

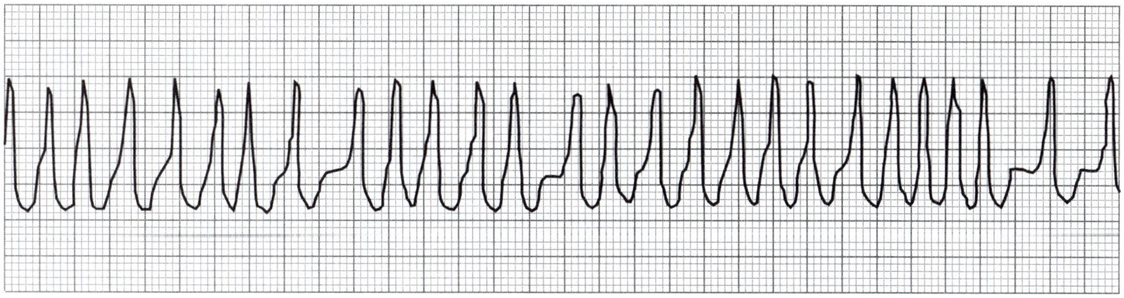

Figure 12-8 A lead II ECG tracing from a patient with diagnosed digitalis toxicity and showing atrial fibrillation using an accessory pathway. Note the broad QRS which, with close inspection, is actually the (+) delta wave on the ascending arm of the QRS, giving the appearance of the broad QRS in ventricular tachycardia. In this tracing, note the irregular ventricular rhythm and very rapid rate.

node and one of the intranodal fibers terminates near the bundle of His (**James fibers**). The major conduction delay in the AV node is circumvented and a short PR interval is recorded of less than 0.12 second. Ventricular depolarization will take place via the normal His-Purkinje system, generating a normal QRS complex. Figure 12-9 illustrates a 12-lead tracing showing the ECG characteristics associated with LGL syndrome.

James fibers
An accessory pathway that connects atrial fibers to the upper part of the AV node. Also referred to as an infranodal bypass tract.

Many patients will be encountered whose ECG displays a short PR interval and a normal QRS complex, but who have no clinical history of tachycardia. Such tracings probably indicate bypass of the AV node by an intranodal fiber, and should be interpreted as consistent with, but not diagnostic of, the Lown-Ganong-Levine presentation.

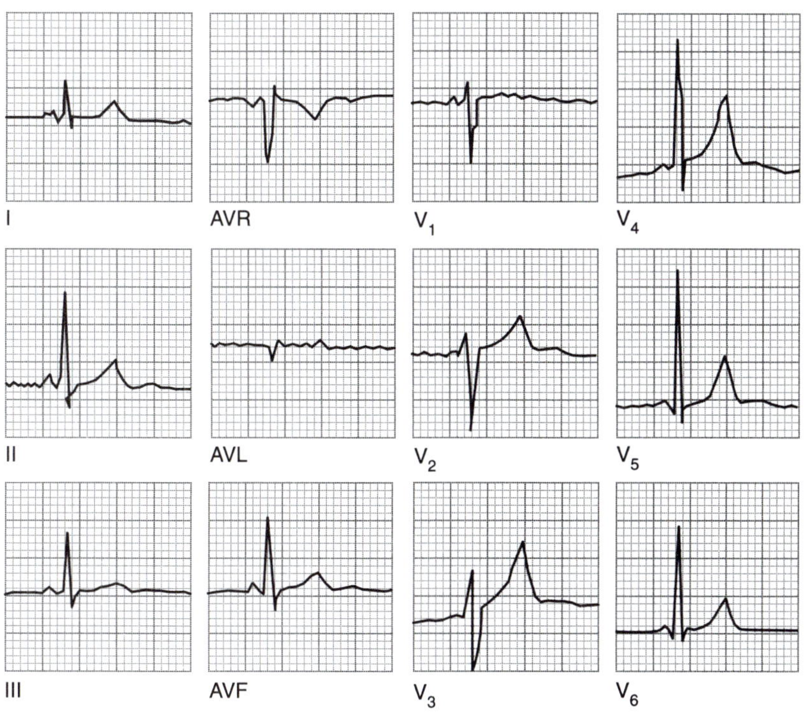

Figure 12-9 A 12-lead ECG showing a short PR interval and narrow QRS complex in a patient with confirmed Lown-Ganong-Levine syndrome.

In summary the three criteria for diagnosis of the Lown-Ganong-Levine syndrome are:

1. short PR interval (0.12 second or less)
2. normal QRS configuration
3. recurrent paroxysmal tachycardia

WOLFF-PARKINSON-WHITE (WPW) SYNDROME

Wolff-Parkinson-White (WPW) syndrome

Ventricular preexcitation by way of an alternate pathway bypassing the AV node. ECG shows a shortened PR interval (less than 0.10 second), slurred upstroke of the QRS complex, and a widened QRS complex.

Wolff-Parkinson-White (WPW) syndrome is a syndrome of preexcitation that occurs using accessory AV pathways (Kent bundles) with tachycardia. WPW occurring without tachycardia is WPW pattern. WPW can occur in healthy hearts. The anatomical presence of the accessory pathway may manifest itself later in life, or with myocardial infarction, or atrial fibrillation.

In WPW, as atrial tissue is depolarized and forms the P wave on the ECG, the depolarizing wave front arrives simultaneously at the crest of the AV node and at the atrial end of the accessory pathway. Conduction through the AV node is normally delayed, but the accessory pathway is capable of very rapid depolarization. Thus, ventricular tissue is depolarized before the AV node has permitted normal conduction to continue through the His bundle.

If all ventricular tissue is depolarized by the impulse using the accessory pathway, the resulting QRS would be different from the sinus-induced QRS. The resulting widened QRS complexes can be confused with bundle branch block or PVCs.

However, as the wave of depolarization slowly spreads out from the prematurely depolarized ventricle, conduction is completed through the AV junction and spreads quickly through the His-Purkinje system.

The result of all of this is a composite of both initial, premature ventricular depolarization (accessory pathway) and later activation of the remaining myocardium using the normal conduction system. The initial aberrant activation generates a slurring of the QRS called the delta wave, explained earlier in this chapter.

The changes that occur with myocardial infarction, bundle branch block, and ventricular hypertrophy will be masked by the WPW pattern. Confident diagnosis of the existence of an accessory pathway must be made by eletrophysiologic testing. Any other conclusion about the electrical conduction system, by simply assessing the QRS, must be discouraged.

The major clinical manifestation of WPW is the recurrent tachycardia. As with LGL syndrome, the accessory pathway supports the circulating, reentrant wave of depolarization. However, unlike LGL, the resulting QRS may be normal or widened depending on the direction of the reentrant wave front.

If the AV node is activated in an antegrade fashion, and the bundle of Kent is activated in a retrograde fashion, the QRS complex will be narrow. However if the bundle of Kent is depolarized in an antegrade fashion, with retrograde depolarization of the AV node, a wide bizarre QRS complex will be recorded. This may mimic ventricular tachycardia.

In summary, the ECG characteristics of a WPW pattern are:

1. short PR interval (0.12 second or less)
2. wide QRS complex

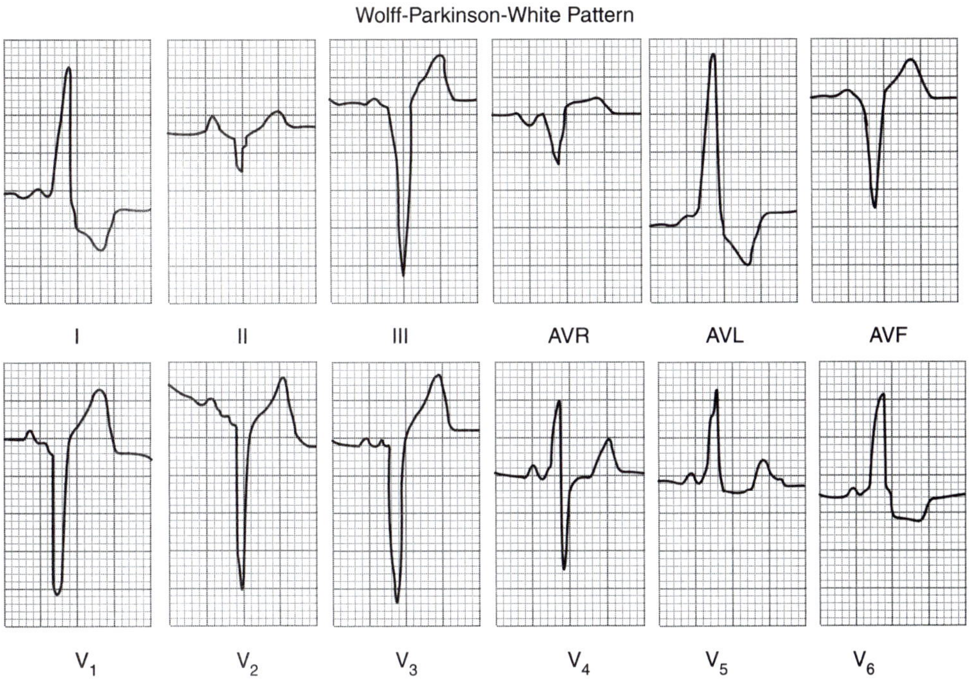

Figure 12-10 A 12-lead ECG showing classic patterns of early activation. Note the short PR interval and the broad QRS complexes. There are (+) delta waves in leads I, AVL, V_4, V_5, and V_6. There are (-) delta waves in all the other leads.

3. delta wave
4. tachycardias with normal QRS
5. tachycardias with wide QRS
6. normal conduction pattern in which the bundle of Kent is not activated and normal pathways of depolarization are followed.

Figure 12-10 is a 12-lead ECG showing classic patterns of early activation.

Patients who persist with complaints for paroxysms of tachycardia should be clinically assessed for the possibility of active AP. Surgery or transvenous radio frequency ablation may be considered in patients who are becoming intolerant of the arrhythmias or have a predilection toward atrial fibrillation. Table 12-1 is the summary of ECG wave forms and characterictics in early excitation using accessory AV bundle, intra-AV nodal bypass tract, and nodofascicular connection.

Summary

Early activation of the ventricular conduction system outside the normal pathways often results in tachycardias that are confused with ventricular tachycardia. The sudden occurance of QRS complexes that are different from the patient's normally occurring QRS complexes is highly suspicious of ventricular tachycardia. However, the ECG tracing must be scrupulously examined for abnormalities in the PR interval and QRS complex for signs of the existence of an accessory path-

Table 12-1 ECG wave forms and characteristics

	Accessory AV Bundle	Intranodal Bypass Tract	Nodofascicular Connection
PR interval	<0.12 second	<0.12 second	normal
QRS duration	>0.11 second	normal*	>0.11 second
Secondary ST-T abnormalities	present	absent	present
Delta waves	present	absent	present
Can mimic myocardial infarction	yes	no*	yes
Can mimic ventricular hypertrophy	yes	no*	yes

*must rule out prior pathology in the bundle branch system

way. For example, the delta wave present when the accessory pathway is active may only be visible during the tachycardia. In contrast, a patient may exhibit delta waves during bradycardia but not during tachycardia.

The frequent occurrence of tachycardia without any overt cardiac disease may be the first sign of the activation of an accessory pathway. Sometimes unexplained tachycardia is the only reported sign heralding pathology in the conduction system. It is important to identify the source of any tachycardia. Conduct diligent and meticulous observation of ECG measurement to ascertain the short PR, delta waves, or other ECG signs of early excitation.

Finally, the ECG in this case can be a valuable tool to be used in conjunction with the available clinical history, and as an evaluation using advanced techniques assessing the electrophysiology of these pathways.

Self-Assessment Exercises

ECG Rhythm Identification Practice

Identify the ECG criterion listed below each 12-lead ECG and check your answers with those in the back of the book.

Figure 12-11

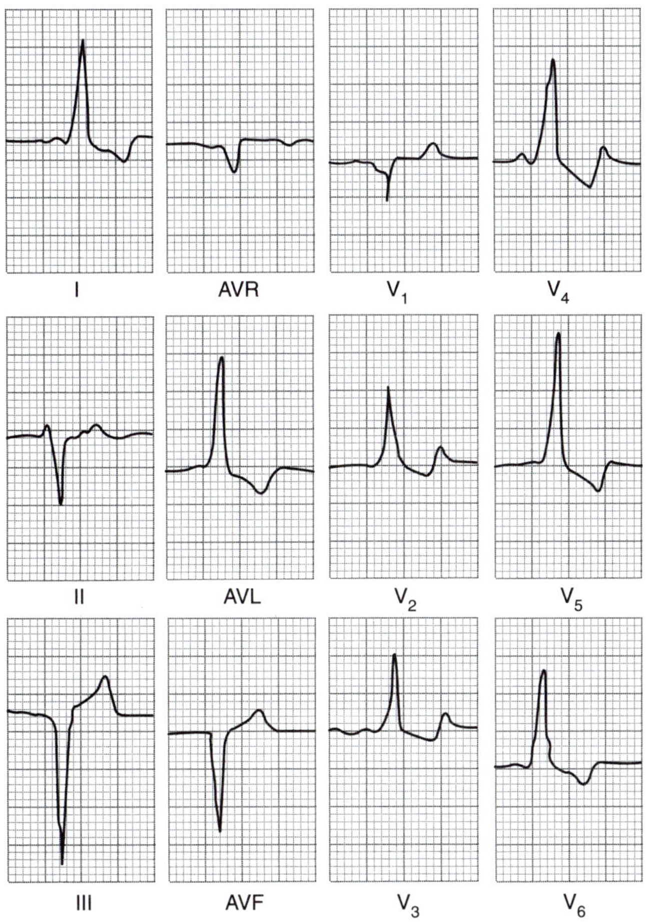

1. What is the underlying rhythm? __________
2. What are the abnormalities? __________

   PRI __________

   QRS __________
3. What is the interpretation? __________

Figure 12-12

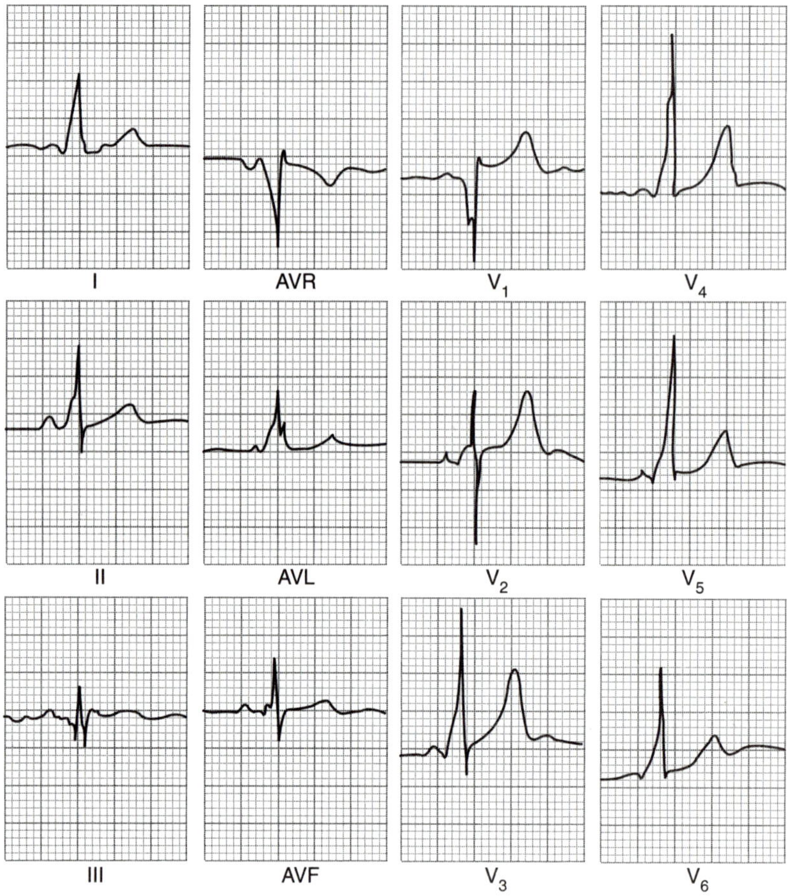

1. What is the underlying rhythm? __________
2. What are the abnormalities? __________

   PRI __________

   QRS __________
3. What is the interpretation? __________

Figure 12-13

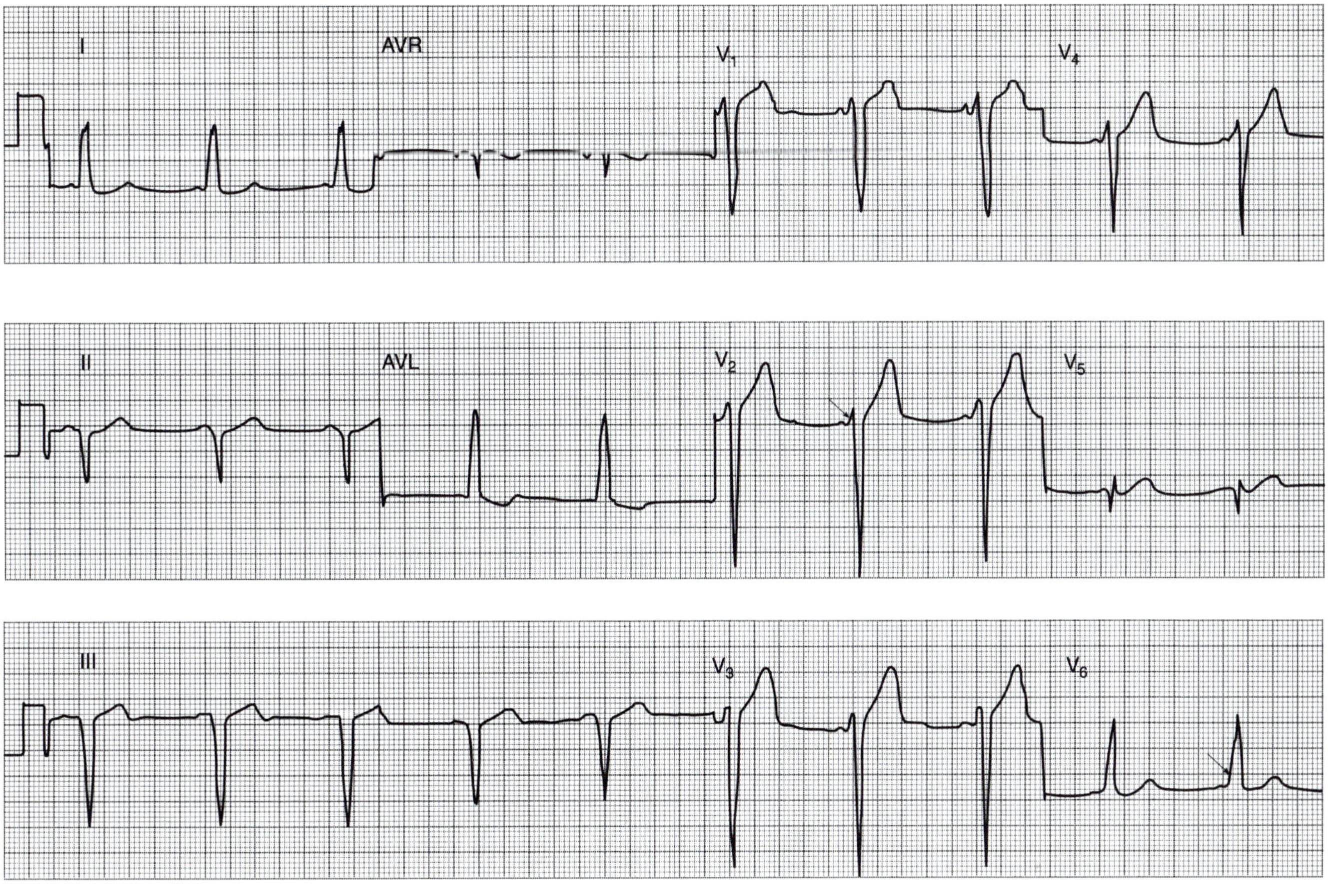

1. What is the underlying rhythm? ______
2. What are the abnormalities? ______
   PRI ______
   QRS ______
3. What is the interpretation? ______

REFERENCES

Conover, M. B. *Understanding electrocardiography: Arrhythmias and the 12-lead ECG* (7th ed.). St. Louis, MO: Mosby-Year Book; 1996.

Conover, M. B. & Wellens, H. J. *The ECG in emergency decision making*. Philadelphia: W. B. Saunders; 1993.

Feola, M., Ribichini, F., Gallone, G., et. al. Analysis of right electrocardiographic leads in 195 normal subjects. *Giorn Ital Clariol*, 24; 376-389; 1994.

Goldberger, E. *Textbook of clinical cardiology*. St. Louis, MO: C. V. Mosby; 1982.

GUSTO, ISIS-4. Collaborative Group, *Lancet* 3, 4, 5, (8591):669.3/18/95.

Langer, A., et. al. Journal of American College of Cardiology, 27(6); 1327. 1996.

Marriott, H. J. *Practical electrocardiography* (8th ed.). Baltimore: Williams and Wilkins; 1988.

Marriott, H. J., & Conover, M. B. *Advanced concepts in arrhythmias* (2nd ed.). St. Louis, MO: C. V. Mosby; 1989.

CHAPTER 13

General Review and Assessment Exercises

ECG Rhythm Identification Practice

For the following ECG tracings, fill in the blanks and then check your answers against those in the back of the book.

Figure 13-1

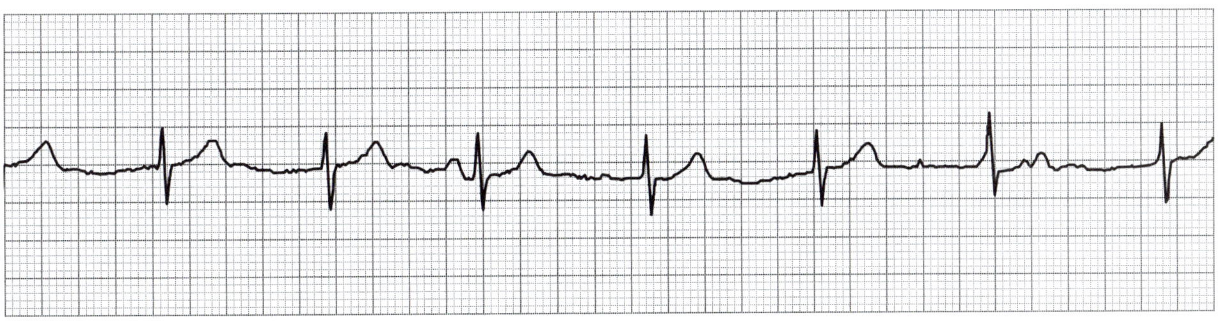

QRS duration ______________ QT ____________

Ventricular rate/rhythm ______________________

Atrial rate/rhythm ________________________

PR interval ____________________________

Identification ______________________________

Symptoms _________________________________

____

Treatment _________________________________

Figure 13-2

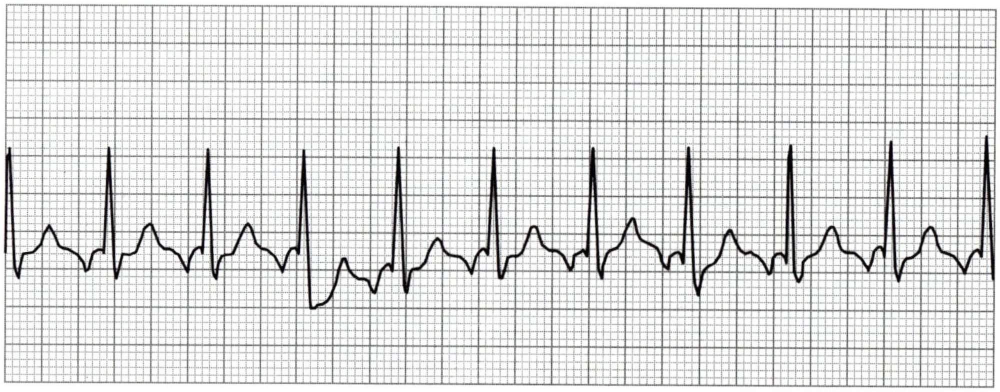

QRS duration ______________ QT ____________
Ventricular rate/rhythm ______________________
Atrial rate/rhythm __________________________
PR interval ______________________________

Identification ______________________________
Symptoms __________________________________
____
Treatment _________________________________

Figure 13-3

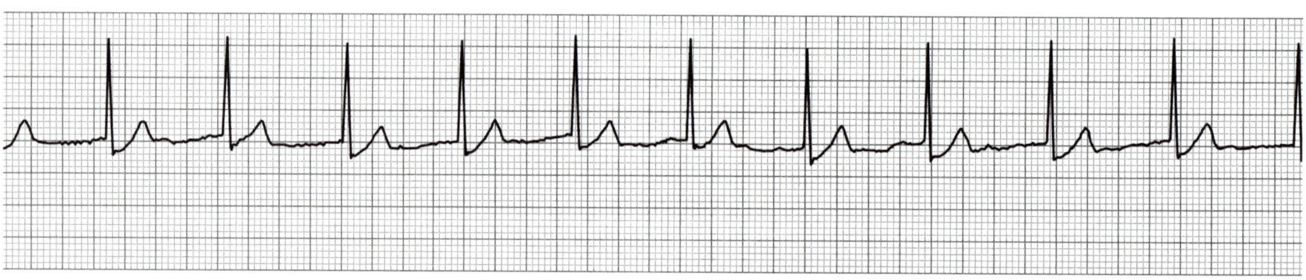

QRS duration ______________ QT ____________
Ventricular rate/rhythm ______________________
Atrial rate/rhythm __________________________
PR interval ______________________________

Identification ______________________________
Symptoms __________________________________
____
Treatment _________________________________

Figure 13-4

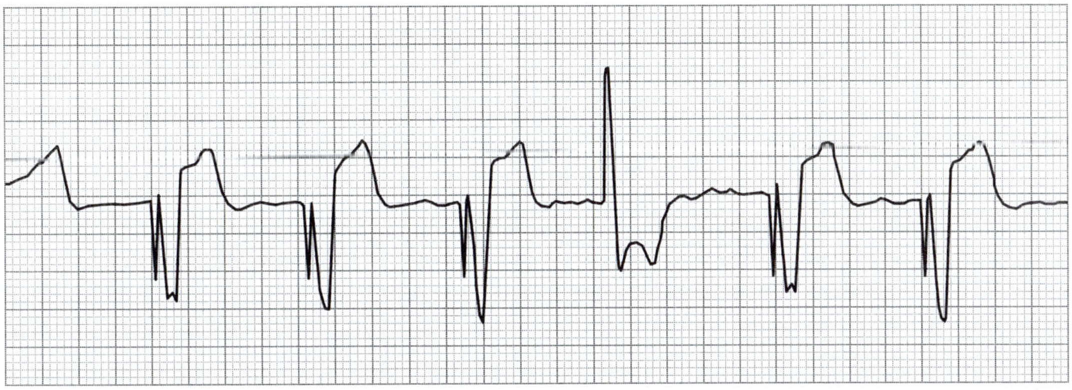

QRS duration ______________ QT ____________

Ventricular rate/rhythm ______________________

Atrial rate/rhythm __________________________

PR interval _________________________________

Identification ______________________________

Symptoms ___________________________________

____

Treatment __________________________________

Figure 13-5

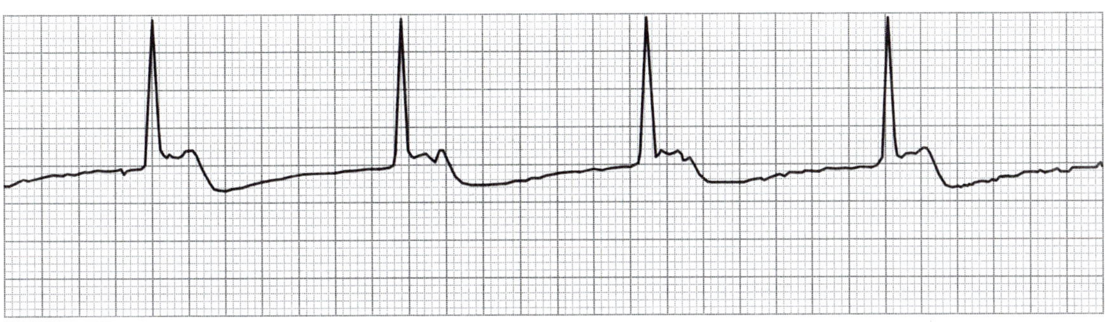

QRS duration ______________ QT ____________

Ventricular rate/rhythm ______________________

Atrial rate/rhythm __________________________

PR interval _________________________________

Identification ______________________________

Symptoms ___________________________________

____

Treatment __________________________________

Figure 13-6

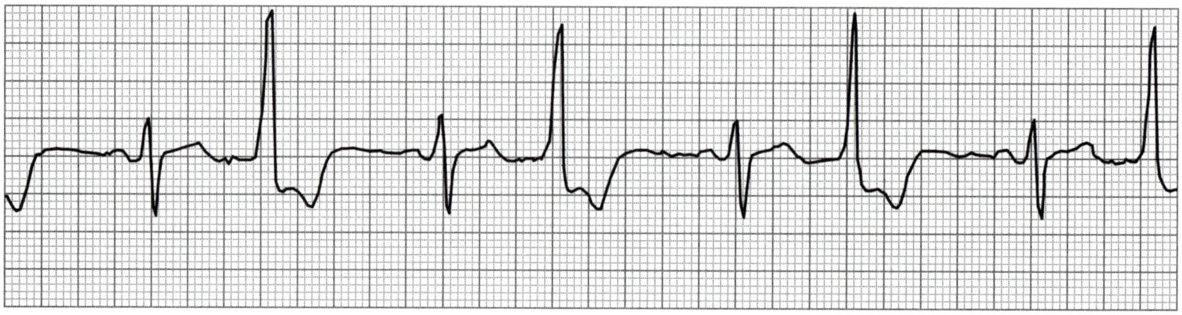

QRS duration ________________ QT ____________

Ventricular rate/rhythm ________________________

Atrial rate/rhythm ____________________________

PR interval __________________________________

Identification ________________________________

Symptoms ____________________________________

____

Treatment ____________________________________

Figure 13-7

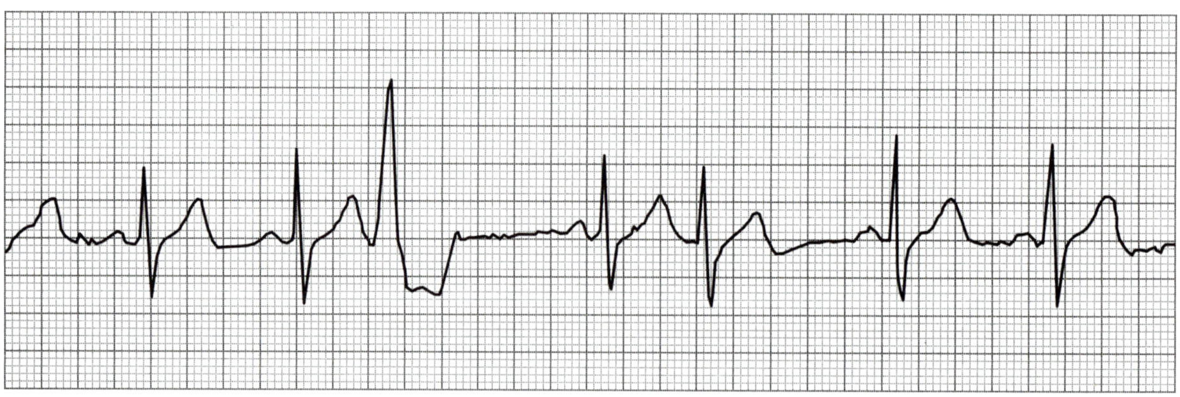

QRS duration ________________ QT ____________

Ventricular rate/rhythm ________________________

Atrial rate/rhythm ____________________________

PR interval __________________________________

Identification ________________________________

Symptoms ____________________________________

____

Treatment ____________________________________

Figure 13-8

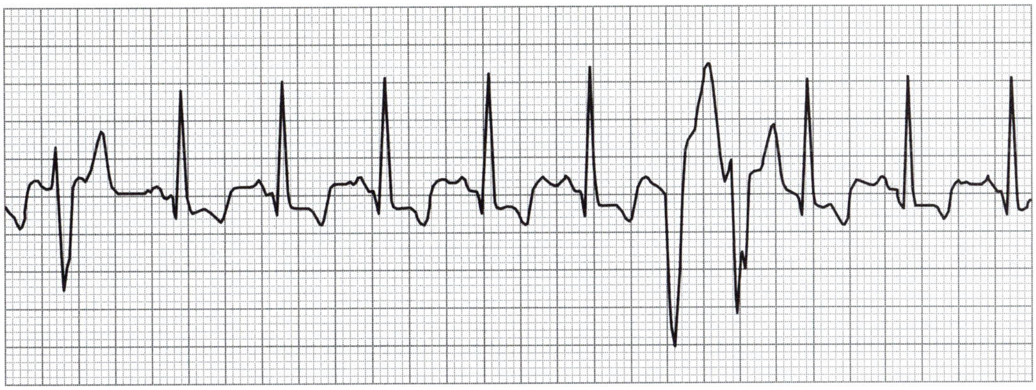

QRS duration ______ QT ______
Ventricular rate/rhythm ______
Atrial rate/rhythm ______
PR interval ______
Identification ______
Symptoms ______
______
Treatment ______

Figure 13-9

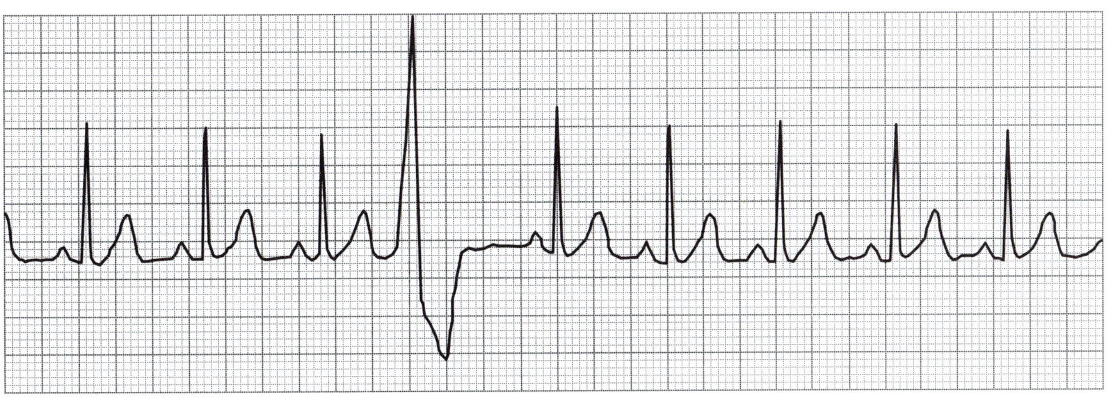

QRS duration ______ QT ______
Ventricular rate/rhythm ______
Atrial rate/rhythm ______
PR interval ______
Identification ______
Symptoms ______
______
Treatment ______

Figure 13-10

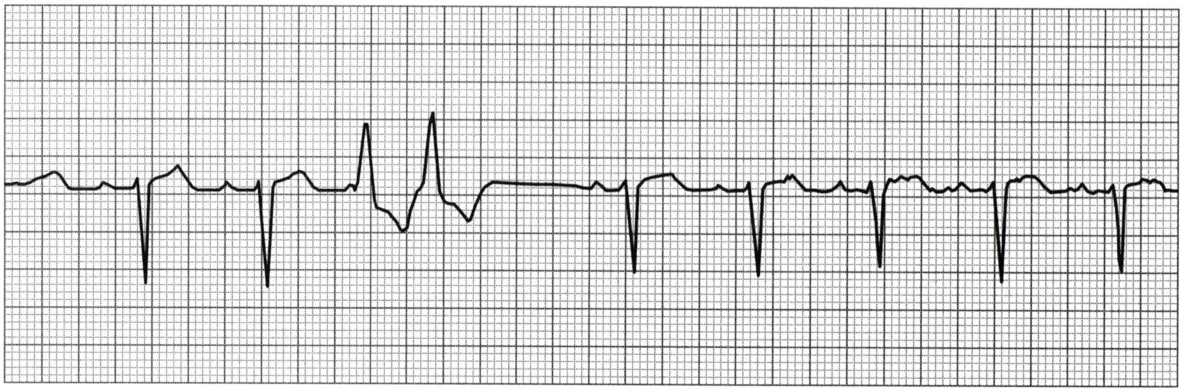

QRS duration ________________ QT ______________

Ventricular rate/rhythm __________________________

Atrial rate/rhythm ______________________________

PR interval ___________________________________

Identification _________________________________

Symptoms ____________________________________

____

Treatment ____________________________________

Figure 13-11

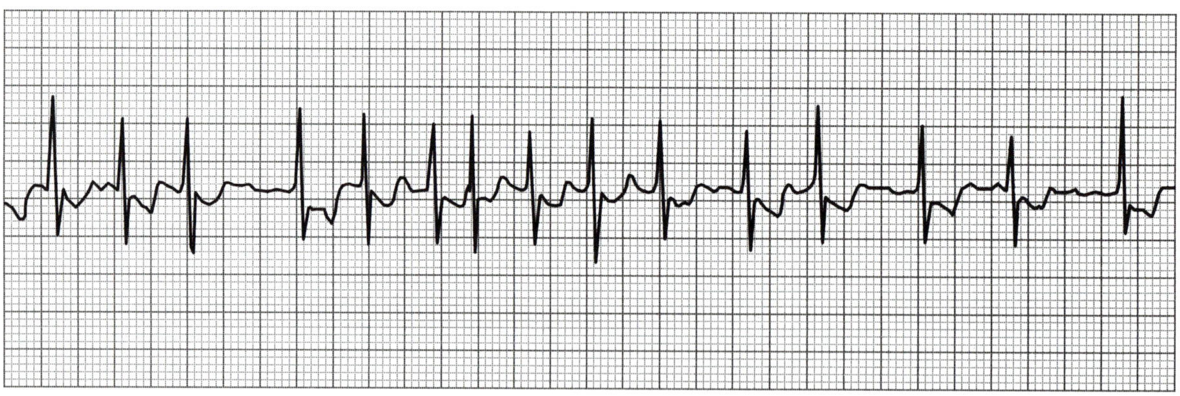

QRS duration ________________ QT ______________

Ventricular rate/rhythm __________________________

Atrial rate/rhythm ______________________________

PR interval ___________________________________

Identification _________________________________

Symptoms ____________________________________

____

Treatment ____________________________________

Figure 13-12

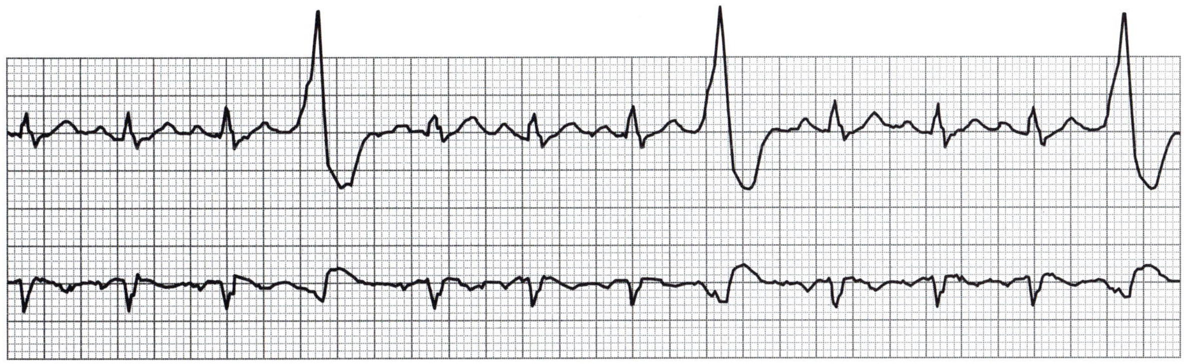

QRS duration ________________ QT ______________

Ventricular rate/rhythm ________________________

Atrial rate/rhythm ____________________________

PR interval __________________________________

Identification __________________________________

Symptoms ______________________________________

____

Treatment ______________________________________

Figure 13-13

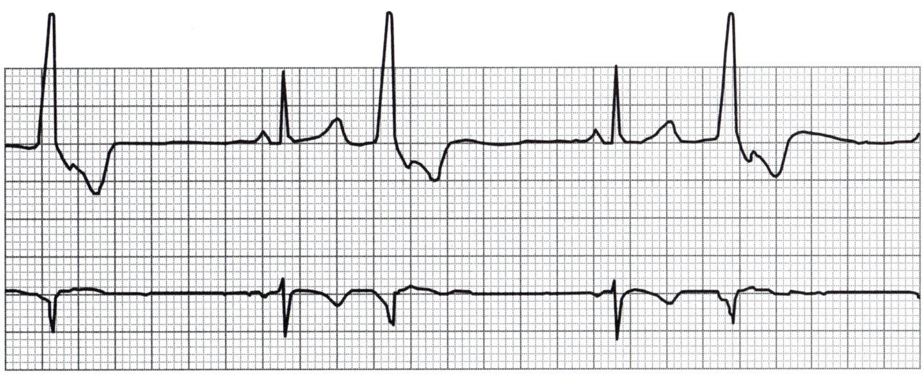

QRS duration ________________ QT ______________

Ventricular rate/rhythm ________________________

Atrial rate/rhythm ____________________________

PR interval __________________________________

Identification __________________________________

Symptoms ______________________________________

____

Treatment ______________________________________

Figure 13-14

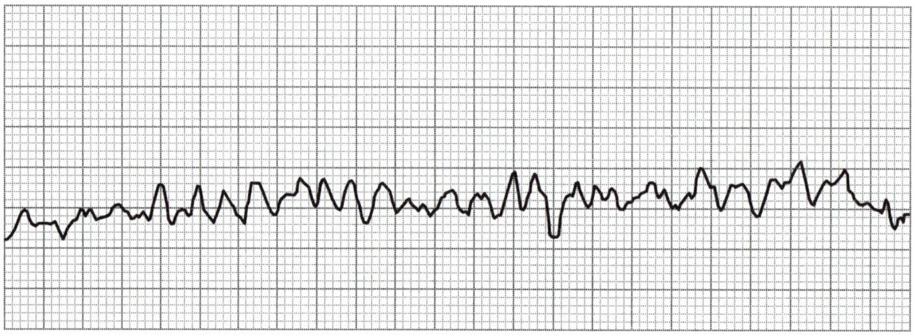

QRS duration ______________ QT ____________

Ventricular rate/rhythm ______________________

Atrial rate/rhythm ___________________________

PR interval _________________________________

Identification ______________________________

Symptoms ___________________________________

____

Treatment __________________________________

Figure 13-15

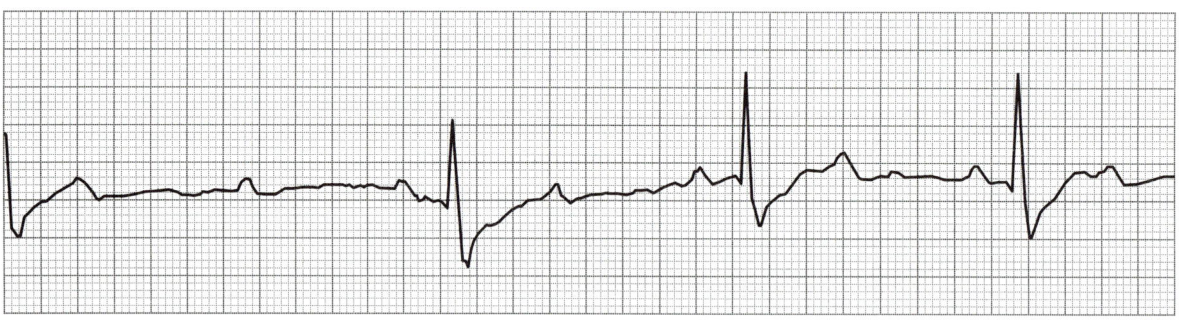

QRS duration ______________ QT ____________

Ventricular rate/rhythm ______________________

Atrial rate/rhythm ___________________________

PR interval _________________________________

Identification ______________________________

Symptoms ___________________________________

____

Treatment __________________________________

Figure 13-16

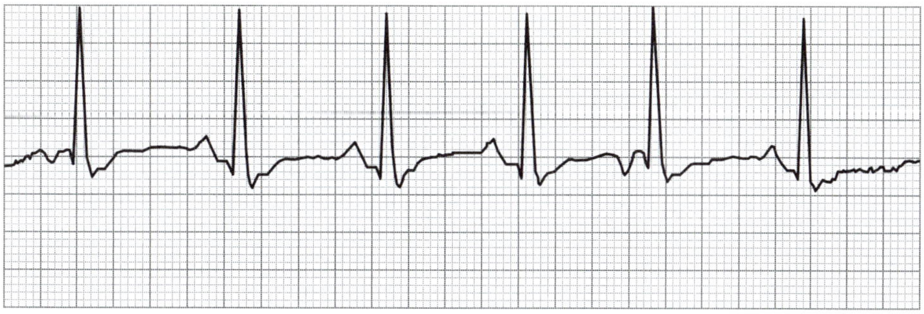

QRS duration ______________ QT ____________

Ventricular rate/rhythm ______________________

Atrial rate/rhythm ________________________

PR interval ____________________________

Identification ____________________________

Symptoms ______________________________

____

Treatment ______________________________

Figure 13-17

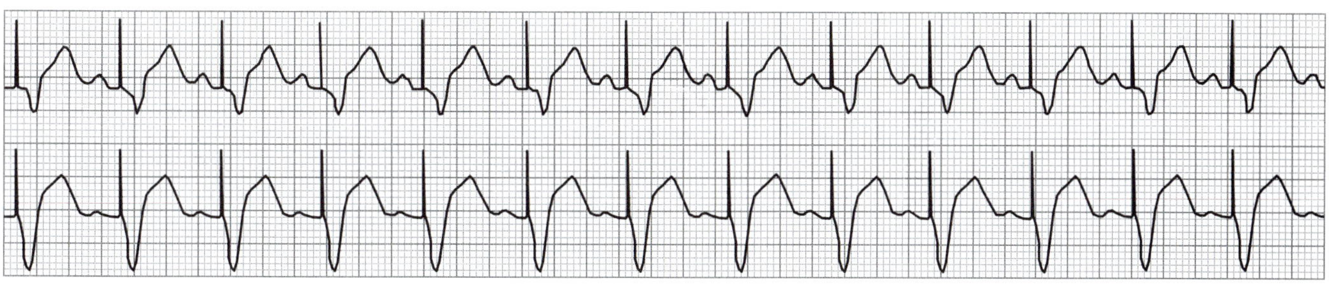

QRS duration ______________ QT ____________

Ventricular rate/rhythm ______________________

Atrial rate/rhythm ________________________

PR interval ____________________________

Identification ____________________________

Symptoms ______________________________

____

Treatment ______________________________

Figure 13-18

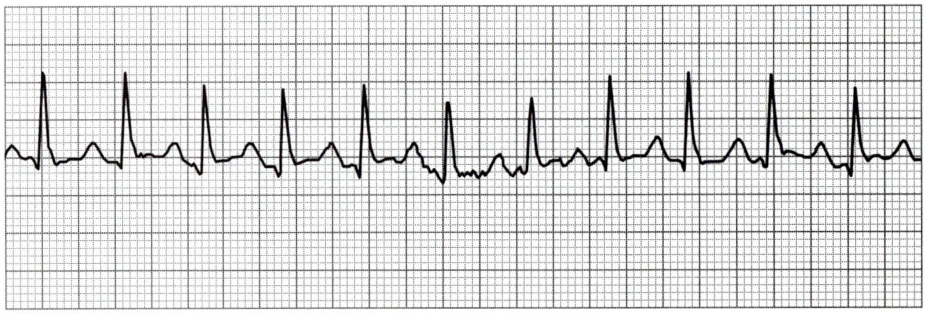

QRS duration ______________ QT ____________

Ventricular rate/rhythm ____________________

Atrial rate/rhythm ______________________

PR interval ___________________________

Identification ___________________________

Symptoms ______________________________

____

Treatment ______________________________

Figure 13-19

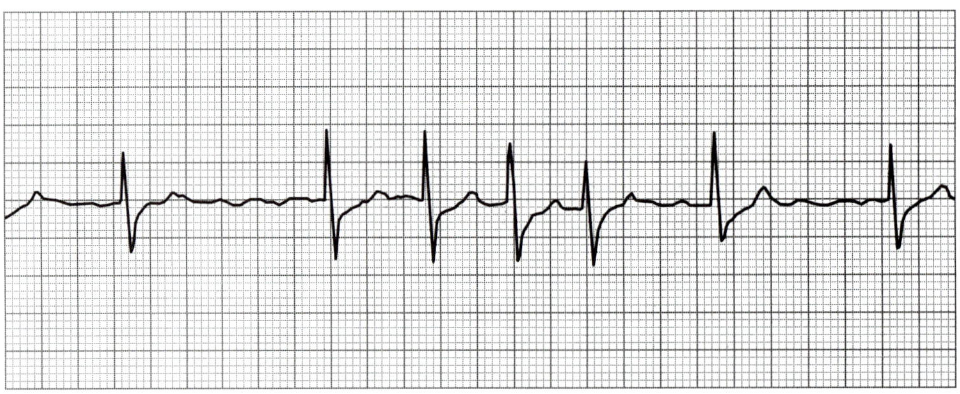

QRS duration ______________ QT ____________

Ventricular rate/rhythm ____________________

Atrial rate/rhythm ______________________

PR interval ___________________________

Identification ___________________________

Symptoms ______________________________

____

Treatment ______________________________

Figure 13-20

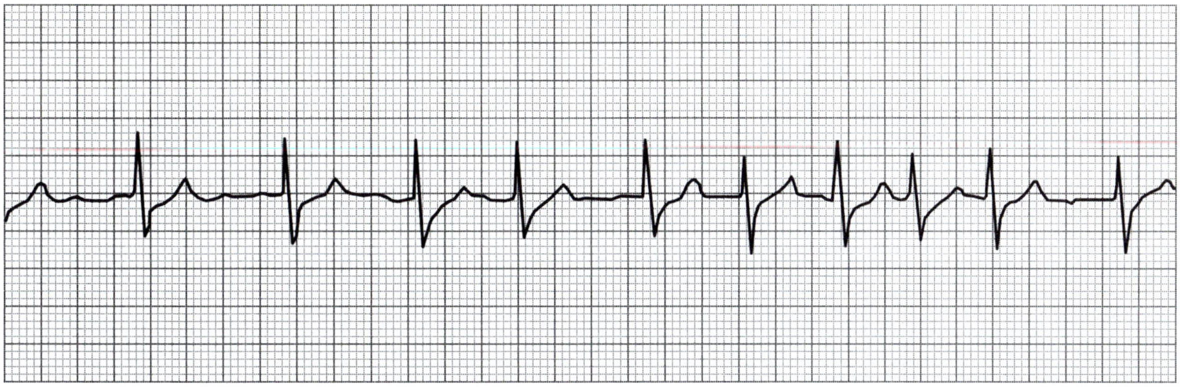

QRS duration ________________ QT _____________

Ventricular rate/rhythm _________________________

Atrial rate/rhythm ______________________________

PR interval ____________________________________

Identification ______________________________________

Symptoms ____

____

Treatment ____

Figure 13-21

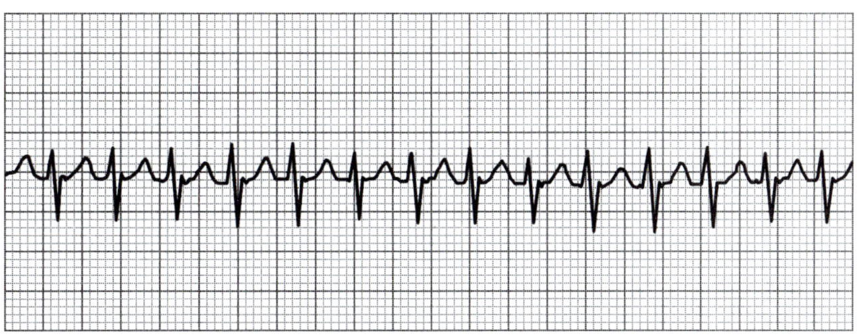

QRS duration ________________ QT _____________

Ventricular rate/rhythm _________________________

Atrial rate/rhythm ______________________________

PR interval ____________________________________

Identification ______________________________________

Symptoms ____

____

Treatment ____

Figure 13-22

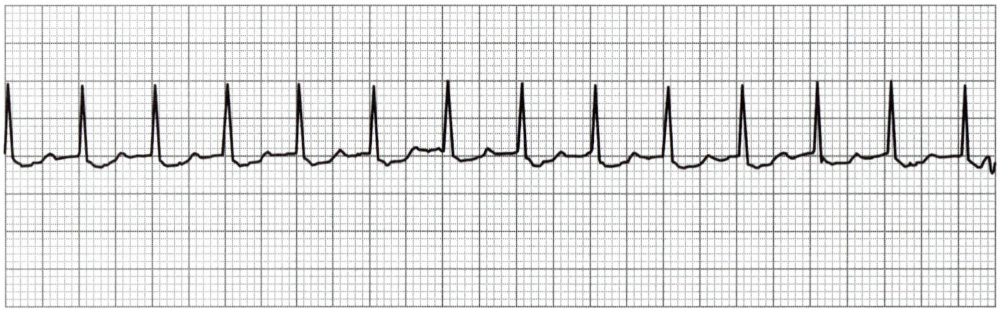

QRS duration ________________ QT ______________

Ventricular rate/rhythm ________________________

Atrial rate/rhythm ____________________________

PR interval ________________________________

Identification ________________________________

Symptoms ___________________________________

____

Treatment __________________________________

Figure 13-23

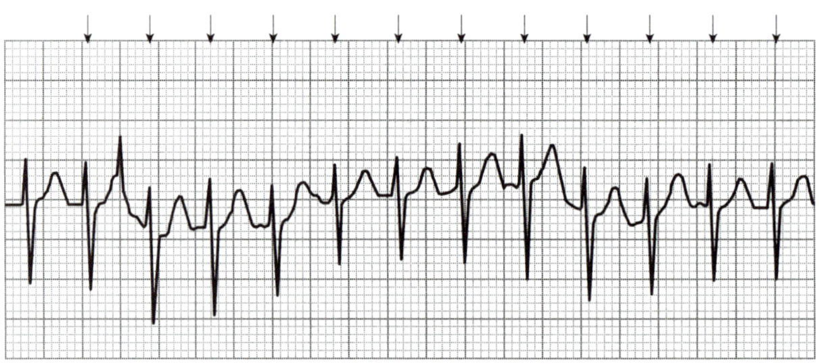

QRS duration ________________ QT ______________

Ventricular rate/rhythm ________________________

Atrial rate/rhythm ____________________________

PR interval ________________________________

Identification ________________________________

Symptoms ___________________________________

____

Treatment __________________________________

Figure 13-24

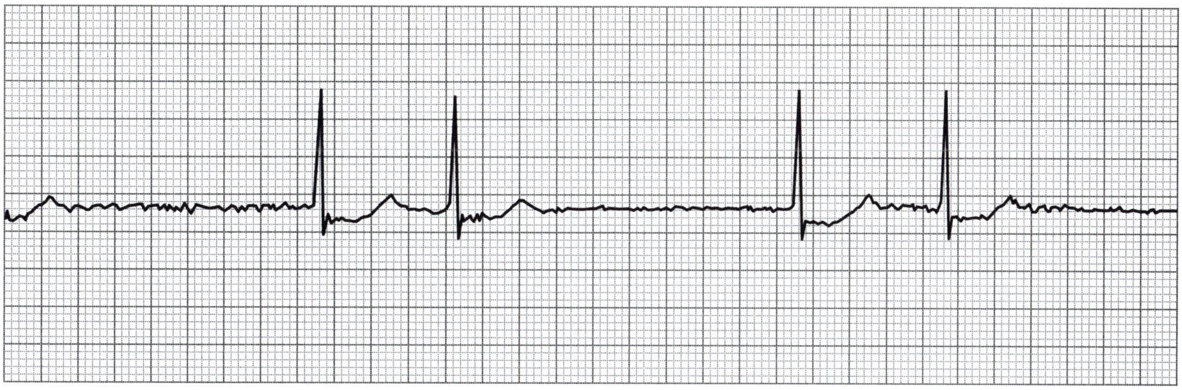

QRS duration ________________ QT ____________

Ventricular rate/rhythm ______________________

Atrial rate/rhythm __________________________

PR interval ________________________________

Identification ______________________________

Symptoms __________________________________

____

Treatment _________________________________

Figure 13-25

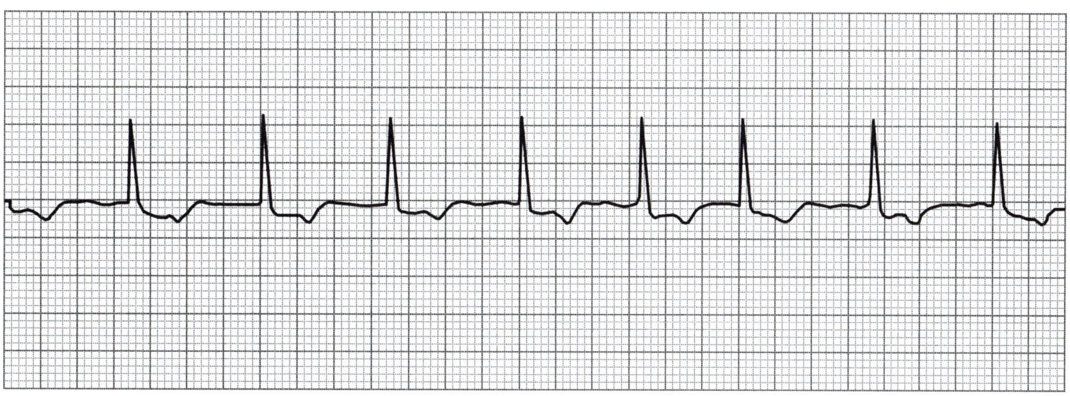

QRS duration ________________ QT ____________

Ventricular rate/rhythm ______________________

Atrial rate/rhythm __________________________

PR interval ________________________________

Identification ______________________________

Symptoms __________________________________

____

Treatment _________________________________

Figure 13-26

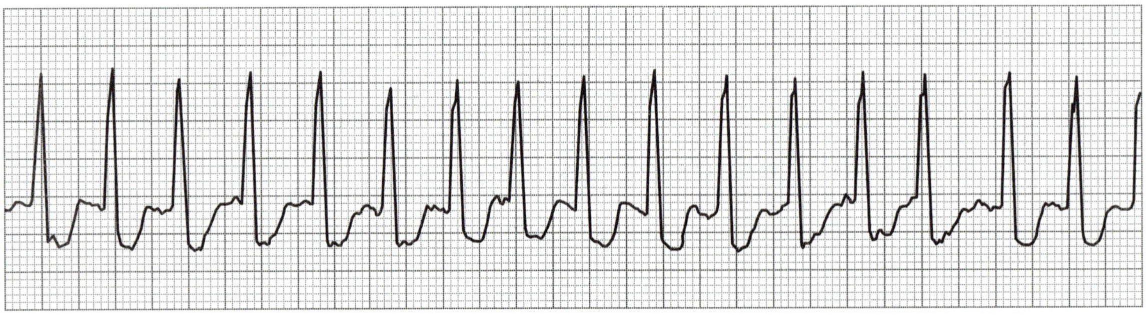

QRS duration ______________ QT ____________

Ventricular rate/rhythm ______________________

Atrial rate/rhythm ______________________

PR interval ______________________

Identification ______________________

Symptoms ______________________

____

Treatment ______________________

Figure 13-27

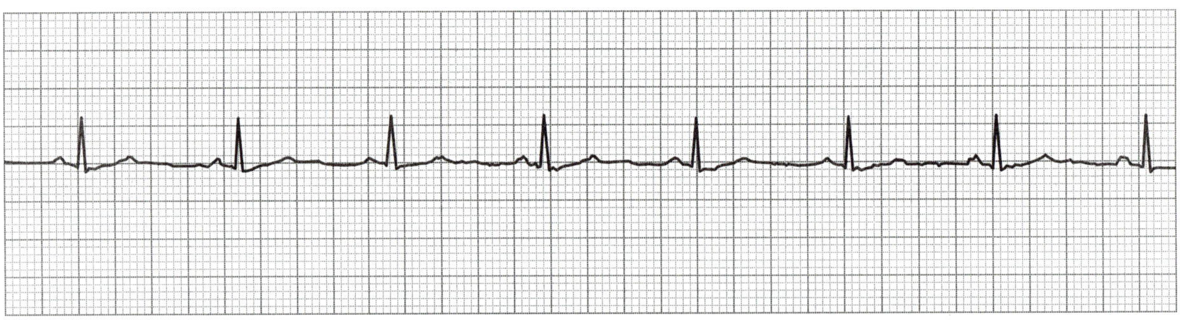

QRS duration ______________ QT ____________

Ventricular rate/rhythm ______________________

Atrial rate/rhythm ______________________

PR interval ______________________

Identification ______________________

Symptoms ______________________

____

Treatment ______________________

Figure 13-28

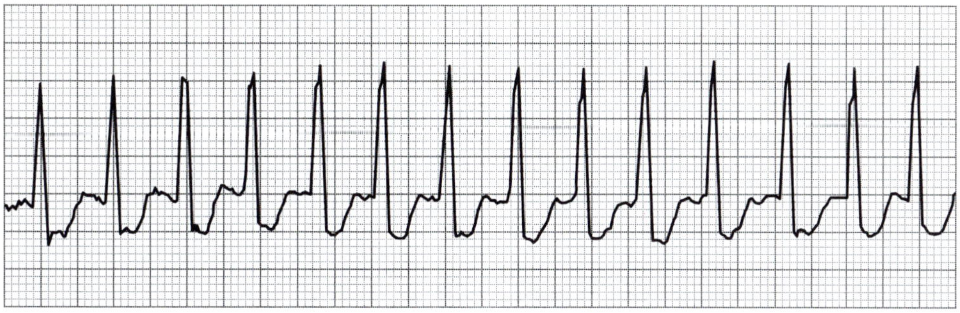

QRS duration ______________ QT ____________

Ventricular rate/rhythm ______________________

Atrial rate/rhythm ______________________

PR interval ______________________________

Identification ______________________________

Symptoms ________________________________

____

Treatment ________________________________

Figure 13-29

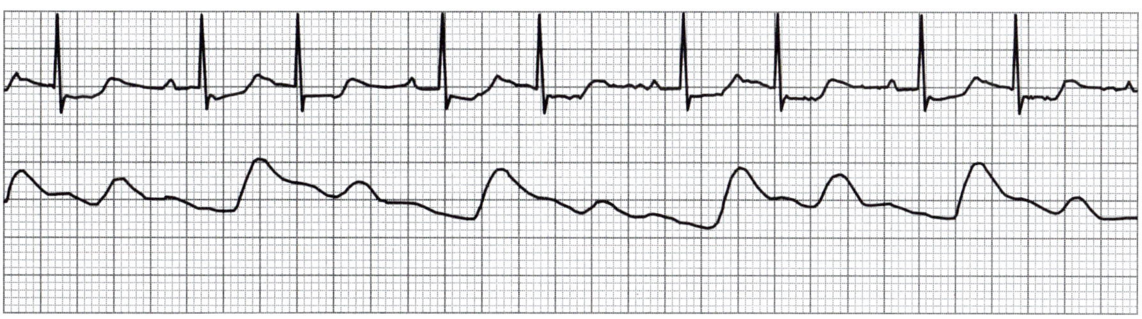

QRS duration ______________ QT ____________

Ventricular rate/rhythm ______________________

Atrial rate/rhythm ______________________

PR interval ______________________________

Identification ______________________________

Symptoms ________________________________

____

Treatment ________________________________

Figure 13-30

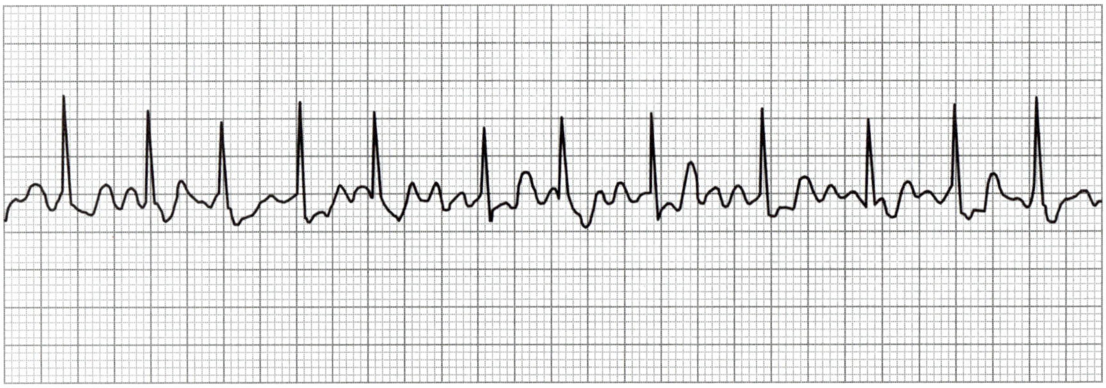

QRS duration ________________ QT ____________

Ventricular rate/rhythm ________________________

Atrial rate/rhythm ____________________________

PR interval ________________________________

Identification ________________________________

Symptoms ___________________________________

____

Treatment __________________________________

Figure 13-31

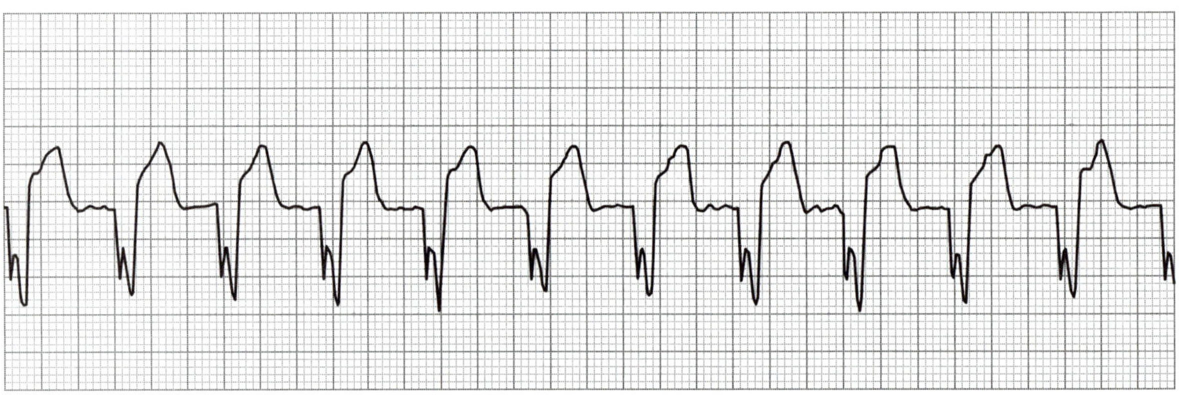

QRS duration ________________ QT ____________

Ventricular rate/rhythm ________________________

Atrial rate/rhythm ____________________________

PR interval ________________________________

Identification ________________________________

Symptoms ___________________________________

____

Treatment __________________________________

Figure 13-32

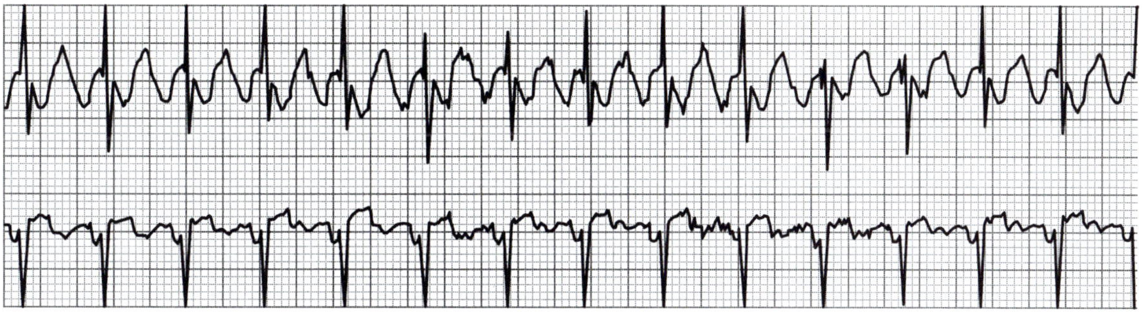

QRS duration ________ QT ________

Ventricular rate/rhythm ________

Atrial rate/rhythm ________

PR interval ________

Identification ________

Symptoms ________

____

Treatment ________

Figure 13-33

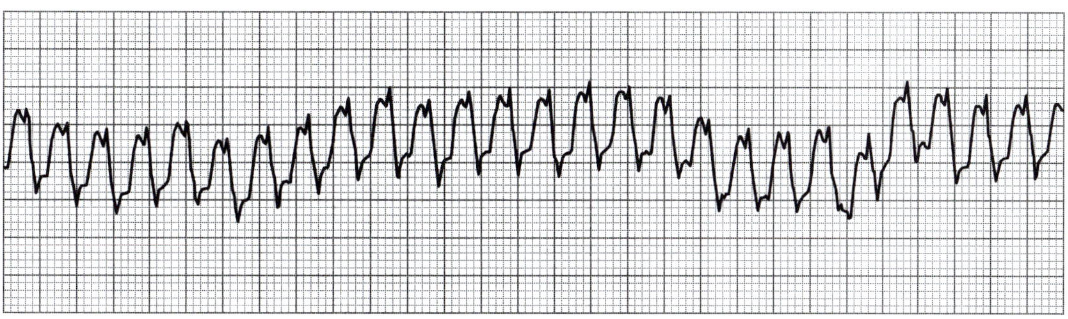

QRS duration ________ QT ________

Ventricular rate/rhythm ________

Atrial rate/rhythm ________

PR interval ________

Identification ________

Symptoms ________

____

Treatment ________

Figure 13-34

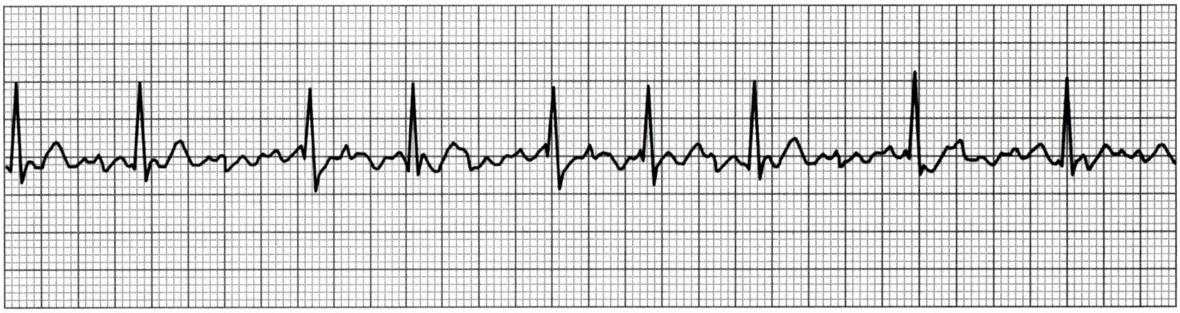

QRS duration ______________ QT ___________
Ventricular rate/rhythm ____________________
Atrial rate/rhythm ________________________
PR interval ______________________________

Identification ______________________________
Symptoms _________________________________
____
Treatment ________________________________

Figure 13-35

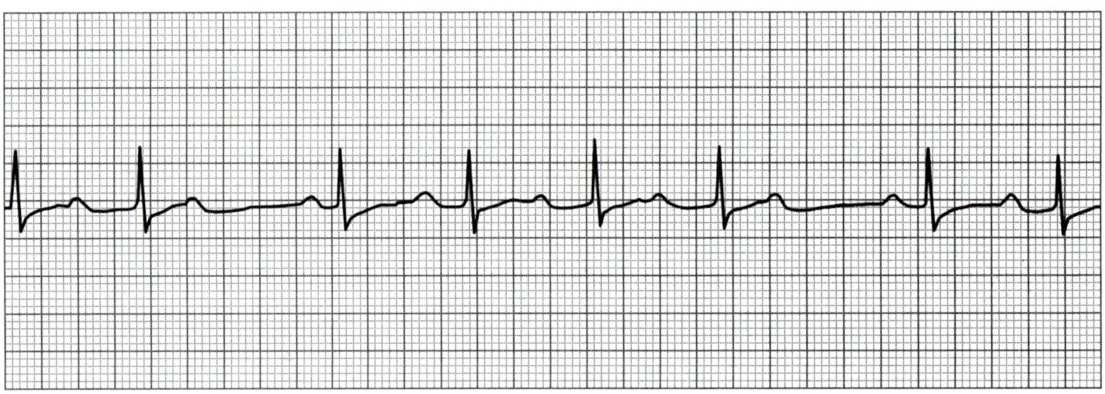

QRS duration ______________ QT ___________
Ventricular rate/rhythm ____________________
Atrial rate/rhythm ________________________
PR interval ______________________________

Identification ______________________________
Symptoms _________________________________
____
Treatment ________________________________

Figure 13-36

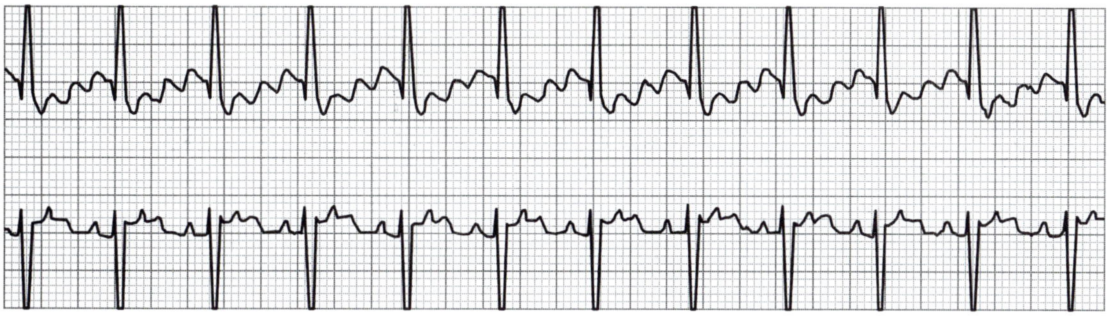

QRS duration ______________ QT ____________

Ventricular rate/rhythm ______________________

Atrial rate/rhythm __________________________

PR interval ________________________________

Identification ________________________________

Symptoms ___________________________________

____

Treatment __________________________________

Figure 13-37

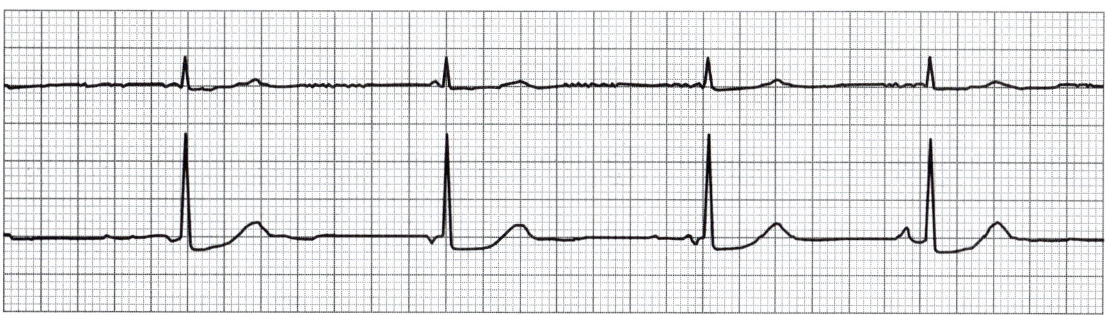

QRS duration ______________ QT ____________

Ventricular rate/rhythm ______________________

Atrial rate/rhythm __________________________

PR interval ________________________________

Identification ________________________________

Symptoms ___________________________________

____

Treatment __________________________________

Figure 13-38

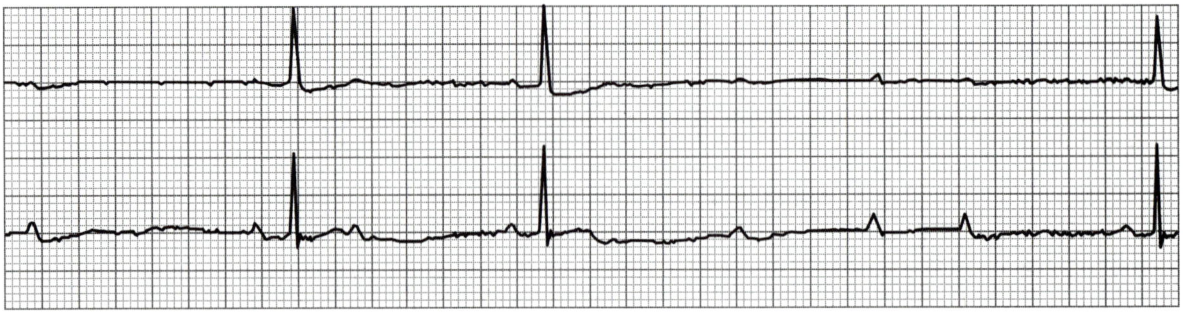

QRS duration ________________ QT ____________

Ventricular rate/rhythm ________________________

Atrial rate/rhythm ____________________________

PR interval ___________________________________

Identification ________________________________

Symptoms ____________________________________

____

Treatment ____________________________________

Figure 13-39

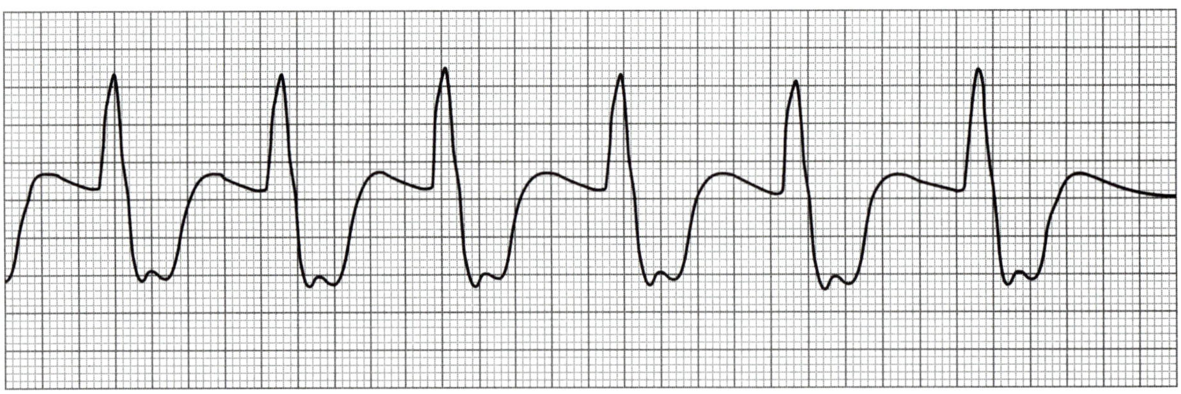

QRS duration ________________ QT ____________

Ventricular rate/rhythm ________________________

Atrial rate/rhythm ____________________________

PR interval ___________________________________

Identification ________________________________

Symptoms ____________________________________

____

Treatment ____________________________________

Figure 13-40

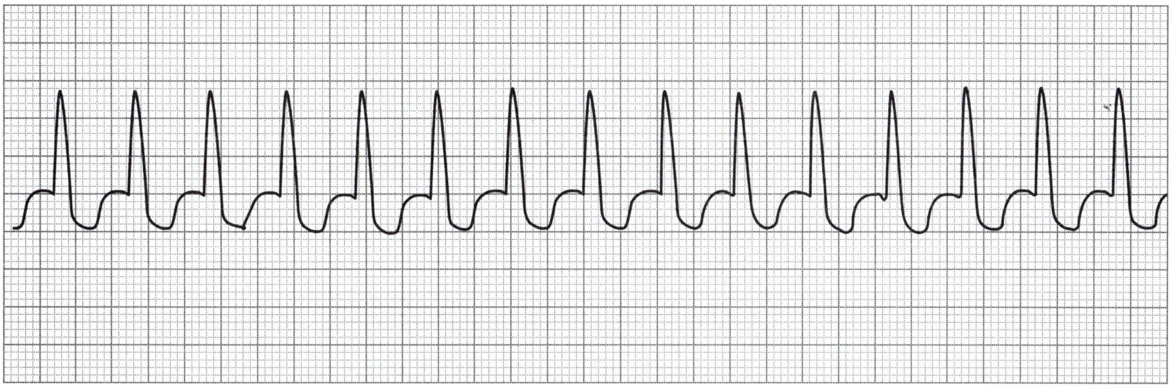

QRS duration ______________ QT ____________

Ventricular rate/rhythm ____________________

Atrial rate/rhythm ________________________

PR interval ______________________________

Identification ______________________________

Symptoms _________________________________

____

Treatment ________________________________

Figure 13-41

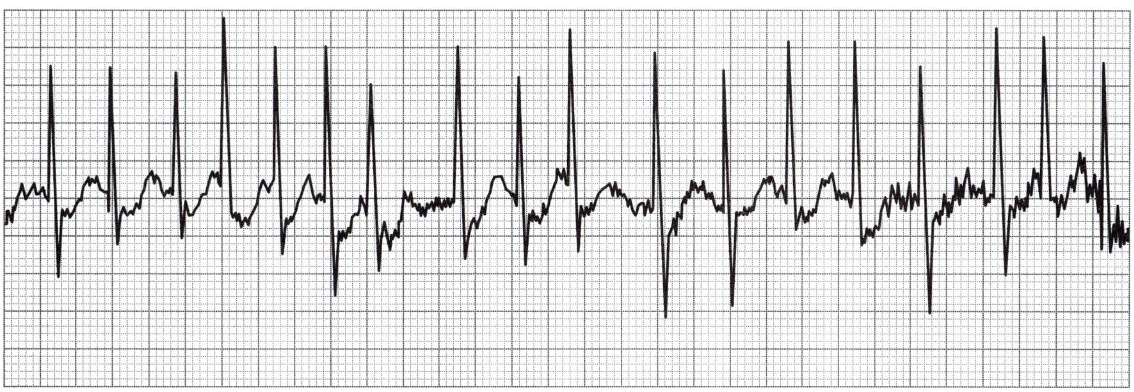

QRS duration ______________ QT ____________

Ventricular rate/rhythm ____________________

Atrial rate/rhythm ________________________

PR interval ______________________________

Identification ______________________________

Symptoms _________________________________

____

Treatment ________________________________

APPENDIX A

Answers to Self-Assessment Exercises

CHAPTER 1 REVIEW OF THE HEART'S ANATOMY AND FUNCTION

Fill in the Blanks

1. function, musculature
2. systemic circulation, lungs
3. oxygenated, lungs, body
4. thicker, systemic circulation
5. tricuspid, right
6. mitral, left
7. pulmonic, lungs; aortic, systemic circulation
8. rotated, anterior; posterior
9. aorta, downward, anterior, posterior; SA, AV
10. septal, bundle of His
11. left anterior descending, left circumflex
12. septum; right bundle branch; left bundle branch
13. circumflex; left posterior fascicle

CHAPTER 2 ELECTROPHYSIOLOGY AND THE ECG RECORDING

Fill in the Blanks

1. electrical, mechanical
2. automaticity
3. excitability
4. conductivity
5. contractility
6. electrical, contraction
7. SA node
8. atrial tissue
9. AV junction
10. AV node, bundle of His
11. right bundle branch
12. left main, left anterior fascicle; left posterior fascicle
13. Purkinje system
14. reciprocal
15. left free wall
16. apical and inferior surface
17. right inferior surface
18. right bundle branch
19. right anterior surface
20. right anterior septal surface
21. left anterior surface
22. left ventricle
23. left lateral surface

CHAPTER 3 WAVE FORMS AND MEASUREMENTS ON THE ECG

Matching

1. T
2. B
3. R
4. I
5. D
6. E
7. L
8. A
9. H
10. N
11. O
12. K
13. C
14. P
15. M
16. S
17. Q
18. F
19. G
20. J

ECG Rhythm Identification Practice

Figure 3-18

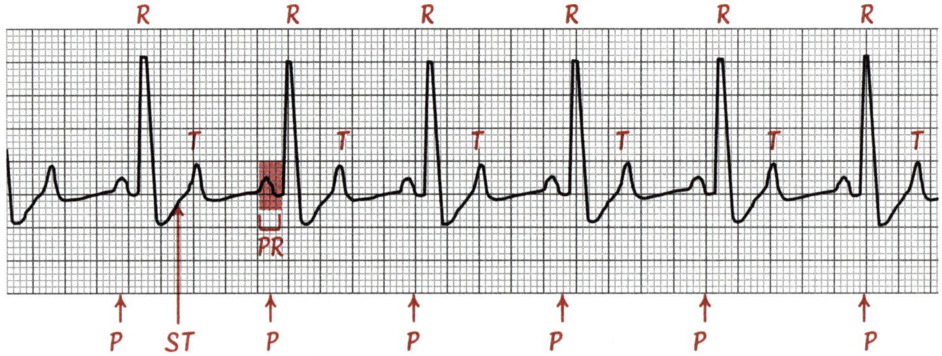

1. There are P, R, and T waves; ST segment is on an angle.
2. The P wave is (+).
3. QRS/ventricular rate/rhythm = 67/minute/regular.
4. P (atrial) rate/rhythm = 67/minute/regular.
5. PR interval = 0.16 seconds and consistent.

Figure 3-19

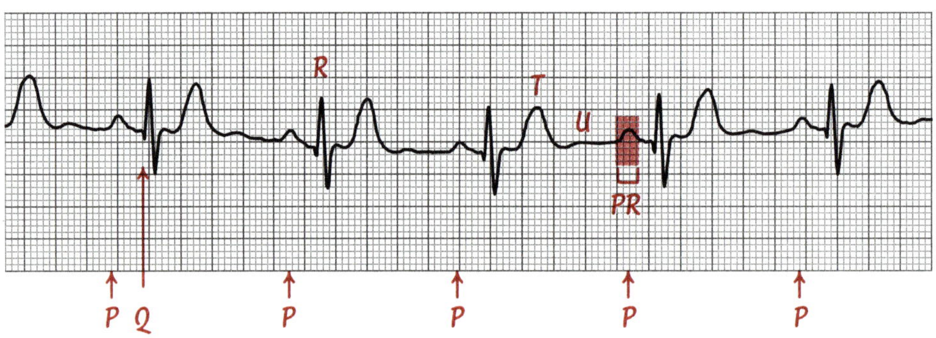

1. There are P, Q, R, S, T, and U waves. ST segment is on the line.
2. The P wave is (+).
3. QRS/ventricular rate/rhythm = 56/min/regular.
4. P (atrial) rate/rhythm = 55/min/regular.
5. PR interval = 0.16 seconds and consistent.

Figure 3-20

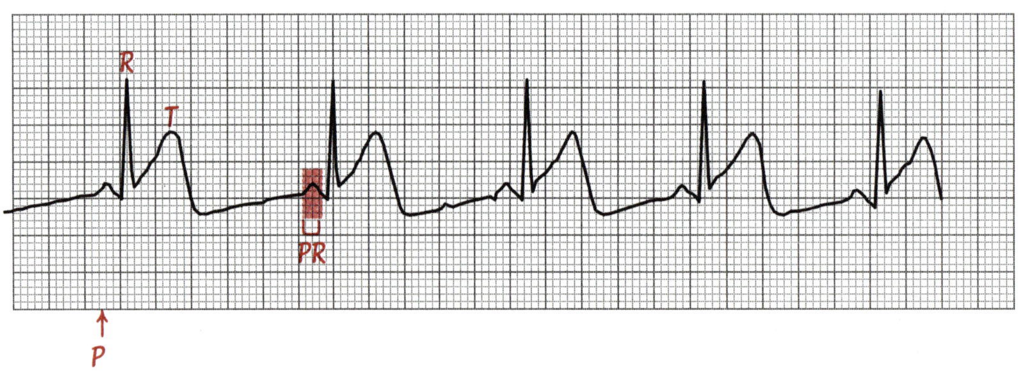

1. There are P, R, and T waves.
2. The P waves are (+).
3. QRS (ventricular) rate = 55/minute/regular.
4. P (atrial) rate/rhythm = 55/minute/regular.
5. PR interval = 0.16 seconds and consistent.

Figure 3-21

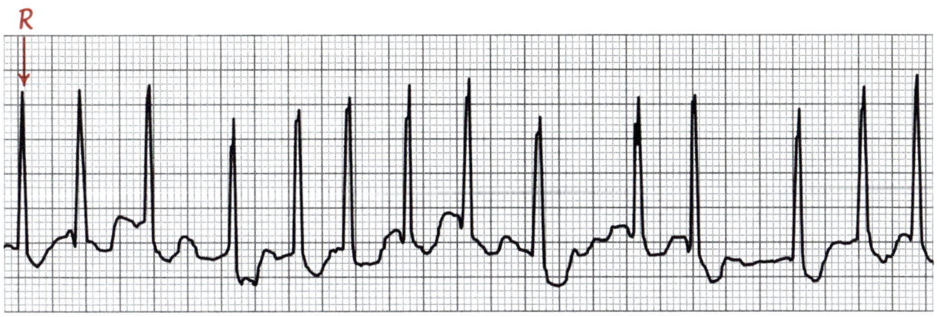

1. The R waves are easily visible; other wave forms are not. ST segment is depressed and varies between 3 and 5 mm.
2. There are no identifiable P waves.
3. QRS (ventricular rate)/rhythm = 100–180 obviously irregular.
4. P (atrial) rate/rhythm = no identifiable P waves.
5. PR interval = none.

Figure 3-22

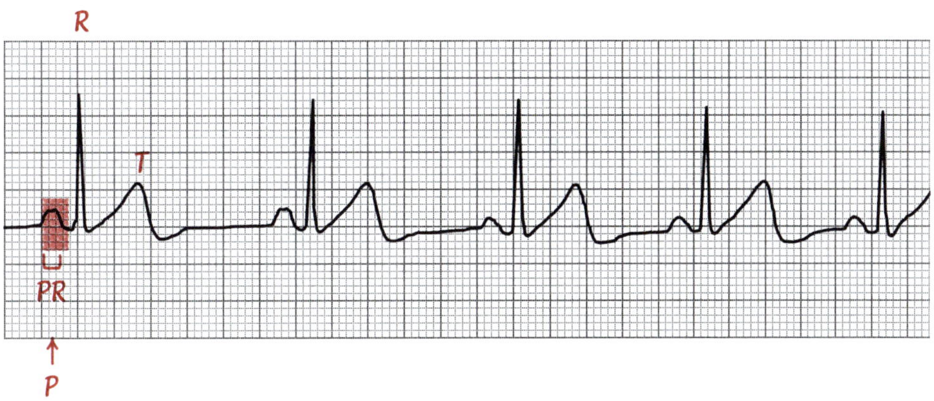

1. There are P, R, and T waves
2. The P waves are (+).
3. QRS (ventricular) rate/rhythm = 53–60/minute irregular.
4. P (atrial) rate/rhythm = 53–60/minute/irregular.
5. PR interval = 0.20 and consistent.

Figure 3-23

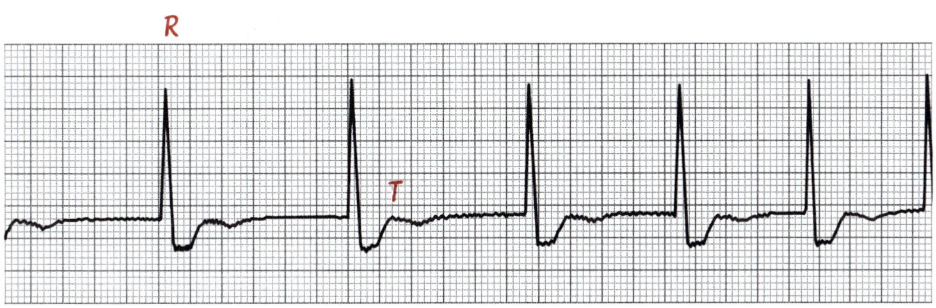

1. There are R and T waves easily visible; ST segment is 4 mm.
2. There are no visible P waves.
3. QRS (ventricular) rate/rhythm = 50–86/minute irregular.
4. P (atrial) rate/rhythm = 50–86/minute/irregular.
5. There are no P waves, therefore, no PR interval.

Figure 3-24

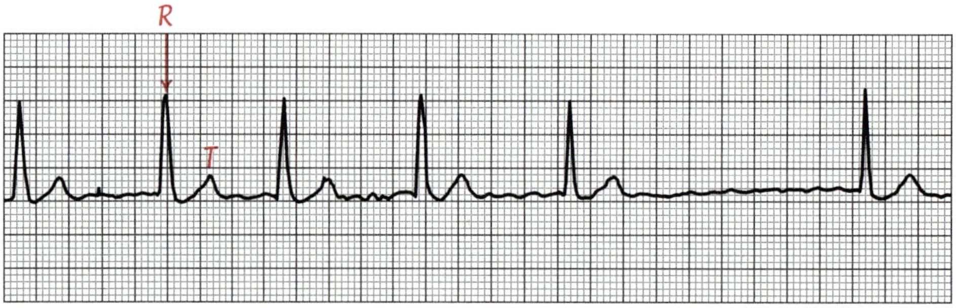

1. There are R and T waves.
2. There are no visible P waves.
3. QRS (ventricular) rate/rhythm = 20–85/minute/irregular.
4. There are no visible P waves; no measurable atrial rate.
5. There are no P waves, therefore, no PR interval.

Figure 3-25

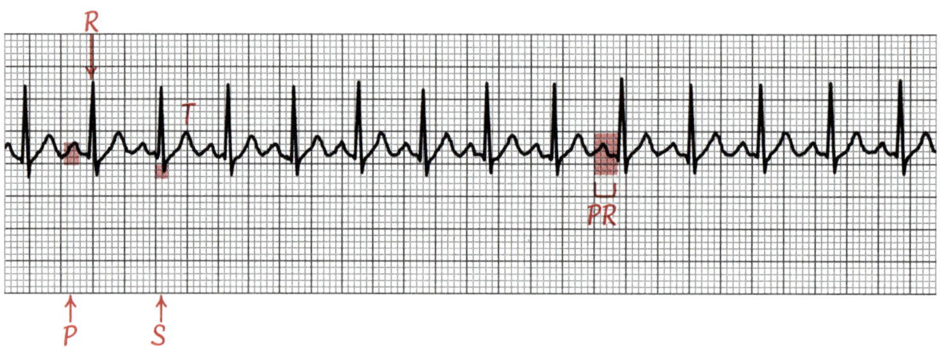

1. There are P, R, S, and T waves.
2. The P wave is (+).
3. QRS (ventricular) rate/rhythm = 150/minute/regular.
4. P (atrial) rate/rhythm = 150/minute/regular.
5. PR interval = 0.16 and consistent.

CHAPTER 4 THE SINUS MECHANISMS

Fill in the Blanks

SINUS RHYTHM	SINUS BRADYCARDIA	SINUS TACHYCARDIA
1 (+) P plus QRS	1 (+) P plus QRS	1 (+) P plus QRS
PRI: 0.12–0.20 second	0.12–0.20 second	0.12–0.10 second
QRS: 0.10 second or less	0.10 second or less	0.10 second or less
RATE: 60–100/minute	< 60/minute	>100/minute
RHYTHM: regular	regular	regular

SINUS RHYTHM	SINUS ARRHYTHMIA	SINUS BLOCK
1 (+) P plus QRS	1 (+) P plus QRS	missing one P wave
PRI: 0.12–0.20 second	1 (+) P plus QRS	n/a
QRS: 0.10 second or less	0.10 second or less	n/a
RATE: 60–100/min	60–100 usually	n/a
RHYTHM: regular	irregular	underlying rhythm usually regular

ECG Rhythm Identification Practice

Figure 4-17

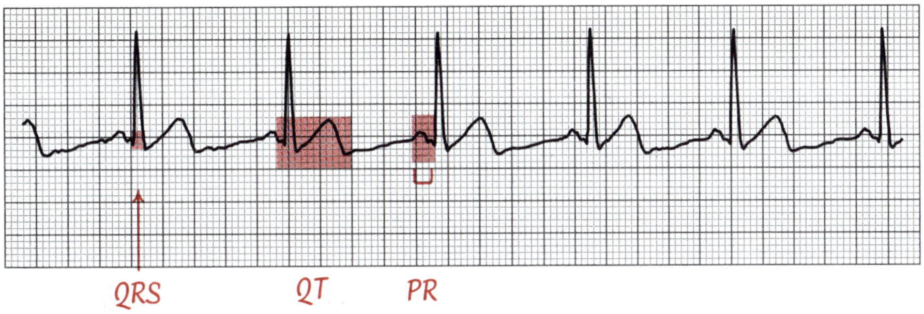

QRS duration 0.10 second **QT** 0.40 second
Ventricular rate/rhythm 86/minute/regular
Atrial rate/rhythm 86/minute/regular
PR interval 0.16 second

Identification sinus rhythm at 86/minute
Symptoms none anticipated
Treatment be supportive

Figure 4-18

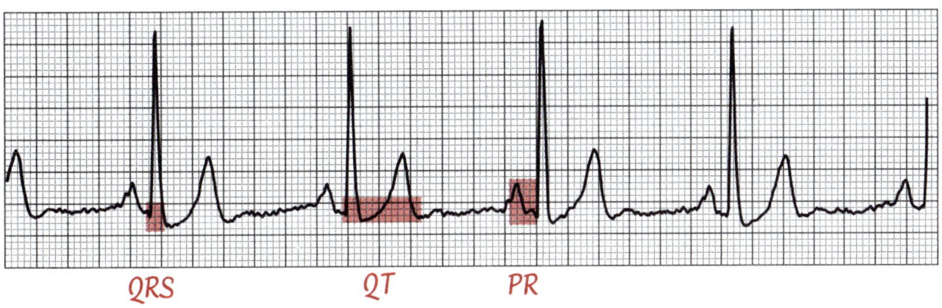

QRS duration 0.08 second **QT** 0.44 second
Ventricular rate/rhythm 41/minute/regular
Atrial rate/rhythm 41/minute/regular
PR interval 0.20 second

Identification sinus bradycardia at 41/min 2-3 mm, ST seg↓
Symptoms ?ALOC, dizziness, s/s hypoperfusion
Treatment if hypotensive and hypoperfusing, ABCs, O_2, (P), IV. ? meds/medical Hx, V/S/allergies: consider Atropine, fluids, dopamine, pace

Figure 4-19

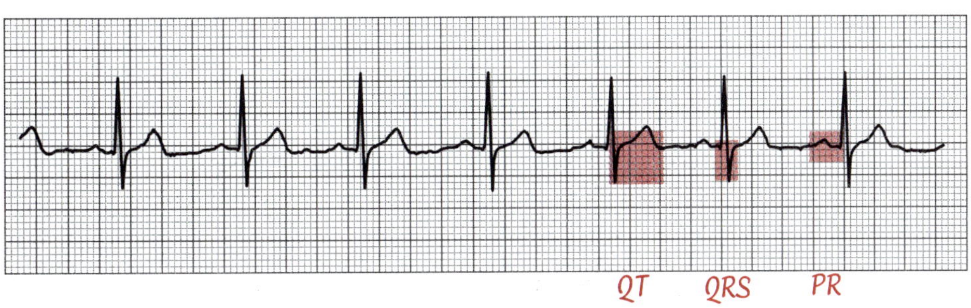

QRS duration 0.08 second **QT** 0.32 second
Ventricular rate/rhythm 75-86/minute irregular
Atrial rate/rhythm 75-86/minute irregular
PR interval 0.16 seconds

Identification sinus arrhythmia at 75-86/minute
Symptoms none anticipated
Treatment be supportive

Figure 4-20

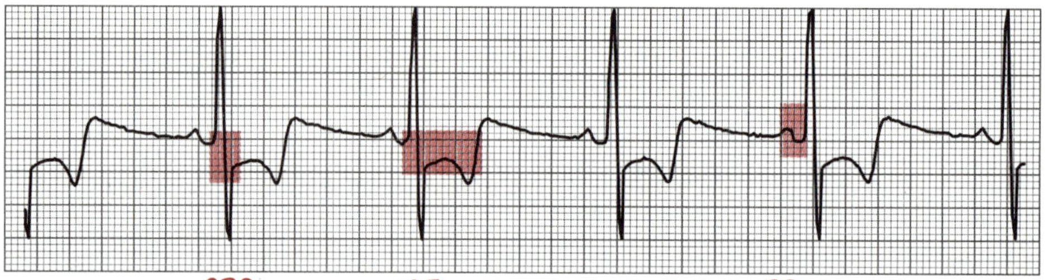

QRS duration 0.10 second QT 0.44 second
Ventricular rate/rhythm 50/minute regular
Atrial rate/rhythm 50/minute regular
PR interval 0.16-0.20 second

Identification sinus bradycardia at 40/min, 3 mm, ST seg ↓ and ↓ T waves
Symptoms ?ALOC, dizziness, s/s hypoperfusion
Treatment if hypotensive and hypoperfusing, ABCs, O_2, (P), IV. ? meds/medical Hx, V/S/allergies: consider Atropine, fluids, dopamine, pace

Figure 4-21

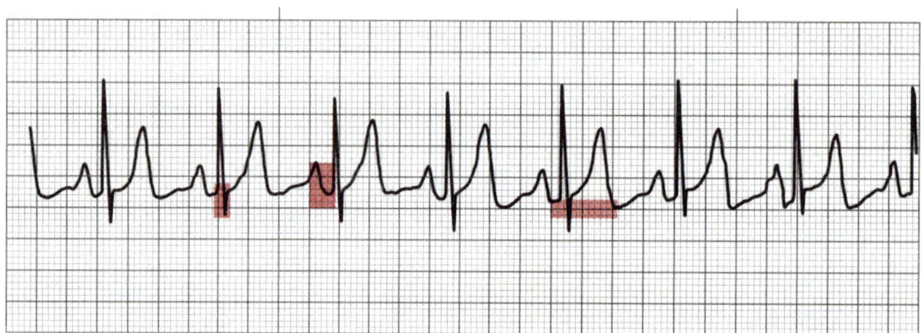

QRS duration 0.06-0.08 second QT 0.32 second
Ventricular rate/rhythm 75/minute regular
Atrial rate/rhythm 75/minute regular
PR interval 0.16-0.20 second

Identification sinus rhythm at 75/minute
Symptoms none anticipated
Treatment be supportive

Figure 4-22

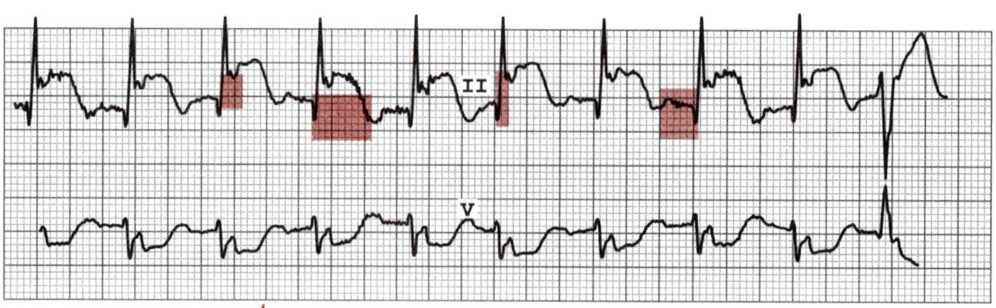

QRS duration 0.08 second QT 0.38 second
Ventricular rate/rhythm 125/minute regular
Atrial rate/rhythm 125/minute regular
PR interval 0.16-0.20 second

Identification sinus tachycardia 125/minute: 3-4 mm
Symptoms ST segment ↓: Q waves
? chest pain, SOB, diaphoresis
Treatment ABCs, O_2, (P), IV, ? meds/medical Hx, V/S/allergies: consider nitro/MS for pain, reassess: ASA, reassess

Figure 4-23

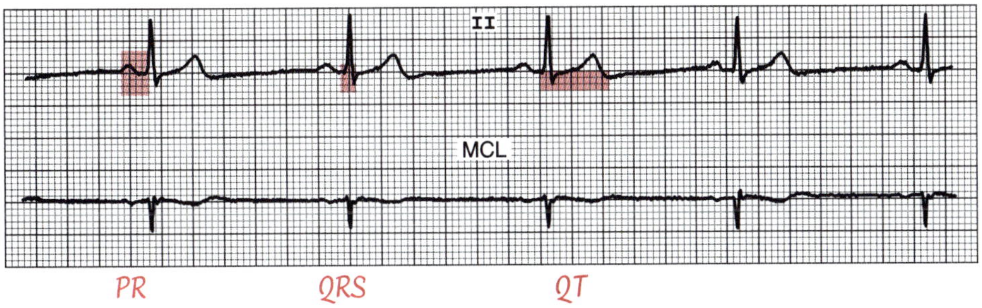

QRS duration 0.08 second QT 0.40 second
Ventricular rate/rhythm 46/minute regular
Atrial rate/rhythm 46/minute regular
PR interval 0.16 second

Identification sinus bradycardia at 46/minute
Symptoms ?ALOC, dizziness, s/s hypoperfusion

Treatment if hypotensive and hypoperfusing, ABCs, O_2, (P), IV. ? meds/medical Hx, V/S/? allergies: consider Atropine, fluids, dopamine, pace

Figure 4-24

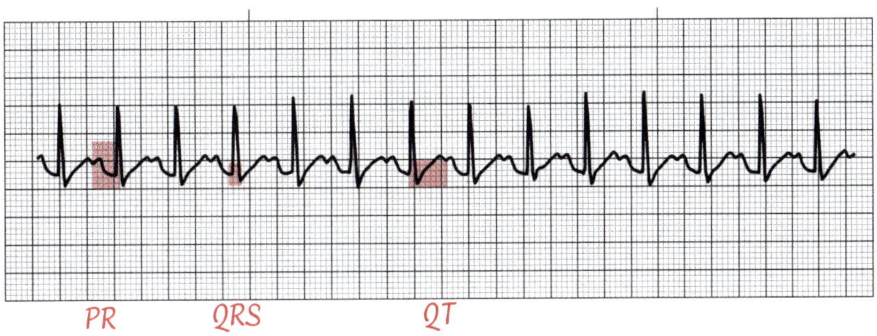

QRS duration 0.08 second QT 0.28 second
Ventricular rate/rhythm 150/minute regular
Atrial rate/rhythm 150/minute regular
PR interval 0.16 second

Identification sinus tachycardia at 150/minute
Symptoms ? fever, anxiety, anger, pain, medications, recreational substances; s/s CHF
Treatment ABCs, O_2, (P), ?IV, ID and Rx the cause:

Figure 4-25

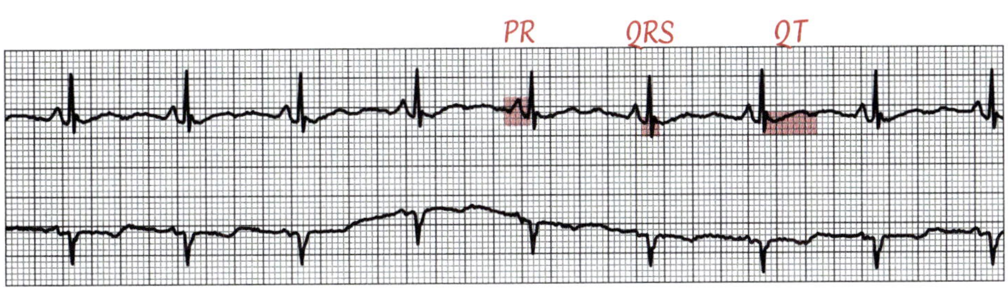

QRS duration 0.06-0.08 second QT 0.38 second
Ventricular rate/rhythm 75/minute/regular
Atrial rate/rhythm 75/minute/regular
PR interval 0.16 second

Identification sinus rhythm at 75/minute
Symptoms none anticipated

Treatment be supportive

Figure 4-26

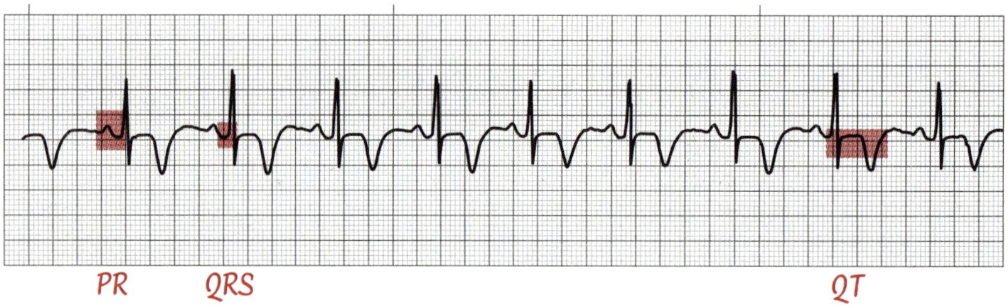

QRS duration 0.08 second **QT** 0.42 second

Ventricular rate/rhythm 75/minute/regular

Atrial rate/rhythm 75/minute/regular

PR interval 0.16 second

Identification sinus rhythm at 75/minute: ↓ T waves

Symptoms none anticipated

Treatment ? med/med Hx. ? pain: circumstances

Figure 4-27

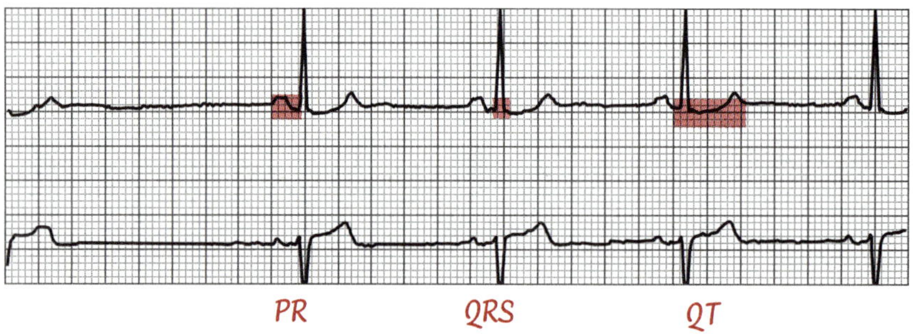

QRS duration 0.04-0.06 second **QT** 0.36 second

Ventricular rate/rhythm 50/minute/regular

Atrial rate/rhythm 50/minute/regular

PR interval 0.16 second

Identification sinus bradycardia at 50/minute

Symptoms ?ALOC, dizziness, s/s hypoperfusion

Treatment if hypotensive and hypoperfusing, ABCs, O_2, (P), IV. ? meds/medical Hx, V/S/? allergies: consider Atropine, fluids, dopamine, pace

Figure 4-28

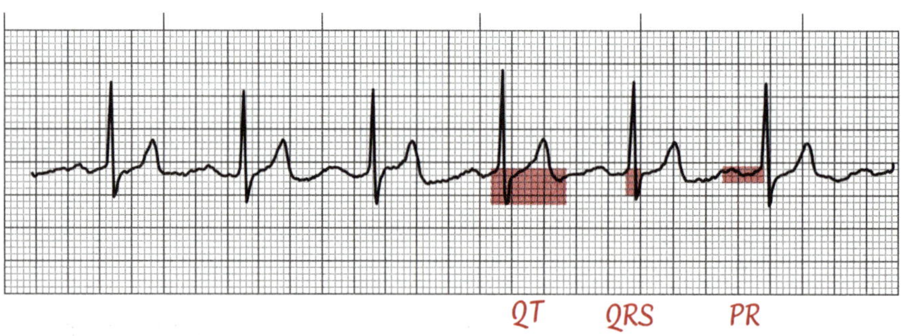

QRS duration 0.10 second **QT** 0.36 second

Ventricular rate/rhythm 75/minute regular

Atrial rate/rhythm 75/minute regular

PR interval 0.20 second

Identification sinus rhythm at 75/minute

Symptoms none anticipated

Treatment be supportive

Figure 4-29

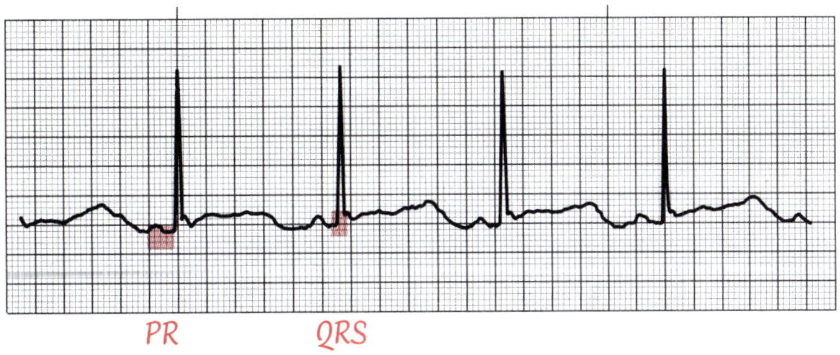

QRS duration *0.06 second* QT *UTD*
Ventricular rate/rhythm *54/minute regular*
Atrial rate/rhythm *54/minute regular*
PR interval *0.16 second*

Identification *sinus bradycardia at 54/minute*
Symptoms *?ALOC, dizziness, s/s hypoperfusion*
Treatment *if hypotensive and hypoperfusing, ABCs, O_2, (P), IV. ? meds/medical Hx, V/S/? allergies: consider Atropine, fluids, dopamine, pace*

Figure 4-30

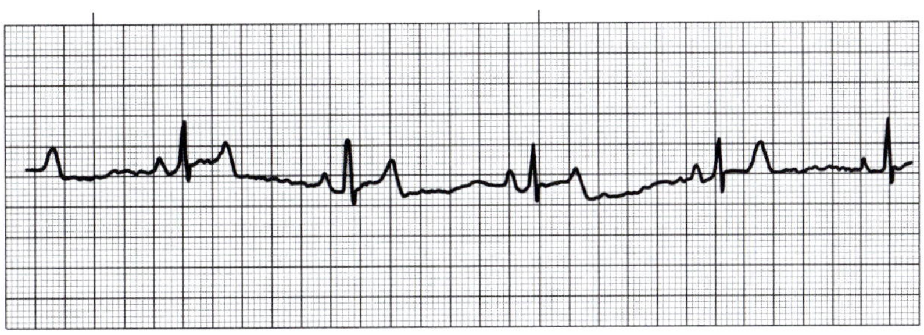

QRS duration *0.08-0.10 second* QT *0.40 second*
Ventricular rate/rhythm *67/minute regular*
Atrial rate/rhythm *67/minute regular*
PR interval *0.16 second*

Identification *sinus rhythm at 67/minute, 1mm ST seg ↑*
Symptoms *? LOC, s/s hypoperfusion: may be "normal" for the patient*
Treatment *be supportive*

CHAPTER 5 THE JUNCTIONAL MECHANISMS

Matching

1. b
2. a
3. c
4. d

Fill in the Blanks

SINUS RHYTHM	SINUS BRADYCARDIA	JUNCTIONAL RHYTHM
1 (+) P plus QRS	1 (+) P plus a QRS	(-) P' or none
PRI: 0.12–0.20	0.12–0.20	0.12 second
QRS: 0.10 or less	0.10 or less	< 0.10 second
RATE: 60–100/minute	<60/minute	40–60/minute
RHYTHM: regular	regular	regular

ECG Rhythm Identification Practice

Figure 5-9

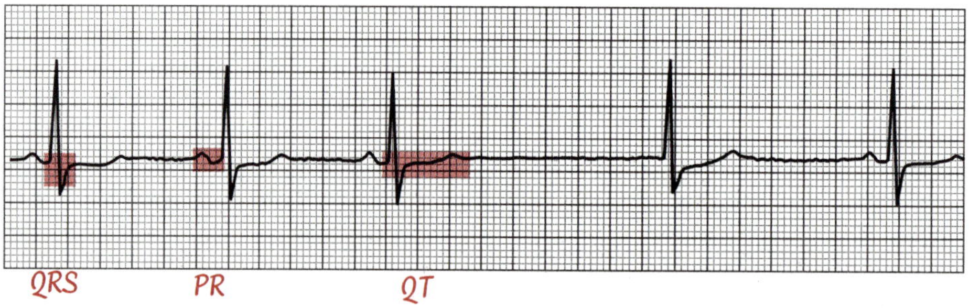

QRS duration 0.08 second **QT** 0.44 second
Ventricular rate/rhythm 55/minute prior to event
Atrial rate/rhythm 55/minute/regular
PR interval 0.16 second

Identification sinus bradycardia at 55/minute, ? SA arrest/block; junctional escape beat → sinus
Symptoms may report syncopal episodes
Treatment if s/s related to brady, intervene as with narrow-complex brady; otherwise, be supportive

Figure 5-10

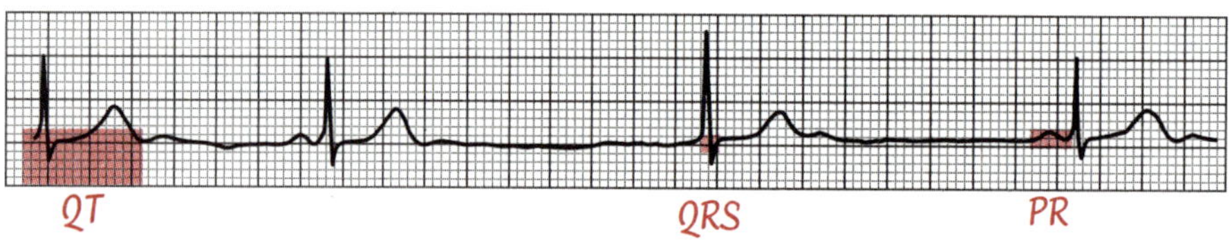

QRS duration 0.08 second **QT** 0.44 second
Ventricular rate/rhythm 47/minute prior to event
Atrial rate/rhythm 47/minute prior to event
PR interval 0.16 second

Identification sinus bradycardia at 47/minute, ? SA arrest or SA block; junctional escape beat → sinus
Symptoms ? LOC, s/s hypoperfusion; may be "normal" for the patient
Treatment be supportive

Figure 5-11

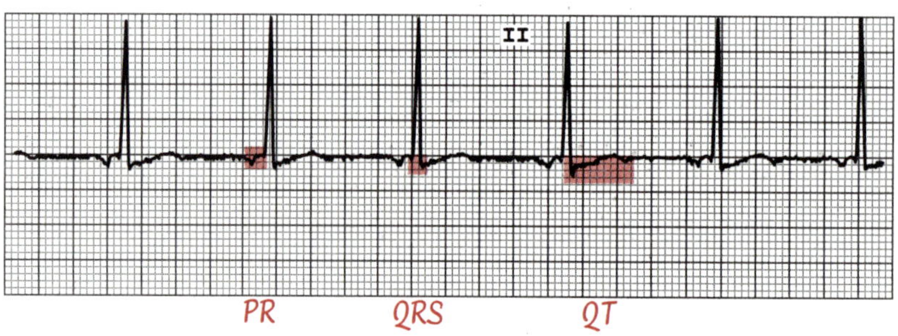

QRS duration 0.08 second **QT** 0.36 second
Ventricular rate/rhythm 67/minute
Atrial rate/rhythm 67/minute
PR interval 0.10-0.12 second

Identification accelerated junctional rhythm at 67/minute
Symptoms none anticipated
Treatment be supportive: ? meds/med Hx

Figure 5-12

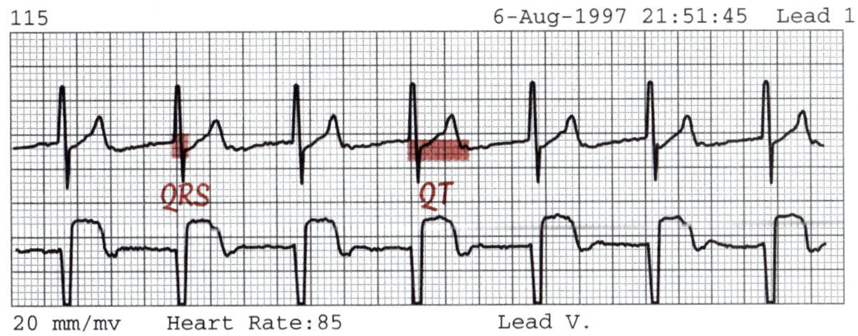

QRS duration 0.08 second **QT** 0.28 second
Ventricular rate/rhythm 86/minute regular
Atrial rate/rhythm UTD
PR interval UTD

Identification accelerated junctional rhythm at 86/minute
Symptoms may report syncopal episodes; ? sudden onset
Treatment be supportive but ALWAYS be concerned; WHY is the sinus not functioning?

Figure 5-13

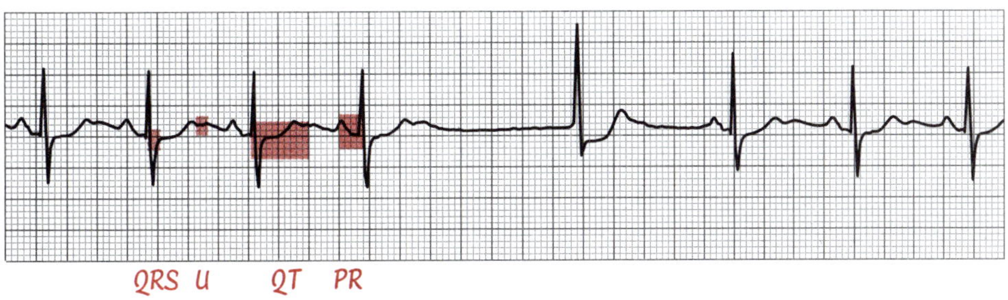

QRS duration 0.08 second **QT** 0.28 second
Ventricular rate/rhythm 75/minute prior to event
Atrial rate/rhythm 75/minute prior to event
PR interval 0.16 second

Identification sinus at 75/minute, U waves, ? SA arrest or SA block; junctional escape beat → sinus
Symptoms ?LOC, s/s hypoperfusion: may be "normal" for the patient
Treatment be supportive

Figure 5-14

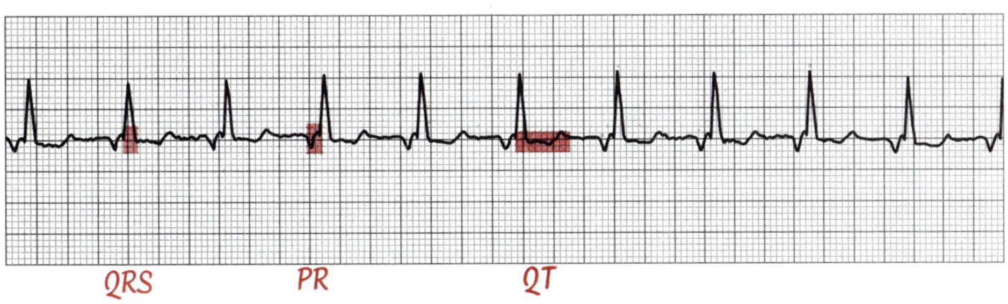

QRS duration 0.08 second **QT** 0.28 second
Ventricular rate/rhythm 96/minute
Atrial rate/rhythm 96/minute
PR interval 0.10 second

Identification accelerated junctional rhythm at 96/minute
Symptoms may report syncopal episodes; ? sudden onset
Treatment be supportive but ALWAYS be concerned; WHY is the sinus not functioning?

Figure 5-15

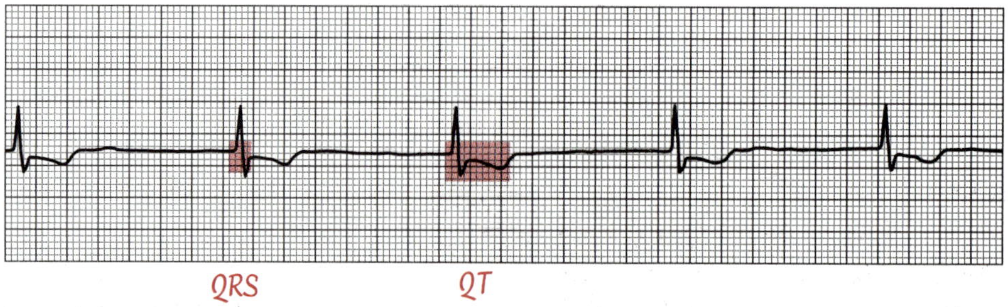

QRS duration 0.08 second **QT** 0.40 second

Ventricular rate/rhythm 46/minute/regular

Atrial rate/rhythm n/a

PR interval n/a

Identification junctional rhythm at 46/minute, ↓T wave

Symptoms ? ALOC, dizziness, s/s hypoperfusion

Treatment if hypotensive and hypoperfusing, ABCs, O_2, (P), IV. ? meds/medical Hx, V/S/ ? allergies: consider Atropine, fluids, dopamine, pace

Figure 5-16

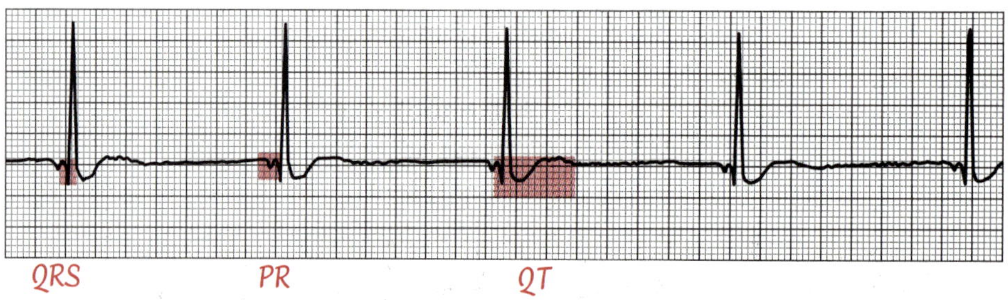

QRS duration 0.08 second **QT** 0.48 second

Ventricular rate/rhythm 46/minute/regular

Atrial rate/rhythm 48/minute/regular

PR interval 0.08 second

Identification junctional rhythm at 48/minute, ↓T wave

Symptoms ? ALOC, dizziness, s/s hypoperfusion

Treatment if hypotensive and hypoperfusing, ABCs, O_2, (P), IV. ? meds/medical Hx, V/S/? allergies: consider Atropine, fluids, dopamine, pace

Figure 5-17

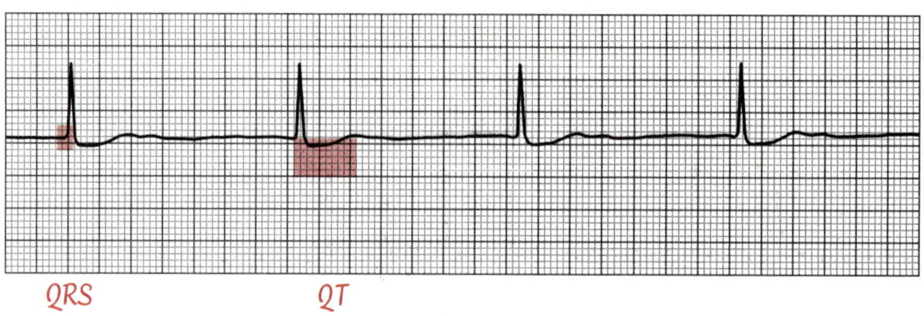

QRS duration 0.04 second **QT** 0.48 second

Ventricular rate/rhythm 43/minute/regular

Atrial rate/rhythm n/a

PR interval n/a

Identification junctional rhythm at 48/minute, ↓T wave

Symptoms ? ALOC, dizziness, s/s hypoperfusion

Treatment if hypotensive and hypoperfusing, ABCs, O_2, (P), IV. ? meds/medical Hx, V/S/? allergies: consider Atropine, fluids, dopamine, pace

CHAPTER 6 THE ATRIAL MECHANISMS

Matching

1. G
2. A
3. C
4. B
5. E

Fill in the Blanks

SINUS RHYTHM
P wave: 1(+) P plus QRS complex
PRI: 0.12–1.20 second
QRS: 0.10 or less
QRS rate: 60–100/min
QRS rhythm: regular

JUNCTIONAL RHYTHM
1 (-)P′ or none
<0.12 second
0.10 or less
40–60/min
regular

PAC
premature (+) P′
may differ from sinus PRI
0.10 or less (usually)
disturbs the sinus cadence
disturbs the sinus rhythm

ATRIAL TACH
P wave: UTD
PRI: UTD
QRS: 0.10 or less
QRS rate: >160/min
QRS rhythm: regular

SINUS TACH
1 (+)P plus QRS complex
0.12–0.20 second
0.10 or less
100–160/min
regular

JUNCTIONAL TACH
(-)P′ or none
<0.12 if P′ is visible
0.10 or less
100–130/min
regular

ECG Rhythm Identification Practice

Figure 6-20

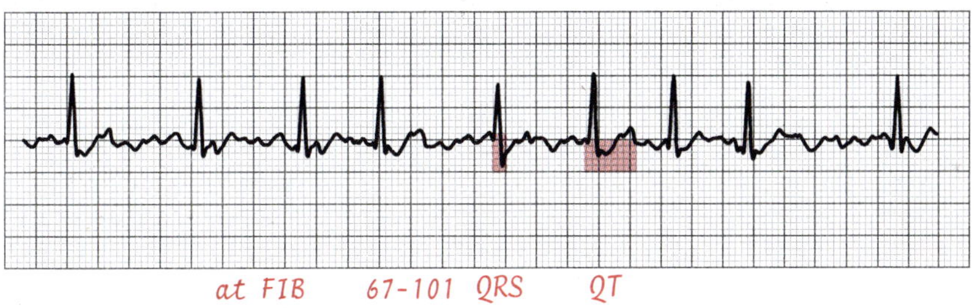

QRS duration *0.08 second* QT *0.32 second*
Ventricular rate/rhythm *67-125/minute*
Atrial rate/rhythm *UTD*
PR interval *none*
Identification *atrial fibrillation ventricular rate 67-125/minute*
Symptoms *none anticipated*
Treatment *? meds, med Hx, be supportive*

Figure 6-21

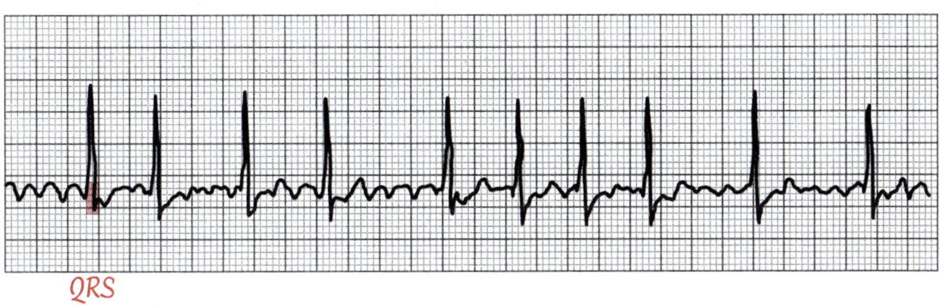

QRS duration *0.08 second* QT *UTD*
Ventricular rate/rhythm *75-150/minute*
Atrial rate/rhythm *UTD*
PR interval *none*
Identification *atrial fibrillation ventricular rate 75-150/minute*
Symptoms *none anticipated*
Treatment *? meds, med Hx, be supportive*

Figure 6-22

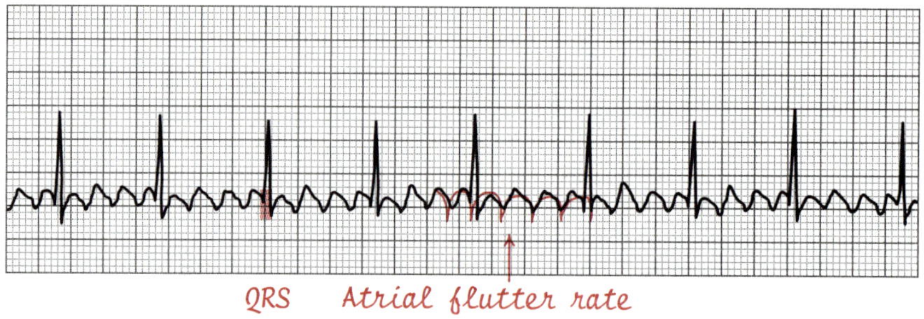

QRS duration 0.04-0.10 second QT UTD

Ventricular rate/rhythm 86-100/minute

Atrial rate/rhythm 300

PR interval none

Identification atrial flutter vent rate 86-100/minute

Symptoms none anticipated

Treatment ? meds, med Hx, be supportive

Figure 6-23

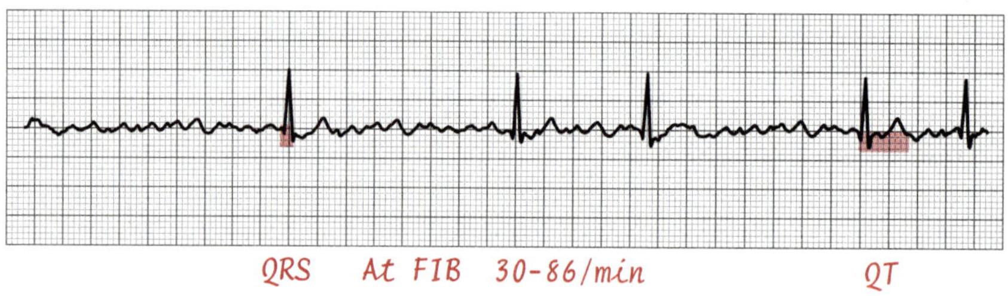

QRS duration 0.08-0.10 second QT 0.38

Ventricular rate/rhythm 30-86/minute

Atrial rate/rhythm UTD

PR interval none

Identification atrial fibrillation vent rate 30-86/minute

Symptoms may be related to slower rates; ? digitalis

Treatment ? meds, med Hx, be supportive; consider fluids/dopamine/pace if s/s hypotension, hypoperfusion

Figure 6-24

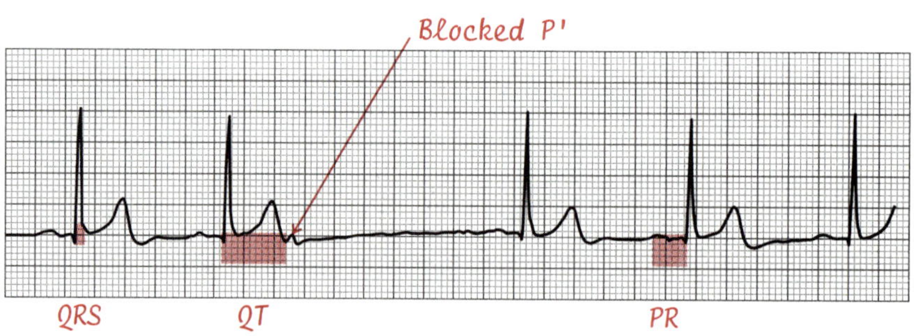

QRS duration 0.10 second QT 0.38 second

Ventricular rate/rhythm 50/minute

Atrial rate/rhythm 50/minute

PR interval 0.20 second

Identification sinus at 60/minute with a blocked PAC (after second QRS)

Symptoms may be related to slow rate

Treatment ? meds, med Hx, be supportive; consider fluids/dopamine/pace if s/s hypotension, hypoperfusion

Figure 6-25

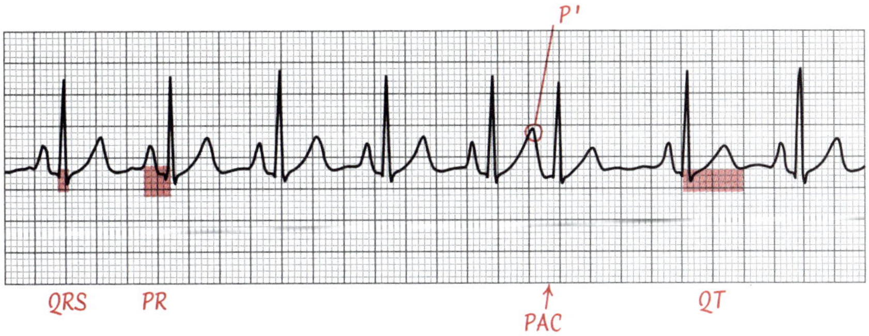

QRS duration 0.06 second QT 0.40 second

Ventricular rate/rhythm 86/minute

Atrial rate/rhythm 86/minute

PR interval 0.16 second

Identification sinus rhythm 86/minute with one PAC (6th complex)

Symptoms none anticipated

Treatment ? meds, med Hx, be supportive

Figure 6-26

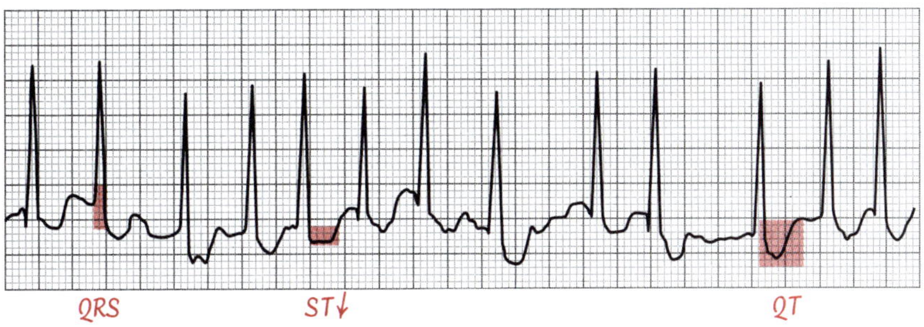

QRS duration 0.08-0.10 second QT UTD

Ventricular rate/rhythm 107-187/minute

Atrial rate/rhythm UTD

PR interval none

Identification atrial fibrillation vent rate 107-180/minute 3-4 mm ST seg ↓

Symptoms may admit to "palpitations" if new onset

Treatment may be asymptomatic: ? meds, med Hx, be supportive; if rapid rates persist and patient is symptomatic, consider verapamil

Figure 6-27

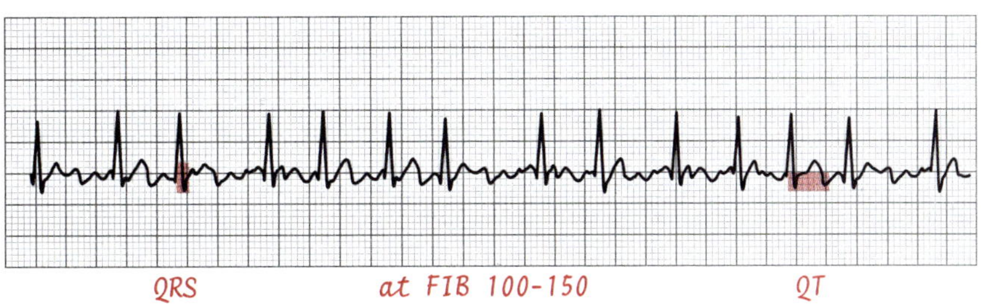

QRS duration 0.10 second QT 0.28 second

Ventricular rate/rhythm 100-150/minute

Atrial rate/rhythm UTD

PR interval none

Identification atrial fibrillation vent rate 100-150/minute

Symptoms may be asymptomatic

Treatment ? meds, med Hx, be supportive

Figure 6-28

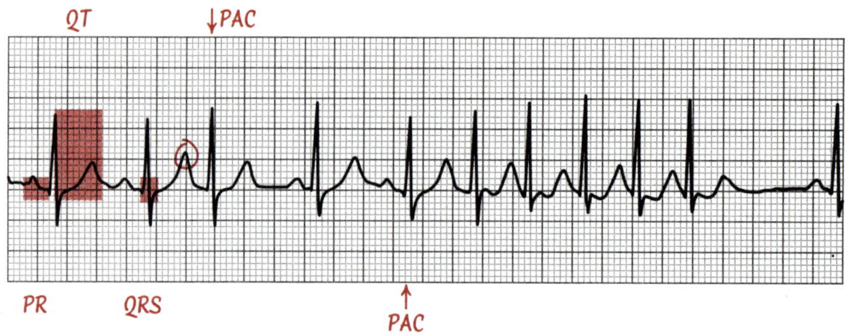

QRS duration 0.08 second QT 0.32 second
Ventricular rate/rhythm 100/minute
Atrial rate/rhythm 100/minute
PR interval 0.16 (sinus)

Identification sinus rhythm at 100/minute, frequent PACs (complex #3 and #6), atrial tach at 150/min → sinus
Symptoms none anticipated, except during bouts of PAT
Treatment ? meds, med Hx, be supportive unless PAT recurs and patient response requires intervention

Figure 6-29

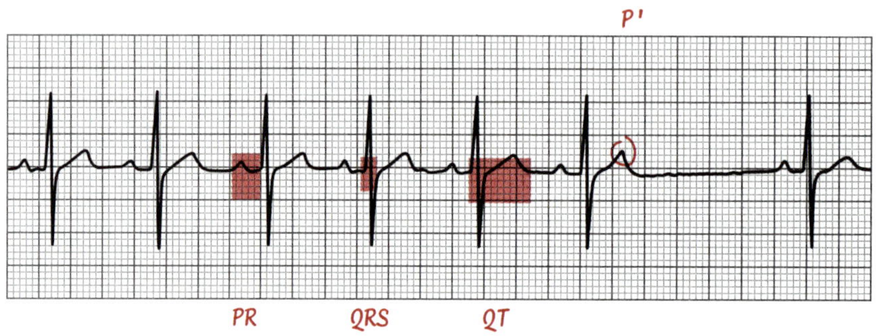

QRS duration 0.08-0.10 second QT 0.38-0.40 second
Ventricular rate/rhythm 40-75/minute
Atrial rate/rhythm 90/minute regular
PR interval 0.16 second

Identification sinus vent rate 90/minute with one nonconducted PAC
Symptoms probably none
Treatment be supportive

Figure 6-30

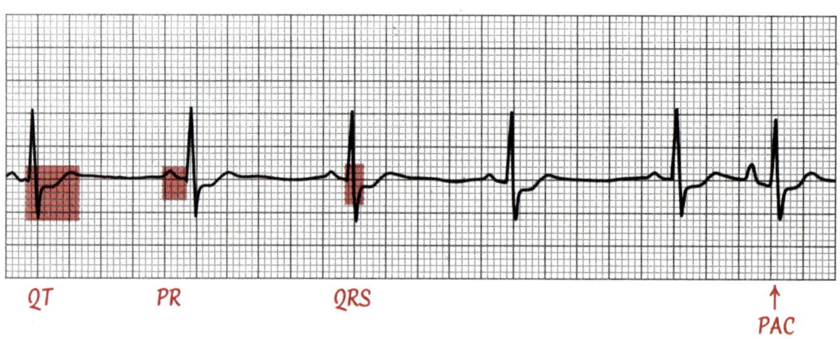

QRS duration 0.08 second QT 0.38 second
Ventricular rate/rhythm 60/minute
Atrial rate/rhythm 60/minute
PR interval 0.16 second

Identification sinus vent rate at 60/minute with a PAC (last complex on the tracing)
Symptoms may be related to slow rate
Treatment ? meds, med Hx, be supportive; consider fluids/ dopamine/pace if s/s hypotension hypoperfusion

Figure 6-31

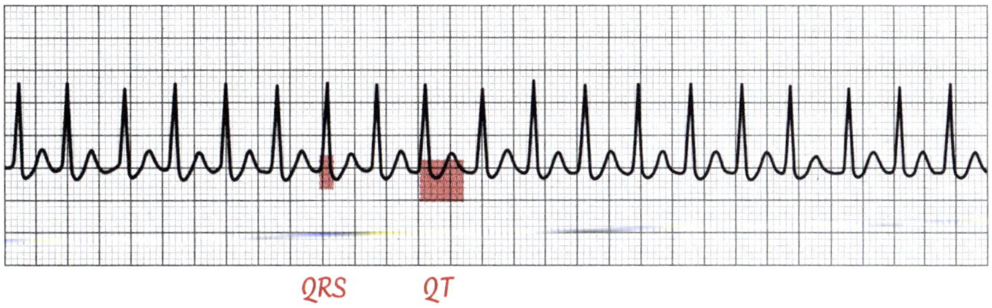

QRS duration 0.08-0.10 second QT UTD

Ventricular rate/rhythm 188/minute

Atrial rate/rhythm UTD

PR interval UTD

Identification SVT vent rate 188/minute

Symptoms ?ALOC, anxiety, feelings of palpitations

Treatment ? meds, med Hx; stable, consider vagal maneuvers, adenosine; unstable, consider synch CV at 50 joules

Figure 6-32

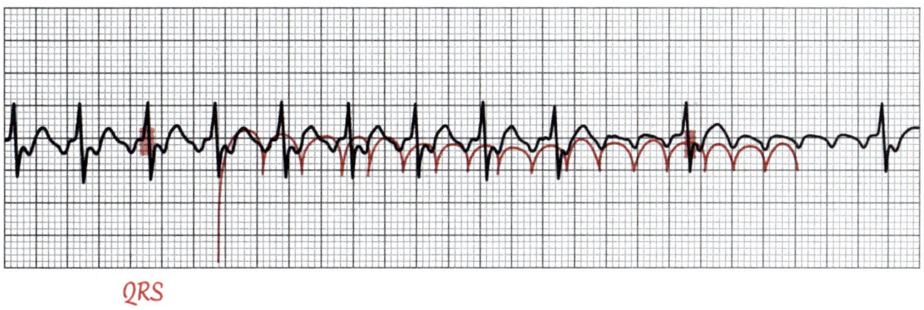

QRS duration 0.08 second QT UTD

Ventricular rate/rhythm 150→50-75/minute

Atrial rate/rhythm f waves at 300/minute

PR interval none

Identification atrial flutter, vent rate 150→50-75/minute

Symptoms may admit to "palpitations"; some patients note the "sudden change"

Treatment may be asymptomatic; ? meds/med Hx; be supportive

Figure 6-33

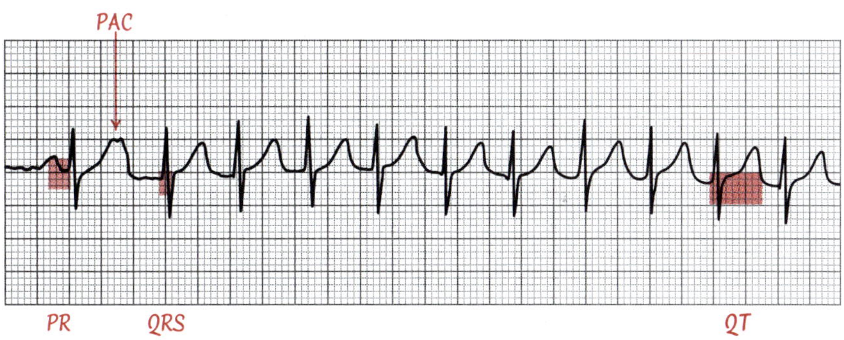

QRS duration 0.08 second QT 0.28 second

Ventricular rate/rhythm 150/minute regular

Atrial rate/rhythm UTD

PR interval 0.16 (sinus beat)

Identification one sinus beat, a PAC→atrial tach at 150/minute

Symptoms may be asymptomatic

Treatment ? meds, med Hx, stable; consider vagal maneuvers, adenosine; unstable; consider synch CV at 50 joules

CHAPTER 7 THE VENTRICULAR MECHANISMS

Fill in the Blanks

SINUS RHYTHM	PJC	PAC	PVC
1 (+) P + QRS	1(-) P' + QRS/or none	premature P'	n/a
PRI 0.12–0.20	<0.12	differs	n/a
QRS 0.10 or less	0.10 or less	0.10 or less	>0.10
QRS rate: 60-100/minute			
QRS rhythm: regular	disturbs sinus cadence	disturbs sinus cadence	sinus cadence *not* disturbed

ATRIAL TACH	SINUS TACH	VENTRICULAR TACH
P wave: may not see	1(+)P + QRS	as with underlying rhythm
PRI: UTD	0.12–0.20 second	UTD n/a
QRS = 0.10 second	0.10 second or less	usually >0.10 second
QRS rate: 150+	100–150	>100/minute
QRS rhythm: regular	regular	regular

ECG Rhythm Identification Practice

Figure 7-27

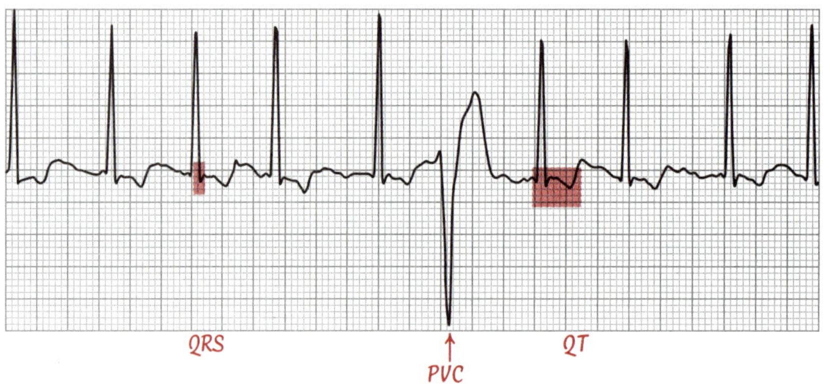

QRS duration 0.06-0.08 second **QT** ±0.28 second

Ventricular rate/rhythm irregular

Atrial rate/rhythm UTD

PR interval UTD

Identification atrial fibrillation vent rate 60-125/minute with a PVC

Symptoms perhaps none

Treatment be supportive; ? meds/med Hx

Figure 7-28

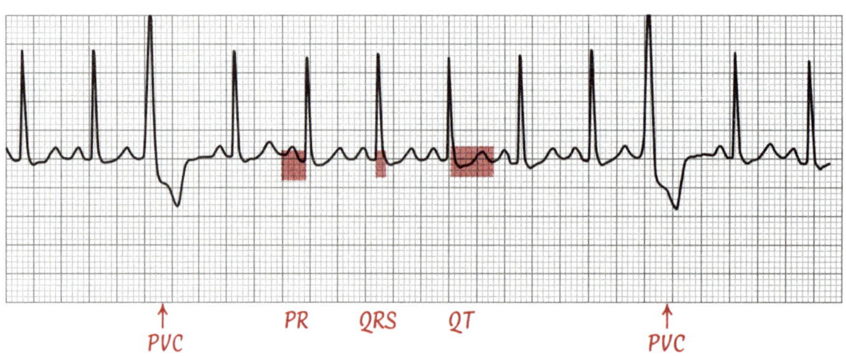

QRS duration 0.06 second **QT** 0.32 second

Ventricular rate/rhythm 125/regular

Atrial rate/rhythm 125/regular

PR interval 0.16 second

Identification sinus trach at 125/regular with freq uniform (u/f) PVCs; assess the underlying sinus rate and rhythm

Symptoms probably none

Treatment be supportive

Figure 7-29

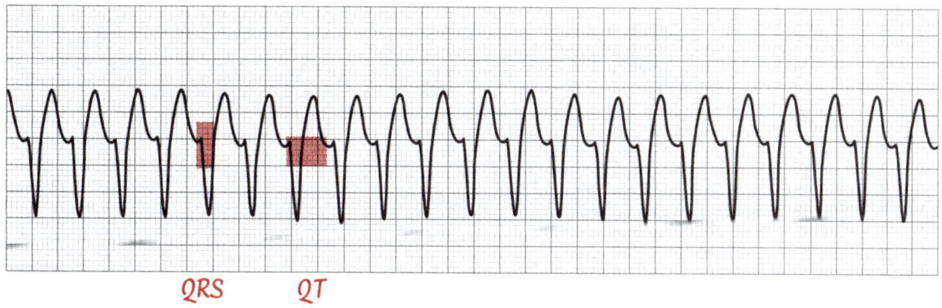

QRS duration 0.12 second **QT** 0.32 second
Ventricular rate/rhythm 168/minute/regular
Atrial rate/rhythm UTD
PR interval UTD

Identification sustained ventricular tachycardia at 168/minute
Symptoms probably useable at this rate
Treatment Consider sedation: cardioversion at 100 joules if the patient has a pulse; 200 joules if the patient is pulseless

Figure 7-30

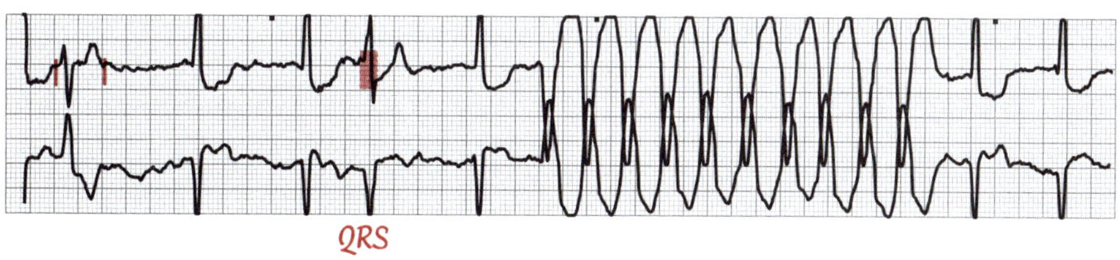

QRS duration 0.08 second **QT** +0.40 second
Ventricular rate/rhythm 75-86(a-fib), 150(v-tach)
Atrial rate/rhythm UTD
PR interval UTD

Identification atrial fib, 75-86/minute with m/f PVCs and a run of V-tach at 150/minute
Symptoms ? symptomatic with V-tach = dizziness, ? syncopal
Treatment ABCs, O_2, (P), IV, consider lidocaine bolus/ infusion

Figure 7-31

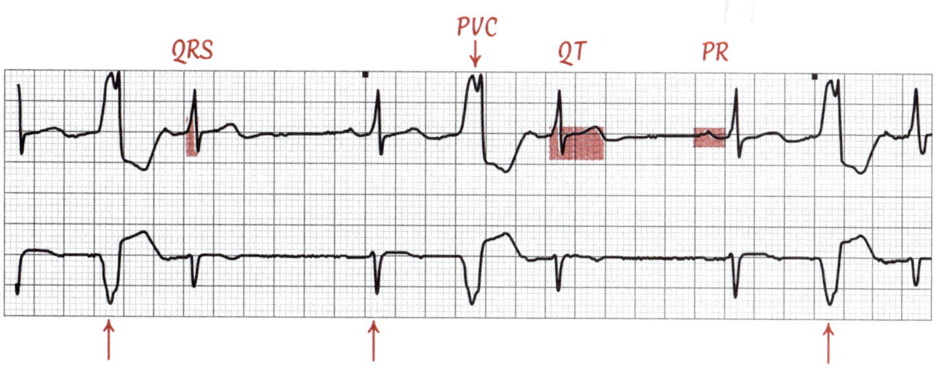

QRS duration 0.08-0.10 second **QT** 0.40 second
Ventricular rate/rhythm 46/minute
Atrial rate/rhythm 46/minute
PR interval 0.16-0.20 second

Identification sinus 48/minute with frequent u/f interpolated PVCs (note how the PVC is sandwiched between normal QRS)
Symptoms may be related to brady, i.e., ALOC, dizziness, etc.
Treatment ? meds especially digitalis, med Hx, vital signs; may consider TCP

Figure 7-32

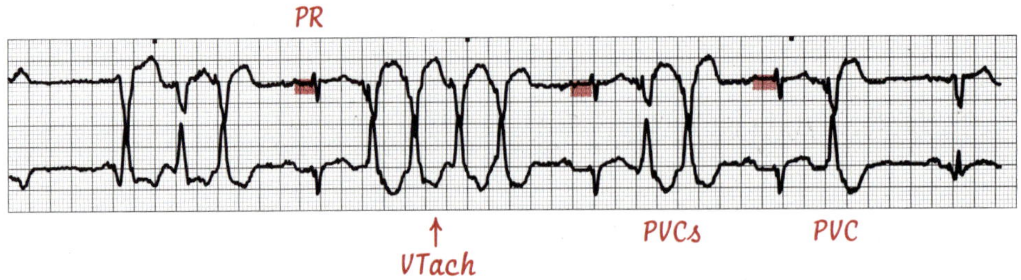

QRS duration 0.08 second (sinus) **QT** 0.38 second
Ventricular rate/rhythm UTD
Atrial rate/rhythm UTD
PR interval sinus 0.16–0.20 second

Identification sinus → freq u/f PVCs; couplets, 3 and 4 beat run of V-tach
Symptoms perhaps with the V-tach
Treatment ABCs, ? meds/med Hx, V/S/ allergies; O_2, (P), IV, consider lidocaine bolus/infusion

Figure 7-33

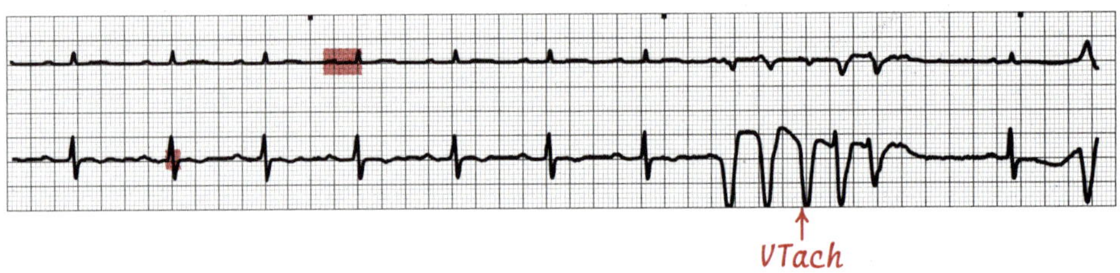

QRS duration 0.06–0.08 second **QT** UTD
Ventricular rate/rhythm 75/regular
Atrial rate/rhythm 75/regular
PR interval 0.28 second

Identification sinus rhythm 75/minute → end diastolic PVC → 5 beat run of V-tach, PRI is 0.28 second
Symptoms perhaps with the V-tach
Treatment ABCs, O_2, (P), IV, consider lidocaine bolus/infusion

Figure 7-34

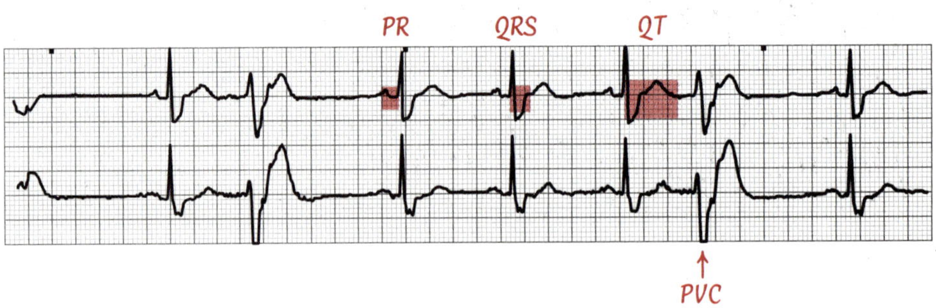

QRS duration 0.16 second **QT** 0.40 second
Ventricular rate/rhythm 67/minute/regular
Atrial rate/rhythm 67/minute/regular
PR interval 0.16 second

Identification sinus at 67/minute with QRS 0.16; frequent u/f PVCs (note the broad S wave) ? RBBB to confirm on 12-lead
Symptoms may be none
Treatment ABCs, O_2, (P), ? meds/med Hx, be supportive

Figure 7-35

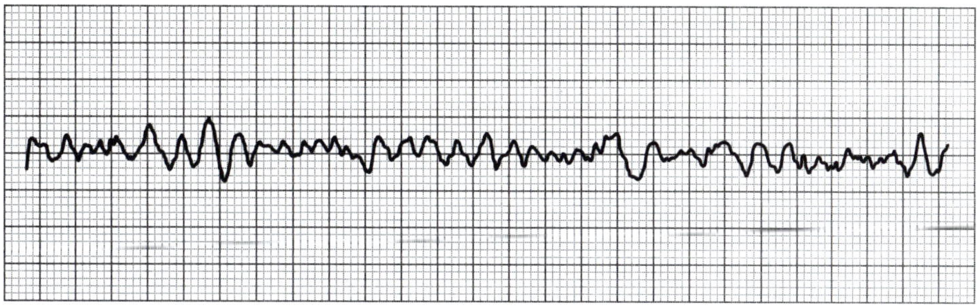

QRS duration: UTD QT: UTD
Ventricular rate/rhythm: UTD
Atrial rate/rhythm: UTD
PR interval: UTD

Identification: ventricular fibrillation; confirm no pulse
Symptoms: pulseless
Treatment: defibrillate at 200 joules initially

Figure 7-36

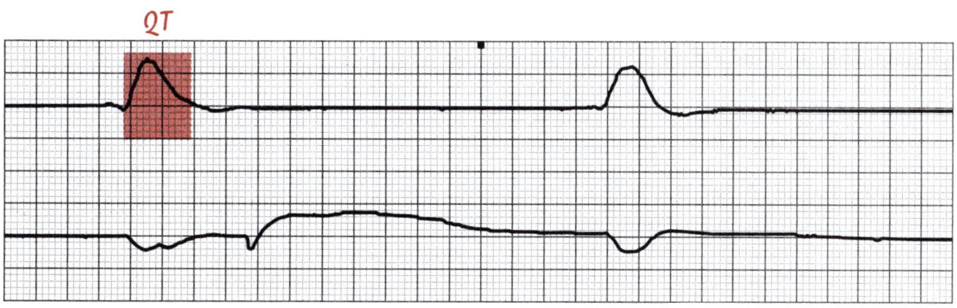

QRS duration: +0.40 second QT: UTD
Ventricular rate/rhythm: 20/minute
Atrial rate/rhythm: UTD
PR interval: UTD

Identification: idioventricular rhythm at 20/minute
Symptoms: ? LOC/pulseless, (? advanced directives)
Treatment: CPR, intubate, IV, fluids, epinephrine, Atropine, TCP

Figure 7-37

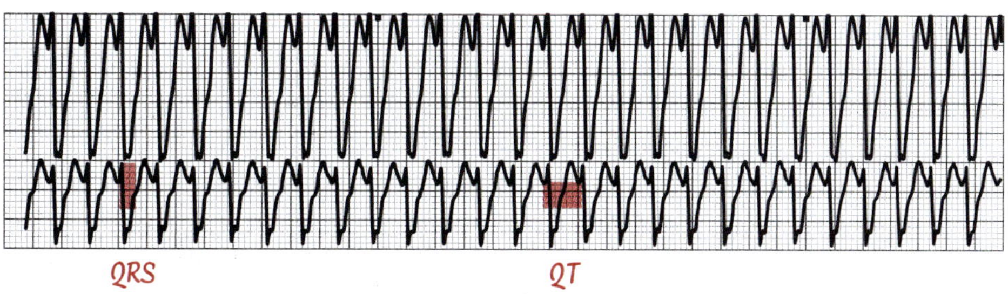

QRS duration: 0.12 second QT: 0.24 second
Ventricular rate/rhythm: 214/regular
Atrial rate/rhythm: UTD
PR interval: n/a

Identification: ventricular tachycardia at 214/minute
Symptoms: ? LOC/pulseless, (? advanced directives)
Treatment: pulseless: defib at 200 initially; if pulse is present, defib at 100 (note: this patient was pulseless)

Figure 7-38

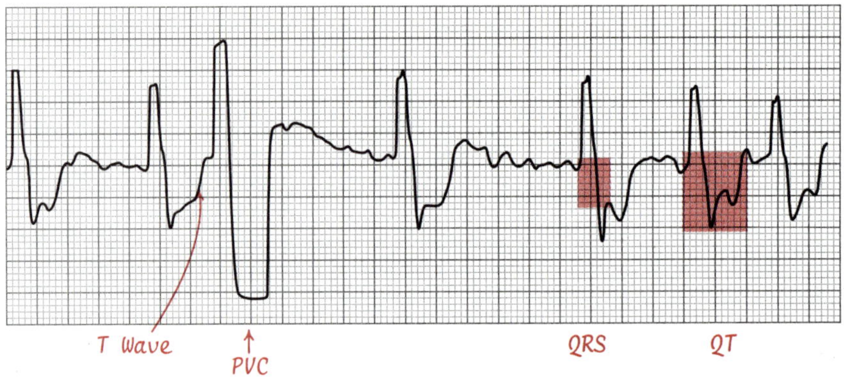

QRS duration 0.16 second QT n/a
Ventricular rate/rhythm 55-100/irregular
Atrial rate/rhythm n/a
PR interval n/a

Identification atrial fibrillation vent rate at 55-100/minute 6 mm ST ↓ and an R on T PVC
Symptoms none noted
Treatment ? meds/med Hx/vitals

Figure 7-39

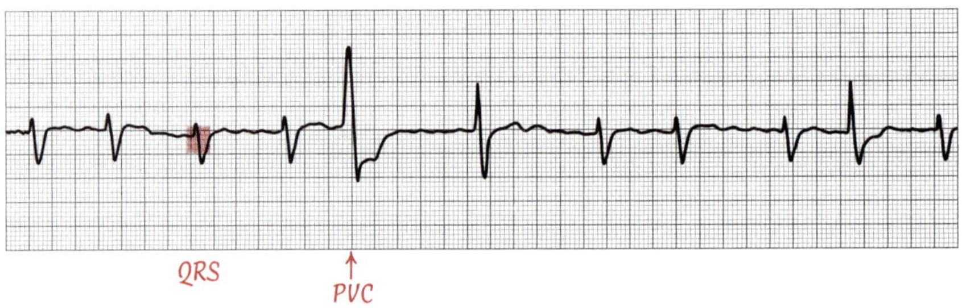

QRS duration 0.12-0.16 second QT UTD
Ventricular rate/rhythm 67-86/minute
Atrial rate/rhythm UTD
PR interval n/a

Identification atrial fibrillation 57-86/minute, PVC QRS 0.12-0.16 second
Symptoms none noted
Treatment ? meds/med Hx, be supportive

Figure 7-40

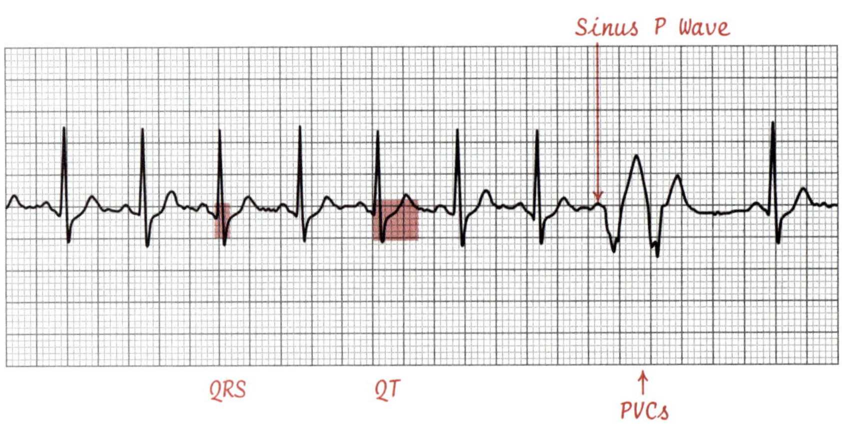

QRS duration 0.08 second QT 0.28 second
Ventricular rate/rhythm 116/regular
Atrial rate/rhythm 116/regular
PR interval 0.16 second

Identification sinus tach at 115 with end-diastolic; paired PVCs
Symptoms ? pain, ? meds/med Hx
Treatment Rx pain and consider lidocaine

CHAPTER 8 AV CONDUCTION DEFECTS

Fill in the Blanks

SINUS RHYTHM	FIRST-DEGREE AV BLOCK	SECOND-DEGREE AV BLOCK TYPE I
P: (+) P for each QRS PRI: 0.12–0.20 second	(+) P for each QRS >0.20 and consistent	(+) P for each QRS sinus P plots thru consistent after the dropped QRS; may progressively prolong as with Wenckebach phenomenon
QRS: 0.10 second or less QRS rate: 60–100 QRS rhythm: regular	0.10 second or less 60–100 regular	0.10 second or less 60–100 May be regular or irregular

SINUS RHYTHM	COMPLETE AV BLOCK	SECOND-DEGREE AV BLOCK TYPE II
P: (+) P for each QRS PRI: 0.12-0.20 second	P wave independent of QRS no consistent PRI	(+) P for each QRS sinus P plots thru consistent after the dropped QRS; may progressively prolong as with Wenckebach phenomenon
QRS: 0.10 second or less	0.10 second if junctional in origin >0.10 if ventricular in origin	>0.10 second may be notched, or an rS, or have a broad, terminal S wave
QRS rate: 60-100	40-60 but regular	60-100, usually slow
QRS rhythm: regular	regular	May be regular or irregular

ECG Rhythm Identification Practice

Figure 8-14

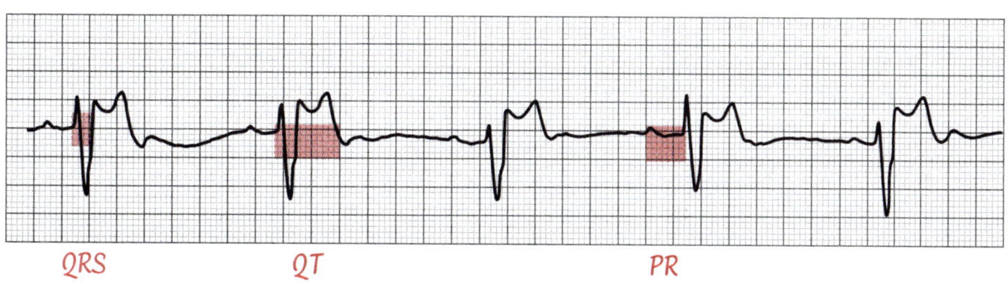

QRS duration 0.12 second QT 0.42 second

Ventricular rate/rhythm 41/minute

Atrial rate/rhythm 41/minute

PR interval 0.28 second

Identification sinus bradycardia, 1° AV block, 2 mm ST↑ QRS 0.12 second

Symptoms associated with bradycardia; dizziness, postural hypotension

Treatment ? meds/med Hx, be supportive; consider Atropine, fluids, dopamine, TCP

Figure 8-15

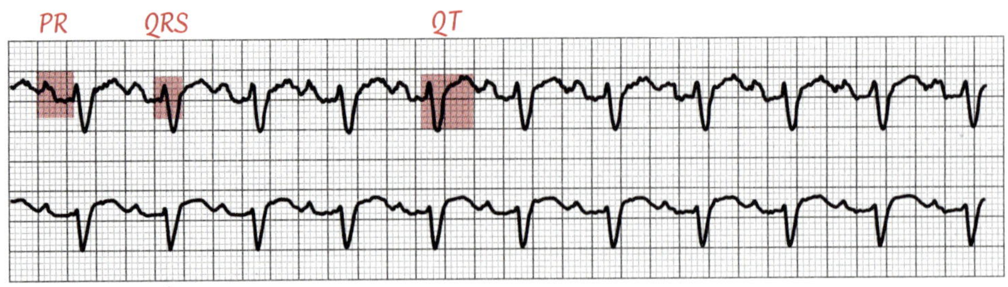

QRS duration 0.12 second QT 0.32-0.36 second

Ventricular rate/rhythm 100/regular

Atrial rate/rhythm 100/regular

PR interval 0.16 second

Identification sinus at 100 with 1° AV block QRS > 0.12 sec, ? 1-2 mm ST ↑

Symptoms pain, ? meds/med Hx

Treatment Rx pain and consider lidocaine

Figure 8-16

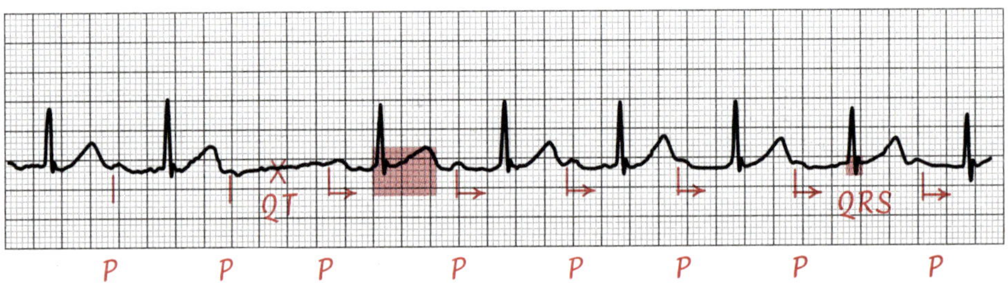

QRS duration 0.08 second QT 0.44 second

Ventricular rate/rhythm 43-75/minute

Atrial rate/rhythm 75/regular

PR interval 0.32, 0.38, 0.40, 0.42

Identification sinus at 75 with 2° AV block probably Type I with Wenckebach

Symptoms none noted

Treatment ? meds/med Hx/vitals

Figure 8-17

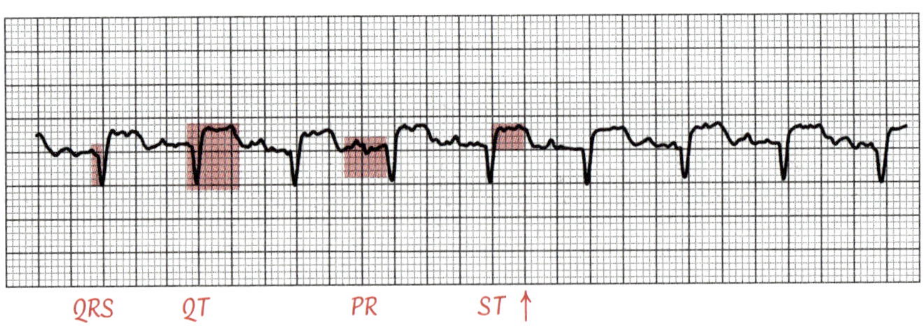

QRS duration 0.04-0.06 second QT 0.28 second

Ventricular rate/rhythm 100/minute

Atrial rate/rhythm 100/minute

PR interval 0.24 second

Identification sinus at 100/minute with 1° AV block with 3 mm ST segment; Q waves 4-5 mm.

Symptoms may have pain

Treatment ? meds/med Hx, be supportive, if pain, Rx the pain

Figure 8-18

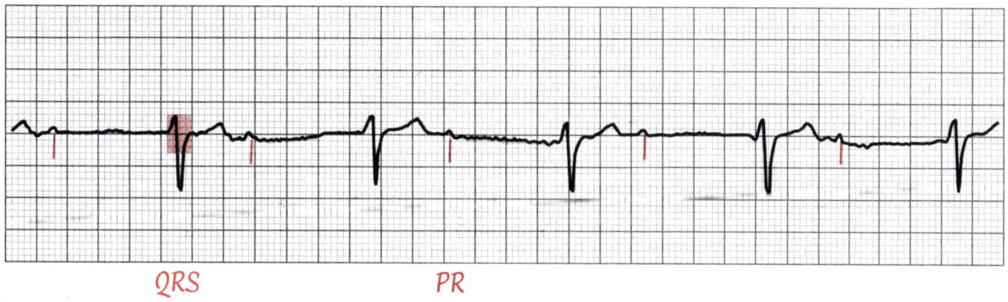

QRS duration 0.10 second QT 0.38 second

Ventricular rate/rhythm 50/minute

Atrial rate/rhythm 50/minute

PR interval 0.78 second

Identification sinus brady at 50/minute with 1° AV block ? isorhythmic AV dissociation

Symptoms associated with bradycardia, i.e., dizziness, postural hypotension

Treatment if symptomatic with bradycardia, consider Atropine, fluids, dopamine, TCP

Figure 8-19

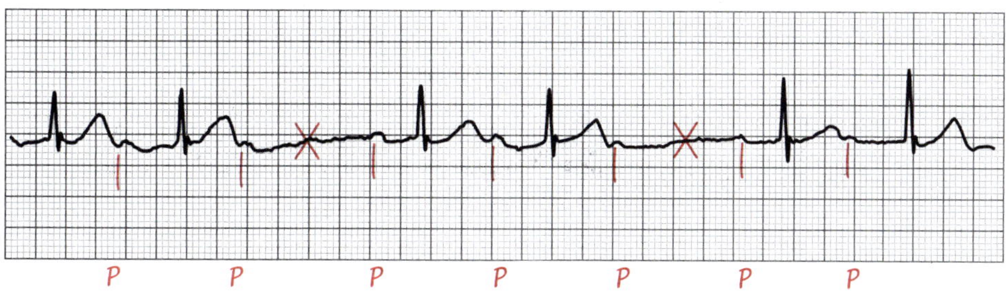

QRS duration 0.08 second QT 0.40 second

Ventricular rate/rhythm 40-75/minute

Atrial rate/rhythm 75/minute

PR interval 0.32, 0.38

Identification sinus at 75 with vent rate 40-75/minute, 2° AV block probably Type I (QRS = 0.08)

Symptoms none noted

Treatment ? meds/med Hx/vitals

Figure 8-20

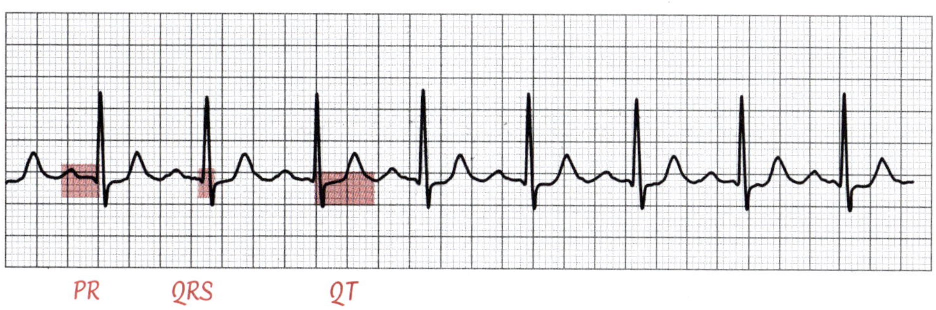

QRS duration 0.08 second QT 0.36 second

Ventricular rate/rhythm 86/minute

Atrial rate/rhythm 75/minute

PR interval 0.24 second

Identification sinus at 86/minute with 1° AV block

Symptoms none noted

Treatment ? meds/med Hx, be supportive

Figure 8-21

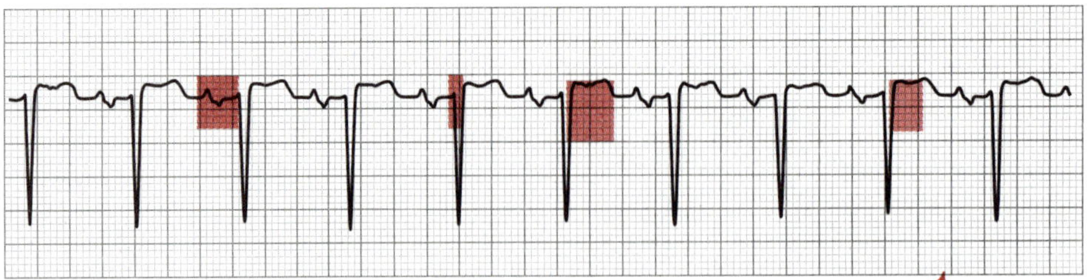

QRS duration 0.06-0.10 second QT 0.32 second

Ventricular rate/rhythm 100/minute

Atrial rate/rhythm 100/minute

PR interval 0.24-0.26 second

Identification sinus at 100 with 1° AV block 2 mm ST seg ↑

Symptoms ? pain, ? meds/med Hx

Treatment Rx the pain, ? meds/med Hx

Figure 8-22

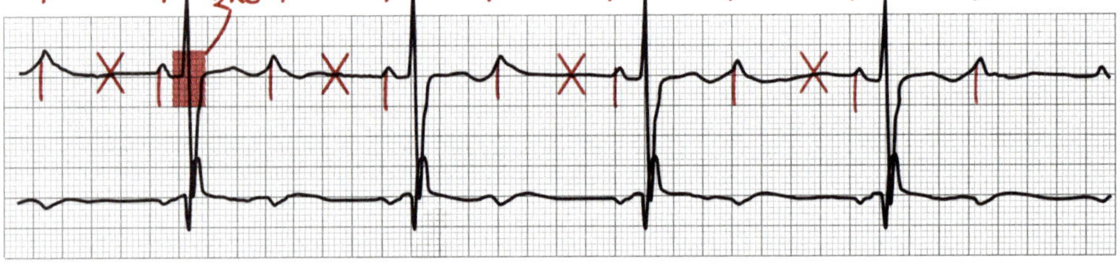

QRS duration 0.12 second QT 0.42-0.44 second

Ventricular rate/rhythm 40/minute

Atrial rate/rhythm 75/minute

PR interval 0.20 second

Identification sinus at 75 with vent rate 40/min, 2° AV block, probably Type II, (QRS 0.16 sec), PR after missed beat is consistent

Symptoms associated with bradycardia

Treatment Rx bradycardia, TCP, may require dopamine for perfusion

Figure 8-23

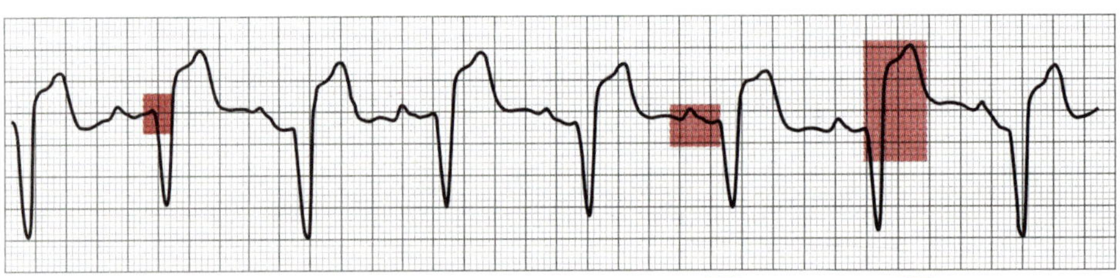

QRS duration 0.12 second QT 0.32-0.36 second

Ventricular rate/rhythm 86/minute

Atrial rate/rhythm 86/minute

PR interval 0.24-0.26 second

Identification sinus arrhythmia at 50-55/min with 1° AV block, 7 mm ST ↑, Q waves 15-17 mm

Symptoms may be associated with chest pain

Treatment ? meds/med Hx, Rx the pain

CHAPTER 9 ELECTRICAL INTERVENTIONS

Matching

1. B
2. J
3. C
4. E
5. G
6. F
7. I
8. A
9. D
10. H

CHAPTER 10 ELECTRONIC PACEMAKERS

Matching

1. H
2. P
3. J
4. N
5. K
6. E
7. C
8. D
9. B
10. T
11. V
12. U
13. Q
14. F
15. L
16. R
17. O
18. G
19. A
20. M
21. I

ECG Rhythm Identification Practice

Figure 10-13

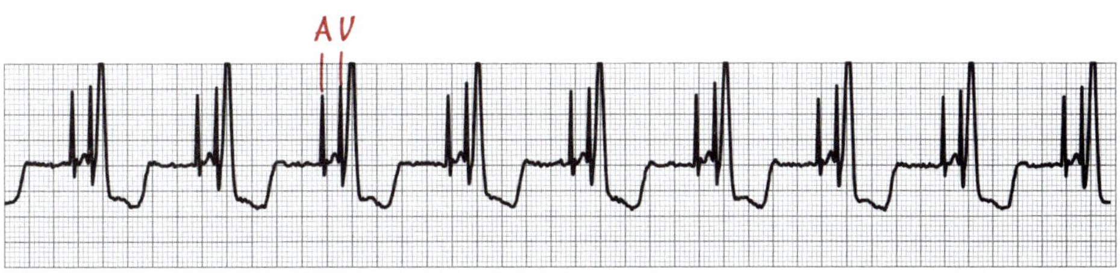

QRS duration 0.20 second QT 0.44 second

Ventricular rate/rhythm 60/minute/regular

Atrial rate/rhythm 60/minute/regular

PR interval none noted

Identification dual-chamber pacer at 60/minute

Symptoms none noted

Treatment be supportive

Figure 10-14

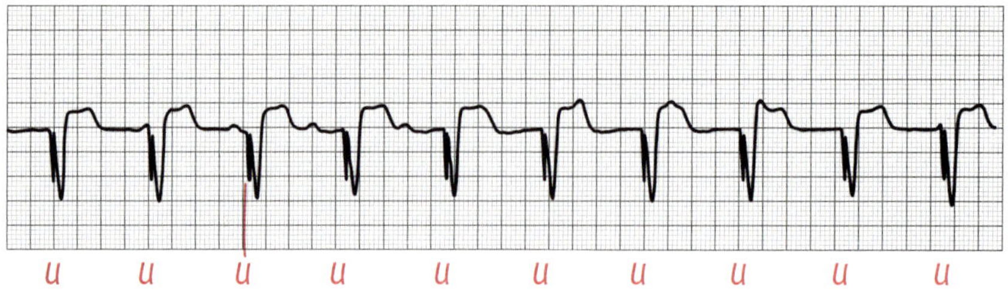

QRS duration 0.16 second QT 0.42 second

Ventricular rate/rhythm 70/minute/regular

Atrial rate/rhythm UTD

PR interval UTD

Identification vent pacer at 70/minute

Symptoms probably none

Treatment be supportive

Figure 10-15

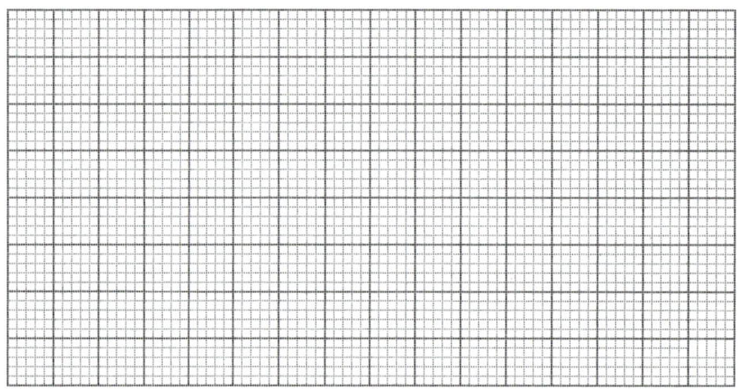

QRS duration 0.16 second QT 0.40 second

Ventricular rate/rhythm 72/regular

Atrial rate/rhythm UTD

PR interval UTD

Identification ventricular demand pacer at 72/minute R-V is consistent

Symptoms probably none

Treatment be supportive

Figure 10-16

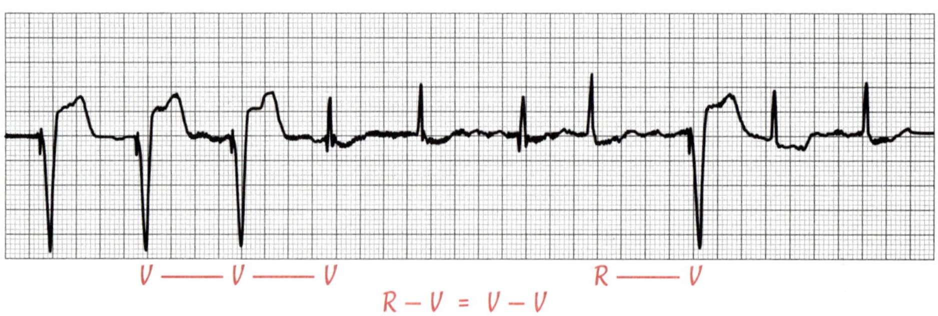

QRS duration 0.04 second QT UTD

QRS pacer = 0.16 QT pacer = 0.44

Ventricular rate/rhythm pacer = 75, a-fib = 67-110

Atrial rate/rhythm 75/regular

PR interval none noted

Identification ventricular demand pacer at 75 with atrial fib 67-110; possible pacer artifacts fused with first QRS of a-fib—at that point the pacer is isorhythmic and there is no problem

Symptoms none noted

Treatment be supportive

Figure 10-17

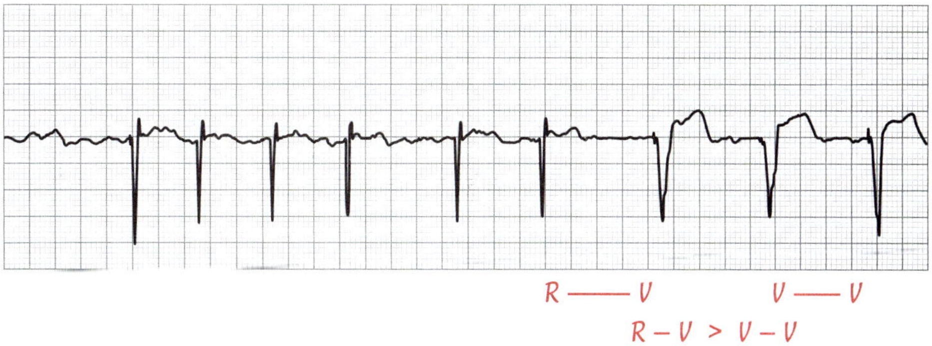

QRS duration 0.08 pacer, 0.16 sec **QT** UTD pacer, 0.44 sec

Ventricular rate/rhythm 75-125 → 75/minute/regular

Atrial rate/rhythm UTD

PR interval UTD

Identification atrial fib 75-125 → vent demand pacer at 75/minute R-V>V-V (0.08 second) ? hysteresis

Symptoms probably none

Treatment be supportive

Figure 10-18

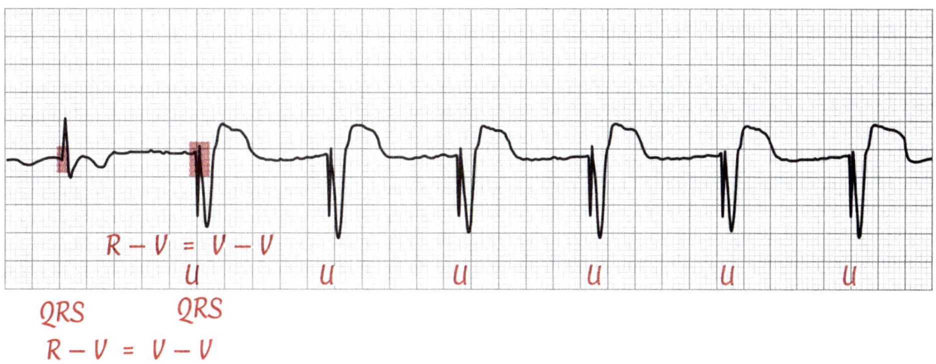

QRS duration 0.08 pacer, 0.16 sec **QT** 0.10 pacer, 0.44 sec

Ventricular rate/rhythm pacer = 61 minute

Atrial rate/rhythm UTD

PR interval UTD

Identification atrial fib 75-125 → vent demand pacer at 61/minute, R-V = V-V

Symptoms probably none

Treatment be supportive

Figure 10-19

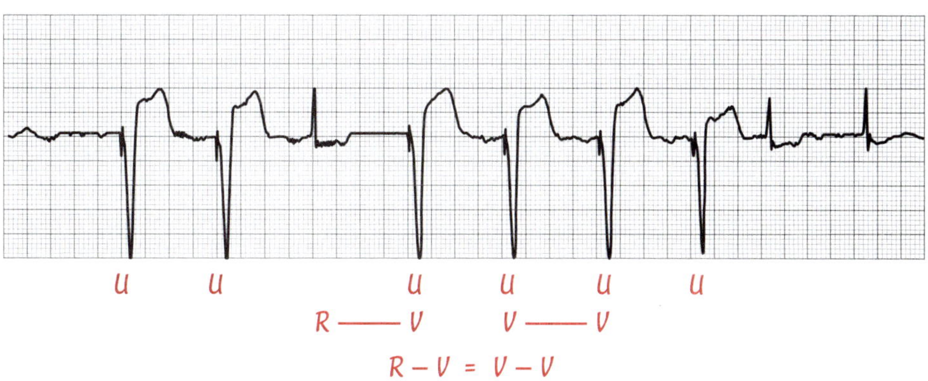

QRS duration 0.08 pacer, 0.16 sec **QT** UTD pacer, 0.44 sec

Ventricular rate/rhythm 75-125 → 75/minute/regular

Atrial rate/rhythm UTD

PR interval UTD

Identification atrial fib 71 → vent demand pacer at 75/minute, R-V = V-V

Symptoms probably none

Treatment be supportive

Figure 10-20

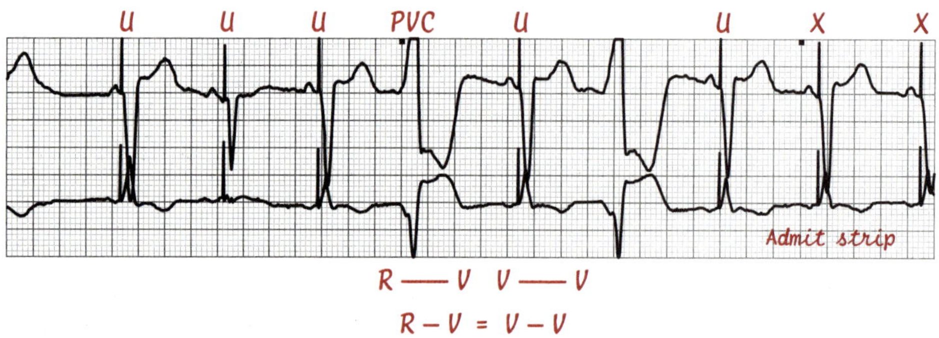

QRS duration pacer = 0.16 sec QT pacer = 0.44 sec

Ventricular rate/rhythm 75/minute/regular

Atrial rate/rhythm 75/minute/regular

PR interval UTD

Identification demand pacer at 75/minute with freq u/f PVCs; escape interval is OK

Symptoms probably none

Treatment be supportive

Figure 10-21

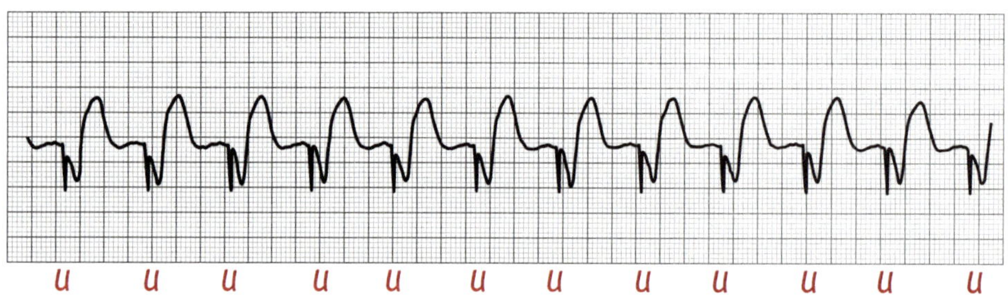

QRS duration 0.16 second QT 0.44 second

Ventricular rate/rhythm 86/minute/regular

Atrial rate/rhythm UTD

PR interval UTD

Identification vent pacer at 86/minute, V-V is consistent

Symptoms probably none

Treatment be supportive

Figure 10-22

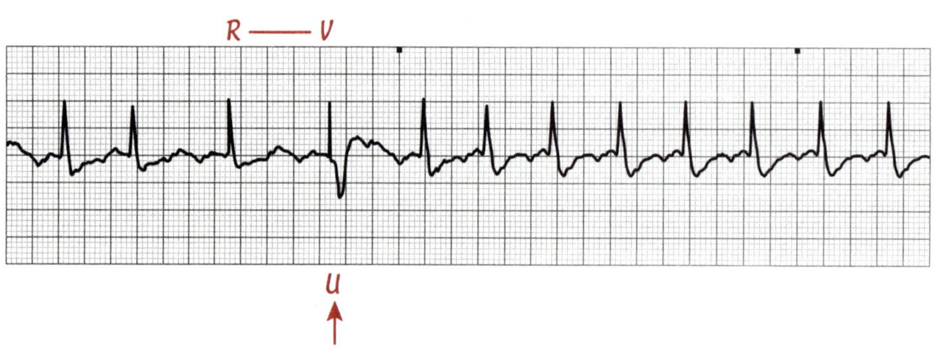

QRS duration 0.10, pacer = 0.16 sec QT pacer = 0.44 sec

Ventricular rate/rhythm 75-110/minute

Atrial rate/rhythm UTD (296-atrial flutter)

PR interval n/a

Identification atrial flutter, 75-110/minute, vent demand pacer

Symptoms probably none

Treatment be supportive

Figure 10-23

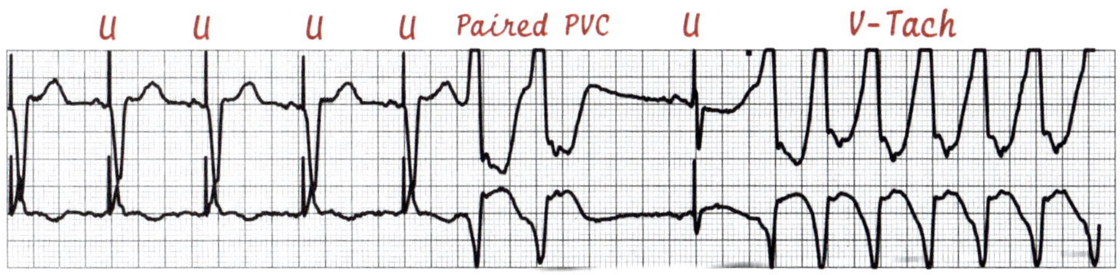

QRS duration pacer = 0.16 sec **QT** pacer = 0.44 sec

Ventricular rate/rhythm 75/minute/regular → 150/minute

Atrial rate/rhythm 75/minute/regular

PR interval n/a

Identification demand pacer at 75/minute, paired PVCs → one paced → beat vent tach at 150

Symptoms associated with v-tach

Treatment Rx the vent tach

CHAPTER 11 THE 12-LEAD ECG

Matching

1. D
2. B
3. C
4. E
5. A

ECG Rhythm Identification Practice

Figure 11-23

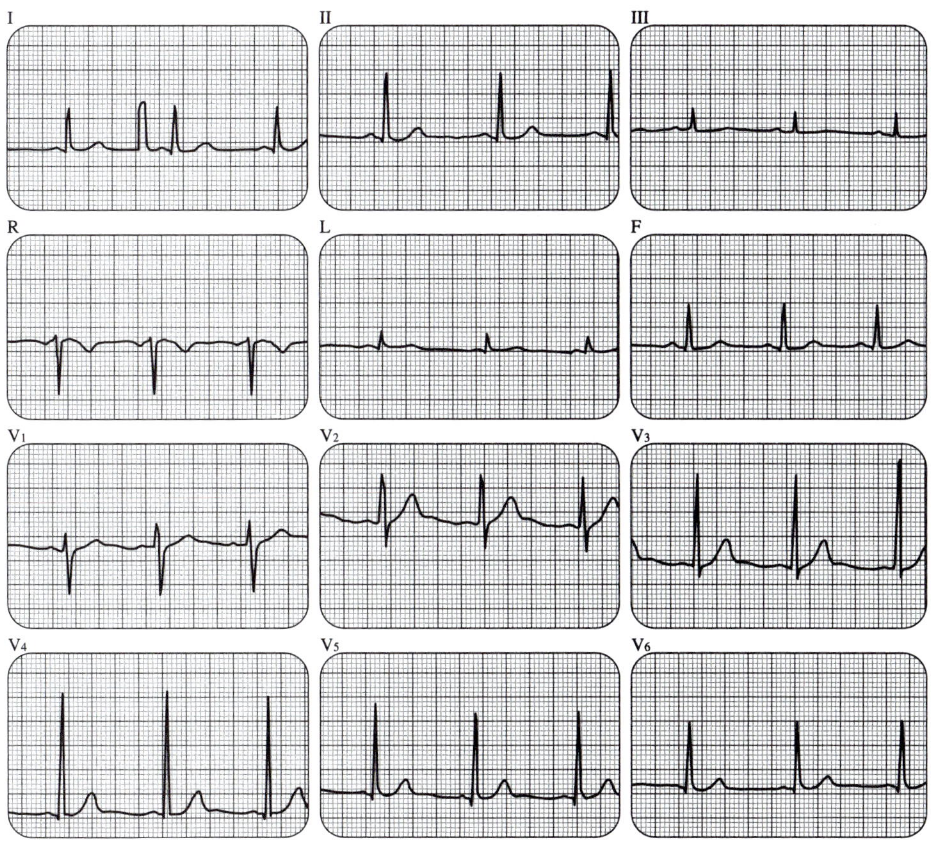

1. **What is the underlying rhythm?**
   Underlying rhythm is sinus at 60/minute.
2. **What are the acute changes?**
   None noted.
3. **What is your interpretation?**
   Interpretation is sinus at 60/minute.
4. **What can happen next?**
   Be supportive.

Figure 11-24

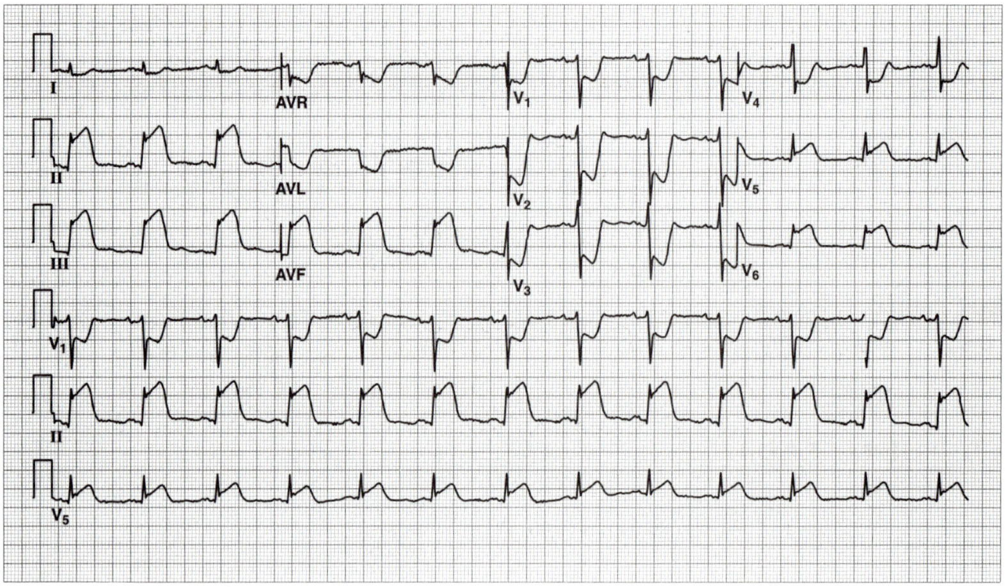

1. **What is the underlying rhythm?**
   Underlying rhythm is sinus at 75/minute.
2. **What are the acute changes?**
   Acute changes are 7 mm ST seg ↑ in II, III, and with reciprocal changes in AVL (ST ↓). There are R waves in $V_2 \rightarrow V_4$ with ST ↓ in V_2, V_3, V_4; ST ↑ in V_5 and V_6.
3. **What is your interpretation?**
   Interpretation is acute infero-posterior wall MI ? Extension to the LL surface?
4. **What can happen next?**
   Observe for SA and AV conduction problems, s/s failure.

Figure 11-25

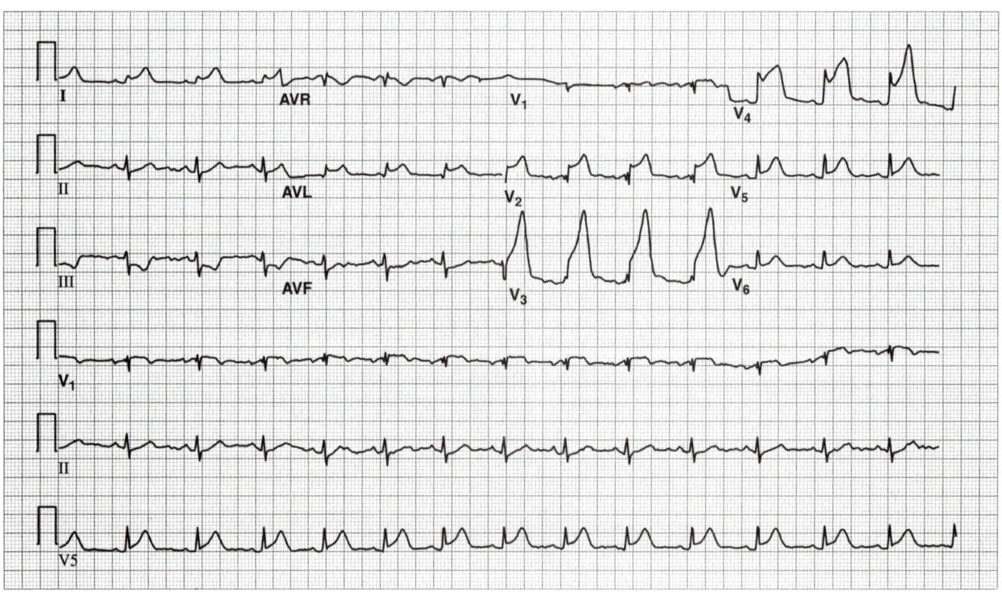

1. **What is the underlying rhythm?**
   Underlying rhythm is sinus at 85/minute.
2. **What are the acute changes?**
   Acute changes are 2mm ST seg ↑ in I, AVL and with reciprocal ST ↓ in II, III, and AVF. There are Q waves in V_1 and V_2. There is progressive ST ↑ in V_2, V_3, and V_4, 2-3 mm ST ↑ in V_5 and V_6.
3. **What is your interpretation?**
   Interpretation is sinus at 85/minute with acute anteroseptal myocardial infarction, extension of injury and ischemia to the antero-lateral surface.
4. **What can happen next?**
   Observe for AV and BB conduction problems, s/s failure.

Figure 11-26

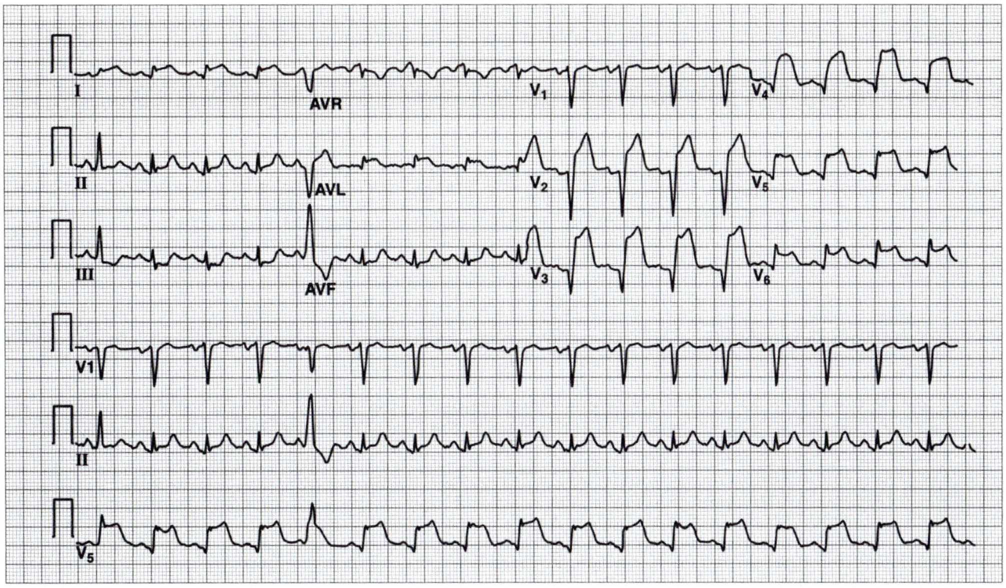

1. **What is the underlying rhythm?**
   Underlying rhythm is sinus at 100/minute.
2. **What are the acute changes?**
   Acute changes are 2 mm ST seg ↑ in I, aVL, and with reciprocal ST ↓ in III and perhaps aVF. There are Q waves in $V_2 \rightarrow V_6$. There is progressive ST ↑ in V_2, V_3, V_4; 5 mm ST ↑ in V_5 and 4 mm ST ↑ in V_6.
3. **What is your interpretation?**
   Interpretation is sinus at 100/minute with acute anterolateral myocardial infarction.
4. **What can happen next?**
   Observe for AV and BB conduction problems, s/s failure.

Figure 11-27

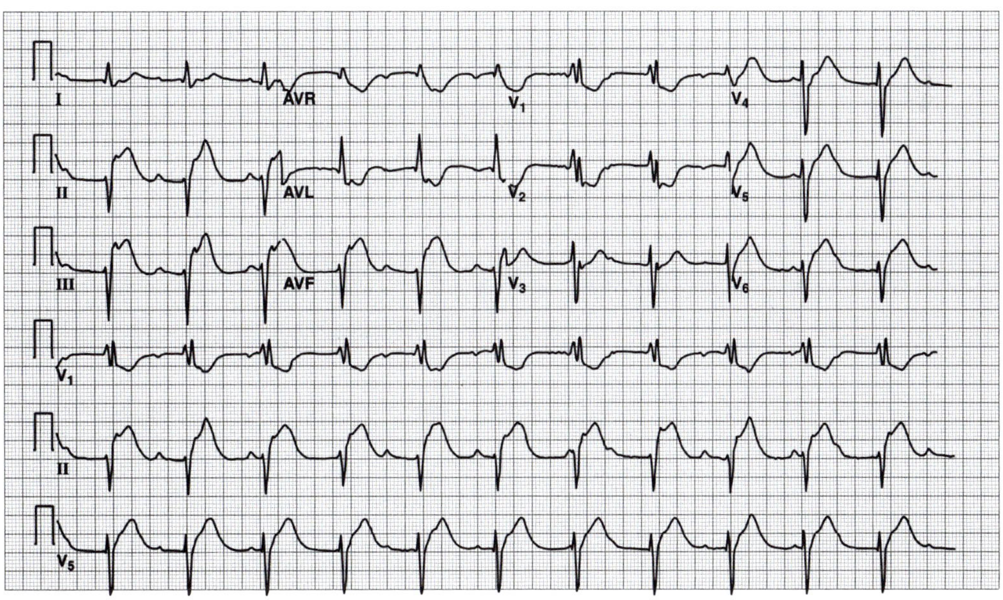

1. **What is the underlying rhythm?**
   Underlying rhythm is sinus at 60 with complete AV block, accelerated junctional rhythm at 67/minute
2. **What are the acute changes?**
   Acute changes are broad S wave in I, AVL; ST ↑ in II, III, and AVF; rS configuration in II, III, and AVF. The QRS in V_1, V_2 and V_3 shows an RSR. There is ST ↓ in V_2, V_3 with ST ↑ in V_4, V_5 and V_6.
3. **What is your interpretation?**
   Interpretation is sinus at 60/minute with acute inferior, possible posterior MI, RBB which may mask the posterior injury pattern.
4. **What can happen next?**
   Observe for BB conduction problems, s/s failure. Consider standby for TCP.

Figure 11-28

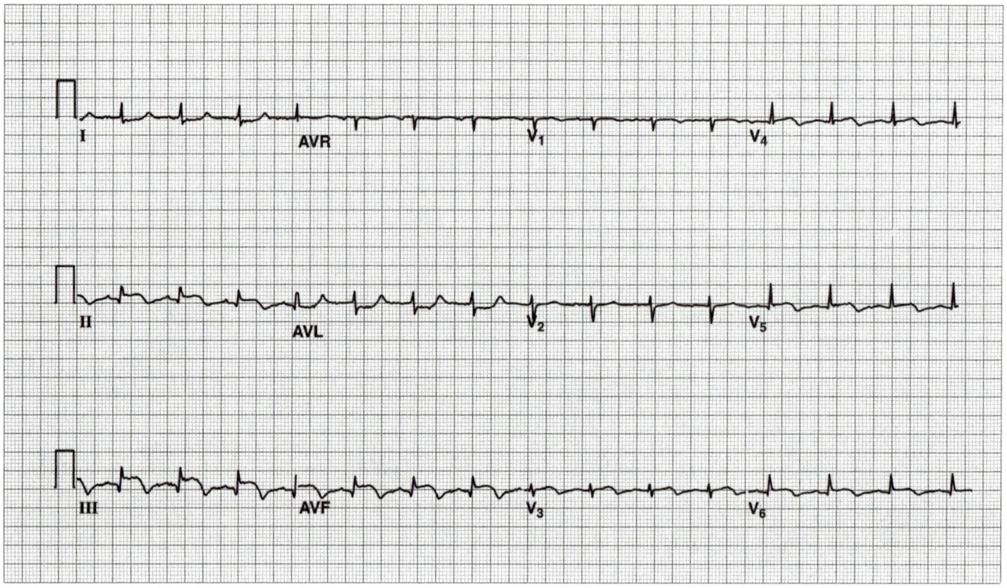

1. **What is the underlying rhythm?**
   Underlying rhythm is sinus at 86, QT 40.
2. **What are the acute changes?**
   Acute changes are small Qs and ST ↑in leads II, III, and AVF reciprocal ST ↓ in I and AVL. T waves in V_4, V_5, and V_6.
3. **What is your interpretation?**
   Interpretation is sinus at 86/minute with inferior myocardial infarction.
4. **What can happen next?**
   Observe for SA and AV conduction problems.

Figure 11-29

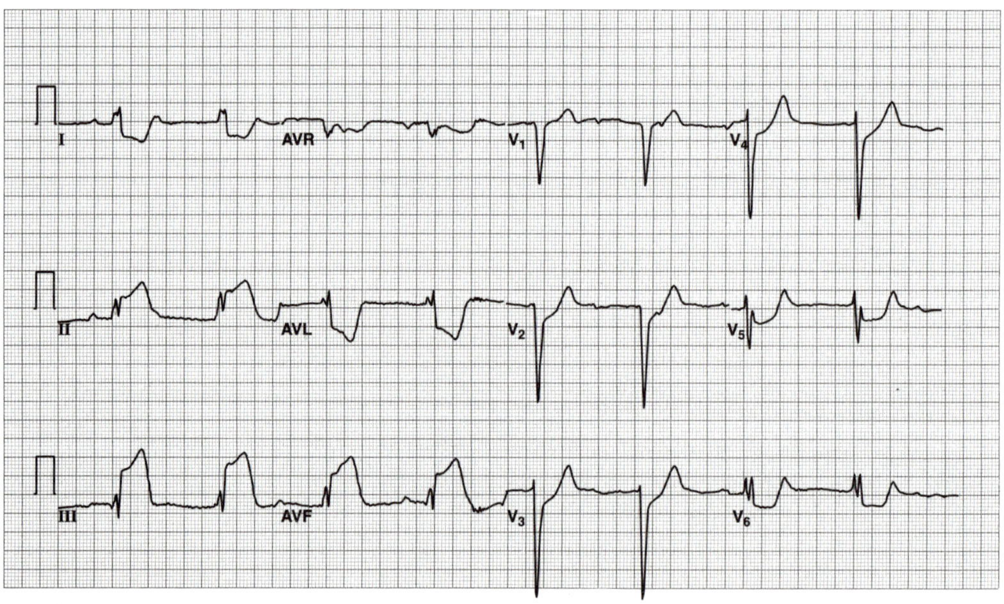

1. **What is the underlying rhythm?**
   Underlying rhythm is sinus at 86 complete AV block with ventricular rate at 50/minute.
2. **What are the acute changes?**
   Acute changes are broad QRS, notched, 14 second in leads I, II, III, and V_6. ST ↑in leads II, III, and AVF; reciprocal ST ↓ in I and AVL. There are deep Qs; ST ↓ in V_2, V_4, V_5, and V_6.
3. **What is your interpretation?**
   Interpretation is sinus at 86/minute with complete AV block; idiojunctional rhythm at 50/minute. Acute anteroseptal MI. Current of injury pattern in II, III, and AVF showing inferior involvement. There is left bundle branch block.
4. **What can happen next?**
   Observe for AV s/s failure; stand by for TCP.

Figure 11-30

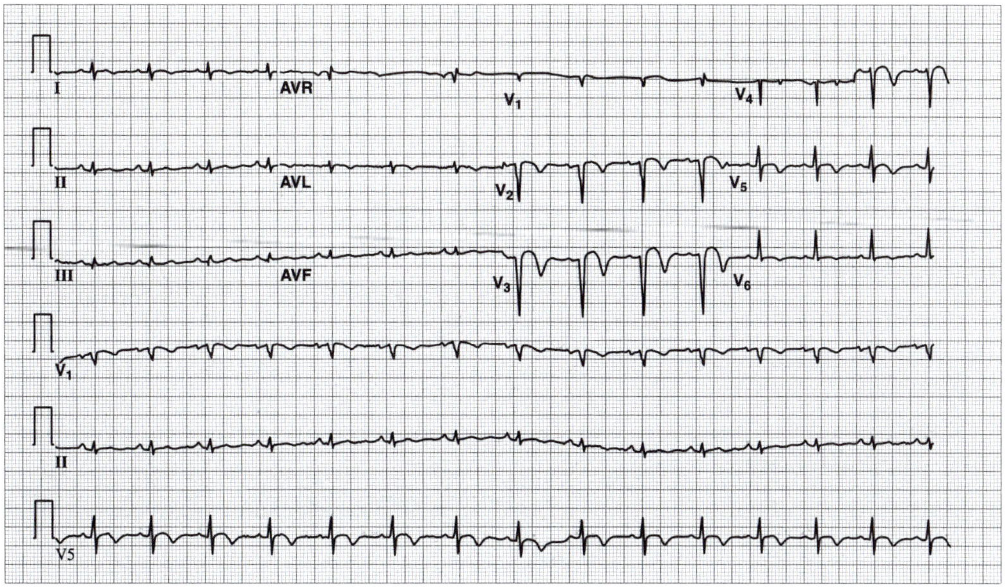

1. **What is the underlying rhythm?**
   Underlying rhythm is sinus at 90/minute.
2. **What are the acute changes?**
   Acute changes are T wave ↓ in I and AVL, $V_1 \rightarrow V_6$; There are deep Qs, ST ↓ in V_2 and V_3; small R waves in V_4.
3. **What is your interpretation?**
   Interpretation is sinus at 90/minute with anteroseptal MI. Current of injury pattern in II, III, and AVF showing inferior involvement.
4. **What can happen next?**
   Observe for s/s failure; stand by for TCP.

Figure 11-31

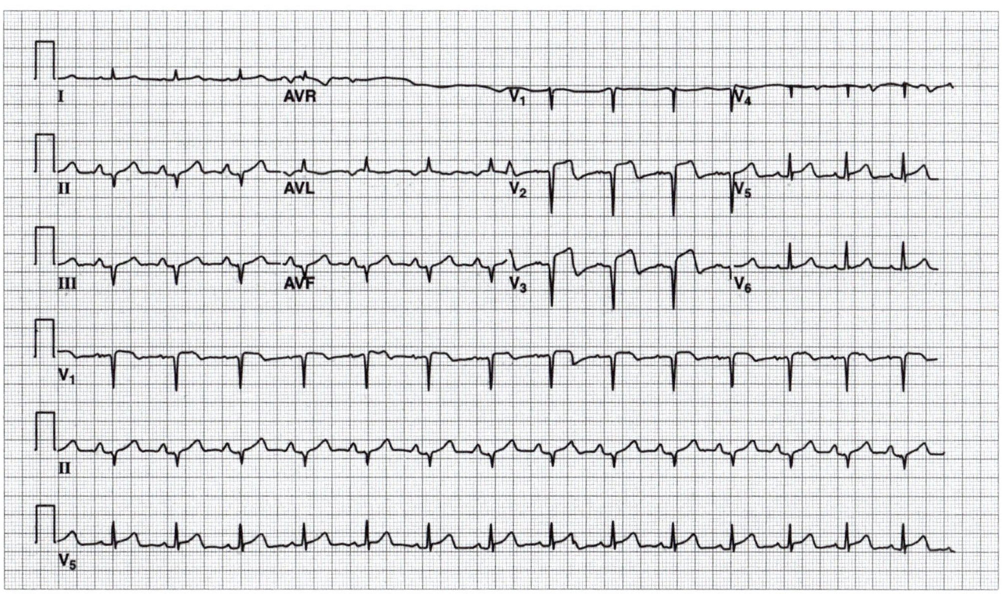

1. **What is the underlying rhythm?**
   Underlying rhythm is sinus at 86/minute
2. **What are the acute changes?**
   Acute changes are rS or QS in II, III, and AVF (no reciprocal changes in I or AVL). Q wave, ST ↑ V_2 and V_5.
3. **What is your interpretation?**
   Interpretation is sinus at 86/minute; acute anteroseptal MI; need serial ECG to clarify presence of Q waves in leads II, III, and AVF.
4. **What can happen next?**
   Observe for AV and/or BB conduction defects.

Figure 11-32

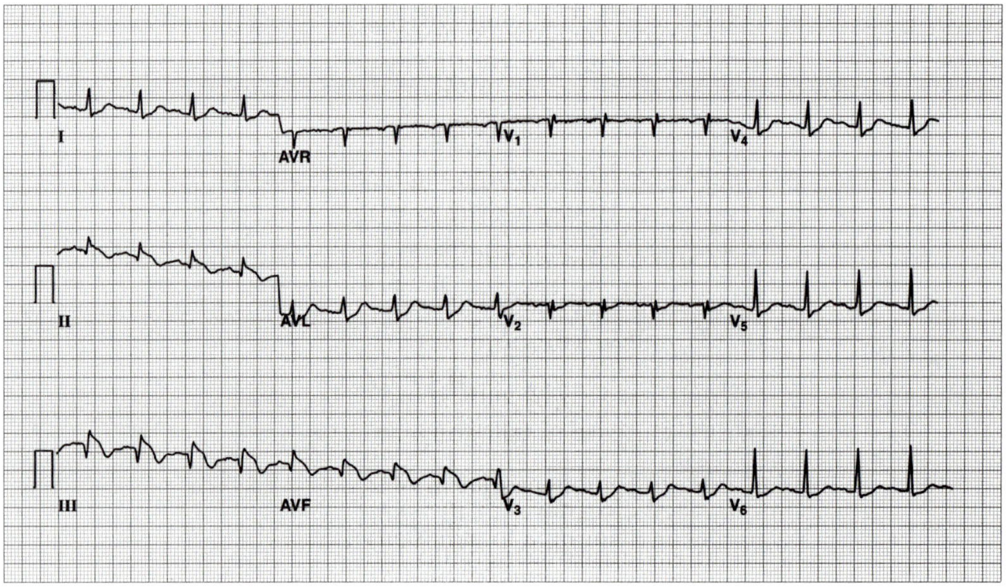

1. **What is the underlying rhythm?**
   Underlying rhythm is sinus at 100/minute
2. **What are the acute changes?**
   Acute changes are Q waves, ST ↑ and T wave ↓ in leads II, III, and AVF; reciprocal ST ↓ in I and AVL; deep Qs, ST ↓ in V_1 and V_2.
3. **What is your interpretation?**
   Interpretation is sinus at 100/minute; acute infero-anteroseptal myocardial infarction.
4. **What can happen next?**
   Observe for SA and AV conduction defects, BB blocks, s/s failure

Figure 11-33

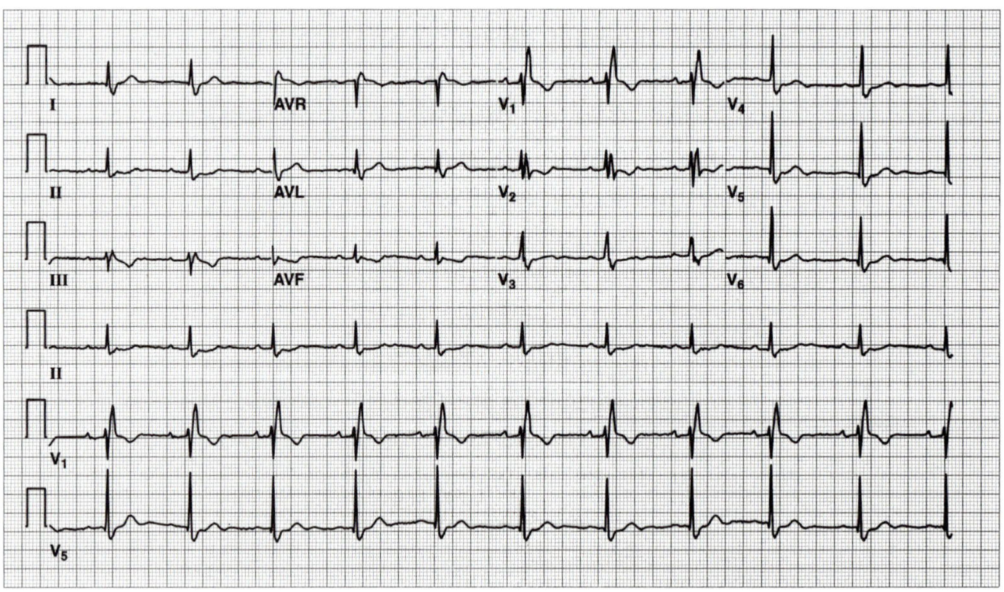

1. **What is the underlying rhythm?**
   Underlying rhythm is sinus at 60/minute. ? 1° AV block (PR = 0.22 second).
2. **What are the acute changes?**
   Acute changes are none. There is a broad terminal S wave in leads I, II, AVF, V_3, V_4, V_5, and V_6. There is RSR in V_1 and V_2. I and AVL: there are deep Qs. ST ↓ in V_1 and V_2.
3. **What is your interpretation?**
   Interpretation is sinus at 60/minute with RBBB, possibly first-degree AV block.
4. **What can happen next?**
   ? meds/med Hx; be supportive.

CHAPTER 12 ARRYTHMIAS DUE TO ABNORMAL CONDUCTION PATHWAYS

ECG Rhythm Identification Practice

Figure 12-11

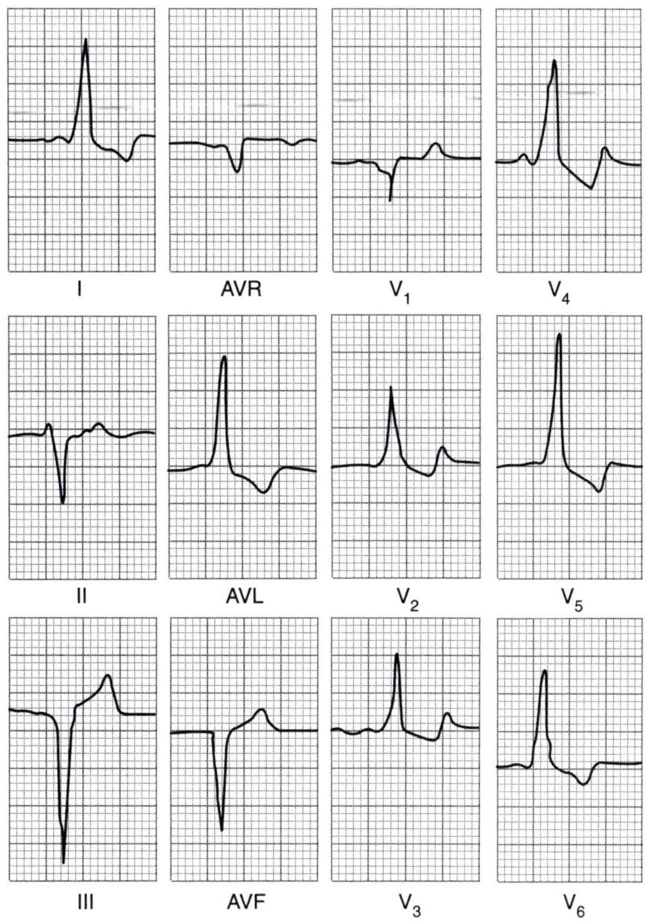

1. What is the underlying rhythm? *Sinus*
2. What are the abnormalities? *rS in lead II, QS in III, AVF, delta in I, AVL(+), III and AVF(-)*

   PRI *0.10 second*

   QRS *0.12 second*
3. What is the interpretation? *Sinus with pattern of preexcitation*

Figure 12-12

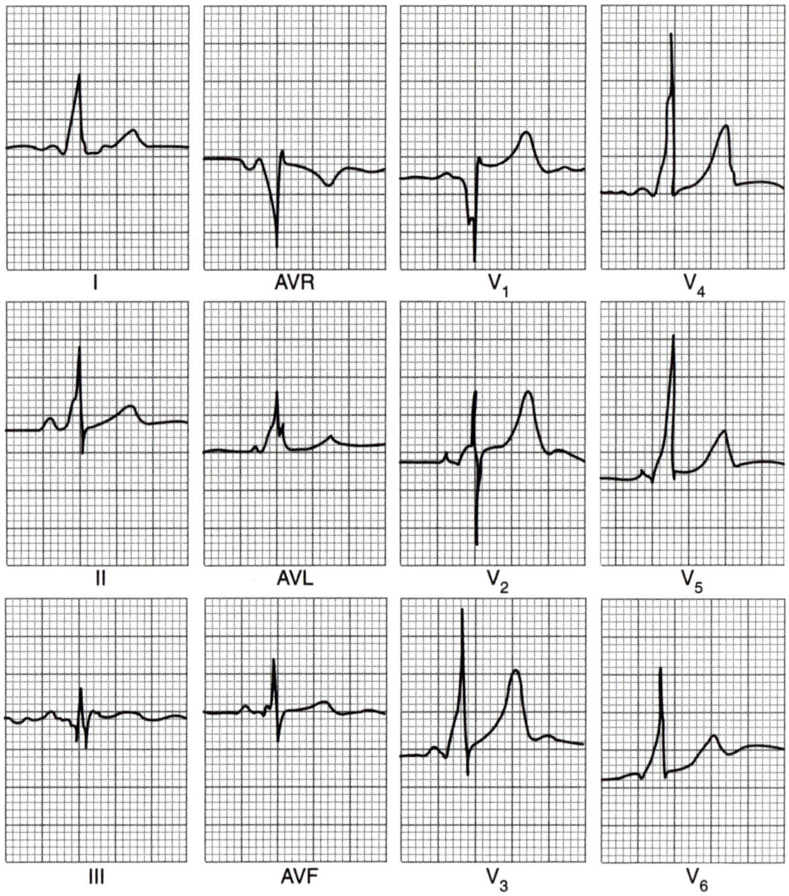

1. **What is the underlying rhythm?** *Sinus*
2. **What are the abnormalities?** *delta in all leads*
   PRI *0.10 second*
   QRS *0.12 second*
3. **What is the interpretation?** *Sinus with pattern of preexcitation*

Figure 12-13

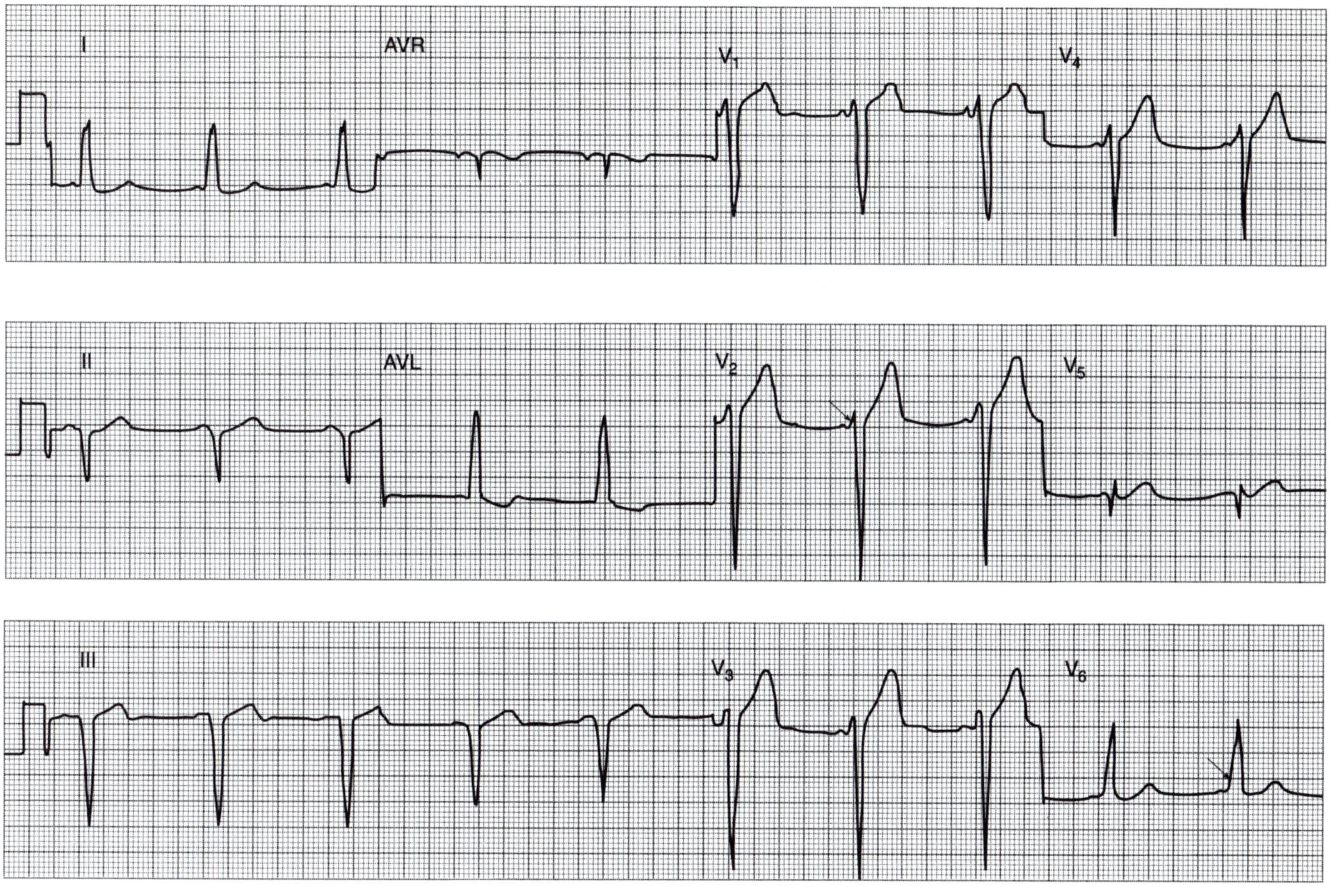

1. **What is the underlying rhythm?** Sinus at 60/minute
2. **What are the abnormalities?** QS in II, III, AVF(+), delta in I, AVL, V_5 and V_6

   PRI 0.08 second

   QRS 0.14 second
3. **What is the interpretation?** Sinus with pattern of preexcitation

CHAPTER 13 GENERAL REVIEW AND ASSESSMENT EXERCISES

Figure 13-1

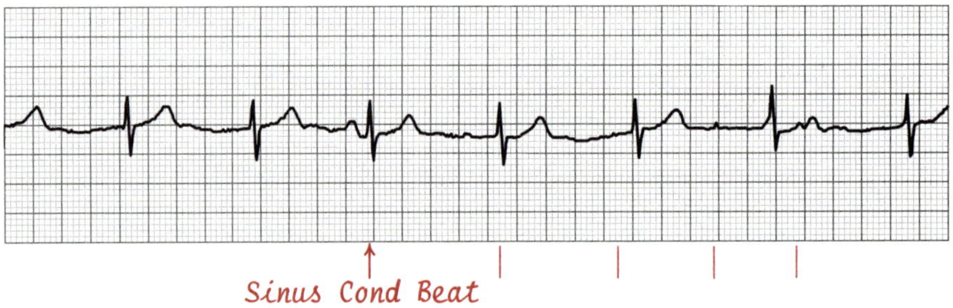

QRS duration 0.08 second **QT** 0.40 second

Ventricular rate/rhythm 67/minute/regular

Atrial rate/rhythm 100/minutes/regular

PR interval none noted

Identification sinus rate 100, complete AV block with accelerated junctional rhythm at 67/minute. There is one sinus conducted beat.

Symptoms ? meds, ? med Hx, ? dizziness s/s hypoperfusion

Treatment stand by for TCP, ? fluids and dopamine for perfusion

Figure 13-2

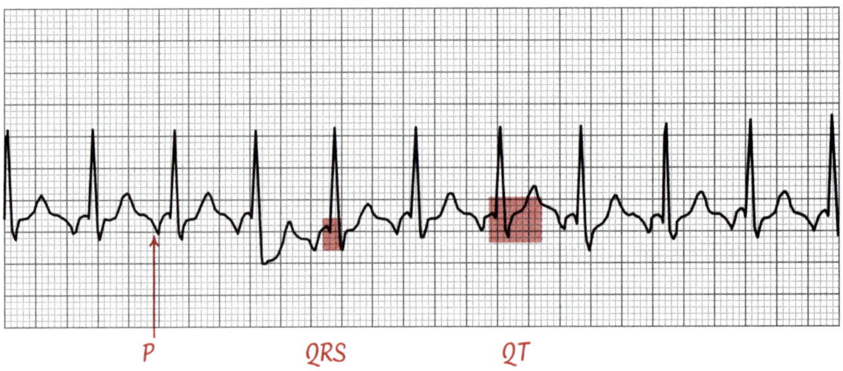

QRS duration 0.10 second **QT** 0.24 second

Ventricular rate/rhythm 110/minutes/regular

Atrial rate/rhythm 110/minute/regular

PR interval 0.12 second

Identification junctional tachycardia vent rate 110/minute.

Symptoms ? dizziness, postural hypotension

Treatment assess for s/s ↓ perfusion; ? why

Figure 13-3

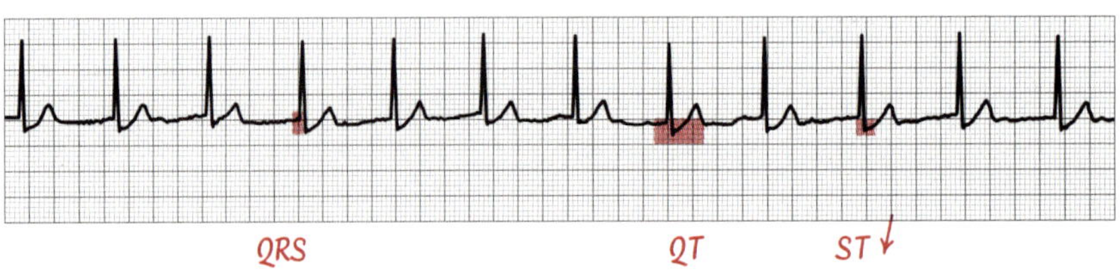

QRS duration 0.04 second **QT** 0.24 second

Ventricular rate/rhythm 75/regular

Atrial rate/rhythm UTD

PR interval UTD

Identification accelerated junctional rhythm at 75/minute.

Symptoms probably none

Treatment ? meds/med Hx; be supportive; ? why

Figure 13-4

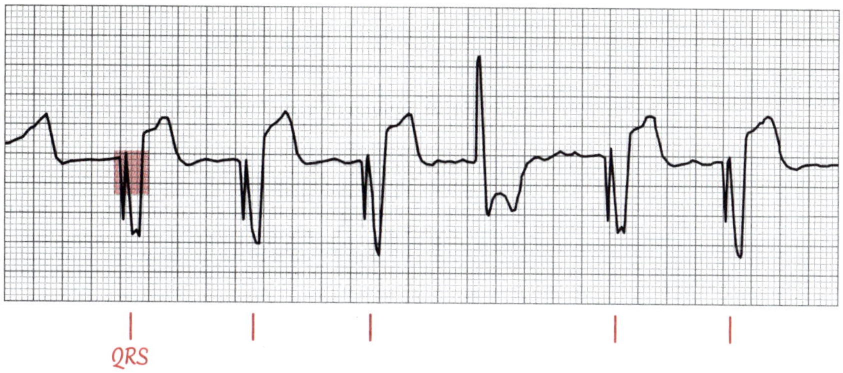

QRS duration 0.16 second QT 0.40 second

Ventricular rate/rhythm pacer at 75/minute (except for event)

Atrial rate/rhythm UTD

PR interval none noted

Identification ventricular demand pacer, a PVC, 75/minute with probably an underlying atrial fibrillation, R-V = V-V

Symptoms probably none

Treatment be supportive

Figure 13-5

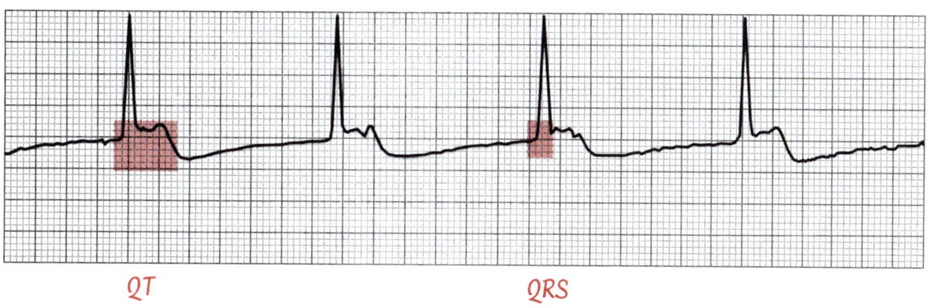

QRS duration 0.10 second QT 0.24 second

Ventricular rate/rhythm 46/minute/regular

Atrial rate/rhythm UTD

PR interval UTD

Identification junctional rhythm, vent rate 46/minute

Symptoms ? dizziness, postural hypotension

Treatment if hypotensive and hypoperfusing, ABCs, O_2, (P), IV, ? meds/med Hx, V/S/ allergies; consider Atropine, fluids, dopamine, pace

Figure 13-6

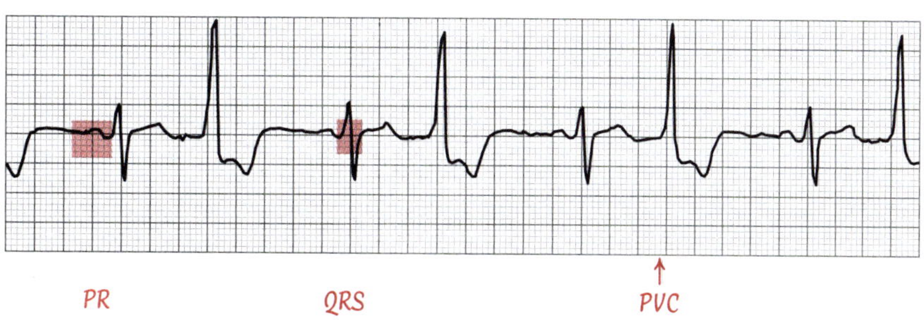

QRS duration 0.12 second QT 0.36 second

Ventricular rate/rhythm 70/bigeminal

Atrial rate/rhythm 35/minute

PR interval 0.16 second

Identification sinus with ventricular bigeminy; overall rate is 70/minute (QRS = 0.12 second rS pattern)

Symptoms probably none

Treatment ? meds/med Hx; be supportive

Figure 13-7

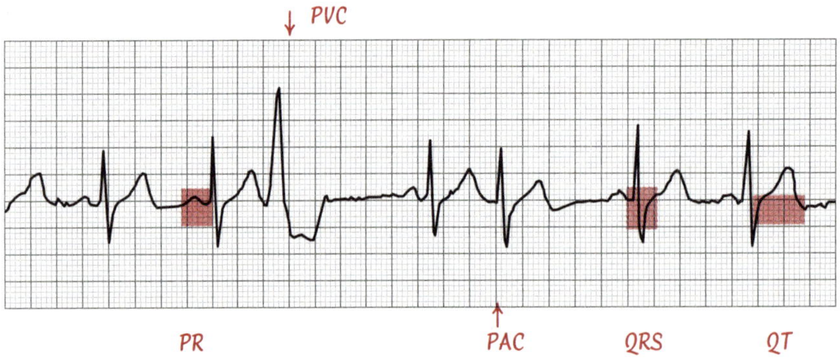

QRS duration 0.10 second **QT** 0.44 second
Ventricular rate/rhythm 67/minute/regular
Atrial rate/rhythm 67/minute/regular
PR interval 0.16 second

Identification sinus at 67/minute with a PAC and an R on T PVC
Symptoms probably none
Treatment ? meds/med Hx; be supportive

Figure 13-8

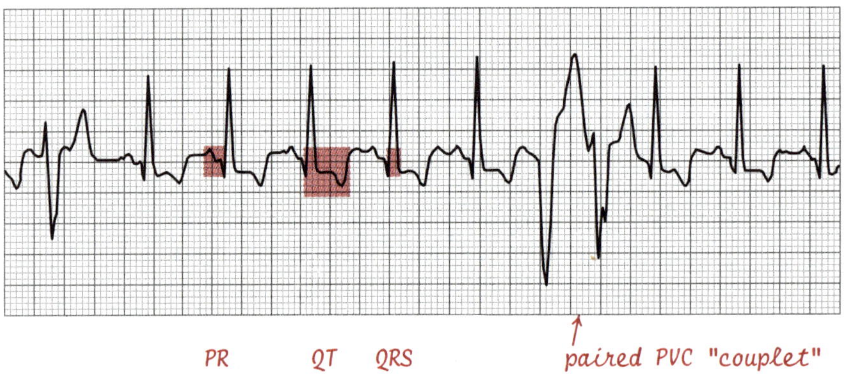

QRS duration 0.10 second **QT** 0.44 second
Ventricular rate/rhythm 100/minute/regular
Atrial rate/rhythm 100/minute/regular
PR interval 0.16 second

Identification sinus at 100/minute with R on T paired PVCs, Q waves, 2 mm ST ↓ and ↓ T waves
Symptoms ? chest pain, meds, med Hx, vital signs, allergies
Treatment Rx pain, reassess, consider lidocaine

Figure 13-9

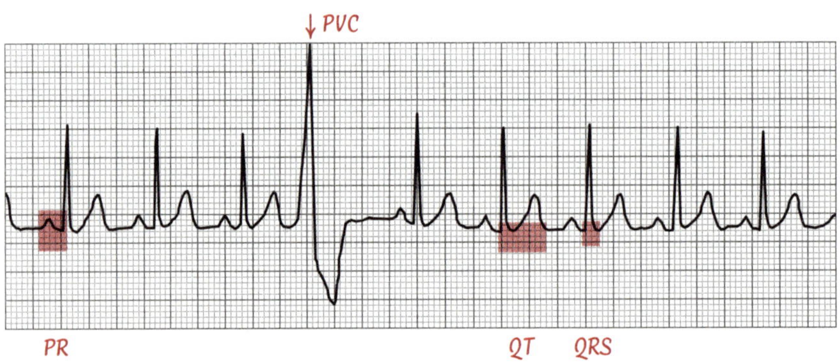

QRS duration 0.08 second **QT** 0.32 second
Ventricular rate/rhythm 100/minute/regular
Atrial rate/rhythm 100/minute/regular
PR interval 0.16 second

Identification sinus at 100/minute with a PVC
Symptoms ? chest pain meds, med Hx, vital signs
Treatment Rx pain, reassess: if PVCs persist or increase in frequency, consider lidocaine

Figure 13-10

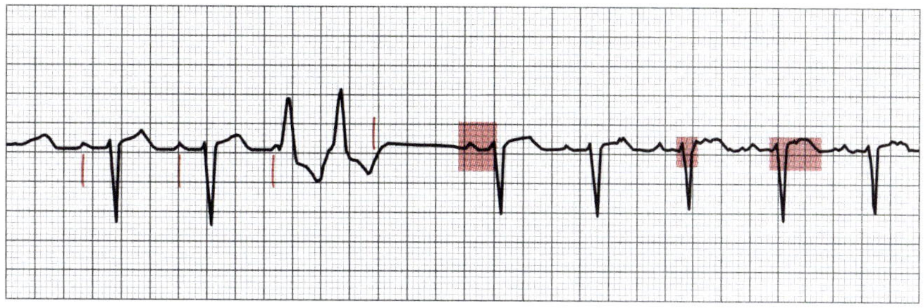

QRS duration 0.08 second QT 0.32 second

Ventricular rate/rhythm 86/minute/regular

Atrial rate/rhythm 86/minute/regular

PR interval 0.16 second

Identification sinus at 86/minute with paired PVCs (note how the P waves plot through the event)

Symptoms ? chest pain meds, med Hx, vital signs, allergies

Treatment Rx pain, reassess, lidocaine

Figure 13-11

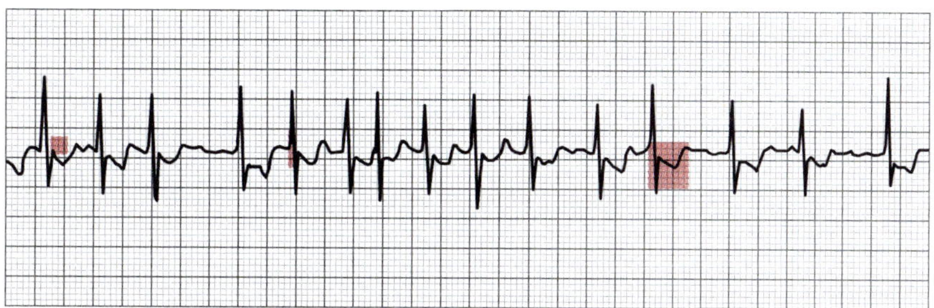

QRS duration 0.06 second QT 0.32 second

Ventricular rate/rhythm 100-296/minute

Atrial rate/rhythm UTD

PR interval UTD

Identification atrial fib 100-296/minute with 2-3 mm ST ↓

Symptoms ? meds/med Hx, vital signs, allergies

Treatment be supportive; if tachycardia persists and patient is symptomatic, may consider verpamil

Figure 13-12

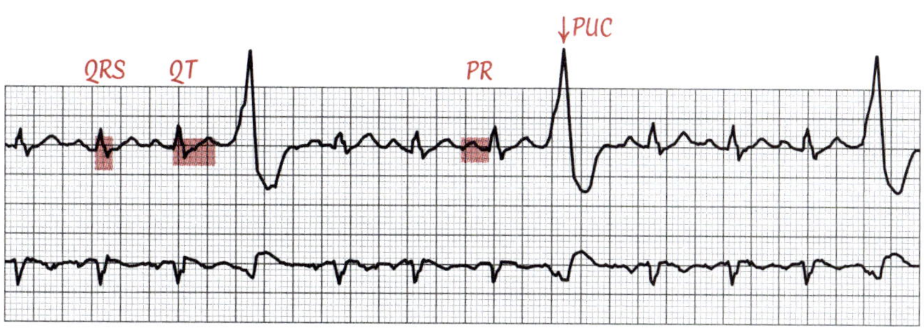

QRS duration 0.10 second QT 0.28 second

Ventricular rate/rhythm 125/regular

Atrial rate/rhythm 125/minute/regular

PR interval 0.16 second

Identification sinus at 125 with freq u/f PVCs (quadrigeminy)

Symptoms ? chest pain meds, med Hx, vital signs, allergies

Treatment Rx pain, reassess, consider lidocaine

Figure 13-13

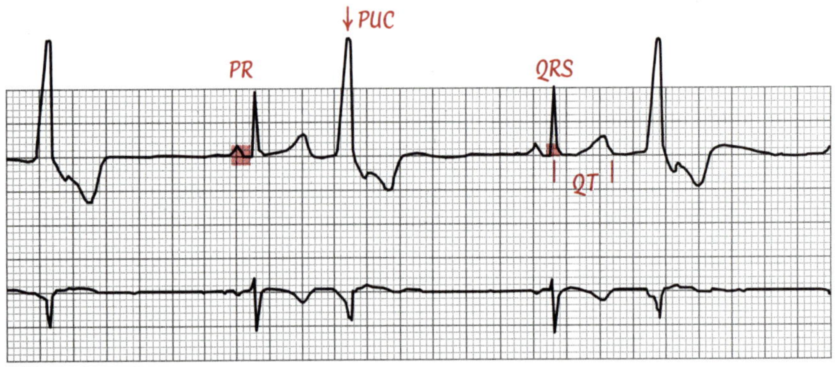

QRS duration 0.08 second **QT** 0.40 second
Ventricular rate/rhythm 80/bigeminal
Atrial rate/rhythm 40/minute/regular
PR interval 0.16 second

Identification sinus at 40 with bigeminal PVCs
Symptoms ? chest pain meds, med Hx, vital signs, allergies
Treatment Rx pain, reassess; if bradycardia persists, consider Atropine, fluids/dopamine/pace

Figure 13-14

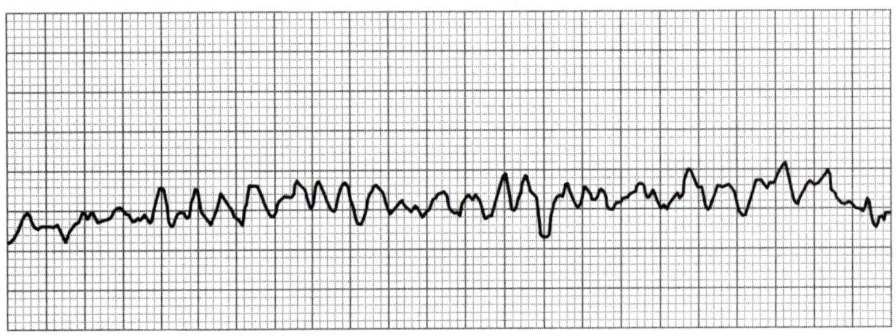

QRS duration UTD **QT** UTD
Ventricular rate/rhythm UTD
Atrial rate/rhythm UTD
PR interval none

Identification ventricular fibrillation confirm no pulse
Symptoms confirm no pulse
Treatment defibrillate 200 to start

Figure 13-15

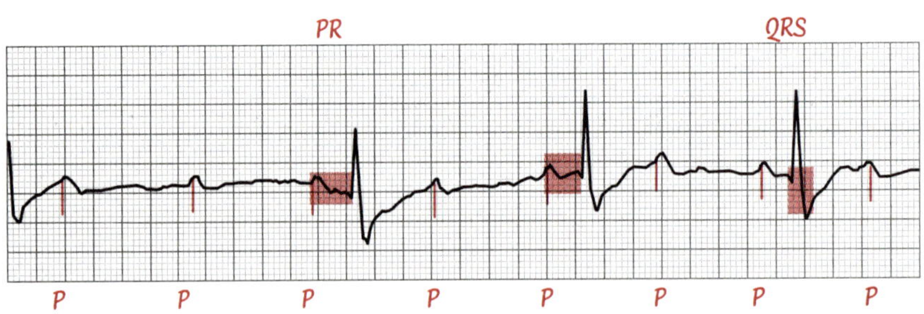

QRS duration 0.16 second **QT** 0.48 second
Ventricular rate/rhythm 18-43/minute
Atrial rate/rhythm 70/minute/regular
PR interval 0.24 second (consistent)

Identification sinus at 70 with high-grade 2° AV block (Type II QRS 0.16 second)
Symptoms ? dizziness, hypotension, ALOC
Treatment ABCs, O_2, (P), IV, ? meds/med Hx, V/S/ allergies; consider fluids, dopamine, pace

Figure 13-16

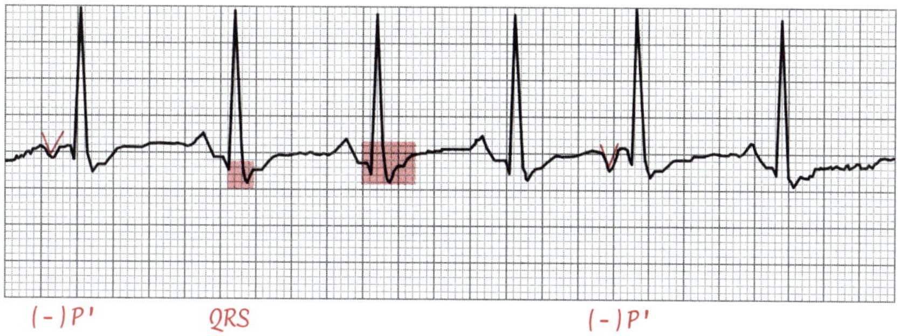

QRS duration: 0.16 second QT: 0.38 second

Ventricular rate/rhythm: 75/regular

Atrial rate/rhythm: 75/regular

PR interval: 0.20 second

Identification: sinus at 75 with a PJC

Symptoms: probably none

Treatment: ? meds/med Hx, V/S/ allergies

Figure 13-17

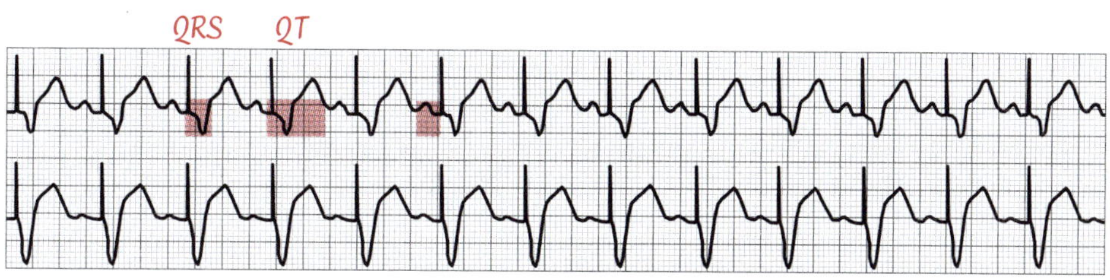

QRS duration: 0.16 second QT: 0.40 second

Ventricular rate/rhythm: 100/minute/regular

Atrial rate/rhythm: 100/minute/regular

PR interval: 0.24 second (consistent)

Identification: ventricular paced rhythm 100/minute ? DVI pacer; V-V consistent

Symptoms: probably none

Treatment: be supportive

Figure 13-18

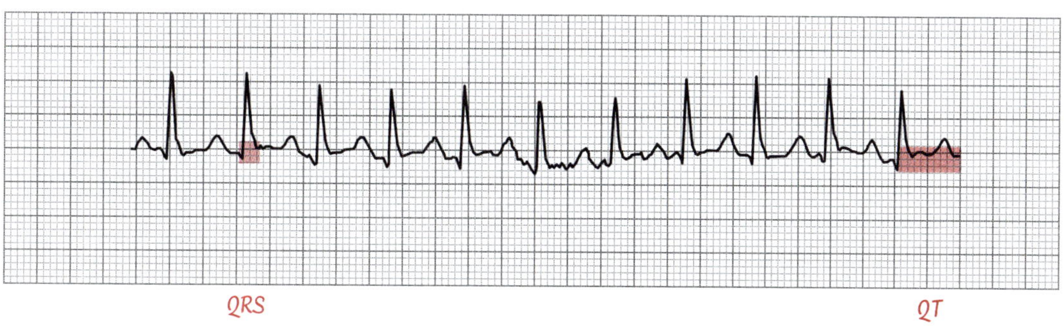

QRS duration: 0.10 second QT: 0.38 second

Ventricular rate/rhythm: 150/minute

Atrial rate/rhythm: UTD

PR interval: UTD

Identification: atrial tachycardia, perhaps atrial flutter (unable to discern P from T; vent rhythm is regular)

Symptoms: ? dizziness, hypotension, ALOC

Treatment: ABCs, O_2, (P), IV, ? med/med Hx, V/S/ allergies; consider vagal maneuvers, adenosine

Figure 13-19

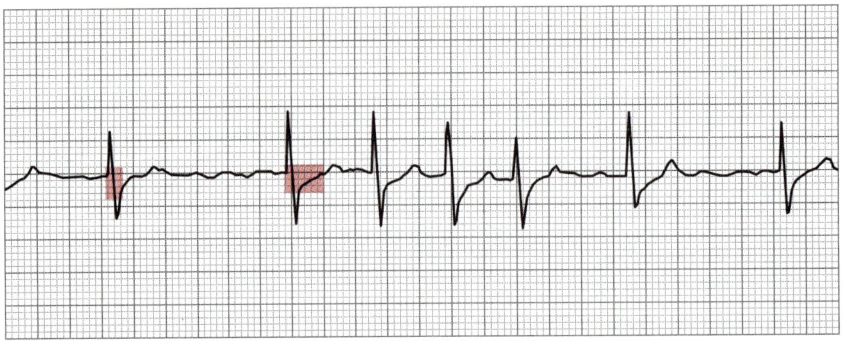

QRS duration 0.10 second QT 0.40 second
Ventricular rate/rhythm 50-150/minute
Atrial rate/rhythm UTD
PR interval UTD

Identification atrial fib vent rate range is 50-150/minute
2 mm ST ↓
Symptoms probably none
Treatment ? meds/med Hx, V/S/ allergies; be supportive

Figure 13-20

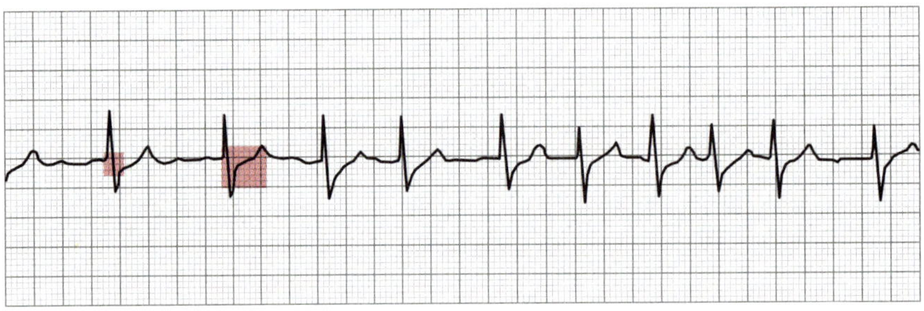

QRS duration 0.10 second QT 0.40 second
Ventricular rate/rhythm 75-150/minute
Atrial rate/rhythm UTD
PR interval UTD

Identification atrial fib vent rate range is 75-150/minute
2 mm ST ↓
Symptoms probably none
Treatment ? meds/med Hx, V/S/ allergies; be supportive

Figure 13-21

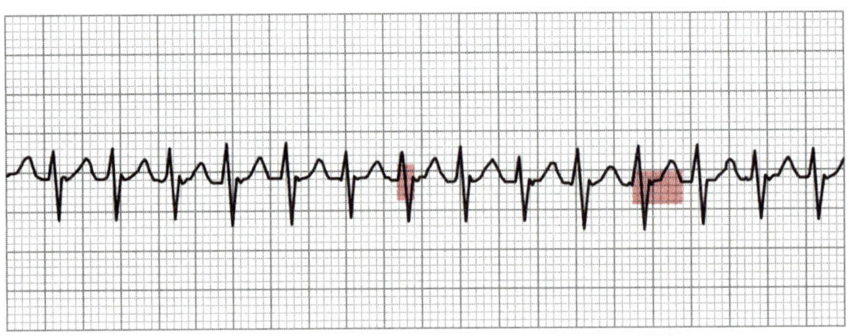

QRS duration 0.06 second QT 0.24 second
Ventricular rate/rhythm 188/regular
Atrial rate/rhythm UTD
PR interval UTD

Identification SVT at 188/minute
Symptoms ? dizziness, hypotension, ALOC
Treatment ABCs, O_2, (P), IV, ? meds/med Hx, V/S/ allergies; consider vagal maneuvers, adenosine

Figure 13-22

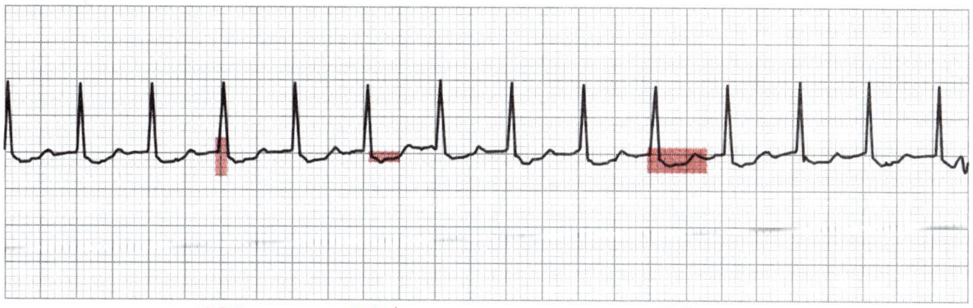

QRS duration 0.04 second **QT** 0.28 second
Ventricular rate/rhythm 150/regular
Atrial rate/rhythm UTD
PR interval UTD

Identification atrial tach at 150/minute
Symptoms ? dizziness, hypotension, ALOC
Treatment ABCs, O_2, (P), IV, ? meds/med Hx, V/S/ allergies; consider vagal maneuvers, adenosine

Figure 13-23

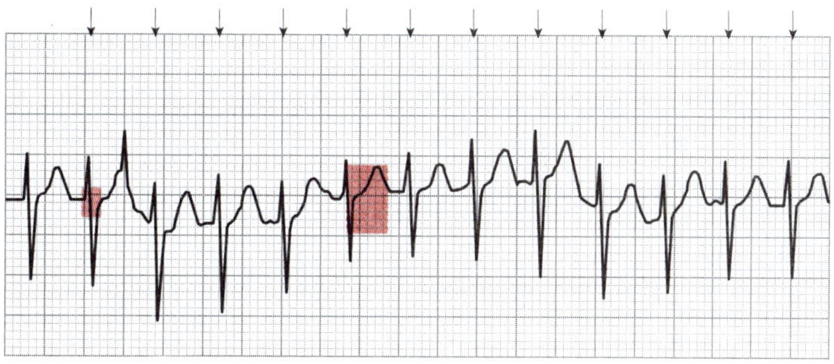

QRS duration 0.08 second **QT** 0.28 second
Ventricular rate/rhythm 188/minute/regular
Atrial rate/rhythm UTD
PR interval UTD

Identification SVT at 188/minute (Note arrows in the top margin; preparations were made for synchronized cardioversion)
Symptoms ? dizziness, hypotension, ALOC
Treatment ABCs, O_2, (P), IV, ? meds/med Hx, V/S/ allergies; consider vagal maneuvers, adenosine

Figure 13-24

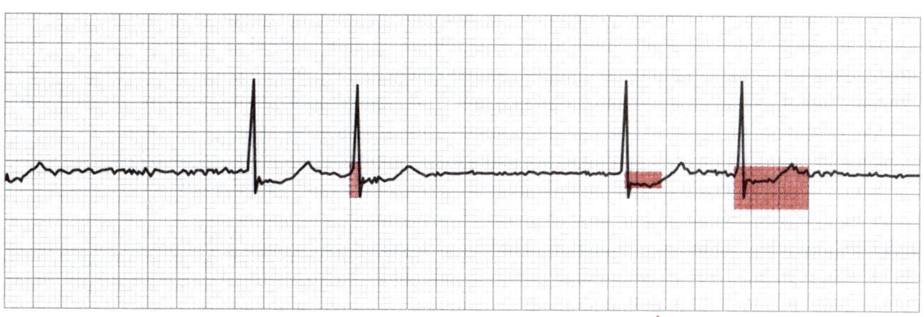

QRS duration 0.10 second **QT** 0.52 second
Ventricular rate/rhythm 31-86/minute
Atrial rate/rhythm UTD
PR interval UTD

Identification atrial fibrillation 31-86 with 2 mm ST ↓; ? possible a-fib with Wenckebach
Symptoms ? dizziness, hypotension, ALOC
Treatment ABCs, O_2, (P), IV, ? meds (dig)/med Hx, V/S/ allergies; consider set up for TCP, ? dopamine for perfusion

Figure 13-25

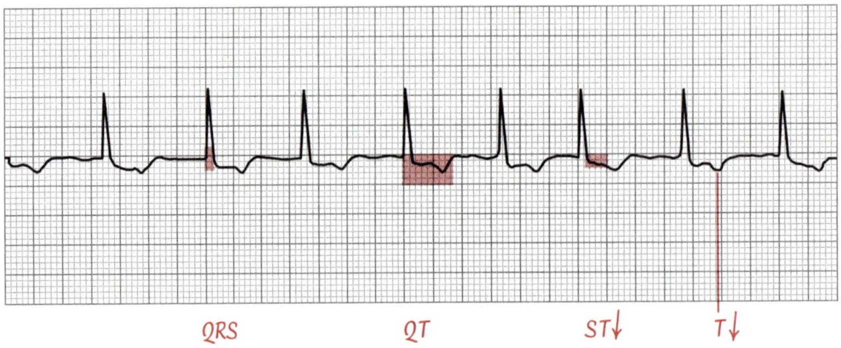

QRS duration 0.08 second **QT** 0.36 second

Ventricular rate/rhythm 86-100/minute

Atrial rate/rhythm UTD

PR interval UTD

Identification atrial fib vent rate range is 86-100/minute with 2 mm ST ↓ and ↓ T wave

Symptoms probably none with rate; ? digitalis Hx

Treatment ? meds/med Hx, V/S/allergies; be supportive; this a-fib is approaching regularity: if so, consider AV block because of dig, ? and consider standby for TCP

Figure 13-26

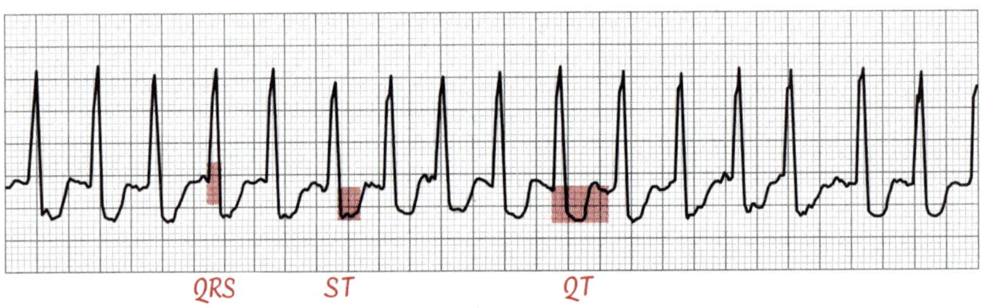

QRS duration 0.10 second **QT** UTD

Ventricular rate/rhythm 136-166/minute

Atrial rate/rhythm UTD

PR interval UTD

Identification atrial fib vent rate range is 136-166/minute with 5 mm ST ↓

Symptoms ? dizziness, hypotension, ALOC

Treatment ABCs, O_2, (P), IV, ? meds/med Hx, V/S/ allergies; consider vagal maneuvers, verapamil, ? synch CV

Figure 13-27

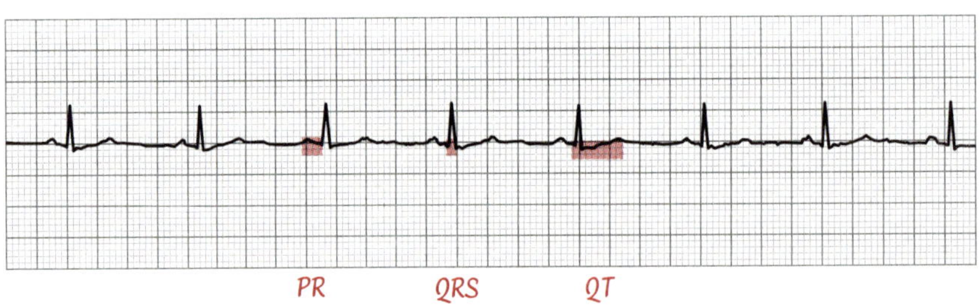

QRS duration 0.06 second **QT** 0.32 second

Ventricular rate/rhythm 67/minute/regular

Atrial rate/rhythm 67/minute/regular

PR interval 0.16 second

Identification sinus rhythm vent rate at 67/minute

Symptoms probably none

Treatment be supportive

Figure 13-28

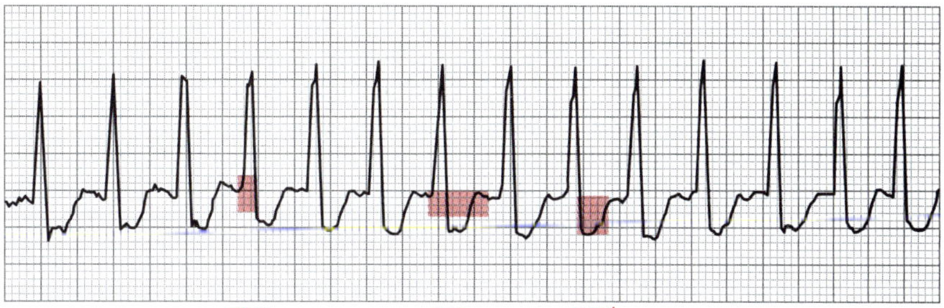

QRS duration 0.10 second QT UTD

Ventricular rate/rhythm 150-188/minute

Atrial rate/rhythm UTD

PR interval UTD

Identification atrial fib vent rate range is 150-188/minute with 4 mm ST ↓

Symptoms ? dizziness, hypotension, ALOC

Treatment ABCs, O_2, (P), IV, ? meds/med Hx, V/S/ allergies; consider vagal maneuvers, verapamil, ? synch CV

Figure 13-29

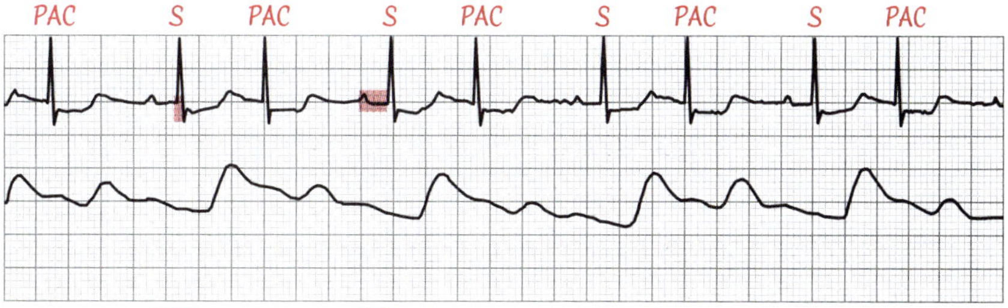

QRS duration 0.06 second QT 0.40 second

Ventricular rate/rhythm 92/bigeminal

Atrial rate/rhythm visible sinus at 46

PR interval 0.16 second

Identification sinus with atrial bigeminy; overall rate is 92 and bigeminal. There is 2 mm horizontal ST seg ↓. Below the ECG is a tracing of the arterial line. Note the diminished systolic pressure with the ectopic. (↑)

Symptoms perhaps none; assess breath sounds

Treatment ABCs, O_2, (P), IV, ? meds/med Hx, V/S/ allergies; assess for s/s CHF

Figure 13-30

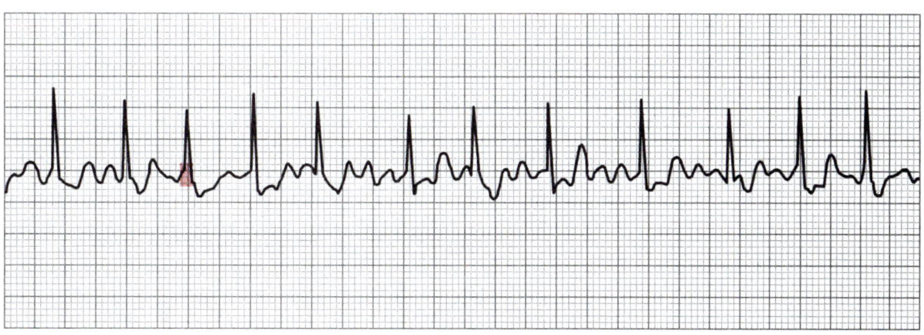

QRS duration 0.04 second QT UTD

Ventricular rate/rhythm 100-150/minute

Atrial rate/rhythm UTD

PR interval UTD

Identification atrial fib vent rate range is 100-150/minute ? 1-2 mm ST ↓

Symptoms ? dizziness, hypotension, ALOC

Treatment ABCs, O_2, (P), IV, ? meds/med Hx, V/S/ allergies; consider vagal maneuvers, verapamil, ? synch CV

Figure 13-31

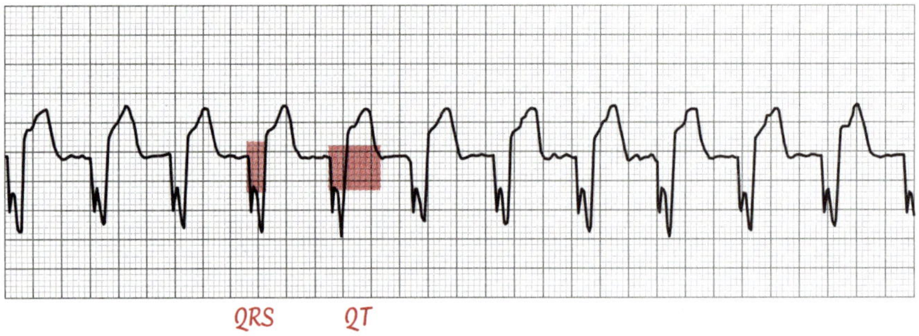

QRS duration 0.12 second **QT** 0.40 second
Ventricular rate/rhythm 100/regular; ? ventricular pacer
Atrial rate/rhythm UTD
PR interval UTD

Identification ventricular pacer at 100/minute (confirmed on patient assessment)
Symptoms none noted
Treatment ABCs, O_2, (P), IV, ? meds/med Hx, V/S/ allergies; be supportive

Figure 13-32

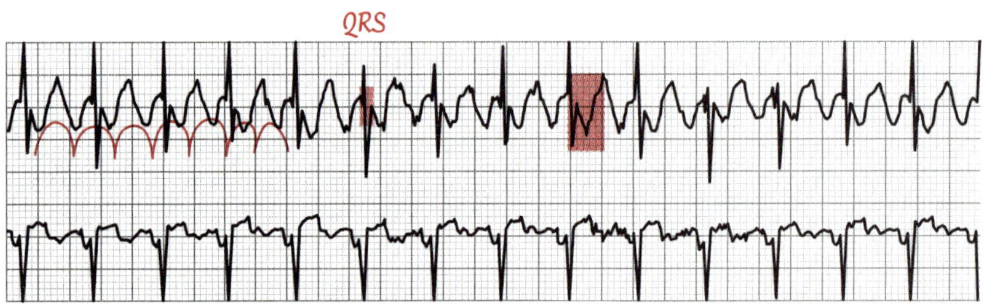

QRS duration 0.06 second **QT** 0.48 second
Ventricular rate/rhythm 167/minute/regular
Atrial rate/rhythm ff 300 regular
PR interval UTD

Identification atrial flutter vent rate range is 167/regular
Symptoms ? dizziness, hypotension, ALOC
Treatment ABCs, O_2, (P), IV, ? meds/med Hx, V/S/ allergies; consider vagal maneuvers, ? adenosine, ? verapamil, ? synch CV

Figure 13-33

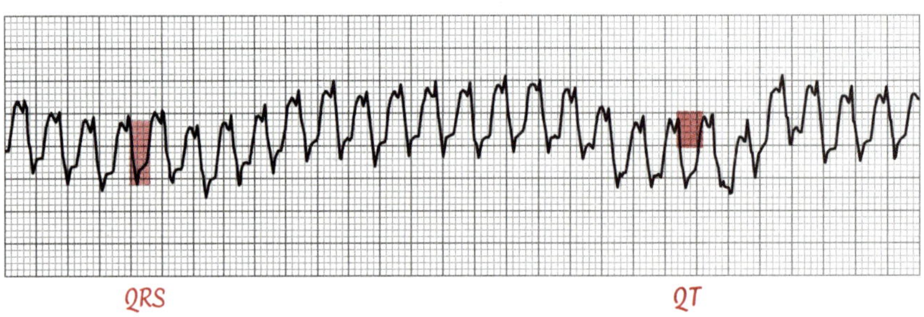

QRS duration 0.16 second **QT** 0.20 second
Ventricular rate/rhythm 250/minute/regular
Atrial rate/rhythm UTD
PR interval UTD

Identification ventricular tachycardia at 250/minute
Symptoms ? pulse, ? stable vs unstable, ? dizziness, hypotension, ALOC
Treatment ABCs, O_2, (P), IV, ? meds/med Hx, V/S/ allergies; pulseless: defib at 200; pulse/unstable–defib at 100

Figure 13-34

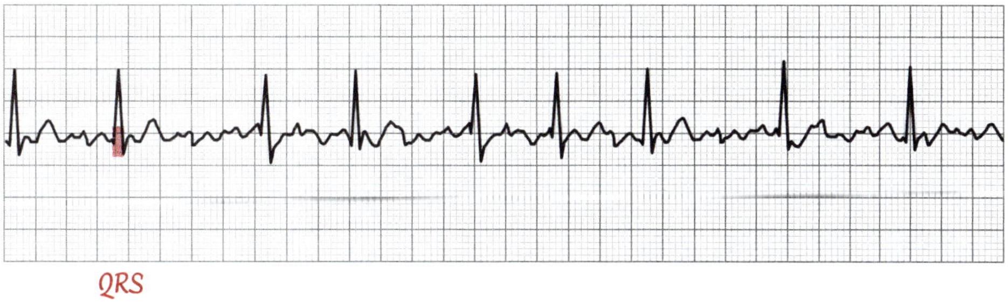

QRS duration 0.08 second **QT** UTD

Ventricular rate/rhythm 67-125/minute

Atrial rate/rhythm UTD

PR interval UTD

Identification atrial fib vent rate range is 67-125/minute

Symptoms probably none with this rate; ? digitalis Hx

Treatment ? meds/med Hx, V/S/ allergies; be supportive; this a-fib may be controlled with meds for this patient

Figure 13-35

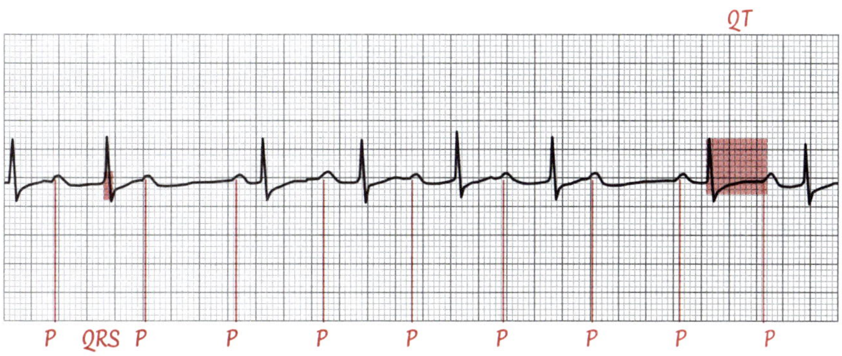

QRS duration 0.08 second **QT** 0.36 second

Ventricular rate/rhythm 55-100/minute

Atrial rate/rhythm 100/regular

PR interval 0.24, 0.32, 0.40 second

Identification sinus at 100; 2° AV block probably Type I (QRS = 0.08), Wenkebach

Symptoms probably none

Treatment ABCs, O_2, (P), IV, ? meds/med Hx, V/S/ allergies

Figure 13-36

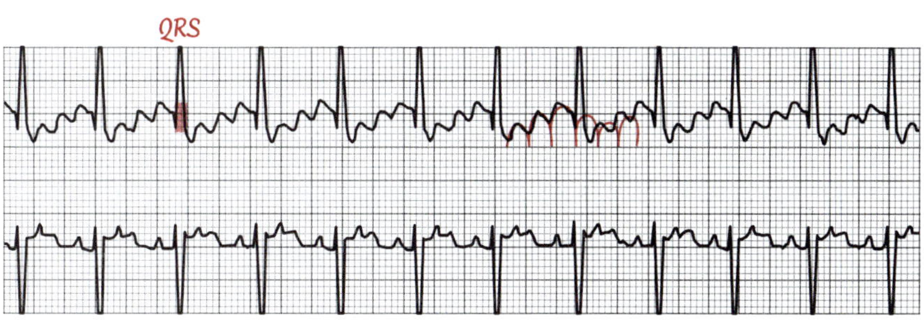

QRS duration 0.10 second **QT** UTD

Ventricular rate/rhythm 125/minute/regular

Atrial rate/rhythm f=300/minute

PR interval UTD

Identification atrial flutter, vent rate 125/minute

Symptoms perhaps none, ? dizziness if new to the patient

Treatment ABCs, O_2, (P), IV, ? meds/med Hx, V/S/ allergies assess for chronic condition

Figure 13-37

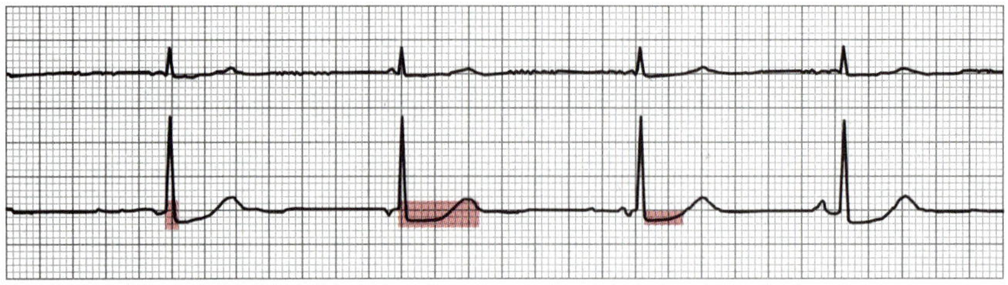

QRS duration 0.08 second **QT** 0.48 second

Ventricular rate/rhythm 67-125/minute

Atrial rate/rhythm sinus = 40, junction = 42

PR interval sinus 0.16, junctional 0.10

Identification sinus at 40→junctional escape at 42/minute→ sinus (note when sinus slows, junction is seen) there is 2 mm ST segment ↓

Symptoms ? dizziness, s/s hypoperfusion, ALOC

Treatment ? meds/medHx, V/S/ allergies; consider Atropine, fluids, dopamine, TCP

Figure 13-38

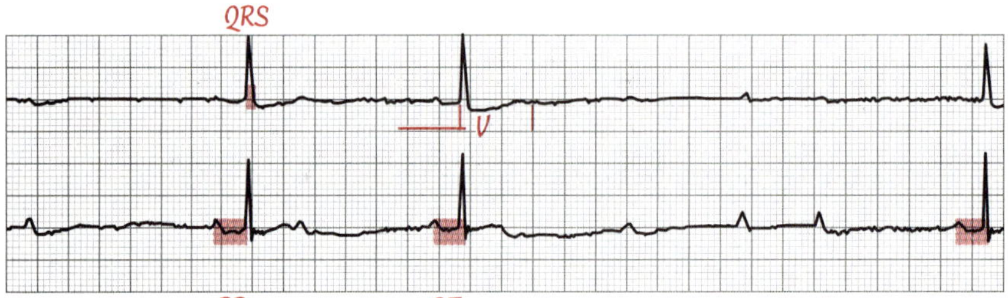

QRS duration 0.08 second **QT** 0.40 second

Ventricular rate/rhythm 17-43/minute

Atrial rate/rhythm P = 50-125

PR interval sinus 0.16, junctional 0.10

Identification sinus P-wave rate varies from 50-125, consistent PR intervals; high-grade 2° AV block, ventricular rate 17-43/min

Symptoms ? dizziness, s/s hypoperfusion, ALOC

Treatment ABCs, O_2, (P), IV, ? meds/med Hx, V/S/ allergies, prepare for TCP ASAP; consider dopamine for perfusion

Figure 13-39

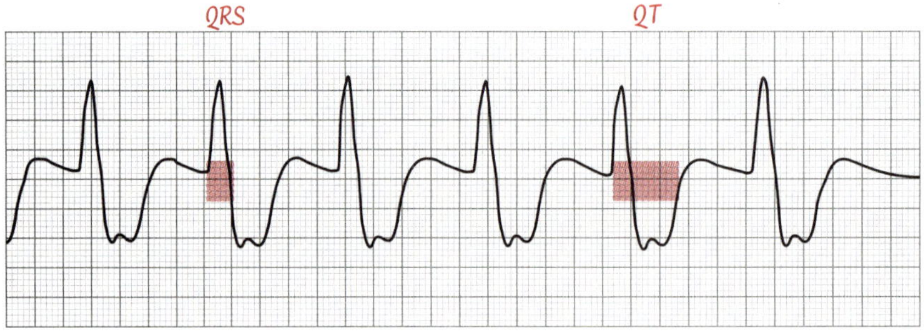

QRS duration 0.16-0.20 second **QT** 0.44 second

Ventricular rate/rhythm 67/minute/regular

Atrial rate/rhythm UTD

PR interval UTD

Identification accelerated ventricular rhythm vent rate of 55/minute

Symptoms ? pulse if pulse present, ALOC

Treatment If pulseless: CPR, intubate, epi/TCP; if pulse is present: consider fluids, TCP ASAP

Figure 13-40

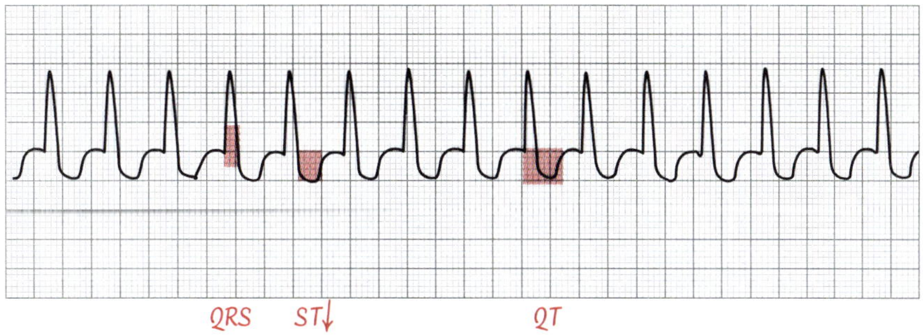

QRS duration 0.10 second **QT** UTD

Ventricular rate/rhythm 150/minute/regular

Atrial rate/rhythm UTD

PR interval UTD

Identification atrial tach at 150/minute; 5 mm ST segment ↓

Symptoms ? dizziness, s/s hypoperfusion, ALOC

Treatment ? meds/med Hx, V/S/ allergies; consider vagal maneuvers, adenosine

Figure 13-41

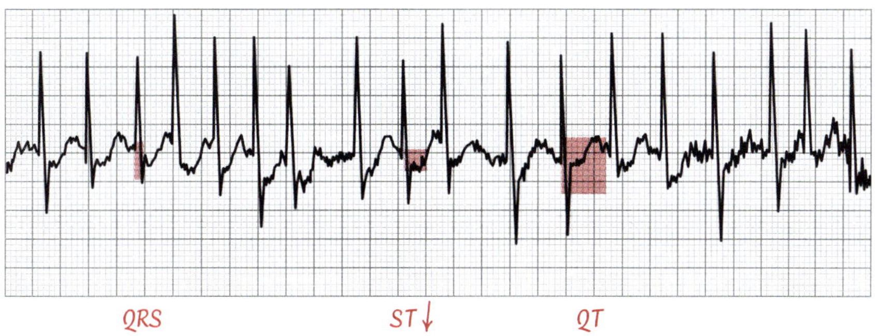

QRS duration 0.06 second **QT** 0.32 second??

Ventricular rate/rhythm 125-296/minute

Atrial rate/rhythm UTD

PR interval UTD

Identification atrial fib with vent rate range 125-296/minute

Symptoms ? dizziness, s/s hypoperfusion, ALOC

Treatment ABCs, O_2, (P), IV ? meds/med Hx, V/S/ allergies, consider vagal maneuvers/verapamil/ ? synch CV

APPENDIX B

Medication Profiles

Premise To know a drug, when to use it, what to expect and most important, when NOT to use it, is a key to the intervention and care of the patient in cardiac compromise.

Introduction

The purpose of this appendix is to review common medications used in the care of patients with cardiovascular disease. This is a quick reference; knowledge of the pharmacokinetics should be maintained with intense study and review of pharmacologic references. Also, practitioners should be aware of standards, guidelines, and oversight that guides patient care in their specific environment.

ACETYLSALICYLIC ACID (ASA)

Generic Name: acetylsalicylic acid (ASA)

Trade Names: Aspirin®, Bayer®, Excedrin®, Bufferin®, Goldline Children's Chewable Aspirin®, others

Classes: platelet aggregator inhibitor, analgesic, antipyretic, anti-inflammatory

Standard Supply: 81 mg (children's flavored chewable tablet) or 325 mg (adult tablet)

Mechanism of Action:

- blocks formation of thromboxane A_2, which prevents platelet clumping and blood clot formation (specifically in the coronary arteries)

Indications:

- chest pain consistent with an acute myocardial infarction
- studies indicate the administration of aspirin in the setting of an acute myocardial infarction or suspected ischemic chest pain has demonstrated significant reduction in mortality comparable to some thrombolytic agents. Aspirin may provide some benefit in management of occlusive/ischemic stroke.

Contraindications:

- bleeding disorders
- known hypersensitivity to the medication

Adverse Reactions:

- gastrointestinal irritation
- gastrointestinal bleeding

Notes on Administration:

Route of Administration:

- oral (chewed or swallowed)

Onset of Action:

- 20–30 minutes

Drug Interactions:

- none in an emergency setting

Adult Dosage:

- 325 mg tablet *or*
- up to four 81 mg children's flavored chewable tablets or
- administer this medication according to current standards and guidelines

ADENOSINE

Generic Name: adenosine

Trade Name: Adenocard®

Classes: antiarrhythmic, endogenous nucleoside

Standard Supply: 6.0 mg/2.0 mL

Mechanism of Action:

- slows conduction of electrical impulses through the SA node and node
- interrupts reentry pathways and can terminate paroxysmal SVT (PSVT)

Indications:

- PSVT, including that caused by Wolff-Parkinson-White (WPW) syndrome refractory to common vagal maneuvers
- wide complex tachycardia of uncertain origin after administering lidocaine

Contraindications:

- second-degree block
- complete (third-degree) block
- Sick-sinus syndrome
- known hypersensitivity to the drug

Adverse Reactions:

- transient flushing of the skin
- chest pain
- dyspnea
- brief period of asystole or bradycardia
- hemodynamic instability

Notes on Administration:

Route of Administration:

- IVP — To be certain adenosine rapidly reaches the central circulation, it should be administered by RAPID intravenous push (IVP) (over a 1–2 second period). Adenosine should be administered into the IV solution intravenous medication port closest to the patient and immediately followed by RAPID 10–20 mL infusion of normal saline.

Onset of Action:

- seconds (adenosine has a 5–10 second half-life)

Drug Interactions:

- concomitant use of methylxanthines may inhibit desired effects
- concomitant use of carbamazepine (Tegretol) can create high degree of AV block
- higher doses may be necessary when theophylline has been taken

Adult Dosage:

- 6.0 mg rapid IVP followed by rapid infusion of normal saline
- if the rhythm does not convert within 2 minutes, administer 12 mg rapid IVP followed by rapid infusion of normal saline
- if the rhythm does not convert within 2 minutes after the second dose, administer 12 mg rapid IVP followed by a rapid fluid infusion of normal saline

ATROPINE SULFATE

Generic Name:	atropine sulfate
Trade Name:	Atropine®
Class:	anticholinergic
Standard Supply:	• 1.0 mg/10 mL • 8.0 mg/20 mL

Mechanism of Action:

- blocks or antagonizes the effects of acetylcholine, thus inhibiting parasympathetic stimulation

Systemic Effects:

- decreases salivary and gastrointestinal secretions/motility
- causes bronchodilation
- decreases mucous production
- decreases urinary bladder tone
- causes mydriasis (pupillary dilation)
- decreases sweat production

Cardiac Effects:

- increases the rate of SA node discharge
- enhances conduction through the node

Indications:

- hemodynamically significant bradycardia
- asystole
- pulseless electrical activity (PEA) with ventricular rate less than 60 per minute
- narrow-complex second degree block
- narrow-complex complete (third-degree) block
- antidote for cholinergic poisonings (e.g., organophosphate and carbamates)

Contraindications:

- wide complex second-degree (Type II) block
- wide complex complete (third-degree) block

Adverse Reactions:

- tachycardia
- anxiety
- palpitations
- headache
- blurred vision

- delirium
- dry mouth
- dilated pupils

Notes on Administration:

Routes of Administration

- IVP
- ET

Onset of Action:

- 1 minute

Drug Interaction:

- sodium bicarbonate inactivates

Adult Dosage:

- for hemodynamically significant bradycardia: 0.5–1.0 mg IVP or 1.0–2.5 mg ET every 3–5 minutes to a total dose of 3.0 mg or 0.03–0.04 mg/kg
- for asystole and slow PEA: 1.0 mg IVP or 2.0–2.5 mg ET every 3–5 minutes to a total dose of 3.0 mg or 0.03–0.04 mg/kg
- for cholinergic poisonings: 2.0–5.0 mg IVP every 5–10 minutes, or administer this medication according to local protocol

NOTE: For adult endotracheal (ET) administration, deliver 2.0–2.5 times the recommended IVP dose and dilute with normal saline according to protocol.

BRETYLIUM TOSYLATE

Generic Name:	bretylium tosylate
Trade Name:	Bretylol®
Class:	antiarrhythmic
Standard Supply:	• 500 mg/5.0 mL • 500 mg/10 mL

Mechanism of Action:

- elevates ventricular fibrillation threshold
- suppresses ventricular ectopy
- may convert ventricular fibrillation or ventricular tachycardia to a supraventricular rhythm

NOTE: Bretylium initially causes a slight increase in heart rate, blood pressure, and cardiac output. These sympathomimetic effects last approximately twenty minutes in the noncardiac arrest setting. Then, norepinephrine release is inhibited which results in an adrenergic blockade. Hypotension may develop, particularly orthostatic hypotension.

The antiarrhythmic effect of bretylium is poorly understood, but it appears to prolong refractory time and increases conduction in the ventricular myocardium.

Indications:

- ventricular fibrillation and pulseless ventricular tachycardia refractory to first-line antiarrhythmics
- ventricular tachycardia with a pulse refractory to first-line antiarrhythmics
- premature ventricular complexes (PVCs) refractory to first-line antiarrhythmics

Contraindication:

- none in the emergency setting

Adverse Reactions:

- hypotension
- nausea and vomiting
- dizziness
- syncope
- seizures
- chest pain
- bradycardia

Notes on Administration:

Routes of Administration:

- IVP
- intravenous infusion

Onset of Action:

- 5 minutes

Drug Interactions:

- digoxin (Lanoxin®) causes increased hypotension
- sodium bicarbonate inactivates

Adult Dosage:

- for cardiac arrest: 5.0 mg/kg IVP to a maximum dose of 35 mg/kg
- for a conscious patient with arrhythmias: dilute the bolus amount in 50 mL or 100 mL of normal saline and infuse over 10–15 minutes

CALCIUM CHLORIDE

Generic Name: calcium chloride
Trade Name: Calcium Chloride®
Class: electrolyte
Standard Supply: 1.0 g/10 mL

Mechanism of Action:

- increases myocardial contractility
- increases ventricular automaticity

Indications:

- calcium channel blocker toxicity (e.g., verapamil, nifedipine)
- acute hyperkalemia (e.g., renal failure with cardiovascular compromise)
- magnesium sulfate toxicity
- acute hypocalcemia
- black widow spider envenomation

Contraindication:

- none in the emergency setting

Adverse Reactions:

- arrhythmias
- hypotension
- syncope
- bradycardia
- nausea and vomiting
- cardiac arrest

Notes on Administration:

Route of Administration:

- IVP

Onset of Action:

- immediate

Drug Interactions:

- sodium bicarbonate inactivates
- thoroughly flush IV tubing with normal saline before and after administration of this medication

Adult Dosage:

- 2.0–4.0 mg/kg IVP
- repeat 2.0–4.0 mg/kg IVP every 10 minutes *or*
- administer this medication according to current standards and guidelines

DIAZEPAM

Generic Name: diazepam
Trade Name: Valium®
Classes: anticonvulsant, sedative
Standard Supply: 10 mg/2.0 mL
Mechanism of Action:

- inhibits neuronal transmission in the central nervous system
- causes muscle relaxation

Indications:

- major motor seizures
- status epilepticus
- sedation before cardioversion or external transthoracic pacing
- skeletal muscle relaxation
- acute anxiety state
- alcohol withdrawal syndrome
- diazepam is a benzodyazepam that is used clinically as a hypnotic

Contraindication:

- known hypersensitivity to the medication

Adverse Reactions:

- hypotension
- respiratory depression or arrest
- blurred vision
- nausea and vomiting
- drowsiness

Notes on Administration:

Routes of Administration:

- immediate (IVP)
- IM and rectal (varies)

Onset of Action:

- IVP
- IM

Drug Interactions:

- incompatible with many medications

Adult Dosage:

- administer under current local standards and guidelines

DOPAMINE

Generic Name:	dopamine
Trade Name:	Intropin®
Class:	sympathomimetic
Standard Supply:	400 mg/5.0 mL 400 mg in a 250 mL bag of D5W (1,600 mcg/mL premixed solution)

Mechanism of Action:
- increases cardiac rate and contractility
- causes peripheral vasoconstriction

Dose-dependent Effects:
- 1.0–2.0 mcg/kg/minute: may dilate vessels in the kidneys and mesentery; may increase urine output; may decrease blood pressure.
- 2.0–10 mcg/kg/minute: increases heart rate and myocardial contractility
- 10–20 mcg/kg/minute: causes peripheral vasoconstriction and hypertension

Indications:
- cardiogenic shock
- hemodynamically-significant hypotension associated with congestive heart failure (CHF)
- hemodynamically-significant hypotension which is unresponsive to IV fluid resuscitation
- hemodynamically-significant hypotension commensurate with the return of spontaneous pulses

Contraindications:
- hypovolemic shock
- pheochromocytoma (a tumor of the adrenal gland)

Adverse Reactions:
- arrhythmias
- tachycardia
- hypertension
- extravasation may cause tissue necrosis
- chest pain
- palpitations
- dyspnea
- headache
- nausea and vomiting

Notes on Administration:

Route of Administration:
- intravenous infusion

Onset of Action:
- immediate

Drug Interaction:
- this medication may be deactivated by sodium bicarbonate

Adult Dosage:
- 2.5–20 mcg/kg/minute: initiate the infusion at 2.5 mcg/kg/min and titrate to effect
- if the patient's blood pressure is less than 70 mm Hg systolic, initiate the infusion at 5.0 mcg/kg/minute
- if the patient's blood pressure is greater than 70 mm Hg systolic, initiate the infusion at 2.5 mcg/kg/minute

EPINEPHRINE

Generic Name: epinephrine
Trade Name: Adrenalin®
Class: catecholamine
Standard Supply:
- 1.0 mg/10 mL (1:10,000)
- 1.0 mg/1.0 mL (1:1,000)
- 30 mg/30 mL (1:1,000)

Mechanism of Action:
- stimulates A-adrenergic receptors
- stimulates β-adrenergic (β_1 and β_2) receptors beta-adrenergic effects of epinephrine are more profound
- A-adrenergic effects
    1. arterial vasoconstriction
    2. increased systemic vascular resistance
- β_1-adrenergic effects
    1. increased heart rate
    2. increased cardiac automaticity
    3. increased cardiac contractility
    4. lowers the threshold for defibrillation
    5. may restore electrical activity in asystole
- β_2-adrenergic effects:
    1. Relaxes bronchial smooth muscle, resulting in bronchodilation

Indications:
- asthma
- reversible bronchospasm associated with COPD
- severe allergic reaction (anaphylaxis)
- hemodynamically significant bradycardia
- cardiac arrest
    1. ventricular fibrillation
    2. pulseless ventricular tachycardia
    3. asystole
    4. pulseless electrical activity (PEA)

Contraindications:
- none in the emergency setting

Adverse Reactions:
- hypertension
- tachycardia
- anxiety
- nausea
- vomiting
- angina
- arrhythmias
- sweating
- palpitations
- headache
- tremors

Notes on Administration:

Routes of Administration:
- IVP

- ET
- IM
- SQ
- intravenous infusion

Onset of Action:
- immediate

Drug Interactions:
- potentiates effects of other sympathomimetic drugs
- may be deactivated by sodium bicarbonate
- may not achieve desired effects in the presence of acidosis

Adult Dosage:
- in cardiac arrest:
    1. 1.0 mg (1:10,000) IVP every 3–5 minutes or
    2. 2.0–2.5 mg (1:1,000) ET every 3–5 minutes
- for anaphylaxis, asthma and reversible bronchospasm associated with COPD:
    1. 0.1–0.3 mg (1:1,000) SQ or IM
    2. 0.2–0.75 mg (1:10,000) ET or IVP if cardiovascular collapse occurs
- as a vasopressor agent: add 1.0 mg into a 250 mL bag of normal saline (4.0 mcg/1.0 mL concentration) and infuse at 2.0–10 mcg/minute (30 gtts–150 gtts/minute)

FUROSEMIDE

Generic Name: furosemide
Trade Name: Lasix®
Class: diuretic
Standard Supply:
- 40 mg/4.0 mL
- 20 mg/2.0 mL

Mechanism of Action:
- causes excretion of large volumes of urine within 5–30 minutes of administration
- inhibits sodium and chloride reabsorption in the kidney
- causes venous vasodilation

Indications:
- fluid overload in congestive heart failure (CHF)
- pulmonary edema

Contraindications:
- hypovolemia
- hypotension
- pregnancy (furosemide has been known to cause fetal abnormalities)

Adverse Reactions:
- dehydration
- electrolyte disturbances
- hypotension
- arrhythmias
- nausea and vomiting

Notes on Administration:

Route of Administration:
- IVP

Onset of Action:
- 5 minutes

Drug Interactions:

- incompatible with diazepam, diphenhydramine, and thiamine
- lithium (may cause toxic levels of this medication)

Adult Dosage:

- 0.5–1.0 mg/kg (usually 20–40 mg) slow IVP

  A patient already taking prescribed furosemide may require a larger dose to achieve desired effects.

LIDOCAINE HCL 2%

Generic Name: lidocaine HCL (2%)
Trade Name: Xylocaine®
Class: antiarrhythmic
Standard Supply:
- 100 mg/5 mL
- 1 g/25 mL
- 2.0 g in a 250 mL bag of D_5W (4.0 mg/mL premixed solution)
- 2.0 g in a 500 mL bag of D_5W (4.0 mg/mL premixed solution)

Mechanism of Action:

- suppresses ventricular ectopy
- increases ventricular fibrillation threshold

Indications:

- ventricular fibrillation
- pulseless ventricular tachycardia
- stable ventricular tachycardia
- wide complex tachycardia of uncertain origin
- premature PVCs:
    1. more than six PVCs per minute
    2. two or more PVCs in a row
    3. multiformed PVCs
    4. R-on-T phenomenon
- post successful defibrillation from ventricular tachycardia or ventricular fibrillation

Contraindications:

- known hypersensitivity to the medication
- ventricular escape rhythm
- idioventricular rhythm
- usually in second degree Mobitz II and complete (third-degree) heart block
- do not administer lidocaine to treat ventricular ectopy if the heart rate is less than 60 beats per minute

Adverse Reactions:

- central nervous system depression, including coma
- seizures
- hypotension
- drowsiness
- paraesthesia
- tremors
- heart blocks
- nausea and vomiting
- cardiac arrest

Notes on Administration:

Routes of Administration:

- IVP
- intravenous infusion
- ET

Onset of Action:

- 1–5 minutes

Drug Interactions:

- none in the emergency setting

Adult Dosage:

- rhythms with a pulse
    1. 1.0–1.5 mg/kg IVP
    2. additional IVP boluses: 0.5–0.75 mg/kg every 10 minutes to a total of 3.0 mg/kg
- rhythms without a pulse (ventricular fibrillation and pulseless ventricular tachycardia):
    1. 1.0–1.5 mg/kg IVP every 3–5 minutes to a total of 3.0 mg/kg
- following the return of pulses: 2.0–4.0 mg/minute intravenous infusion

  For adult endotracheal (ET) administration, deliver 2.0–2.5 times the recommended IVP dose and dilute with normal saline.

  NOTE: The dosage may need to be decreased for the elderly patient as well as those patients with liver disease.

MAGNESIUM SULFATE

Generic Name: magnesium sulfate
Trade Name: Magnesium Sulfate®
Classes: electrolyte, anticonvulsant, antiarrhythmic
Standard Supply: 1.0 g/2.0 mL

Mechanism of Action:

- stabilizes muscle cell membranes by interacting with the sodium/potassium exchange system
- alters calcium's effect on myocardial conduction
- depresses the central nervous system
- causes smooth muscle relaxation

Indications:

- obstetrical
    1. pregnancy-induced hypertension
    2. seizures associated with preeclampsia
    3. pre-term labor
- cardiac arrhythmias
    1. Torsades de Pointes
    2. ventricular fibrillation/pulseless ventricular tachycardia

  There is growing support in advanced cardiac life support for use of magnesium sulfate as a first-line agent in the treatment of myocardial ischemia, myocardial infarction, and cardiac arrhythmias.

Contraindications:

- heart blocks
- respiratory depression
- kidney failure

Adverse Reactions:

- hypotension
- respiratory depression or arrest
- cardiac arrest
- hypotension
- drowsiness
- arrhythmias

NOTE: Calcium chloride should be administered as an antidote to magnesium sulfate if respiratory depression occurs.

Notes on Administration:

Routes of Administration:

- IVP
- IM
- intravenous infusion

Onset of Action:

- immediate

Drug Interactions:

- none in the emergency setting

Adult Dosage:

- for seizures associated with preeclampsia:
    1. 3.0–6.0 g IVP or infusion delivered over 10–15 minutes
    2. repeat bolus 2.0–4.0 g IVP or infusion over 10–15 minutes
    3. if intravenous access cannot be established: 2.0–4.0 g IM

  Because of the volume of this medication, the IM dose should be divided in half and administered IM at separate sites (usually each gluteus). An infusion may be prepared by adding the medication to a 50 mL or 100 mL bag of normal saline.
- for pre-term labor:
    1. 4.0–6.0 g IVP or infusion delivered over 10-15 minutes
    2. follow initial bolus with 2.0 g per hour infusion which may be continued until uterine contractions are reduced to one or less every 10 minutes
- for cardiac arrhythmias:
    1. 1.0–2.0 g IVP or infusion delivered over 1–2 minutes
- for Torsade de Pointes:
    1. 1.0–2.0 g IVP or infusion delivered over 1–2 minutes
    2. follow initial bolus with 1.0–2.0 g infusion delivered over 1 hour

MORPHINE SULFATE

Generic Name: morphine sulfate
Trade Name: Morphine Sulfate®
Class: narcotic analgesic
Standard Supply: 10 mg/1.0 mL
Mechanism of Action:

- provides relief of pain
- causes central nervous system depression
- causes peripheral venous dilation (↓preload)
- decreases systemic vascular resistance (↓afterload)

Indications:

- chest pain in myocardial infarction
- pain associated with burns
- pain associated with musculoskeletal injuries

- pain associated with kidney stones
- pulmonary edema

Contraindications:

- known hypersensitivity to the medication
- acute bronchospasm or asthma
- respiratory depression
- head injury
- abdominal pain of unknown etiology
- hypotension

Adverse Reactions:

- central nervous system depression
- hypotension
- nausea and vomiting
- respiratory depression
- respiratory arrest
- constricted pupils

Notes on Administration:

Routes of Administration:

- IVP
- IM

Onset of Action:

- immediate

Drug Interactions:

- central nervous system and respiratory depression can occur when administered with antihistamines, sedatives, hypnotics, barbiturates, antidepressants, and alcohol
- effects of this medication can be reversed by administration of naloxone (Narcan)

Adult Dosage:

- for relief of pain: 2.0–10 mg slow IVP or IM
- for cardiogenic chest pain: 1.0–3.0 mg IV

  Additional doses of 2.0 mg every 2–10 minutes may be administered to titrate for relief of pain.
- for pulmonary edema: 1.0–3.0 mg IVP or according to protocol

NITROGLYCERIN

Generic Name: nitroglycerin
Trade Names: Nitrostat®, Nitro-Bid®
Classes: vasodilator, antianginal
Standard Supply: 0.4 mg tablet
Mechanism of Action:

- relaxes vascular smooth muscle resulting in
  1. coronary artery vasodilation
  2. relief of chest pain by dilating coronary arteries
  3. decreased return of blood to the heart (preload)
  4. decreased myocardial oxygen demand
  5. decreased workload on the heart
  6. decreased systemic vascular resistance (afterload)

Indications:

- signs and symptoms associated with angina pectoris

- signs and symptoms associated with myocardial infarction
- congestive heart failure with pulmonary edema

Contraindications:

- the patient already has taken the maximum prescribed dose of the medication
- hypotension
- shock
- head injury

Adverse Reactions:

- hypotension
- headache
- dizziness
- bradycardia
- weakness
- fainting
- tachycardia
- flushing and feelings of warmth
- nausea and vomiting
- bitter taste
- burning or tingling sensations in the mouth

Notes on Administration:

Route of Administration:

- SL

Onset of Action:

- immediate

Drug Interactions:

- increased effects with other vasodilators
- alcohol (may cause severe hypotension)
- beta-adrenergic blockers (may cause orthostatic hypotension)
- Viagra (concomitant use may cause severe hypotension)

Adult Dosage:

- 0.4 mg SL
- 0.4 mg SL may be repeated after 5 minutes, and then again after 5 more minutes, for a total of 3 doses (1.2 mg)

  NOTE: Nitroglycerin must be protected from light and expires quickly once the bottle has been opened.

OXYGEN

Generic Name: oxygen
Trade Name: Oxygen®
Class: natural gas

There is 21% oxygen present in atmospheric air. Arterial partial pressure is represented by the abbreviation *Pa*. The normal arterial partial pressure for oxygen (PaO_2) = 100 Torr (range = 80–100 Torr).

Standard Supply:

- Oxygen is stored in steel-green or aluminum gray cylinders

  under pressure of 2,000–2,200 psi.
- Oxygen cylinders are designated by letters to identify their size. D, E, and M cylinders are the most common in emergency care.

- Oxygen flow from a cylinder is controlled by a regulator that reduces high pressure and controls liter (L) flow.

Mechanism of Action:

- rapidly diffuses across the alveolar walls and binds to hemoglobin in the red blood cells
- reverses deleterious effects of hypoxemia on the brain, heart, and other tissues in the body
- increases arterial oxygen tension (PaO_2)
- increases hemoglobin saturation
- is necessary for the efficient breakdown of glucose into a usable energy: adenosine triphosphate (ATP)

This process is known as *aerobic metabolism*, metabolism that occurs in the presence of oxygen.

Indications:

- any condition in which systemic or local hypoxemia may be present, including
  1. dyspnea or respiratory arrest from any cause
  2. chest pain
  3. shock
  4. cardiopulmonary arrest
  5. unconsciousness
  6. any submersion accident
  7. toxic inhalations
  8. stroke
  9. head injury
  10. seizures
  11. any critical patient, including all forms of trauma and medical emergencies

Contraindications:

- none in the emergency setting
- There is concern that patients with chronic obstructive pulmonary disease (COPD) may experience respiratory depression with the administration of high flow oxygen. COPD patients' respiration tends to be regulated by a *hypoxic drive* in which respiration is stimulated by the brain's perception of a low oxygen level, rather than by a high carbon dioxide level, as in normal patients. High flow oxygen administration to the COPD patient does not have a clinically significant effect on respiration during the brief time it is used in an emergency setting.

Adverse Reactions:

- none in the emergency setting

Notes on Administration:

Routes of Administration:

- inhalation
  1. nasal cannula
  2. simple face mask
  3. nonrebreather mask
- ventilation
  1. any ventilatory device (e.g., bag-valve-mask, automatic transport ventilator, pocket mask with oxygen inlet)

Onset of Action:

- variable

Drug Interaction:

- none in the emergency setting

Oxygen Delivery Devices:

Device	Flow Rate	% of O_2 Delivered
nasal cannula	1-6 L/minute	24-44%
simple face mask	8-10 L/minute	35-60%
nonrebreather mask	15 L/minute	95%

NOTE: Other oxygen delivery systems include the pocket mask, bag-valve-mask (BVM), flow-restricted oxygen-powered ventilation device, and automatic transport ventilator (ATV).

SODIUM BICARBONATE

Generic Name: sodium bicarbonate
Trade Name: Sodium Bicarbonate®
Class: alkalinizing agent
Standard Supply: 50 mEq/50 mL

Mechanism of Action:

- increases pH (alkalinization) in the blood and urine
- acts as buffering (neutralizing) agent for acids in the blood and interstitial fluid
- increases tricyclic antidepressant excretion from the body in an overdose setting (by making the urine more alkaline)

  NOTE: Controlled studies have shown that sodium bicarbonate is ineffective in the management of acid/base imbalance associated with cardiac arrest. Once considered the cornerstone of advanced cardiac life support (ACLS), it has been linked to many adverse reactions, including paradoxical intracellular acidosis.

Indications:

- severe acidosis refractory to ventilation
- tricyclic antidepressant overdose
- documented metabolic acidosis
- considered after 10 minutes in resuscitation of cardiac arrest

  NOTE: Ventilatory management, prompt defibrillation, and the administration of epinephrine and lidocaine should always proceed use of sodium bicarbonate. Because these therapies take at least 10 minutes to carry out, sodium bicarbonate should rarely be administered in the first 10 minutes of cardiac resuscitation.

Contraindications:

- none in the emergency setting

Adverse Reactions:

- paradoxical intracellular acidosis
- metabolic alkalosis

  NOTE: Sodium bicarbonate transiently raises arterial PCO_2. Administration of this medication must be accompanied by efficient ventilation to blow off excess carbon dioxide.

Notes on Administration:

Route of Administration:

- IVP

Onset of Action:

- immediate

Interactions:

- inactivates sympathomimetic medications (e.g., epinephrine, dopamine, and isoproterenol when they come in contact, i.e., when given together)

- may produce a chalky precipitate of calcium carbonate when administered together with calcium chloride, calcium gluconate, atropine, morphine sulfate, aminophylline, and magnesium

Adult Dosage:

- 1.0 mEq/kg IVP
- repeat every 10 minutes: 0.5 mEq/kg

VERAPAMIL HCL

Generic Name: verapamil HCl
Trade Names: Calan®, Isoptin®
Class: calcium channel blocker
Standard Supply: 5.0 mg/2.0 mL

Mechanism of Action:

- causes vascular dilation
- selectively inhibits slow calcium channels in cardiac tissue
- slows conduction through the AV node
- inhibits reentry during paroxysmal supraventricular tachycardia (PSVT)
- decreases the rate of ventricular response associated with atrial fibrillation and atrial flutter
- reduces myocardial oxygen demand
- causes coronary artery vasodilation
- causes peripheral vasodilation

Indications:

- narrow-complex PSVT refractory to administration of adenosine
- atrial fibrillation with rapid ventricular response
- atrial flutter with rapid ventricular response

Contraindications:

- hypotension
- cardiogenic shock
- wide complex tachycardia
- ventricular tachycardia
- Wolff-Parkinson-White (WPW) syndrome
- sick-sinus syndrome
- beta-blocker medications

Adverse Reactions:

- bradycardia
- hypotension
- headache
- dizziness
- heart block
- congestive heart failure with pulmonary edema
- nausea and vomiting
- asystole

Notes on Administration:

Route of Administration:

- slow IVP (over 1–2 minutes)

Onset of Action:

- 1–10 minutes

Drug Interactions:

- beta-blocker medications
- calcium chloride may be administered to prevent hypotensive effects in the management of a calcium channel blocker overdose

Adult Dosage:

- 2.5–5.0 mg slow IVP
- repeat in 15–30 minutes: 5.0–10 mg IVP up to a maximum of 30 mg in 30 minutes

APPENDIX C

Emergency Cardiac Care Guidelines

The following tables include the Emergency Cardiac Care Guidelines based on the American Heart Association's *1997–1999 Handbook of Emergency Cardiovascular Care for Health Care Providers.* These are guidelines for possible interventions for the patient who presents with cardiac compromise. Regardless of the clinical setting, the provider must be aware of protocols and guidelines that affect and govern treatment modalities. Now, more than ever, changes in treatment, drugs, and drug dosages occur frequently.

This appendix is not meant to be prescriptive, merely a baseline for assessment and a memory-jogger for the more common approaches to patient care. It is the responsibility of the provider to maintain commitment to the knowledge and implementation of patient care standards in a specific work environment.

Advanced Cardiac Life Support Algorithms

Ventricular Fibrillation and Pulseless Ventricular Tachycardia	Asystole	Pulseless Electrical Activity (PEA)
• ABCs • Perform CPR until defibrillator available • VF/VT present on defibrillator ↓ Defibrillate up to 3 times if needed for VF/VT @ 200J, 200-300J, 360J ↓ Persistent or recurrent VF/VT ? ↓ CPR If No Pulse Intubate at once Establish IV Access (at least 16G) ↓ Epinephrine 1:10,000 **1.0 mg q 3-5 min** IVP ↓ • Defibrillate with up to 360 Joules* within 30-60 seconds after dose of medication ↓ Lidocaine **1.5 mg/kg IVP q 3-5 min** to a total dose of 3 mg/kg 4 ↓ Bretylium 5 mg/kg IVP. Repeat in 5 minutes at 10 mg/kg (Consider Bicarb 1 mEq/kg) ↓ Defibrillate 360 J, 30-60 seconds after each dose of medication (Consider Magnesium sulfate for refractory VF) * May use stacked shocks of 200J, 200-300J, 360 J.	• Continue CPR • Intubate at once • Obtain IV Access • Confirm Asystole in 2 leads 4 ↓ Consider Possible Causes **H(x4)AD** **H**ypoxia, **H**yperkalemia, **H**ypokalemia, **H**ypothermia, **A**cidosis, **OD** ↓ Consider Immediate Transcutaneous External Pacing (TCOP) ↓ Epinephrine 1:10,000 **1.0 mg q 3-5 min** IVP ↓ Atropine **1 mg IVP, repeat every 3-5 min** up to a total of .04 mg/kg ↓ May consider Bicarb 1 mEq/kg with consideration to patient's clinical situation ↓ Consider termination of efforts Per local protocol and policy	*PEA Includes*: EMD, Pseudo-EMD, Idioventricular, Ventricular Escape Rhythms, Bradyasystolic Rhythms ↓ • Continue CPR • Intubate at once • Obtain IV Access ↓ Consider Possible Causes **PATCH(4) MD** **P**ulmonary **E**mbolism, **A**cidosis, **T**ension **P**neumothorax, **C**ardiac **T**amponade, **H**ypovolemia, **H**ypoxia, **H**ypothermia, **H**yperkalemia, **MI**, **D**rug Overdose ↓ Epinephrine 1:10,000 **1.0 mg q 3-5 min** IVP ↓ Consider 250 ml Fluid Bolus ↓ If absolute bradycardia (HR <60) or relative bradycardia, give Atropine **1 mg IVP q 3-5 min** up to a total of 0.04 mg/kg

Sustained Ventricular Tachycardia With a Pulse	Wide-Complex Tachycardia of Uncertain Type	Bradycardia (HR < 60 beats per min)
Stable: Heart Rate < 150 Without Compromise • Assess ABCs • High-flow Oxygen • Obtain IV Access • Attach to Monitor and Assess Vital Signs ↓ Lidocaine **1-1.5 mg/kg IVP** Rebolus @ 0.5-0.75 mg/kg IVP Every 5-10 min until VT resolves, or until a total dose of 3 mg/kg is given ↓ Procainamide 20-30 mg/min, max total 17 mg/kg Bretylium 5-10 mg/kg over 8-10 min, to a max of 30 mg/kg total dose ↓ **Synchronized Cardioversion 100J, 200J, 300J, 360J** **Unstable: Heart Rate > 150 and Compromised** ABCs, 0_2, IV Consider Brief Trial of Medications ↓ **Unsynchronized Cardioversion** if patient is unconscious, hypotensive, or presents with pulmonary edema. May **attempt** synch cardioversion with sedation, but not to delay therapy. **100J, 200J, 300J, 360J**	**If patient is unstable (HR > 150) now or becomes unstable - Perform** **Synchronized Cardioversion @ 100J, 200J, 300J, 360J** ↓ **STABLE:** Assess ABCs, High-flow Oxygen, Obtain IV Access, Assess Vital Signs ↓ Lidocaine 1-1.5 mg/kg IVP, may rebolus @ 0.5-0.75 mg/kg IVP to a total of 3 mg/kg ↓ Adenosine 6 mg, rapid IVP over 1-3 sec, if no response in 1-2 minutes, then ↓ Adenosine 12 mg, rapid IVP over 1-3 sec, may repeat once in 1-2 minutes ↓ Procainamide 20-30 mg/min, max total 17 mg/kg ↓ Bretylium 5-10 mg/kg over 8-10 minutes, maximum total 30 mg/kg ↓ **Synchronized Cardioversion 100J, 200J, 300 J, 360J**	• Assess ABCs, Secure Airway • High-flow Oxygen • Obtain IV Access • Attach Monitor and Assess Vital Signs ↓ **Rate Too Slow?** ↓ **Serious Signs and Symptoms?** ↓ **NO Sign/Symptoms** ↓ Observe and Transport If patient presents with Type II second-degree or third-degree AV block, be ready to use Transcutaneous External Pacing (TCP). If delayed or unavailable, give **Atropine 0.5-1.0 mg IVPq 3-5 min to a total dose of 0.03-0.04 mg/kg** **YES Signs/Symptoms** **Atropine 0.5-1.0 mg IVP**, may repeat every 3-5 minutes up to a total of 0.03-0.04 mg/kg (May use up to 3 mg total for severe cases) ↓ Transcutaneous External Pacing (TEP) ↓ Dopamine 5-20 mcg/kg/min (For **BP < 70** start at 5 mcg/kg/min and for **BP > 70** start at 2.5 mcg/kg/min) ↓ Epinephrine Infusion 2-10 mcg/min

NOTE: When preparing for synchronized cardioversion, premedicate the patient whenever possible. Some possible choices might include ciazapam or morphine sulfate. This will be a clinical based on patient presentation and urgency of the situation.

Supraventricular Tachycardia	Atrial Fibrillation and Atrial Flutter	Polymorphic Ventricular Tachycardia
Unstable: (Heart rate > 150) ABCs, O_2, IV ↓ **Prepare for Synchronized Cardioversion (Consider Sedation)** • Synchronized Cardioversion at 50 Joules, 100J, 200J, 300J, & 360J ↓ Reassess **Stable:** Vagal Maneuvers ↓ Adenosine **6 mg, rapid IVP over 1-3 sec** If no response, may give a bolus of 12 mg, rapid IVP over 1-3 sec May repeat 12 mg bolus in 1-2 minutes ↓ **• Consider Complex Width:** **NARROW COMPLEX → Normal or ↑ BP** Verapamil 2.5-5 mg IVP Verapamil 5-10 mg IVP (in 15-30 minutes) **NARROW COMPLEX → Low or Unstable BP** Synchronized Cardioversion **WIDE COMPLEX** Lidocaine 1-1.5 mg/kg IVP Procainamide 20-30 mg/min, maximum total 17 mg/kg Synchronized Cardioversion	Assess ABCs, High-flow O_2, Obtain IV Access, Attach Monitor, and Assess Vital Signs ↓ Unstable - Synchronized Cardioversion @ 100J, 200J, 300J, 360J* Stable → Consider use of the following: Diltiazem, β-Blockers, Verapamil, Digoxin, Procainamide, Quinidine, Anticoagulants *In cases of **atrial flutter** and **PSVT**, the energy required for synchronized cardioversion begins with 50J.	ABCs, O_2, IV ↓ **Electrical** treatment of choice is unsynchronized cardioversion in sustained tachycardia Transcutaneous (overdrive) pacing ↓ **Magnesium Sulfate 1-2** grams over 1-2 minutes, followed by the same amount infused over 1 hour **UNSTABLE:** Assess ABCs ↓ O_2, IV access ↓ Unsynchronized cardioversion @ 200J 200-300J, 360J ↓ If the patient becomes pulseless, treat as ventricular fibrillation.

Shock, Hypotension, and Pulmonary Edema

• Assess ABCs, High-flow O_2, Obtain IV Access, Attach Monitor, and Assess Vital Signs

↓

WHAT IS THE NATURE OF THE PROBLEM?

RATE: Go to the Tachycardia or Bradycardia Algorithm

VOLUME: Administer Fluids, Cause-specific Interventions, Consider Vasopressors, AND

↓

PUMP: **WHAT IS THE BLOOD PRESSURE?**

↓

Systolic BP<70	**Systolic BP 70-100**	**Diastolic BP>110**
1. 250-500 ml Fluid Challenge 2. Norepinephrine (0-5-30 mcg/min) 3. Dopamine (5-20 mcg/kg/min)	1. Dopamine	1. Nitroglycerin (10-20mcg/min) 2. Nitroprusside (0.1-5.0mcg/kg/min)

Systolic BP >100

1. Dobutamine (2-20 mcg/kg/min)

↓

Consider Other Actions, Especially for Patients in Pulmonary Edema

↓

First Line: Lasix IV 0.5-1.0 mg/kg; Nitroglycerin SL; Morphine IV 1-3 mg; Oxygen/Intubate PRN

Second Line:
Nitroglycerin IV (if BP > 100)
Nitroprusside IV (if BP > 100)
Dopamine IV (if BP < 100)
Dobutamine IV (if BP > 100)
PEEP, CPAP

Third Line: Amrinone 0.75 mg/kg, then 5-15 mcg/kg/min
Consider Aminophylline, Thrombolytics, & Digoxin

Acute Myocardial Infarction

Community Emphasis on "Call First/Call Fast, Call 911'

↓

• EMS System

Oxygen-IV-cardiac monitor (1 2-Lead)-vital signs

• Nitroglycerin

Pain relief with narcotics
Notification of Emergency Center
Rapid Transportation and Prehospital Screening for Thrombolytic Therapy
Initiation of Thrombolytic Therapy

↓

• Emergency Center

"Door-to-Drug" team protocol approach with rapid triage of patients with chest pain and clinical decision maker established (emergency physician, cardiologist, etc.)

↓

Time interval in emergency center not to exceed 30-60 minutes to receive thrombolytic therapy

↓

Assessment Immediate:	*Treatments to consider if there is evidence of coronary thrombosis:*
Vital Signs Oxygen Saturation Start IV 12-lead ECG Brief History/Physical Decide on eligibility for thrombolytic therapy *As soon as possible:* Chest X-ray Blood Studies Consult	High-flow Oxygen Nitroglycerin-SL, BP > 90 Morphine IV Aspirin PO Thrombolytic Agents *Nitroglycerin IV* β-Blockers Heparin IV PTCA Prophylactic use of lidocaine is not recommended for all AMI patients, only if symptomatic

APPENDIX D

Quick Review of Assessment and Interventions for Patients and Arrhythmias

APPROACH TO PATIENTS

Once attention to ABCs and oxygen therapy has begun, securing an IV for possible administration of fluids and medications is usually the next step. Assessing and documenting vital signs and initial ECG analysis should follow.

In cases where more than one advanced life support (ALS) provider is present, there is almost simultaneous assessment, history taking, noting of the physical environment, and detailed physical examination. Questions should be appropriate to assess the chief complaint, history of present illness, medical history, any medication history, and allergies that may contribute to patient care decisions.

The patient's statements describing signs and symptoms are documented in the patient's own words. Clinical assessment, vital signs, and reassessment are done after each intervention. For example, if the patient received pain medication, the reassessment would include the patient presentation, vital signs, effect on the ECG rhythm, and the effect on the ectopics if applicable.

Following are guidelines for possible interventions for the patient who presents with cardiac compromise. Regardless of the clinical setting, the provider must be aware of protocols and guidelines that affect and govern treatment modalities. Now, more than ever, changes in treatment, drugs, and drug dosages occur frequently.

This section is not meant to be prescriptive, merely a baseline for assessment and a memory-jogger for the more common approaches to patient care. It is the responsibility of the provider to maintain commitment to the knowledge and implementation of patient care standards in a specific work environment.

Suggested guidelines for approach to care in the patient with suspected cardiac compromise.
(It is the responsibility of the provider to maintain commitment to patient care standards in a specific work environment.)

For Slow Rates in the Patient Is Hypotensive and Hypoperfusing	For the Narrow QRS Tachycardia	For the Wide QRS Tachycardia
Narrow QRS: *Consider* Atropine for rate Dopamine for perfusion Pacemaker Epi infusion (clinical) **Wide QRS:** *Consider* Pacemaker Dopamine for perfusion Pacemaker Epi infusion (clinical) **AV Block with Narrow QRS and rapid sinus rate:** *Consider* Dopamine for perfusion Pacemaker Epi infusion	**Stable:** Goal: To slow down AV conduction and provide a better perfusing ventricular rate *Consider* Vagal Maneuvers Adenosine Verapamil (first line for A-fib) **Unstable:** Patient is hypotensive and hypoperfusing Goal: To depolarize the ectopic Synch CV beginning at 50J A-Fib @ 100J	**V Tach Stable:** Goal: To make the irritable ventricular cells more refractory *Consider* Lidocaine Bretylium or Procainamide **V Tach Unstable:** Patient is hypotensive and hypoperfusing Sync CV beginning at 100J **V Tach Torsade** Defibrillation beginning at 200J **V Tach Pulseless** Defibrillation beginning at 200J
For Ventricular Fibrillation	**For Asystole**	**For Pulseless Electrical Activity**
Confirm "no pulse" Goal: To depolarize the fibrillating myocardium Defibrillation beginning at 200J Epinephrine Lidocaine Bretylium ? Magnesium	**Confirmed in a second lead** Goal: To maintain the patient and try to support an underlying escape rhythm CPR, Intubation Epinephrine Atropine Pace Consider causes **DO NOT DEFIBRILLATE!**	**Identify the rhythm** Goal: To identify any mechanical impairment to pulse and cardiac output CPR (assess for pulses; ? MI tamponade/rupture) Intubate (assess breath sounds; ? pneumothorax) IVs (Fluid Challenge; ? hypovolemia) Epinephrine IV/ET Atropine if there is a bradycardia As you treat, reassess; assessment contributes to determining the cause.

Glossary

Aberrant conduction: Abnormal impulse transmission causing the ECG waves to leave a distorted shape. Often used when referring to a PAC or SVT with aberration, meaning that the QRS complex, instead of being narrow, is wide and distorted.

Absolute refractory period: The phase of refractoriness when the cells are unresponsive to a stimulus.

Accelerated AV junctional rhythm: Ectopic AV junctional pacemaker discharging at a rate above 60 per minute but below 100 per minute.

Accelerated idioventricular rhythm: Ectopic ventricular pacemaker discharging at a rate above 40 per minute but under 100 per minute. Often incorrectly referred to as "slow ventricular tachycardia."

Accelerated rhythm: An ECG rhythm that occurs at a rate faster than the usual intrinsic rate of depolarization for a specific focus. For example, an ectopic pacemaker originating in the ventricles at a rate of 75 per minute would be considered accelerated because the usual rate of spontaneous discharge (automaticity) for such a focus is in the range of 20 to 40 per minute.

Accessory bundle (or AV pathway): Alternate muscular connection between the atria and ventricles that bypasses the AV node.

Action potential: Abrupt phasic changes in the electrical charges of the cell membrane, including polarization, depolarization, and repolarization.

After-depolarization: Small electrical impulses, occurring following action potentials, which can cause dysrhythmias if they are large enough to reach threshold.

Agonal rhythm: ECG rhythm recorded from a dying heart; asystole with several idioventricular complexes.

Akinesis: Lack of motion.

Amplitude: The maximum departure of the wave from the average value.

Anoxia: Absence of oxygen.

Antegrade: Flowing in a forward direction (anterograde).

Antidromic: Reentry tachycardia that uses the accessory pathway in an antegrade fashion and the AV node in a retrograde direction.

Antidysrhythmic drugs: A variety of different types of agents, including oxygen, digitalis, lidocaine, and propranolol, used to correct disordered cardiac rhythms and rates.

Arrest: Cessation of activity. Sinus arrest: failure of SA node to discharge. Cardiac arrest: cessation of heart activity.

Arrhythmia: Disorder of heart rate or rhythm.

Arrhythmogenic: Capable of causing dysrhythmias; examples include ischemia, hypoxia, acidosis, and certain drugs.

Artifact: An artificial disturbance of the ECG signal, commonly caused by electrical (60-cycle) interference or muscular activity.

Artificial pacemaker: An electrical pulse generator that can provide a substitute on a temporary or permanent basis. An electronic method for providing a minimum heart rate.

Asynchronous: A pacemaker current generated at a fixed, preset rate.

Asystole: Lack of cardiac electrical activity reflected by a flat (isoelectric) line on the ECG and accompanied clinically by absent pulse. Cardiac arrest.

Atrial depolarization: Activation of atrial tissue. Seen on ECG as a P wave.

Atrial extrasystole: Premature atrial depolarization. Seen on ECG as a P′.

Atrial fibrillation: A tachydysrhythmia characterized by chaotic atrial activity at a rate above 350 per minute.

Atrial flutter: Tachydysrhythmia characterized by regular atrial wave forms about 250 to 350 per minute. Rate of conduction to the ventricles is dependent on AV refractoriness.

Atrial kick: The amount of blood added to ventricular diastole with atrial contraction.

Atrial repolarization: The process in which the atrial tissues return to their resting state following depolarization. Atrial repolarization is not usually reflected on the ECG since the larger QRS complex overshadows the activity. Occasionally, there is distortion of the QRS that may reflect atrial repolarization.

Atrial tachycardia: A tachyarrhythmia where an ectopic focus generates a rapid impulse that is transmitted to the ventricles. It is characterized by a sudden start and stop.

Atrioventricular (AV) block: Disturbance in conduction at or below the AV node. Impulses can be delayed temporarily or unable to activate the ventricles because they are blocked.

Atrioventricular (AV) dissociation: Independent activation of atria and ventricles.

Atrioventricular (AV) junction: Tissue at the junction of the atria and ventricles. Consists of the AV node and the bundle of His, which possesses automaticity.

Atrioventricular (AV) Node: Small mass of conducting tissue lying in the posterior floor of the right atrium connecting the atria and ventricles. Capable of delaying impulses being transmitted to the ventricles.

Automated external defibrillation: A defibrillator computer that evaluates patient ECG rhythm and confirms the need for defibrillation. A fully automated defibrillator operates without action by the operator except to apply and turn on the power. A semi-automated defibrillator uses a voice prompt to advise the operator of the steps to take based on the analysis of the patient's ECG rhythm.

Automaticity: The ability of a cell to generate spontaneously an impulse without being externally stimulated. Cells that possess automaticity at a predictable rate serve as pacemakers. Cells that possess automaticity in competition with pacemakers are called "ectopics."

Available energy: The amount of actual energy that is delivered to a patient with an impedance of 50 ohms.

A-V interval: In pacemaking, the distance between the paced atrial wave form and the paced ventricular wave form.

Axis : The mean flow of electrical current.

Axis deviation: The direction of the mean flow of electrical current outside the normal limits.

Beat: One complete electrical and mechanical cardiac cycle that results in a pulse.

Bigeminy: An ECG rhythm where every other beat is an ectopic.

Biphasic: Having positive and negative components.

Block: A delay in conduction that can be complete or incomplete.

Bradycardia: A slow heart; a disorder in heart rate where the ventricular rate is below 60 beats per minute.

Bundle branch block: A conduction disorder in one or more of the bundle branch fascicles.

Bundle branches: The continuation of the AV bundle that divides into right and left conducting branches or fascicles.

Bundle of His: Continuation of AV nodal fibers that spreads downward into the ventricles. Also known as the AV bundle.

Bypass tract: An abnormal bundle of muscle connecting the atria and ventricles but bypassing the AV node. The AV node no longer controls the rate of ventricular stimulation because the atrial impulses follow an alternate pathway.

Cardiac cycle: The electrical (P waves, QRS complexes, T waves) and mechanical events (systole and diastole) that compose a single heartbeat.

Cardiac output: The product of heart rate and stroke volume.

Cardiac standstill: *See* asystole.

Cardioversion: Delivery of an electrical discharge used to terminate dysrhythmias that are refractory to drugs, or, to cause an immediate conversion to sinus rhythm.

Carotid sinus massage (CSM): Application of digital pressure to the neck region just lateral to the trachea, thereby stimulating the vagus and causing a discharge of parasympathetic impulses to slow tachycardias and convert them to a slower heart rate.

Chest pain: The term used by patients to describe pain, discomfort, burning, pressure, tightness, heaviness, aching, fullness, or difficulty in breathing or getting one's breath.

Compensatory pause: The period following a PVC that compensates for the premature impulse so that the interval between the R wave before the PVC and the one after the PVC is equal to twice the normal R-R interval.

Complex: A group of wave forms.

Conductivity: The property of cardiac muscle that describes the ability to transmit an impulse.

Contractility: The property of cardiac muscle that describes the ability of the heart to react to electrical conduction with organized response. The mechanical response to depolarization.

Couplet: Paired PVCs; two PVCs that occur in succession.

Coupling: The time between the normal beat and the ectopic complex.

Current of injury pattern: The ST-segment elevation that occurs following the insult.

Defibrillation: Delivery of electrical current in an effort to terminate a life-threatening arrhythmia.

Deflection: Movement of the ECG stylus from the baseline caused by changes in transmembrane potential.

Delivered energy: The amount of joules administered to a patient.

Delta wave: Initial slurring of the QRS complex. This is seen in preexcitation states such as the Wolff-Parkinson-White pattern. As a result, the P-R interval is shortened. It does not have to be seen in all leads.

Demand mode: When an artificial pacemaker senses intrinsic cardiac activity and does not discharge. This prevents competition between the artificial pacemaker and sinus activity. The pulse generator has a timing mechanism and discharges only when it senses an R-R interval that is longer than the preset rate.

Depolarization: Electrical activation of the heart tissue due to spread of the electrical impulse.

Diastole: The period during which rest, relaxation and filling of blood takes place. The term applies to atrial and ventricular relaxation and filling; however, when the term stands alone, by convention, it refers to ventricular relaxation and filling.

Diastolic filling time: Amount of time available for the chambers of the heart to fill with blood between systoles. As the heart rate increases the diastolic filling time decreases, causing a fall in cardiac output.

Dissociation: Isolation of electrical and/or mechanical activity.

Dropped beat: A QRS that is missing. Usually refers to a "missing" QRS because of AV node refractoriness.

Duration: The time it takes for a wave to begin and end.

Dyskinesis: The paradoxical bulging during ventricular systole.

ECG: Abbreviation for electrocardiogram.

Ectopic: Originating from a site other than the sinus node (e.g., atrial, junctional, or ventricular); also called "extrasystole."

Ectopic focus: Cells that compete with pacemaker cells; occur early, or premature, in the cardiac cycle.

Ectopy: Complexes of ectopic origin; when cells compete with pacemaker cells; occurs early in the cardiac cycle.

Electrical alternans: Variation in the size of every other QRS complex; often seen in chronic lung disease and pericardial effusion.

Electrocardiogram (ECG): Graphic record of electrical activity of the heart.

Electrode: The conductor used to establish electrical contact with the body.

Electromechanical association: Normal state in which ECG events are coordinated with a pulse and cardiac output.

Electromechanical dissociation (EMD): (also known as pulseless electrical activity) Pathologic state in which an action potential does not result in systole. Organized ECG activity is not accompanied by cardiac contraction.

Electronic capture: A pacer spike directly associated with ECG complex.

Elevation: The height of the wave; deviation of the ST segment above the baseline.

End-diastolic: A PVC occurring at the end of, or just after a sinus P wave.

Endocardium: The inner lining of the heart, consistent with the inner lining of the arterial vascular system. The most electrically sensitive area of the endocardium is the right ventricular septal endocardium.

Enhanced automaticity: Increased excitability of pacemaker tissue.

Epicardium: The outer layer of the heart.

Escape beat: The development of latent pacemakers to stimulate the heart when there is sinus node slowing or arrest. The atria, AV junction, or ventricles may be the site of a single complex or a sustained escape rhythm.

Escape interval: The preset amount of time from the last sensed beat to the first pacer spike.

Excitability: The ability of a cell to become depolarized when stimulated.

Exit block: Failure of stimulus to activate surrounding structures. For example, in sinus exit block, the sinus impulse is unable to spread to the atrial tissue.

Extrasystoles: Ectopic complexes.

Failure to capture: A pacer spike with no associated ECG complex.

Failure to sense: Malfunction of an electronic pacemaker where the normal QRS complexes are not sensed.

Fascicular block: Interruptions in conduction delaying activation of the ventricular septum on the wall of the ventricle.

ff Waves: Fibrillatory waves characteristic of atrial fibrillation.

Fibrillation: Chaotic electrical cardiac activity that is unable to stimulate coordinated cardiac contractions. As a result, the pumping activity of the atria and/or ventricles is lost. The ECG inscribes an irregular and wavy baseline.

First-degree AV Block: A delay in AV conduction reflected in a P-R interval greater than 0.20 second.

Flutter: Rapid ectopic electrical activity that stimulates cardiac chambers in a rapid, yet organized fashion.

Focus: Site of impulse formation. "Unifocal" refers to one site of origin, as opposed to "multifocal," which describes more than a single site.

Fusion beat: A complex produced by the simultaneous discharge of two pacemakers as with an atrial and ventricular focus. As a result, the two waves collide within the ventricles or atria, and the two forces somewhat blend or cancel each other, producing a smaller or narrower complex than normal. The resulting complex shows some characteristics of the ectopic and the sinus beat.

F waves: Flutter waves characteristic of atrial flutter.

Heart rate: The number of contractions, or how fast the heart beats.

His Bundle: That portion of conducting pathway that is a continuation of AV nodal fibers that travel into the ventricles and then divide into bundle branches. It channels sinus impulses to the ventricular muscles and is capable of pacemaker control. It is also known as the "pacer in a pinch."

His-Purkinje network: Portions of the intraventricular conduction system composed of the tissues of the His bundle, including the fibers of the terminal Purkinje pathways.

Hypoperfusion: Deficiency in circulation of oxygenated blood.

Hypoxia: Low oxygen content.

Hysteresis: A delay mechanism on some permanent pacemakers to allow programming of prolonged intervals used to promote normal intrinsic function as long as possible.

Idio-: Prefix meaning "from within." An idioventricular rhythm arises in the ventricle and controls only the ventricle. An idiojunctional (nodal) rhythm arises in the AV junction and controls only the ventricles.

Impedance: Interference to the flow of energy (resistance).

Infranodal: Below or inferior to the AV node /His bundle.

Infranodal bypass tract: An AP that connects atrial fibers to the upper part of the AV node.

Inhibited: Restrained from firing.

Interpolated beat: An ectopic beat occurring so early that it activates the ventricle and repolarizes by the time the next sinus impulse arrives. There is no compensatory pause as the complex is sandwiched between two normal beats.

Interval: A measurement on the ECG equal to a wave form plus a segment.

Intraventricular conduction defect (IVCD): Abnormal conduction due to disease or dysfunction in one or more of the ventricular fascicles. Causes a bizarre QRS complex or prolonged QRS duration.

Inverted: Turned upside down or reversed; a negative wave form.

Irritability: Increased automaticity, commonly caused by ischemia or hypoxia.

Ischemia: Inadequate blood supply, resulting in decreased supply of oxygen relative to demand; leads to anaerobic metabolism. Deficiency in perfusion of oxygenated blood.

Isoelectric line: Flat ECG line found between the waves or cycles.

Isorhythmic AV dissociation: The atria and ventricles beat independently because the rates of the pacemakers are very close to one another. No actual AV block is present, yet sinus slowing permits the AV junction to discharge and compete for control.

James bundle: An accessory pathway that connects atrial fibers to the upper part of the AV node. Also referred to as an infranodal bypass tract.

Joules: Unit of energy equal to approximately 0.7375 foot-pounds.

J (junction) point: Point at which the QRS complex merges with the ST segment.

Junctional rhythm: The point at which the bundle of His is able to sustain the role of back-up pacemaker when the sinus node is blocked or has failed.

Junctional (AV) tachycardia: An ectopic rhythm originating from the AV junction at a rate above 100 per minute.

Kent bundles: Accessory AV pathways that connect the atrium to the ventricles.

Lead: An electrical picture of the heart's surface.

Lown-Ganong-Levine (LGL) syndrome: A combination of a short PR interval, normal QRS configuration, and recurrent supraventricular tachycardias. With this condition, the intranodal fibers bypass the crest of the AV node and one of the intranodal fibers terminates near the bundle of His.

Mahaim's fibers: AP that connect the AV node and the ventricle, or the bundle of His and the bundle branch nodofascicular, or the bundle branch and the fascicular ventricle.

Milliampere: One thousandth of an ampere.

Millivolt: One thousandth of a volt.

Mobitz Type II AV block: Second-degree AV block, characterized by QRS complex greater than 0.10. Implies a conduction defect below the level of the AV node and involving the penetrating portions of the bundle branch system.

Mode of pacemaker response: The vibration pattern of the pacemaker's shock wave.

Modified (bipolar) chest lead (MCL): System that simulates the pattern found with unipolar leads. For example, $MCL_1 = V_1$, and $MCL_6 = V_6$.

Multifocal: More than one focus or site.

Multifocal atrial tachycardia (MAT): A disordered atrial rhythm where the atria are discharging at a rate over 100 per minute and present two or more differently shaped P waves; associated with pulmonary disease.

Multiform: Ectopic beats with different shapes; presumed to result from different origins. May be a single focus but following a different pathway when activating the ventricles.

Myocardial cells: Cells that make up the bulk of the heart's muscle and are the actual contractile units of the heart. These cells must be able to respond to electrical stimulus.

Myocardium: The middle layer of muscle in the heart.

Negative: A wave inscribed below the baseline.

Nonrefractory phase: The final phase of refractoriness when all cells are repolarized and ready to respond in a normal fashion.

Nontransmural: A myocardial infarction confined to the subendocardium or inner aspects of the myocardium.

Orthodromic: Reciprocating tachycardia that conducts down the normal AV conduction system, but reenters the atria through the accessory pathway.

Overdrive suppression: Pacing at very rapid rates to overcome an ectopic.

Oversensing: The pacemaker's sensing of interference as if it were a depolarization wave form.

PAC: Premature atrial complex.

Pacemaker: The site that controls the heart rate because it has the fastest rate of automaticity.

Pacemaker identification code: A five-letter code designed to explain the operation of a pacemaker.

Paroxysm: An abrupt start or stop; occurs in bursts or spasms, as in paroxysmal supraventricular tachycardia, in which the onset and termination are always abrupt.

Paroxysmal atrial tachycardia (PAT): A tachycardia that results from an atrial ectopic. More correctly termed "paroxysmal supraventricular tachycardia."

Perfusion: The distribution of oxygenated blood through blood vessels in the body.

Physiologic (rate-adaptive): A pacemaker that has physiologic sensors and alters pacing functions according to the changes noted.

PJC: Premature junctional complex.

Polarized state: An electrically responsive state in which a cell is able to respond to a stimulus by becoming depolarized.

Positive: A wave inscribed above the baseline.

P-P interval: Distance between consecutive P waves.

P′ (P Prime) wave: Any ectopic P wave, that is, other than a sinus impulse.

Precordial: The area of the anterior surface of the chest, overlying the heart.

Precordial thump: An unsynchronized, mechanical shock delivered by a forceful blow to the precordium.

Preferential conduction: The method of depolarization of atrial tissue from the SA node through the geometric arrangement of right atrial muscle bundles to the AV node.

Premature atrial complex (PAC): A discharge of an atrial ectopic focus that causes earlier than normal atrial depolarization. Represented on the ECG by a P′.

Premature junctional complex (PJC): A discharge of an ectopic focus from the area of the bundle of His that causes premature depolarization of the atria (inverted P wave) and the ventricles. Morphology of the QRS is usually similar to a QRS of sinus origin.

Premature ventricular complex (PVC): A discharge of a ventricular ectopic focus that causes earlier than normal ventricular depolarization. Represented on the ECG by a QRS complex that is distorted. The QRS is opposite in polarity from its T wave.

P-R interval: Period from the beginning of atrial depolarization (P wave) to ventricle activation (the QRS).

Programmed upper rate limit (PURL): The fastest rate at which the pacer is programmed to function. The pacer cannot exceed a programmed number of pacing impulses.

Purkinje fibers: The distal portion of the ventricular conduction system that penetrates ventricular tissue.

P Wave: The wave form of atrial depolarization. Can be positive (+) when generated by a sinus and most atrial ectopic foci; is usually negative (-) when the atria are depolarized in a retrograde fashion from the AV junction.

QRS complex: That portion of cardiac cycle corresponding to depolarization of the ventricles. Made of any combination of the Q, R, and S wave forms.

QRS duration: Measured from the beginning of the Q or R wave (whichever is present) to the end of the R or S wave (whichever is present). Corresponds to the time of ventricular activation.

Q-T interval: The period from start of the QRS complex until the end of the T wave; corresponds to ventricular depolarization and repolarization.

Quadrigeminy: Grouping of four beats, usually three sinus beats and a PVC.

Q wave: Initial negative deflection of the QRS complex. Q waves are considered pathologic when they are new to the patient and/or greater than 0.04 second. Considered indicative of a myocardial infarction.

Rate-adaptive (physiologic): A pacemaker that has physiologic sensors and alters pacing functions according to the changes noted.

Reentry mechanism: The ability of an impulse to reexcite the same region though which it has previously passed.

Refractoriness: The ability of myocardial tissue to reject an impulse. This capability exists in various stages or degrees.

Refractory period: The time during which a cell is unresponsive to a stimulus.

Repolarization: The process by which a cell, after being discharged, returns to its state of readiness.

Resistance: Opposition to the flow of energy (impedance).

Retrograde atrial depolarization: The reverse direction; inferior to superior.

Rhythm: Recurring movement or fluctuation pattern.

R-on-T phenomenon: A PVC occurring so prematurely that it lands on the prior T wave (the ventricle's vulnerable period of repolarization). Ventricular fibrillation may result.

R-R interval: Period between consecutive QRS complexes.

R wave: The first positive deflection of the QRS complex.

SA arrest: An event caused by a sudden failure of the SA node to initiate a timely impulse.

SA block: An event in which the SA node initiates the impulse, but the propagation over atrial tissue is blocked, so the atria are not depolarized.

SA node: Sinoatrial, or sinus, node; the normal pacemaker for the heart.

Second-degree AV block: A form of heart block characterized by a missing QRS; a disorder in which one or more of the sinus impulses are not conducted along the AV pathway. One or more sinus impulses are blocked and are unable to stimulate the ventricles.

Sensitivity: The ability of a pacemaker to process the heart's intrinsic signals.

Sinus arrest: A disorder where the sinus fails to generate an impulse.

Sinus block: A disorder where the atria are unable to respond to the sinus stimulus.

Sinus bradycardia: A disorder where the sinus is the pacemaker but the ventricular response is less than 60 per minute.

Sinus node: The dominant pacemaker site of the heart; small bundle of tissue in right atrium that has the fastest rate of automaticity.

Specialized cells: Cells with four specific properties that govern their function: automaticity, excitability, conductivity, and contractility. These cells make up the heart's electrical conduction system.

Stokes-Adams syndrome: Syncope caused by bradycardia associated with SA arrest or block and with AV conduction defects.

Stored energy: Amount of joules available in the defibrillator's capacitor.

Stroke volume: The amount of blood ejected with each heartbeat.

ST segment: The line between the QRS and the T wave. Represents early ventricular repolarization. Ventricular systole takes place at the junction of the S wave and the ST segment.

ST-segment deviation: Abnormality in repolarization of the ventricles that shifts the ST segment above or below the baseline. Elevation in a lead reflects ischemia in the surface of the heart facing the positive (+) electrode of that lead.

Supraventricular: A site above the ventricles, that is, the SA node, atria, or AV junction.

Supraventricular Tachycardia (narrow QRS-complex tachycardia): A dysrhythmia originating from an ectopic focus above the bifurcation of the AV bundle. Generally, such beats have narrow QRS complexes unless aberrant conduction is present. This also refers to a group of tachyarrhythmias arising from above the AV bundle bifurcation, including sinus tachycardia, PSVT, atrial flutter and fibrillation, and AV junctional tachycardia.

S wave: The last negative deflection of the QRS complex. Represents completion of ventricular depolarization. A wave is usually less than 0.04 second in duration and less than 0.5 mV in depth. S waves that are greater than 0.04 second and 1.0 mV in depth may be indicative of myocardial hypertrophy.

Synchronized: Delivery of an electrical discharge programmed simultaneously to the patient's QRS complex.

Systole: Muscular contraction of the heart. The term applies both to atrial and ventricular contraction; however, when the term stands alone, by convention, it refers to ventricular contraction.

Tachycardia: Heart rate greater than 100 beats per minute.

Threshold: The least amount of energy needed to generate a response.

Torsade de Pointes: A form of ventricular tachycardia in which the QRS complexes change configuration.

Trabeculae: Extensions of myocardial muscle that provide turbulence of blood and boost ejection during systole. Specialized trabeculae are papillary muscles that connect with chordae tendinea to the AV valves.

Transmural: A myocardial infarction with necrosis, where there is fibrosis of the full thickness of the myocardial wall.

Trigeminy: Grouped beating where every third beat is an ectopic. The ectopic can be atrial or ventricular in origin.

T wave: The wave form corresponding to ventricular repolarization.

Undersensing: The ability of a normally-operating pacemaker to sense depolarization.

Uniform: Similar in appearance, size, and amplitude.

Unstable: Signs of cardiopulmonary dysfunction that may jeopardize life.

Unsynchronized: No use of a sensing mechanism to deliver shock current.

U wave: A wave sometimes observed following the T wave; thought to be related to late repolarization of the ventricles. Sole presence or absence of the U wave often is used incorrectly to infer problems with electrolyte imbalance.

Vagal maneuvers: A number of actions aimed at increasing parasympathetic tone. Some examples are carotid sinus massage, sudden immersion of the face into cold water, and the Valsalva maneuver.

Vasovagal attack (syncope): Sudden episode of hypotension and hypoperfusion due to increased parasympathetic (vagal) tone, leading to bradycardia and vasodilation. Referred to as a "simple faint," this condition will correct itself if the patient is allowed to assume a supine position, thereby correcting the transient hypotension.

Ventricular aneurysm: A condition where a portion of the infarcted myocardial tissue does not contract or expand normally causing the myocardium to bulge outward.

Ventricular ectopy: *See* PVC.

Ventricular fibrillation: Life-threatening dysrhythmia characterized by absent cardiac cycles (PQRST complexes) and a chaotic pattern on ECG. It is the most common cause of cardiac arrest.

Ventricular flutter: An accelerated form of ventricular tachycardia. It resembles a continuous sine wave and is observed just before ventricular fibrillation.

Ventricular standstill: Cessation of QRS activity.

Ventricular tachycardia: A disorder caused by the discharge of an ectopic ventricular ectopic at a rate of over 100 beats per minute. It is characterized by abnormal, often broad, QRS complexes. Depending on the ventricular rate, P waves may be seen independent of the QRS complexes.

Vulnerable period: Phase of cardiac cycle corresponding to upstroke of T wave; period when the heart is vulnerable to initiating serious ventricular dysrhythmias if a PVC occurs.

Wandering atrial pacemaker (WAP): An ambivalent term used to describe the period when the sinus node temporarily loses pacing function to an ectopic atrial or junctional focus; the ECG shows P waves of different shapes and varying P-R intervals.

Wenckebach phenomenon: Progressive prolongation of conduction time. Seen in atrial flutter, atrial fibrillation, SA block, and AV conduction defects.

Wolff-Parkinson-White (W-P-W) syndrome: Case of ventricular preexcitation by way of an alternate pathway that bypasses the AV node. ECG shows a shortened P-R interval (less than 0.10 second), slurred upstroke of the QRS complex, and a widened QRS complex. The patient usually has a history of tachycardia.

Index

Note: page number in **bold type** reference non-text material.

A

Q